Sleep and Wakefulness

Sleep
and Wakefulness

by Nathaniel Kleitman

REVISED AND ENLARGED EDITION

 THE UNIVERSITY OF CHICAGO PRESS
CHICAGO & LONDON

International Standard Book Number: 0-226-44073-7

Library of Congress Catalog Card Number: 63-17845

The University of Chicago Press, Chicago 60637
The University of Chicago Press, Ltd., London

Acknowledgments

To Professor A. J. Carlson, in whose laboratory I have worked since 1921—first as a student and later as a member of the staff—goes my profound gratitude for the innumerable kindnesses he has shown me during all these years.

Within the past few years the pace of my work has been markedly accelerated through generous grants made for that purpose by the trustees of the Rockefeller Foundation. In the previously published papers, referred to in this book, acknowledgment of the aid received from the Foundation has been made in each instance. I wish to enumerate some of the problems worked on, the results of which are reported in this book for the first time—not only to indicate my obligation to the Rockefeller Foundation but also to name my collaborators in each case so that, if they so desire, they may claim credit for their part of the co-operative effort. If these results had been published in scientific journals, the individuals mentioned would undoubtedly have shared authorship with me. Incidentally, abstract and review journals may be particularly interested in the unpublished material.

The work on the electrical skin resistance (chap. iii) was done mainly by S. Titelbaum, aided by N. Porte (chap. xvi); the blood-composition and blood-volume studies (chaps. iv and xxi) were made with the help of N. R. Cooperman and the late Arnold Robinson, and more recently by B. H. Richardson; the variation in intracranial pressure in wakefulness and sleep (chap. vi) was studied by H. Hoffmann; the diurnal temperature and motility curves in the feeble-minded (chaps. xv and xxviii) were obtained by M. W. Rubenstein, F. J. Mullin, and S. Titelbaum; the diurnal variations in "blocking" (chap. xvi) were established with the aid of S. Titelbaum and R. M. Beavers; the diurnal curve of phosphate excretion (chap. xvii) was investigated with the help of A. I. Doktorsky and S. Platt; the modifiability of the diurnal temperature and motility cycle (chap. xviii) was determined with the assistance of S. Titelbaum, Y. T. Oester, B. H. Richardson, and H. Schamp; the data on seasonal variation in motility during sleep (chap. xix) were analyzed with the aid of N. R. Cooperman, S. Titelbaum, and P. Feiveson; motility during sleep in psychopathic and mentally retarded individuals (chap. xxviii) was followed by N. R. Cooperman and S. Titelbaum; the effects of benzedrine on blocking and on the ability to remain awake (chap. xxix) were studied with the aid of S. Titelbaum, R. M. Beavers, and more recently of J. Schreider. I am also indebted to F. R. Stauffer, T. Lomangino, T. Engelmann, and A. Joslyn for considerable help in various studies, but most particularly to F. J. Mullin, N. R. Cooperman, and S. Titelbaum for supervising the work of others and relieving me of the burden of attending to many details in the various projects undertaken.

Many thanks are due to Drs. P. E. Bucy, E. L. Compere, R. R. Grinker, J. H. Masserman, W. L. Palmer, F. W. Schlutz, and D. Slight, all of the University of Chicago Clinics; to Dr. M. Sherman and staff of the Orthogenic School; and to Dr. F. A. Causey and staff of the Lincoln State School and Colony, for enabling us to utilize the facilities of their respective departments or establishments and for their active co-operation to that end. We are greatly obliged to Mr. W. W. Thompson and his associates of the Mammoth Cave Properties for placing at our disposal all their facilities to enable us to make observations (chap. xviii) at Mammoth Cave.

Thanks are extended to the many unnamed subjects of the different experiments whose faithful carrying-out of instructions and whose willingness to remain awake for long periods of time or to follow some unusual routine of sleep and wakefulness made possible the gathering of necessary data in which the individuals figured as mere statistical units.

The manuscript was read part by part as it was being written by Drs. A. J. Carlson and F. C. McLean. They have put a great deal of time and effort toward improving the style of, and removing ambiguities in, the presentation and toward shortening the text. The whole manuscript was very carefully and critically read by Dr. P. Bassoe, and portions of it were read by Drs. P. Bailey, E. M. K. Geiling, R. W. Gerard, L. N. Katz, and C. P. Miller, all of the University of Chicago. Dr. A. B. Luckhardt placed his extensive library at my disposal, and most of the historical references were obtained from his books, often at his suggestion. All of these gentlemen are entitled to the reader's thanks, in addition to my own, for greatly bettering the quality of the manuscript. It was, of course, beyond their power to remove all the defects and to smooth all the unevennesses, and toward the remaining shortcomings I invite the reader's indulgence.

Since my own reading ability is limited to French, German, Italian, and Russian, I was fortunate in securing the assistance of B. B. Lifschultz, whose knowledge of the Scandinavian languages, as well as of Dutch and Spanish, was of invaluable help to me in gathering and classifying the bibliographical material.

To Dr. D. R. Hooker, managing editor of the *American Journal of Physiology* and the *Physiological Reviews,* I am very thankful for permission to quote from the articles from our laboratory that have appeared in these publications, and also to reproduce Figures 2–8 [8.1–8.4, 9.1, 10.1 and 10.2 in revised edition], 13 [15.3], 16–20 [16.1–16.4], 29 [20.1], and 32 which originally appeared in the *American Journal of Physiology*. I am also indebted to Mr. C. C Thomas, publisher, for permission to quote from Kanner's *Child Psychiatry* and from an article by Blake and others that appeared in the *Journal of Neurophysiology*, and to reproduce Figures 1, 11, and 31 from that article. Thanks are also due to the Oxford University Press for permission to quote from Pavlov's *Conditioned Reflexes*.

Lastly, I want to thank my wife for the patience she has shown during the writing of this book. She not only read and helped to correct the first draft of the manuscript but read the proofs and aided in the compilation of the Bibliography and the indexes.

N. K.

University of Chicago
March 1939

The 1939 edition has been out of print for many years, and secondhand copies have become increasingly scarce. Insistent quests for available copies induced several publishers to inquire into the feasibility of issuing reprints of *Sleep and Wakefulness*. I was reluctant to authorize a mere reproduction of the original, since the Bibliography was hopelessly out of date, the text itself obsolete, and significant new findings had led to the modification of my views concerning (*a*) a basic rest-activity cycle; (*b*) evolutionary changes in sleep, as well as in wakefulness; and (*c*) separation of the concept of consciousness from that of wakefulness.

During the years spent in bibliographical research, I was ably assisted by Mr. Theodore G. Engelmann. Unstinted and cheerfully rendered help was received from the staffs of the libraries of the University of Chicago, the University of California (Berkeley, San Francisco, and Los Angeles), Columbia University, the New York Academy of Medicine, the Royal Society of Medicine (London), the John Crerar Library of Chicago, and the National Library of Medicine of Washington, D.C. (now Bethesda, Maryland). To the staff members of all these libraries go my profound and heartfelt thanks.

For permission to reproduce figures and tables not included in the 1939 edition I am grateful to the Elsevier Publishing Company for Figures 11.2 and 11.3 from *Electroencephalography and Clinical Neurophysiology;* to J. B. Lippincott Company for Figure 15.6 from *Endocrinology;* to the American Physiological Society for Figures 11.1, 15.1, 15.2, 16.5, and 18.5 and Tables 13.1 and 15.1 from the *Journal of Applied Physiology;* to the American Psychological Association for Figure 22.1 from the *Journal of Experimental Psychology;*

to Professor Edward J. Murray, Department of Psychology, Syracuse University, for furnishing me with the body-temperature data from which Figure 22.1 was constructed; and to the Naval Medical Research Institute, Bethesda, Maryland, for Figures 30.1 and 30.2.

My wife, Paulena, and my daughters, Hortense and Esther, helped me without measure in the writing, typing, retyping, copyediting, proofreading, and indexing; and, prior to the actual writing, in the many time-consuming chores involved in collection, classification, and analysis of the three thousand new bibliographical items. For them, it was a labor of love, and any words I might use to express my indebtedness to them would be as inadequate as they are unneeded.

N. K.

Santa Monica, California
October 1962

Contents

Part 1

Functional Differences between Sleep and Wakefulness

Chapter 1

Introduction: Definition of Terms

Sleep is commonly looked upon as a periodic temporary cessation, or interruption, of the waking state, which is the prevalent mode of existence for the healthy human adult. While a satisfactory short definition of sleep is lacking, Piéron (3192) considered it a suspension of sensory-motor activities characterized by an almost complete absence of movement and an increase in the thresholds of general sensitivity and of reflex irritability. Piéron further qualified his definition by the requirement that the suspension of activity be dependent upon internal necessity and not on external conditions, thus distinguishing it from temporary inactivity of plants and animals resulting from environmental influences. Another qualification is the preservation of the ability to be aroused or awakened, differentiating sleep from many sleeplike states, such as coma, anesthesia, and trance.

Although it is a daily recurring phenomenon, often taken for granted as part of the routine of life, sleep has always aroused speculation on its nature, cause, effect, and whether or not it is a necessary evil. Because the waking state in adults is of longer duration than sleep, and also because it constitutes the only period when overt activities are carried on, the average individual is likely to consider it the sole portion of his existence that "counts" in any way, sleep appearing as "time out" from the game of living. This popular view of sleep as the antithesis of wakefulness has been traditional since the days of Aristotle (125), who declared:

> First, then, this much is clear, that waking and sleep appertain to the same part of the animal, inasmuch as they are opposites, and sleep is evidently a privation of waking. For contraries, in natural as well as in all other matters, are seen always to present themselves in the same subject, and to be affections of the same: examples are—health and sickness, beauty and ugliness, strength and weakness, sight and blindness, hearing and deafness.

A similar attitude was evidenced by Philip (3176), who stated:

> We can perceive no final cause of the alternation of watchfulness and sleep, but such as has its origin in the imperfection of our nature. The end of life is

enjoyment, and . . . sleep, if we may not regard it as a positive evil, prevents uniformity in the accomplishment of this end.

In other words, wakefulness is good and desirable, sleep is bad, although perhaps unavoidable.

One could go on quoting statements of this type, picturing sleep as a disturber of the "natural" waking state, but this attitude is too well known to require reiteration. It will be my object to prove that, far from being the opposite of wakefulness, sleep is in reality a complement to the waking state, the two constituting alternate phases of a cycle, the one related to the other as the trough of a wave is related to the crest. Instead of an abrupt descent from the high plateau of waking efficiency to a uniformly low level of existence during sleep, followed by a sudden ascent again to the waking level at the end of so many "wasted" hours, there are curvilinear phases for both wakefulness and sleep. The wave need not be sinusoidal—it may be complex and skewed—nor does each of the two phases necessarily comprise one-half of the wave. There are gradations with respect to length, amplitude, shape, and subdivisions of the wave, but the cyclic character of the alternation of sleep and wakefulness is preserved, the two phases accentuating each other. Without wakefulness sleep cannot be said to exist, although as a pathological phenomenon the sleep phase may become very nearly continuous.

It is not my intention to claim originality for the treatment of sleep and wakefulness as alternate phases in the cycle of existence. Very little can be said about sleep that has not been said already, not only by scientists but by philosophers and poets as well. Books of "familiar quotations" contain large sections devoted to pertinent and often pungent remarks on the subject by Shakespeare (610, 673) and others. While some speak of wakefulness and sleep as life and death (and even of death itself as a sort of sleep), there are others who see periodicity in a variety of natural phenomena, astronomical as well as biological, and who refer to winter and spring, for instance, as the sleep and awakening of nature.

The word "sleep" is short and its meaning in everyday discourse unambiguous, but there is no satisfactory word in English for denoting the state of being awake. Vigilance, and adjectives suffixed by "ness"—alertness, attentiveness, watchfulness, sleeplessness—have been equated with wakefulness and often used to indicate a state of being "wide-awake." "Wake" (796) is short, but has several specialized meanings unrelated to sleep; the coined term "awakeness" (3028, 3847) has been proposed but not generally accepted. I shall, therefore, use "wakefulness," long and awkward as it may be, for "not being asleep." A term sometimes incorrectly used as synonymous with wakefulness is consciousness (2191). Sleep and wakefulness, as states, can be objectively observed and to some extent measured. They can be compared and contrasted, and, like ice and water, distinguished from each other by simple inspection. The melting point of ice or freezing point of water thus corresponds to the drowsiness level or intermediate stage between wakefulness and sleep. As liquid water may be near the freezing point or close to the boiling point, so may alertness vary from semi-wakefulness to manic hyperactivity ("boiling mad"). Conversely, the depth of sleep, like the coldness of ice, may be close to the transition state or near coma. In consciousness, however, the sleep-wakefulness dichotomy is absent: there is only one variable, whose criteria are partly objective, but mainly subjective, with the observer making only inferences. These criteria are: (*a*) critical—as against stereotyped—reactivity, involving an analysis of incoming impulses in the light of one's individual experience, and the elaboration of appropriate reactions (thinking), and (*b*) subsequent spontaneous or evoked recall of events (memory). The level of consciousness fluctuates; at any moment it is determined by the degree of one's ability to utilize the past and contribute to the future. Further details of the levels of consciousness are considered in Chapter 4, in connection with the discussion of cortical activity.

My own work on sleep was carried on at first along conventional lines. To answer the question of the "why and how" of sleep, I studied the effects of prolonged deprivation of sleep, as well as the concomitants of the deep sleep that follows such an experimental period of wakefulness. From the beginning I was struck by the fact that the effects of staying awake for several days did not manifest themselves in a continuously increasing physiological deterioration of the subjects, but that, instead, there was in the downward trend a waxing and waning with the succession of days and nights. One was less sleepy on the afternoon of the third day of sleep deprivation than in the middle of the second night. I also noted that the higher cortical functions seemed to be most markedly depressed by lack of sleep and that muscular activity was a decisive factor in enabling the person or animal to remain awake for a longer time than usual. These and other observations, in addition to previously reported facts and ideas advanced by other investigators, led to the elaboration of a tentative working hypothesis (2176, 2179) for which I do not claim exclusive authorship.

Sleep is a topic on which almost everyone considers himself an authority because of personal interest and firsthand experience. It is customary to preface articles and books on sleep by the statement that, although sleep is a familiar phenomenon, nothing, or almost nothing, is known about it. Then the writer proceeds to explain sleep on a very simple basis, unhesitatingly defines good (restful, refreshing, restorative) sleep, and usually concludes with an infallible recipe for attaining the best kind of sleep. There has thus accumulated a vast literature on the physiology of sleep, much of it purely discursive in character; and it often takes a good deal of hunting through the haystack before one becomes convinced that the proverbial needle is not even there.

The Bibliography of more than 4,000 references comprises a great diversity of contributions—observational and experimental, on animals and human subjects, young and old, normal and abnormal, factual and theoretical—making it difficult to allot them appropriate space in the treatment of the several aspects of sleep and wakefulness. No significance at all should be attached to whether or not name or names accompany the number in parentheses that refers to a particular publication. Failure to mention a reference by name or number in the text may mean that it was impossible to pinpoint the contents of the particular item, or that the paper (often the book) contained nothing of interest. The reason for including such references is to indicate that they were not omitted inadvertently. The absence of a numerical reference to some of the findings made in our laboratory means that they have not been published. Combinations of capital letters are used to indicate frequently employed overlong words (EEG for electroencephalogram) or word groupings (BSRF for brain stem reticular formation). Such abbreviations are explained when first introduced and are spelled out in the Index.

In arranging the material presented in this book, I have endeavored to proceed from the observational through the experimental and pathological to the theoretical. The initial chapters are devoted to the functional differences between wakefulness and sleep, what have been called the concomitants of sleep. The next part deals with the course of events in a single sleep period, more properly the sleep phase of the cycle. In the third division are treated activities extending over both phases of the cycle and exhibiting periodic or rhythmic characteristics. The next two parts comprise artificial (experimental) interference with, and spontaneous (pathological) changes in, the sleep-wakefulness rhythm. The sixth and seventh parts pertain to means of influencing sleep and wakefulness through pharmacological, therapeutic, and hygienic measures, and to states resembling sleep—hypnosis and hibernation. The final part of the book contains an analysis of existing theories and a further development of my previously advanced working hypothesis, which emphasizes the wakefulness phase of the sleep-wakefulness alternation.

The mixture of sense and nonsense that makes up the conception of the nature of sleep in any age may be illustrated by the following excerpt from Hartley's (1654) *Observations on Man: His Frame, His Duty, and His Expectations,* first written in 1748:

> Here I observe, first, that new-born children sleep almost always. Now this may be accounted for by the doctrine of vibrations, in the following manner: The fetus sleeps always, having no sensation from without impressed upon it, and only becomes awake upon its entrance into a new world, viz. by means of the vigorous vibrations which are impressed upon it. It is reasonable therefore to expect, that the new-born child should fall back into its natural state of sleep, as soon as these vibrations cease, and return again to a state of vigilance, only

from the renewal of vigorous impressions; and so on alternately, agreeably to the fact.

Secondly, even adults are disposed to sleep, when the impressions of external objects are excluded, and their bodies kept in a state of rest, for the same reasons as those just mentioned in the similar state of young children. However, they incline more to vigilance than children, partly because their solids and fluids are more active, and less compressible, i.e. more susceptible and retentive of vibrations; and partly, because association brings in perpetual trains of ideas, and consequently of vibrations, sufficiently vivid to keep up vigilance in common cases.

Thirdly, having presented the reader with the two foregoing observations, which are of a very obvious kind, I will now inquire with more minuteness, into the intimate and precise nature of sleep. It appears then, that, during sleep, the blood is accumulated in the veins, and particularly in the venal sinuses which surround the brain and spinal marrow; and also, that it is rarefied, at least for the most part. For as the actions of the muscles squeeze the blood out of the veins during vigilance, so their inactivity during sleep suffers the blood to lodge in the veins; and the recumbent posture, which is common to animals in sleep, suffers it to lodge particularly in the venal sinuses of the brain and spinal marrow. . . . It follows therefore, that the brain and spinal marrow will be particularly compressed during sleep. . . .

What advances have been made toward the understanding of the "intimate and precise nature of sleep" within the last 214 years?

Chapter 2

Position of the Body: Skeletal Musculature

One recognizes the state of sleep in a person or animal by the immobility of the body and the abolition, in most cases, of what is known as the normal upright posture. The tonic reflexes of proprioceptive, labyrinthine, and visual origin that are responsible for righting the body and maintaining the normal position are, with a few exceptions, inoperative during sleep; the body is allowed, even before the onset of sleep, to assume a dorsal or lateral position, which depends almost entirely on gravity for its preservation. Among the special muscular conditions associated with sleep are the closed eyelids and the deviation of the eyes upward and outward, as well as a powerful contraction, or at least resistance to forcing from inside, of the anal and vesicular sphincters. Muscular relaxation is a notable concomitant of sleep, in itself leading to decreased metabolic activity and to recovery from muscular fatigue. The latter is due not only to overt muscular acts but also to the maintenance of a continuous state of muscle tonus, since the tonic contraction of certain muscle groups is required for the retention of the standing and walking position of the body against the force of gravity.

Various recumbent positions of the human body during sleep have been described (1057, 1093), with the assertion that the majority of sleepers assume a definite position (1804, 1806) or that there is no fixed position (3936). Stradling and Laird (3842), for 161 right-handed and 31 left-handed persons, determined that both groups assumed the right-side position in slightly more than half of the cases. Boynton and Goodenough (437), on the other hand, noted that those individuals in whom handedness was well developed were somewhat more likely to assume a position which allowed the preferred hand to be free.

In an extensive photographic study of several subjects, Johnson and co-workers (2003) found that most sleepers had a dozen or more favorite positions, some or all of which they might assume during a single night's sleep. According to these authors, all the positions that "are maintained for fairly long periods are contorted; in particular, the spinal column is always curved laterally, and usually bowed backward, and also twisted. . . . All the postures that are favored require some supporting strain, which is often exerted against the shoulder joint and hip joint of one side, the femur and humerus being used as props. Even in a dorsal position the sleeper does not lie flat but disposes one leg so as to prevent rotation and to throw more of his weight on the other side. The posture that requires the least effort for maintaining it is a prone position." Under conditions conducive to sprawling, one of their subjects assumed thirty-three different postures during one night's sleep.

The findings of Johnson and associates did not prevent further expressions of opinion concerning the significance or desirability of a particular sleep posture (250, 1824, 2609, 3098). Schuetz (3598) noted that each person had his own characteristic sleeping position, and Leak (2387) stated that "a normal healthy person usually lies on the right side." In McDonnell's opinion (2750), lateral recumbency is the one correct sleep posture. Niemi and co-workers (3010), in checking the midnight sleeping position of 433 persons, found one-half of them lying on one side, with legs bent.

Observations made on infants and young children led to the conclusion that they are less completely relaxed while asleep than older children and adults. Wagner (4095) studied the sleeping posture of ninety-five newborn infants and found more variations than had been suspected. In deep sleep, when the respiration was regular, the most frequent position was flexion of arms and legs, with mouth closed. The positions assumed varied from one infant to another, and for the same infant at different times, during the first ten days of life. It is doubtful, however, if infants are capable of rolling over till they are about five to six months old (107). They are usually placed in the prone position, as this position appears to be more acceptable to them (103), and they often fold their legs under them (3178). Abnormal sleeping positions of infants, if continued, may cause permanent distortions of the limbs (3920), but this seldom happens. Indeed older infants usually sleep in the supine position, with their arms in the air (2131), or held symmetrically above their shoulders (2689).

The frequency with which different positions were selected by fifty-six preschool children during an afternoon nap of an hour's duration was reported upon by Boynton and Goodenough (436, 437). The preferred position was the right side, followed by the left side, the abdomen, and the back, with the corresponding percentages of time that these different postures were assumed 31, 29, 27, and 13. Scott (3631), in a similar study on twenty-nine children between the ages of one and four and a half years, also found that the right-side position was the favorite one, accounting for 44 per cent of the total observations, and the left next with 38 per cent. Despert (924) noted that thumb-suckers preferred the prone position.

Sleeping positions of animals have been described by several authors. Fernberger (1157) found rats asleep while hanging by their upper teeth from the wire mesh covering the top of their cage when many of them were crowded together. That the perching of sleeping birds may require the maintenance of tonus in certain muscle groups was shown by Hondelink (1828), who studied the effect of certain hypnotic drugs on small birds that habitually slept on perches. With a small dose of the drug the bird would be found sitting on its perch fast asleep, but, if the dose was increased, the animal would lie on the floor of the cage. This method enabled the author to distinguish between sleep-producing and narcotizing doses of one or another hypnotic. According to Eckstein (1029), canaries sleep in one of four different positions.

A very thorough investigation of the sleeping position of the horse, an animal that "traditionally" sleeps standing, was made by Steinhart (3798). The six hundred army horses observed assumed four resting and sleeping positions: (*a*) standing, head held free, (*b*) standing with head resting on manger or stall partition, (*c*) lying on belly, and (*d*) lying on side. Horses can stand without leaning when lightly asleep, less frequently when moderately so, but never when deeply asleep. In most cases of light and moderate sleep they either lie down or rest their heads against some supporting structure. When deeply asleep, they are always in the lying position, more frequently side than belly. The side position when lying down was assumed in 85 per cent of the cases. Steinhart stated that all healthy horses lie down at least once daily, the great majority more than once; also that, while there is a great divergence in the proportion of sleep in the lying position to that standing up, some animals sleep mostly lying down.

Another ungulate—the cow—has been observed to lie down from 6 to 12 hours, usually during the night (659), preferring one position over another (916). The question has been raised, however, whether the cow sleeps at all, as judged by behavioral criteria (189, 542). The role of gravity in the proper functioning of the reticulo-rumen requires the upright position of the thorax, resulting in the characteristic ventral position of the body, with the legs tucked under; the frequent belching and rumination tend to keep the cow awake. On the other hand, very young calves "have been observed on occasion to go into what appears a state of torpor from which it is difficult to arouse them, and, when lifted bodily, remain limp though the eyes are open" (542).

A fine collection of photographs showing the sleeping positions of a great variety of vertebrates was published by Hediger (1677).

Certain sleeping positions may lead to abnormalities of structure and function, and some pathological conditions are conducive to particular sleeping postures. That some people do have single favorite positions during sleep is indicated by the studies of Stallard (3777) on the role of sleeping postures in the etiology of malocclusions and other jaw abnormalities. There are pictures of sleeping postures of children: the head so placed on the pillow as to exert a considerable pressure against the face; hand under the pillow with the knuckles against the cheek; the palm against the maxillary arch; pressure directed against the mandible, resulting in mandibular contraction (the inbite) and opposite retraction; and the influence of thumb-sucking, with pillowing on the back of the hand. Mansbach (2653, 2654), referring to similar findings by Schwarz (3626), added her own observations on sixty-three children, in whom she determined the habitual posture of head, body, and limbs during sleep. In general, she confirmed the earlier results with respect to the mandible but not to the upper jaw. She disagreed with Schwarz, who held that the dorsal decubitus position was responsible for mouth breathing, and that thumb-sucking was an etiological factor in orthodontic anomalies. Spitzer (3771) also called attention to the possible injurious effect of certain sleeping postures on the jaws and on the teeth system. The various effects of pressure on nerves and blood vessels from certain sleeping postures are discussed in connection with other sleep abnormalities (p. 285).

Zacks and co-authors (4304) found no "natural" tendency to occupy one side position in relation to the more affected lung in pulmonary tuberculosis; nor is it clear whether, after a lung had been collapsed, it is more beneficial to sleep in one position or the other (2609, 3349). Pain in one side of the body may cause the sleeper to favor the opposite side position (1824). Cardiac patients usually sleep on the right side, if they have pain (3598, 4098), or on the left side if the insufficiency is mild (2387). The normal hypotonia of the diaphragm leads to "oppressive effects" on the heart and lungs in cases of meteorism (1151). Respiratory infections may cause children to sleep in the prone position, which affords postural drainage (103).

The condition of the extrinsic eye musculature is of significance because ocular activity is related to normal sleep and ocular symptoms are prominent in pathological sleep. The closed eyelids are one of the most characteristic signs of behavioral sleep, but physiological lagophthalmos has been reported (98), and about 5 per cent of five hundred Chinese students were observed to sleep with the eyelids open 1–4 mm (1318). Mathis and Fischgold (2712) had two comatose patients whose eyes remained continuously open.

For eye positions, Pietrusky (3195) investigated three hundred subjects, from nurslings to old people. The orbicularis muscle is usually relaxed. Sometimes the lids are not completely closed. The most frequent position of the eyes is divergence upward, accounting for 46 per cent of the cases. Least frequent positions are divergence downward (3 per cent) and convergence upward (4 per cent). In our experience the eyes were found nearly always in the position of outward divergence, the most frequent of Pietrusky's positions, but would sometimes return to the middle position when the eyelids were spread apart.

In puppies, however, the eyes are generally rolled inward and downward

(2178), and in the cat Bremer (479) observed a downward rotation of the eyeballs during sleep.

The outward divergence of the eyeballs probably represents a resting state, brought about by the absence of centrifugal influences from the central nervous system (CNS). It can be acquired in the waking state as a result either of alcoholic intoxication or of prolonged wakefulness, and is characterized by double vision.

Concerning the intrinsic eye muscles, Pietrusky (3195) found the pupil small in proportion to the depth of sleep. In all but one of our subjects the pupils were also constricted during sleep (2176). Byrne (598) ascribed the pupillo-constriction during sleep to an inherent tonus of the third nerve, to be looked upon as a release phenomenon, like decerebrate rigidity, to which it is related functionally and developmentally. In this connection it should be mentioned that Bremer (478), in transecting the brain stem of the cat, immediately behind the emergence of the third pair of cranial nerves, obtained a progressive pupilloconstriction. At the end of 30 minutes the myosis was very marked, with the pupils reduced to mere slits. This delay in the development of myosis Bremer thought was due to the powerful sympathetic stimulation and particularly to the hyperadrenalemia, caused by the etherization of the cat prior to the transection. The same operation, when performed on two cats previously entirely sympathectomized, led to a complete pupilloconstriction in less than 5 minutes. Bremer considered the myosis simply an expression of a diminution of the cortically originating pupillodilator effects.

Although the skeletal musculature is relaxed during sleep, there is a variation in the tonus of different muscle groups. Infants often hold their fists very tightly closed, but their body musculature is quite limp. Froment and Chaix (1306), referring to the greater tonus in the limb than in the trunk musculature during sleep in children, looked upon it as a real dissociation in muscular activity, similar to that observed in certain states following encephalitis. A much simpler explanation is that the greater limb tonus is an atavistic survival of the arboreal existence of our ancestors, when the ability of the young to hold on tightly to a branch of a tree during sleep meant survival. Anyone who has seen very young monkeys clutch their mothers, as the latter climb upon a tree or jump from branch to branch, has undoubtedly been struck by the tenacity of their hold. During the waking state also one can see much more activity in the hands and fingers of an infant than in its arms.

Max (2718) recorded action potentials of various skeletal muscles in normal persons and in deaf-mutes during sleep and wakefulness. There was a progressive diminution of action potentials during sleep in both deaf and hearing subjects, but more so in the deaf. However, even in the deaf, a complete absence of muscular activity was rare. In most instances the muscle potentials either diminished progressively to a minimum of 0.1–0.9 microv or remained above that microvolt level throughout the period of sleep. These residual action potentials were more prominent in the arm than in the leg muscles.

Pakhanov (3080) developed a complex hydrodynamic system of tubes for measuring the tonus of the flexor of the fingers and found that the tonus varied with the depth of sleep.

By the use of myography to measure stretch-resistance, Schaltenbrand (3544) showed that in a patient with a total transection of the spinal cord the spasticity of the legs was decreased during sleep. Friedlander (1296) noted that "the slow tremor of basal ganglion disease disappears during sleep, but is replaced by a tremor of similar rate to that seen in normals during sleep."

Jouvet and co-workers (2033, 2046) observed a marked decrease in the tonus of the neck muscles of the cat during the "paradoxical" or "rhombencephalic" phase of sleep (p. 212).

Thus, the relative inactivity and muscular relaxation associated with the assumption and maintenance of the sleeping position are not all-or-none conditions. Variations appear with respect to species, age, muscle group, state of health, and time—related, no doubt, to the functions of the several other systems that operate in the sleeping organism. Most immediately involved, and to be considered next, is the nervous system, upon which the skeletal muscles depend for their tonic and phasic contractions in the regulation of static and kinetic activity.

Chapter 3

The Nervous System

CHRONAXIE

The time element in excitability has been applied to the study of muscles, nerve fibers, and neurones. In a series of papers, Kisselev and Mayorov (2166–68) confirmed earlier findings (426) concerning a rise in motor chronaxie during sleep. Mayorov (2727, 2728) traced the changes in absolute and relative values of the chronaxies of flexors and extensors through successive "phases" of sleep. Korotkin and Kryshova (2242, 2243, 2291) noted the peculiarities of chronaxie changes during sleep in infants, and Saper (3518), in old persons. The most ambitious attempt to link chronaxie to sleep was made by Chauchard (682–85), utilizing the notions about heterochronism and isochronism and chronaxies of constitution and subordination. According to Chauchard, in wakefulness there is isochronism of cortical and peripheral neurones, with the former much lower and the latter somewhat lower than their corresponding constitutional chronaxies. During sleep, peripheral subordination is lost, and heterochronism manifests itself in a slight rise of the peripheral neuronal chronaxie to its constitutional level and a great rise of the central neuronal chronaxie above even its high constitutional value. It should be pointed out that Rosenthal and Filipova (3411) felt that chronaximetric changes observed during sleep might be an artifact produced by displacement of surface electrodes, and Bonvallet and co-authors (405) counselled "prudence" in evaluating Chauchard's data.

REFLEX EXCITABILITY

Strange as it may seem, there is no agreement concerning the effect of sleep on reflex excitability. Piéron (3192) listed eight reports of increased and six of decreased reflexes during sleep, showing the complexity of the phenomena studied and differences of interpretation. Tarchanov (3906) determined the effect of sleep on tendon reflexes in two puppies whose spinal cords had been cut. There was a decrease in reflex irritability in the region above the transection and no change below. Tarchanov concluded that during sleep there was a greater inhibitory influence from the brain on the portion of the cord with which it was still connected, but no evidence of "spinal cord sleep." It will be recalled, however, that Schaltenbrand (3544) did observe a decrease in the spasticity of the legs during sleep in a patient with a transected spinal cord (p. 13).

Concerning the tendon reflexes, commonly represented by the knee jerk, it is usually stated that they either disappear or are greatly diminished during sleep (540, 1476, 3734). We (2400) worked under very favorable conditions because our subject was often extremely sleepy, as a result of prolonged wakefulness. When no special effort was made to keep him awake, after he settled down in the comfortable chair to which the recording device was attached, he would fall asleep in a minute or so. It was then possible to alternate sleep and wakefulness in one test any number of times, and each time the onset of sleep was accompanied by a gradual disappearance of the knee jerk. The subjects of Tuttle (3995) were probably less sleepy, and the knee jerk did not always disappear, even though it was invariably diminished, in sleep. There seemed to be some degree of correlation between the magnitude of the reflex and the depth of sleep. Just as it is possible to preserve a weak knee jerk during sleep, this reflex has been seen to disappear completely in the waking state (1939). It was accomplished by voluntary muscular relaxation, with or without special training, so that, while still awake, the subject attained a "degree of neuromuscular tonus lower than that of light sleep." The knee jerk decreased in proportion to the development of the relaxed state.

Puppies in the dorsal position, paws up in the air, preserved good homolateral and crossed knee jerks, even when deeply asleep (2178). Here, as in the case of young infants sleeping with their arms directed upward, one may be dealing with a special phenomenon related to the age of the animal or subject.

Cutaneous reflexes are variously affected by sleep, depending upon the type of reflex, the depth of sleep, and the species studied. In the dog, for instance, the scratch reflex may disappear, while the reflex contraction of the eyelids and movements of the skin of the lips, when the snout is scratched, persist even in deep sleep. In man, too, reflexes that do not disappear are weakened, and the reflex time is lengthened. Occasionally, complex responses follow cutaneous stimulation, as shown in our laboratory (2176). Brushing the sleeper's cheek with a piece of paper, from the ear to the corner of the mouth, often elicited a facial grimace and a movement of the hand, apparently intended to scratch the stimulated area. There was no strict homolaterality about this response. Ordinarily, the right hand would respond when the right cheek was stimulated, but, if this hand was under cover, the left hand would be used instead. The response was usually slow in developing. Piéron (3192) reported a lengthening in the cutaneous reflex time of a sleeping child, from the usual fraction of a second to 2–5 seconds.

The pupillary reflex is preserved in sleep, as a rule. Although the pupil is small, it can be made smaller by shining a light into the eyes after gently spreading the eyelids apart. The pupillary reflex time is lengthened, often by several seconds (2176). Pietrusky (3195) observed a weakening of the pupillary light reflex with the increase in the depth of sleep in human beings, and Byrne (598) reported a complete disappearance of the response, in both animals and man, during deep sleep. In puppies I always obtained a pupillary response, irrespective of the depth of sleep. On the other hand, Pietrusky (3195) and Peiper (3135) noted a widening of the pupils in adults and children following stimulation of a variety of receptors other than the eyes. Strong illumination of the eyes through the closed eyelids usually produces a contraction of the orbicularis muscle.

Max (2718) obtained action potentials in the skeletal musculature of the deaf after the application of various stimuli. Steinhart (3798) could elicit responses to olfactory and visual stimuli in horses during any but the soundest sleep. While the responses were still obtainable, there was a lengthening of the reflex time with the increase in the depth of sleep.

Labyrinthine responses to rotation were studied by Di Giorgio (1453) in seven infants, after allowing them to fall asleep in a rotating chair, head and trunk held erect by means of bandages. Deep sleep was indicated by the immovable position of the eyeballs when the lids were lifted. The infants were usually rotated for 1 to 4 minutes at a uniform rate of 10 to 40 turns per minute, then suddenly stopped. There was never any postrotatory nystagmus, but, instead, a marked deviation—like the slow component of nystagmus—first in one, then in the opposite, direction. The reactions differed in duration and division of phases with the rate and duration of rotation, as well as from one infant to another, but a certain type of stimulation always called forth the same response in a particular infant. In puppies, when they were fast asleep, I noticed a complete abolition of the labyrinthine righting reflexes exerted on the position of the head (2178). Holding the sleeping animal in the air, belly up, its head could be allowed to dorsiflex until the snout pointed straight downward without causing awakening. The abolition of the vestibular response is, of course, consistent with the animal's assuming a sleep position in which there is no need for the maintenance of equilibrium.

One of the most characteristic phenomena that in healthy adults appears only during sleep or anesthesia is the toe-extension response to scratching of the sole of the foot, otherwise known as the positive Babinski sign. This peculiar sleep reflex was described by Rosenbach (3406) in 1880, sixteen years before Babinski (168) discovered its significance as a diagnostic sign indicative of a break in the pyramidal pathways from the cerebral cortex to the lower part of the spinal cord. Babinski (169) also noted the presence of his positive sign in normal newborn infants, but never seemed to connect it with sleep. It remained for Bickel (330) and Goldflam (1468) to discover, several years later, that a positive Babinski sign could be elicited in normal adults during sleep, as well as in ether and chloroform anesthesia, and to interpret it as a functional break between cortex and spinal cord.

In our experience (2176) a person must be deeply asleep before a dorsiflexion, or curling-up of the big toe, can be obtained through stroking the sole of the foot. When elicitable, it can be evoked any number of times, provided a suitable interval (15–20 seconds) is allowed to elapse between stimulations. If the sole is scratched at shorter intervals, several extensor responses are followed by extension and flexion, later by flexion of the toe and either an attempt to rub the stimulated sole with the other foot or a flexion of the leg upon the thigh. There also appear other signs of a decrease in the depth of sleep, and, if stimulation continues, an awakening of the sleeper.

Elliott and Walshe (1069) observed the appearance of a positive Babinski sign, apart from organic disease of the pyramidal tract system, in a variety of toxic states, usually characterized by a comatose condition. The dorsiflexion of the toes does not occur in diabetic coma or in uremic coma, except when the latter is associated with epileptiform fits, but may appear in coma due to the impairment of metabolic functions of the liver brought about by acute or chronic liver disease, even without epileptiform convulsions.

The relation of the positive Babinski sign to functional depression of the nervous system was brought out by the observation of Tournay (3960) of a periodic alternation of the toe-extension and flexion phenomenon, parallel with the alternating phases of Cheyne-Stokes breathing, in a semi-comatose patient suffering from nephritis, with hypertension, complicated by uremia: during the polypnea phase the Babinski sign was negative; during the apnea, positive. Likewise, in one case of cardiac insufficiency there was a positive Babinski response, changing to a negative after cardiotonic medication.

Geyer (1414) tested ten identical and ten fraternal pairs of twins. There was a greater frequency of the positive Babinski sign appearing in both identical twins than in the fraternal ones. The children were healthy, none showing the toe-extension phenomenon in the waking state. The author concluded that there had to be a constitutional cause for the presence or absence of the Babinski sign in sleep.

Taking into consideration that the individual must be deeply asleep before the toe-extension response can be elicited, it is not surprising that it cannot be demonstrated with ease in every sleeper. As stated, the toe-extension response, when present in sleep, can be easily reversed. The significance of this reversible phenomenon for the complete understanding of the nature of sleep is discussed in Chapter 33. In so far as other reflexes not peculiar to sleep are concerned, their deportment during sleep is what one would expect on the basis of a general muscular relaxation, assumption of the horizontal position, and raising the threshold of irritability of the CNS.

SWEATING AND ELECTRICAL SKIN RESISTANCE

The function of sweating properly belongs among the visceral activities of the organism and is related, in general, to muscular work and body-temperature control. There are certain skin areas where sweating serves a special purpose. They are the hairless thick-skinned palmar and plantar surfaces, well adapted for their function of gripping. A certain amount of perspiration on these surfaces minimizes sliding and is therefore produced in a variety of situations that involve danger to the individual and may be looked upon as a preparation for meeting emergencies. Kuno and Ikeuchi (2304) have demonstrated that palmar and plantar sweating in man is only of incidental significance in temperature regulation, since it does not increase with a rise in atmospheric temperature that leads to increased sweating in the remainder of the skin. Kuno (2302) referred to the special palmar sweat-gland activity as "mental sweating." Attempts to solve mathematical problems caused a great increase in the sweating of the palms but not, for instance, of the forehead. Kuno concluded that, "if this [mental] sweating has any physiological significance, it may conceivably be in some relation to mental stress which is its most adequate cause." Kosuge (2250), employing Kuno's method, measured the secretion of sweat on the palm of the hand and on the chest. He made two hundred tests on ten healthy men in a room that was kept "gloomy and quiet" so that the subjects could sleep easily. With the room temperature at 19°–20° C., palmar sweating decreased during sleep and recovered after awakening, both changes being prompt and marked when the palmar sweating was high prior to the onset of sleep. At this room temperature there was no change in chest sweating. When the room temperature was raised to 29° C. (during the winter), chest sweating started moderately in about 30 minutes and stopped on awakening. With still higher room temperatures, 30°–35° C., chest sweating increased without exception, in some cases markedly, at once or after a delay. There were minor changes in rectal temperature but not enough to account for the increased sweating during sleep. Chest sweating represents the perspiration of the whole body, as shown by weight-loss figures obtained by Sauter's balance. The loss in weight is larger, sometimes twice as large, during sleep than during wakefulness. Kuno (2303) has found, further, that even chest sweating may be under the control of the cerebral cortex, inhibited during wakefulness and released in sleep.

Darrow (822) offered definite proof that changes in electrical skin resistance (ESR) are due to variations in the activity of the sweat-glands; one should expect to get an increased palmar ESR during sleep, together with changes in either direction in the ESR elsewhere, and that is exactly what happens. Likewise, any situation which involves accelerated mental activity should lead to a lowering of the palmar resistance, and this is also true. The change in resistance is known variously as the psychogalvanic reflex, psychogalvanic response, or galvanic skin response (GSR), and is sometimes expressed as a decrease of resistance in ohms, or, reciprocally, an increase of conductance in mhos. It has been used for different purposes, among others for "lie detection," with variable results, on the assumption that the mental conflict resulting from attempts to deceive will cause an increase in palmar sweating and therefore a drop in ESR.

Peiper (3134) stated that the GSR can be obtained in children older than one year but not in younger ones. It can be elicited by sensory stimulation during light sleep but disappears in deep sleep. Farmer and Chambers (1139) observed a rapid increase in the ESR at the beginning of sleep, with a peak shortly before getting up, and a rapid fall on awakening. Richter (3337) measured the ESR of sixteen subjects during sleep, with electrodes applied either to the palms or to the backs of the hands, thus determining the resistance to the passage of a galvanic current through the body from hand to hand. As the main part of the body's electrical resistance lies in the skin, he measured substantially the resistance of the two skin surfaces in contact with non-polarizable electrodes. In the palm-to-palm conduction the ESR rose, in one case, from a waking value of 70,000 ohms to as high as 1,400,000 ohms during sleep, while the back-to-back ESR increased in some subjects and decreased in others. Richter further stated that persons in whom sleep produced a great increase in ESR slept soundly and were hard to awaken; the opposite was true of individuals with only small rises in ESR. Landis (2360) severely criticized these findings (1139, 3337). He noted that "non-polarizable" electrodes became polarized, that the drying of the paste between the electrodes and the skin led to an increase in resistance, and that only one-fifth of the body resistance was due to the skin. He failed to observe a rise in ESR during sleep but, on the contrary, obtained a gradual fall to a low level at which the resistance remained. He did not explain how all the defects in the method produced a fall in ESR on awakening, as reported by the authors whose sleep data he held to be artifacts. Forbes and Piotrowski (1239) found no relationship between the Richter type of ESR curves and sleep. They noticed that the ESR, as measured by Richter's method, showed greater variability than when determined by the Wheatstone bridge method. Freeman and Darrow (1273), using the Wheatstone bridge, obtained an increased ESR in the palm, but not on the back of the hand, during sleep.

The work of Titelbaum (3948) consisted of a systematic study of variations in palmar, and at times of back-of-wrist, ESR in a number of subjects during wakefulness, sleep, and periods of sleep deprivation. He used the Darrow photopolygraph, which, among other devices, contained a Behavior Research resistance box (822) and a highly sensitive, quick-acting galvanometer. The circuit employed in this resistance-box Wheatstone bridge had high resistances, and high external potentials were therefore necessary. When 4.5 v were applied to the circuit, 0.0409 milliamperes passed through the body of the subject. For each 1,000 ohms resistance change, either way from the balance, within the recording range, there was a variation in current of less than one millionth of an ampere. The arrangement provided for automatic balancing of the bridge, precluding the possibility of significant changes in the measuring current, thus meeting objections to the use of direct current for measuring ESR. Zinc electrodes were strapped to the dorsum of the wrist and the palm of the hand. The electrodes were cylindrical cups filled with absorbent cotton soaked in a 3 per cent solution of $ZnSO_4$. Prior to applying the "indifferent" electrode, the skin on the wrist was vigorously rubbed with "redux" electrode paste to produce an abrasion and make certain that the resistance measured was mainly that of the palmar skin area in contact with the "different" electrode. In some experiments five electrodes were used, two on each hand, as indicated, and one on the plantar surface of the right foot. By means of a switching panel board and dial any two of the five electrodes could be connected to the resistance box, and the ESR determined for (*a*) right palm, (*b*) left palm, (*c*) right sole, (*d*) palm to palm, and (*e*) back to back. Simultaneously with the resistance changes, and on the same moving photographic paper, records were made of respiration and motility, and in some cases the rectal temperature was continuously recorded by an electrical resistance thermometer.

A total of thirty-four complete night records of ESR were made on eight adult subjects. The ESR was tested every 20 minutes or oftener. The room was completely dark, except for a small shielded light over the apparatus, and the sleeper was only rarely disturbed by the operation of the photopolygraph. Mean ESR levels for successive tenths of the sleep period for each subject were tabulated, eliminating distortions of the composite values due to the effects of differences in the hour of going to bed, and in the duration of sleep, that occur even in the same subject. The pre-sleep ESR levels of the subjects varied from a mean of 19,000 at one extreme to 60,000 ohms at the other. The mean ESR values of the group, with the mean pre-sleep ESR as 1.00, were, for successive tenths of the sleep period, 1.40, 1.50, 1.50, 1.60, 1.76, 1.94, 2.34, 1.87, 1.87, 1.21.

Fluctuations in the ESR appeared from time to time, apparently spontaneously, and persisted for from $\frac{1}{2}$ to 40 minutes. These fluctuations were more likely to occur during sleep that followed prolonged wakefulness than in an ordinary night's sleep. They were not found to be related to the ESR level or to the hour of the night. A body movement was usually accompanied by a fall in ESR but was almost always followed by a sharp rise. In two subjects there was occasionally a synchronicity between the ESR variations and the phases of the respiratory cycle. The ESR increased with inspiration and decreased during expiration. That those fluctuations were not artifacts, resulting from movements of the hand placed on the chest, was shown by their simultaneous presence in the other palm and the sole. Incidentally, the ESR of the left palm was almost invariably lower than that of the right, and the plantar

ESR was higher than the sum of both palmar ESRs as it exceeded the level resulting from a palm-to-palm hookup.

Substantially the same ESR findings were reported by others (1669, 2467, 3298, 3300, 3301). Kamiya (2069) noted a steady all-night increase in ESR, without any terminal decline.

Regelsberger (3299), in a study of vegetative correlations during sleep, made simultaneous records of ESR and the CO_2 content of alveolar air. The two variables followed the same course, and their parallel curves had a serrated appearance (*Zackenbild*), with 4 peaks 55 to 120 minutes apart. Regelsberger referred to this periodicity as *kleine rhythmische Schwankungen* or *Kurz-rhythmen* and suggested that they are a part of the vegetative regulations of the organism.

It may be concluded that during sleep there is a distinct rise in the ESR of the palmar surface, related to some extent to the depth and duration of sleep, following a fairly definite though somewhat fluctuating course during the night. As will be shown later, the ESR increases while the body temperature falls and the movements become more frequent, but the trough of the body-temperature curve precedes and the peak of body motility follows the maximum of the ESR.

THE CEREBRAL CORTEX

The contributions of the various parts of the CNS in producing the functional differences between wakefulness and sleep are discussed in Chapter 21, in which the effects of lesions and stimulations are considered. The question of the necessity of the anatomical presence of the cerebral cortex for the alternation of these two states was answered in 1892, when Goltz (1474) succeeded in keeping a completely decorticated dog alive to observe his behavior. Goltz often found his dog asleep, with eyes closed, and breathing regular. He could be awakened, but stronger than usual stimuli were required. During his waking hours the decorticated dog was hyperactive, walking aimlessly for long periods of time, generally in a circle. After he was fed, he made a few turns, then lay down and fell asleep. His rest and sleep were usually of short duration. Deprivation of food increased the animal's restlessness.

Rothmann (3455) not only found that his decorticated dog slept after the manner of a normal animal but also detected in him a sense of time (*Zeit-gefühl*). The dog slept at night and remained awake in the daytime. He apparently knew when he was going to be fed, because at the proper time he would "of his own choice" place himself by the door of his cage and wait for his food. He was hyperactive at times, particularly prior to micturition and defecation, or when he was hungry.

Dresel (978) kept a dog alive for three months after removing his cerebral cortex and striatum. That dog also was very active before micturition and before feeding, but manifested no regular night-sleep habit. Rademaker and Winkler (3256) noted that their decorticated dog "lived in two alternately varying periods. In one it was restless, it tried to make walking movements and to lift itself. In the other it seemed to sleep." They did not state what relation, if any, to day and night the "two alternately varying periods" had.

All the foregoing investigators seemed to agree that their dogs slept after removal of the cerebral cortex. But does a decorticated dog sleep most of the time, or is his period of wakefulness longer than that of sleep? Do the periods of rest and activity alternate regularly? To answer these and other questions, we (2192) studied four decorticated dogs. The completeness of decortication was verified in each case by postmortem examination, and later confirmed by histological studies. The cortex was removed in two stages 4 to 6 weeks apart. The decorticated animals were blind and would bump into obstacles, or into a wall, when allowed to run free in a room. However, they had good pupillary and corneal reflexes. Reflex responses to touch were not only preserved but exaggerated. Touching any part of the dog's body called forth struggling and attempts to bite. In snapping, the dog usually turned to the right or to the left, depending upon which side of the body was stimulated. The movements produced were, aside from correctness of direction, disorderly and quite ineffective.

In general, decorticated dogs, no matter how stimulated, always reacted as if they were displeased. The only temporary failure, or inhibition, of this type of response could be seen during feeding. The eagerness with which the dogs ate was the nearest approach to the manifestation of pleasure. The dogs might struggle as they were picked up to be fed, but, once the feeding commenced, not only were they docile but tickling or pinching was without any effect.

Even casual inspection left no doubt that decorticated dogs slept. When asleep, they lay curled up or sprawled on the floor, eyes closed, their breathing quiet and regular. Upon awakening, they nearly always stretched and yawned. It was easy to follow the various stages of drowsiness prior to the onset of sleep. Through the semiclosed eyelids one could observe how the eyes rolled downward and the nictitating membrane crept over them. There was a marked lowering of reflex irritability during sleep. To obtain a response, one had to apply the stimulus repeatedly at short intervals or increase its intensity.

Once asleep, the dogs did not wake up spontaneously for from 30 minutes to several hours, but most frequently they slept 1 to 2 hours. When awake, they generally walked about, sometimes incessantly, sometimes with short rest periods interspersed. As a rule, the walking was in a circle. We utilized this fact in making the dogs record their activity by means of an inverted hand centrifuge, suspended in the air about 3 feet from the floor. A four-foot rope connected the axis of the centrifuge with the dog's collar. The dog's walking in a circle caused the rope to become twisted, and the slightest twist of the rope was sufficient to rotate the centrifuge. At each such turn an electric contact was made, and this was recorded on a very slow-moving kymograph by means of a signal magnet. In this manner continuous records of activity were obtained. No recording over a certain period did not necessarily mean that the dogs were asleep, although this was generally the case. The continuous records revealed that the decorticated dogs were at rest or active without regard to day and night. On the average, the animals spent from 10 to 45 minutes of every hour walking, the figures varying in different dogs, or in the same dog on successive days. The longest recorded period of incessant walking was 6 hours and 40 minutes. As a rule, there were about 5 or 6 periods of rest and sleep in each 24 hours. Unlike other observers, we did not notice any marked increase in motility at the time when the dogs could be expected to be hungry. On the other hand, satiety did result in a temporary decrease in activity. After they were fed, the dogs usually walked for a while, often urinated and defecated, then lay down and slept for a hour or two. From motility records of our first dog for 17 days it was determined that after feeding he walked for from 5 to 60 minutes (mean, 29 minutes), then slept from 30 minutes to 6 hours (mean, 2 hours and 11 minutes).

Jouvet and Michel (2035, 2036) reported an alternation of sleep and wakefulness in decorticated cats, but the sleep differed from that of intact cats (p. 213).

Karplus and Kreidl (2084) removed the cerebral hemispheres in seventeen monkeys in two stages. Five survived the second operation for from 8 to 26 days. The animals could not be said to have recovered from the operation, but, as long as they lived, they showed an alternation of a more somnolent state and one of being more widely awake. In the sleepy state they made no spontaneous movements, uttered no cries, kept their eyelids closed and hardly responded to external stimuli.

On the clinical side there are the older observations of Edinger and Fischer (1040) and the later reports of Gamper (1347) and Monnier and Willi (2870). The anencephalous child studied by Edinger and Fischer died when he was nearly four years old. From birth on the boy slept but would stir and cry when hungry, thirsty, or soiled. His eyes, when opened, were turned upward. He never learned to recognize his mother either by sight or by the sound of her voice. The authors likened the child to a newborn infant who is also practically without a functioning cerebral cortex. Gamper's paper dealt with the week-long study of an infant who could be classed as a "midbrain" animal, to use the terminology of Magnus. Some posterior periventricular gray around the third ventricle was preserved, but the infant had no temperature control and had to be kept in an incubator. She was also blind. She manifested distinct periods of sleep and wakefulness, but the alternation of these phases was not regular and had no detectable relation to day and night. At times the infant behaved like an ordinary nursling with respect to sleep; at others she remained asleep for 1 to 2 days and had to be aroused to be fed; at still other times she was awake for as long as 12 hours. When awake, she kept her eyes open. During sleep her eyelids were closed and eyes turned up. She could stretch and yawn and was quite active when awake, although she moved little in sleep. Gamper stated that there was no question in anyone's mind that the infant slept at certain times and was awake at others. Nielsen and Sedgwick (3006) described the behavior of an anencephalous infant who lived for 85 days. The infant "would sleep after feeding and awaken when hungry, expressing hunger by crying," and yet had no anatomical structures higher than mesencephalic level—"not even recognizable thalami."

It thus appears certain that dogs, cats, monkeys, and infants are capable of alternating wakefulness and sleep even in the absence of the cerebral cortex. However, they either lose or never develop the ability to adapt their cycle of existence to the 24-hour period of day and night.

Chapter 4

Brain Potentials

Action potentials accompany, or are a part of, every excitatory event in living cells; their patterns have been utilized to record and analyze many physiological processes. The brain, made up of billions of cells, receiving, transmitting, and discharging a great variety of impulses, does not yield a simple bioelectric pattern in active wakefulness. During repose, with the body musculature relaxed, and influx of afferent impulses reduced to a minimum, a "natural" electric beat—an electroencephalogram (EEG)—can be obtained from almost any part of the brain surface, reflecting orderly potential fluctuations. Berger (301) was the first to record EEGs, using non-polarizable Ag-AgCl electrodes, placed epidurally, but since then a variety of electrodes have been developed and are now placed on the skin of the scalp, usually in a number of places permitting potentials to be led off interchangeably from different regions of the head. Berger described several types of potential magnitude and frequency, among them the alpha pattern of about 10/sec, which he considered "an expression of the psycho-physical processes taking place in the brain."

Sleep has been, from the start, one of the conditions studied by the EEG method (27, 28, 301). The refinement of the EEG technique, particularly the employment of permanently implanted electrodes for experimental purposes, has led to an accumulation of significant data on the onset, course, and termination of sleep, dreaming, individual variations, ontogenetic development and decay, and perhaps even more on the levels of consciousness than on the states of sleep and wakefulness.

The pioneer work in classifying EEG patterns was done by the Davis-Harvey-Loomis group (841, 1658, 2559–61), who designated the successive stages in the passage from wakefulness to deep sleep by the first five letters of the alphabet: *A,* or interrupted alpha pattern, 9–11/sec, about 60 microv, seen in wakefulness, perhaps slight drowsiness, on lying down, relaxed, eyes closed; *B,* or low voltage pattern, in which the alpha rhythm has been re-

placed by small undulations, characterized by a sensation of "floating," passing into definite sleep; *C,* or spindle pattern, which includes the appearance
of trains of waves of 14–15/sec, 20–40 microv, superimposed on an irregular
pattern of slower waves; *D,* or spindles-plus-random pattern, with additional
delta waves of about 1/sec, and as high as 300 microv; *E,* or random pattern,
made up of still slower and larger delta waves, with the spindles usually gone.
The letter *K* was used by these authors to denote a sharp diphasic change of
potential, about 1 second in duration and 200–300 microv in magnitude,
which is superimposed on the *B* or *C* pattern, following an auditory stimulus
of effective intensity (842, 843, 3447).

The alphabetical classification stood the test of time, though other schemes
have been proposed periodically (365, 366, 876, 2347, 3709, 4173–75). Dement
(901) simplified the categorization of sleep EEGs on the basis of the presence
of spindling, suggesting four stages: 1, or modified alpha, somewhat irregular, and a fraction of a cycle slower than the waking alpha pattern, but no
spindling, corresponding to late *A* and *B;* 2, or spindling, with low-voltage
background activity, and an admixture of some 3–6/sec waves, very much
like *C;* 3, delta with spindling; and 4, slower delta without spindling, the
equivalents of *D* and *E.* K-complex can be seen in stage 2 (901, 2047).

A shift in the region of maximal EEG activity from the parieto-occipital
area in wakefulness to the frontal one during sleep has been noted (463, 1542).
Continual changes in EEG pattern in the course of a night's sleep, in connection with body motility (366, 467, 2560), as well as in complete immobility,
were also recorded (467, 1542, 2560, 3683). The occurrence of regular cyclic
oscillations in the sleep EEG pattern, at 85- to 90-minute intervals, each time
reaching the modified alpha stage 1 pattern (901), has been linked with the
dreaming process and is discussed in Chapter 11. As will be seen, the EEG
periodicity has been discerned in sleep records of a great variety of sleepers, in
different locations, but its existence has also been denied (663, 1550). In any
case, during the emergent stage 1 EEG it was much harder to awaken the
sleeper than in the initial stage 1 EEG—an example of the inadequacy of the
EEG alone as a criterion of the depth of sleep, and, as will be shown, of sleep
itself.

In animal studies, differences between wakefulness and sleep EEGs were
followed almost exclusively in cats, starting with the earlier observations of
Klaue (2172) and Bremer (473–78), who described the peculiarities character-
izing these two states. Derbyshire and associates (917) noticed the occasional
presence of "small rapid waves, as in the alert wake state" in the cat's sleep
EEG, and Hess and co-workers (1729), in comparing behavioral and EEG
signs of sleep in the cat, concluded that "stages comparable to the human *B*
stage and *E* stage cannot be identified with certainty, and spindles are not a
reliable indication of the depth of sleep." It remained for Dement (899), how-

ever, to discover a regular alternation of periods of slow waves and spindles, or high-voltage slow activity (HVSA), lasting about 10 minutes at the first onset of sleep, and equal-length periods of low-voltage fast activity (LVFA) in the cat's sleep EEG. Dement designated the latter as activated sleep which, mainly on the basis of the EEG, had to be called "light." Hubel (1850), in confirming Dement's EEG findings, classified the sleep as "deep," because the threshold of arousal was much higher during the LVFA EEG than it was in the HVSA phase. On account of the conflict between EEG pattern and behavioral depth of sleep indicators, Jouvet and co-workers (2033, 2047) coined the term "paradoxical phase" (p.p.), later changed to "rhombencephalic phase" sleep (r.c.s.) when they placed the origin of the cortical activation in the pons (p. 212). Several other investigators observed the alternation of the two EEG patterns in the cat's sleep (1624, 1834, 2082, 3425, 4288), with the concomitant twitching movements of the limb and face musculature, noticed by Dement, and the complete relaxation of the nuchal muscles emphasized by Jouvet and co-workers. Despite differences in results and interpretations, it may be considered as established that in the cat there exists a short-term periodicity in the EEG and other concomitants of sleep which is probably related to a similar basic rest-activity periodicity in other animals and man.

The ontogenesis of the EEG has been followed from birth on, with several observations on premature infants (1430, 1862, 2634, 2766, 3047, 3596), the most extensive ones by Dreyfus-Brisac and associates (980–87), who found some non-rhythmic activity at the fetal age of five months but could distinguish quantitatively between the EEG of frank wakefulness and that of drowsiness at six to six and a half months, with definitely qualitative differences appearing at the fetal age of eight and a half months, or close to term. Smith (3738) was the first to report that in neonates there is no EEG in the occipital region, but that some 4–5/sec activity can be seen in the motor area, and there during sleep only. Other observers (985, 1067, 1862–64, 2127, 2634, 2766, 3794) also underlined the non-occipital location of activity, and the presence of spindles in some cases during sleep (1067, 2127), with a flattening of the tracings following a spontaneous movement (1065). Smith (3738, 3739) also demonstrated that a distinct EEG pattern appears in the occipital area during the third or fourth month of extrauterine life, and this finding was confirmed by many others (460, 985, 1067, 1430, 2125–27, 2162, 2268, 2523–25, 2839), with minor differences concerning the age and the frequency range. The age of ten to fourteen weeks, at which a regular EEG appears in the occipital area, marks the termination of cortical blindness and ushers in a new orientation to the environment (p. 134).

In studies of the EEGs of animals, Kornmueller (2238) found the newborn rabbit's cortex to be electrically silent, but EEG activity appeared at the age of several days. Gokhblit (1467) followed the increase in the EEG frequency of puppies from 10–14/sec at birth, through 16–18/sec at the age of eighteen days, to 35–45/sec at three months. Sleep-wakefulness bioelectric differences could not be seen in puppies before they were eighteen to twenty days old, and at three months their sleep EEG changes were similar to those of adult dogs. In young pigs, however, Pampiglione (3086) recognized EEG sleep-wakefulness differentiation and the K-complex at the age of one week, with full maturation of the EEG at three to four weeks, and in the macaque monkey Cavennes (665) recorded drowsiness rhythms of 4–5/sec and spindle activity during light sleep at the age of one day, and slow $1\frac{1}{2}$–3/sec waves in deep sleep by the end of the first week.

Systematic studies of the evolution of the alpha EEG pattern in older infants, children, and adolescents, pioneered by Smith (3738, 3739), Lindsley (2523–25), and Bernhard and Skoglund (314), and reinvestigated by Kellaway (2125, 2126), Fois (1221), and others (460, 1430, 3597), dealt with the progressive demarcation between the EEGs of sleep and wakefulness, as well as the increase in the frequency of the alpha pattern with age. Smith's figures showed that the central area alpha frequency remains unchanged at 7/sec till the end of the first year, while the occipital 3–4/sec pattern, after its belated appearance, rapidly increases in frequency, almost catching up with the central alpha at the age of one to two and a half years, the two thereafter increasing in a parallel manner, with the occipital pattern 1/sec behind the central one. The curves of the alpha frequencies plotted against age differ somewhat, but frequencies of 8–9/sec have been seen in children of three to five years of age, and the adult alpha pattern is reached in some children at the age of eight years (3738).

At the other end of the age scale, it has been reported that in normal persons there is a slowing down of the alpha pattern (3036). In senile depression there is a reduction in the frequency of the alpha pattern to as low as 6.5–7.5/sec, and a rise to 9–11/sec with improvement in condition (1158). In senile dementia there is a reduction in alpha content of the EEG (2948), with the remaining alpha pattern below 8/sec (2154).

The terms "alpha index" and "alpha content" have been used to indicate the percentage of time in which the alpha pattern dominates the EEG. According to Rubin (3468), the alpha index in the occipital region is not only high but very stable and reproducible, whereas in the frontal region—another area of maximal alpha activity—the index is variable, fluctuating from day to day and hour to hour. Knott and co-workers (2219) detected no obvious sleep EEG differences between five subjects with alpha indices of over 65 per cent and five who had an alpha index of less than 5 per cent. Brazier and Beecher (467) noted a decrease in alpha content of the sleep EEG, after the administration of sedatives, and an anticipatory increase in alpha content a few seconds prior to bodily movement. Lemere (2424) related the ability to produce a good alpha pattern to the affective capacity of the person. Among the psychopaths, mildly manic or depressed patients gave good alpha waves, whereas schizophrenics did not. Saul and co-authors (3527) also found a correlation between character traits and the alpha index, high values shown by "passive" individuals and low ones by women with strong masculine trends. Davis and Davis (839) reported a striking similarity of alpha patterns in each of fifteen pairs of identical twins, but no relation of EEG to intelligence. Lindsley (2524) saw no correlation between ascendance-submission and emotional stability of subjects of varying ages and their alpha indices.

Abnormal EEGs have been related to certain types of brain damage (1222, 2124, 2165, 2576, 2577, 2678), with the sleep EEGs in hydrocephalus sometimes appearing bilaterally asynchronous (1223). Much higher than normal percentages of low-voltage activity in the sleep EEGs of psychotics, with greater variations in sleep EEG stages, have been reported (932, 2586, 2587), and the employment of the sleep EEG for diagnostic purposes was advocated by many investigators (259, 1458, 2982, 2983, 3698–700, 3797, 4103, 4130, 4176).

Alpha amplitude, according to Stennett (3803), is related to the level of palmar conductance, the curve resembling an inverted U, with low microvoltages at the two extremes and maximum at 73 micromhos. Coleman and associates (739, 740) noted that EEG amplitude during sleep was positively correlated with reaction time and inversely related to the duration of immobility.

Discriminative behavior during sleep was demonstrated with the aid of EEG and conditioning. Christake (698) elicited both behavioral and EEG arousal in sleeping rats by presenting them with meaningful, but not with neutral, auditory stimuli. Rowland (3460) was able to get EEG desynchronization without behavioral arousal in cats by presenting them with a "positive" auditory conditioned stimulus. Toman and co-workers (3953) repeatedly delivered verbal stimuli to sleeping subjects, whose EEG pattern was modified more easily by "loaded" words (the subject's nickname) than by physically equivalent "non-loaded" words. This discriminatory phenomenon was also reported by others (1962, 3071). Buendia and co-workers (561) found that cats discriminated learned sound frequencies during sleep, but that the reactivity was more markedly reduced in the LVFA phase than during the "classical" HVSA phase. Like Rowland, they noted that the EEG change was often the first, or only, response, behavioral manifestations appearing later or not at all. Granda and Hammack (1498) studied "operant" behavior of sleepers, who could, and did, avoid unpleasant electric shocks by pressing a key oftener than every three seconds during all EEG stages of sleep, but mostly during deeper levels of stage 1 EEG.

The dissociation between behavioral and EEG responses to stimulation during sleep raises a question of the adequacy of the EEG pattern for differentiating between wakefulness and sleep. Wikler (4207) recorded EEG sleep patterns in dogs after injections of atropine, and yet the animals were unmistakably awake. Similar results were obtained in cats and monkeys by Bradley and Elkes (444, 445). Hamoen (1621) and Roth and Šimek (3443) saw sleep EEGs in waking patients with a variety of nervous or mental ailments. Other examples could be given (112, 120, 171, 1122, 1185, 1186, 3620), but it is clear that the EEG by itself not only fails to gauge the depth of sleep but the very presence of behavioral sleep. It does not mean that the EEG is not a useful tool when coupled with other concomitants of sleep, and where there is a conflict between the different indices, behavioral signs must be given preference over EEG patterns.

What has been indicated with respect to the level of consciousness, associated with sleep or wakefulness (p. 4), also seems to apply to the EEG. In relaxed wakefulness children and adults maintain a certain degree of alertness, coupled with a regular alpha pattern. A newborn infant, even when definitely awake, is not conscious and shows no regular EEG. Before attempting to equate the level of consciousness with the frequency of the alpha pattern (admitting that "non-alpha" persons can reach a high level of consciousness), it may be well to consider further the meaning of the term consciousness. There has been a tendency to evade the difficulty of defining the term by declaring that "consciousness is an abstraction, and cannot as such be the object of scientific investigation" (2293); that "introduction to physiology of such concepts as consciousness . . . is unnecessary and sometimes misleading" (3207); or that "consciousness has no meaning without its contents" (3560). Nor will it do to avoid the subject of consciousness because it "is a psychologic problem" (3143). Physiological or psychological, the problem of consciousness has been the topic of conferences (4, 875), and numerous publications were devoted mainly, or exclusively, to the consideration of its various characteristics (592, 1161, 1519, 2190, 2191, 2293, 2420, 2526–28, 3017, 3143–47, 3207, 3214, 3560, 4033, 4108, 4135). As used here, the term consciousness stands for critical reactivity, with the level of consciousness the degree to which an animal or person is capable of critical reactivity—analyzing incoming information in the light of previous experience and integrating a response directed to certain goals. Judging by the behavior of a wakeful neonate, or an older anencephalous infant, or a decorticated dog, their level of consciousness is extremely low. Conscious processes require the operation of neural circuits involving the cerebral cortex. The fact that one can remove any area of the cerebral cortex without abolishing consciousness (3146) does not mean that one can dispense with the entire cortex and still retain the usual level of consciousness. To say also that "the indispensible substratum of consciousness lies outide the cerebral cortex, probably in the diencephalon" (3143), or that the "system essential to crude consciousness is located where the mesencephalon, subthalamus and thalamus meet" (3926, 3927), is simply to indicate that the cortex deprived of afferent and efferent connections cannot carry out its analyzing and integrating activities. Dandy (819) placed the conscious (also sleep) center in the corpus striatum, as permanent loss of consciousness was produced in patients whose anterior cerebral arteries were ligated, but Meyers (2798) challenged Dandy's conclusions. Watson and Adams (4128) considered the relation of consciousness and responsiveness to lesions confined to the brain stem as a result of a thrombotic occlusion of the basilar artery. The list of authors who emphasized attention or awareness, or some other favorite aspect of consciousness, linked to one or another structure from the cortex downward, is almost endless (12, 54, 96, 452–54, 485, 590, 878, 993, 1002, 1160, 1386, 1391, 1660, 1672–74, 1919, 1953, 2053, 2054, 2215, 2298, 2300, 2367, 2368, 2372, 2509, 2541, 2695, 2697, 2745, 2761, 2799, 2822, 2836, 2923, 2969, 3007, 3057, 3148, 3227, 3272, 3440, 3443, 3469, 3533, 3549, 3967, 4205). It is to be understood that the arguments and exercises in semantics presented in the publications referred to only by number are not different, in any material respect, from those whose authors were named.

To return to the alpha EEG pattern, it is not the alpha content, index, percentage, or magnitude that characterize the level of consciousness, but its frequency and regularity, granted that the conditions are conducive to the recording of the EEG. The ontogenesis and eventual decay of the alpha pattern in man parallel his cortical capacities. Each "alpha" person has his own frequency range and mean, and, as shown by Ellingson and associates (1068), there is no correlation between alpha frequency and intelligence. It is rather the deviation from one's usual frequency pattern that is indicative of a change in the level of consciousness (1769). It is significant that in "intense attention" there was no change in the alpha mode in the occipital area, but in the motor region the peak alpha frequency shifted from 9.4/sec to 10.2/sec (584). Conversely, boredom resulting from sensory isolation for 96 hours caused the alpha frequency mode to shift from 10/sec to 9/sec in two subjects and to 8/sec in a third (1716). Acute alcoholic intoxication also brought on a decrease in alpha frequency (848, 1086, 1087), by a fraction of a cycle to over 2/sec. Chronic alcoholism has not been found to affect the EEG (848, 1014), probably because no "normal" frequency was available for comparison. Anoxia leads to errors in performance and eventual loss of consciousness (1811), but milder oxygen lack (equivalent to 14,000 to 16,000 feet elevation) causes a decrease in alpha frequency, as does a blood sugar reduction to hypoglycemic levels in man (847, 1085, 1087) and dog (1791). By contrast, inhalation of 100 per cent oxygen or an injection of glucose shifts the alpha frequency upward (1085). Hyperthermia raises the alpha frequency (1513, 1789, 1790), though not always (2259); mental confusion at the height of the fever may slow down the EEG (2517); and delirium from a variety of causes has also been reported to shift the alpha mode into much lower frequencies, in proportion to the disturbance of consciousness (3399). In ten patients with congenital hypothyroidism, ages ranging from a few weeks to thirty-three years, Nieman (3009) reported the dominant EEG frequency to be lower than that of normal individuals of corresponding ages. Thyroxin therapy led to behavioral improvement and an increase in the alpha frequency. In a four-year-old girl, the dominant occipital alpha was shifted from 3.5–4.0/sec to 8–9/sec after thyroxin. Conversely, in hyperthyroidism, the alpha frequency was higher than in pre-morbid recordings, the increase, in some cases, showing a relation to the change in the basal metabolic rate (BMR) (2154). It appears, then, that the level of consciousness, as expressed by the regularity and frequency of the alpha pattern, may be an index of the metabolic activity of the cerebral cortex during muscular relaxation and a minimum of sensory influx. The bearing of the character of the alpha pattern on the level of consciousness is further discussed in connection with the physiology of dreaming (Chapter 11).

Davis and associates (844) reported that "no correlation could be detected between the stage of sleep and the D.C. potential differences or changes in D.C. potential observed between chest and head, scalp and mastoid region, frontal and occipital regions, or right and left sides of the head." Burge and Vaught (576) and King (2157) did record a smaller difference in potential between the forehead and other parts of the body during sleep than in wakefulness. Caspers and Schulze (650, 653) obtained similar results in freely moving rats, with implanted electrodes, recording D.C. potential differences between the surface of the cortex and the nose.

Of greatest significance are the findings of Evarts and associates (1116, 1119, 1120) on the rate of spontaneous discharge of single neurones in the visual cortex of the cat, recorded by implanted electrodes. The rate is higher during sleep, particularly during the LVFA phase. They also found that "neurons which discharge rapidly during sleep tend to discharge more rapidly during waking, whereas neurons with relatively low rates of discharge during sleep tend to have reduced spontaneous activity during waking." Thus, sleep is not associated with generalized inhibition of cortical activity, as maintained gratuitously by Pavlov (3122), and uncritically echoed by a host of his "hero-worshippers" (p. 344).

The brain potentials discussed in this chapter represent spontaneous activity in normal intact animals and human subjects, with an emphasis on the differences between wakefulness and sleep. Many other bioelectric manifestations are considered in connection with the events of a night's sleep, periodicity, interference with, and spontaneous changes in the sleep-wakefulness cycle, in succeeding parts of this book. It will be seen that the most important advances in the understanding of sleep, wakefulness, and consciousness were made by recording spontaneous and evoked electrical changes in the CNS.

Chapter 5

The Blood

Although Piéron (3192) devoted a not inconsiderable portion of his monograph to the discussion of the effect of sleep deprivation on the composition of the blood, he did not mention blood changes that are concomitant with normal sleep. However, many extensive studies have since been made on this topic, some resulting from, others leading to, strange notions and theories concerning the physiology of sleep. Foremost among these is the view that calcium partially disappears from the blood and retreats into, or is taken up by, the brain during sleep.

It is hard to take up the topic systematically because there is an interrelationship among the various blood constituents, some changes depending on others and becoming understandable only in the light of these other changes. For instance, most of the constituents studied show a decreased concentration during sleep. If it could be demonstrated that there is an increase in the circulating blood volume, these changes would naturally follow a dilution of the blood and would not as such be connected with the state of sleep. If, further, it should be demonstrated that the recumbent position by itself led to an increase in the volume of blood, sleep would appear to produce such a change only because the person or animal usually assumed a horizontal position while asleep. The reader should keep these possibilities in mind as the findings of various blood changes during sleep are discussed.

With the development of pH-determination methods several observers successfully measured differences in hydrogen-ion concentration of the blood in wakefulness and sleep. Collip (745) found no change or a slight decrease in the alkali reserve of the blood as a result of sleep, comparing samples obtained before retiring at night with those drawn after getting up in the morning. The hydrogen-ion concentration was increased slightly during sleep. This finding was confirmed by others (1075, 1653). Kunze (2306) gave the mean blood pH values for twelve subjects as 7.62 in wakefulness and 7.58 during sleep, and corresponding figures obtained by Robin and associates (3376) on thirteen persons were 7.43 and 7.40.

Amsler (56), in discussing the blocking effect of sleep on the development of inflammation, saw the cause of this phenomenon as residing in changes produced in the tissues by sleep. These changes involve cell-alkali fixation and lead to sleep acidosis. Conversely, during the waking state there is an alkalosis.

In natural sleep Endres and Lucke (1080) observed a rise in blood sugar from 98–99 mg per cent to 111–124 mg per cent. After awakening, the blood sugar was found to be as low as, or lower than, it was the night before. It is not certain, according to these authors, whether or not the rise is produced through a modification of central nervous blood-sugar regulation. They advanced as a probable explanation the shift in reaction of the blood to the acid side during sleep. Trimble and Maddock (3976) made hourly determinations of the capillary blood-sugar concentrations of nine normal young men. Sleep produced no change in the sugar values. A third possibility—that the blood sugar is decreased during sleep—was reported by Dienst and Winter (935), according to whom, not only is there a decrease of blood sugar during sleep, but hypoglycemia, whether produced by insulin or phlorizin or otherwise, itself produces sleep, as experiments on dogs and men convinced them. Sleep resulting from barbiturates closely resembled natural sleep insofar as changes in blood chemistry were concerned, while alcohol and its derivatives produced hyperglycemia. Buondonno and Fiore (566) also found a decrease in blood sugar during sleep, the means for thirty subjects changing from 80 mg per cent to 58.

Chieffi and Rosselli del Turco (694) followed the blood-sugar curves in twenty-eight children, ranging in age from one and a half months to eight years. The blood sugar increased in sleep, the more so the better nourished the children and the deeper their sleep.

Heilig and Hoff (1681) noted that giving 100 gm of sugar by mouth to a person suddenly awakened and then permitted to fall asleep again led to a greater rise in blood sugar than it did when the subject stayed awake.

Hopkins (1832) reported a low blood cholesterol, and Chieffi and Rosselli del Turco (694) a decreased blood fat in sleep. Jones (2009) studied a case of a woman, twenty-two years old, who suffered from attacks of prolonged sleep of 1 to 6 days' duration. The most striking biochemical finding was a low blood cholesterol, 75–105 mg per cent, which the author compared with figures obtained on a narcoleptic patient whose blood cholesterol fell from 200 mg per cent to 100 or less during sleep.

Gollwitzer-Meier and Kroetz (1473) found no changes in the potassium, calcium, and bicarbonate ions of the plasma in sleep but an increase in chloride and acid-soluble phosphorus; Rubino (3471), however, noted decreases in serum calcium and magnesium during sleep. Haldane and co-workers (1603) detected an increase in organic phosphates in the blood not only during sleep but also as a result of breathing CO_2. Collip (745) in six cases out of nine noted a definite increase in plasma bicarbonate and in the remaining three no change.

Heilig and Hoff (1681) perfused blood drawn from a waking person through frog blood vessels and obtained a certain degree of vasoconstriction. Blood taken from the same individual while asleep had a weaker vasoconstricting effect than did the first blood sample. However, Renton and Weil-Malherbe (3321) found that the adrenalin content of the plasma was about 40 per cent higher during sleep than it was immediately on getting up in the morning, with no significant changes in nor-adrenaline content. Perkoff and associates (3158) ascribed the 24-hour variation in plasma 17-hydroxycorticosteroids to the abrupt rise that occurs during sleep. There is a decrease in serum cholinesterase content in the majority of human subjects (3471), as well as in hens (1310), during sleep.

Cloetta's view (721) that during sleep calcium passes from the blood into the brain has given rise to a number of investigations. Unlike Gollwitzer-Meier and Kroetz (1473), who reported no change in plasma calcium, Demole (908) noted a decrease, and Heilig and Hoff (1681) an increase. Fischer (1175) obtained a decrease in blood calcium in cats, narcotized by somnifen. Cerebral excitation, produced by betatetrahydronaphthylamine, he found, on the contrary, led to a rise in blood calcium. Fischer stated that this shift of calcium into and out of the blood is independent of the cerebral cortex, as it still occurs after decortication, but it fails completely after decerebration. The regulation of blood calcium, then, according to Fischer, resides in the brain stem, presumably in the diencephalon. Potassium and calcium are antagonistic to each other, and in sleep and narcosis with a fall in serum calcium there is a rise in potassium. As in the case of calcium, the regulating center for potassium is in the diencephalon. Later Cloetta and co-authors (723), by the use of special methods, found that there was a fall in both calcium and potassium of the plasma in man during natural sleep, or sleep following hypnotics, and also in dogs and rabbits put to "sleep" by the injection of calcium into the infundibular region. However, if the hypnotics did not produce sleep, but, as in certain psychopaths and in cats, hyperexcitability, there was no decrease in plasma calcium or potassium. Although the conclusion was again made that entrance of calcium into the diencephalon is a feature of the onset of sleep, the authors realized that the amount of calcium thus taken up could not account for all the calcium that presumably disappeared from the blood; so the muscles were postulated to take up the bulk of both calcium and potassium during sleep, just as they are supposed to release these two ions into the circulation during activity. Cloetta (721), in reviewing his twelve-year study of the chemical basis of the alternation of sleep and wakefulness, elaborated the facts and fancies previously published, going on record as holding that there is a 6 to 10 per cent fall in plasma calcium and potassium but no change in sodium and magnesium. Katzenelbogen (2092) could not detect any difference in the calcium concentration of any part of the brain, including the hypothalamus, between wakefulness and narcosis produced in cats by diallylbarbituric acid, thus refuting Cloetta's contention about the passage of calcium into the diencephalon. However, Katzenelbogen, too, found a suggestion of a decrease in blood calcium of these cats, although the proportion of the calcium concentration of the blood to that of the cerebrospinal fluid remained unchanged.

As about one-half of the total calcium of the plasma is protein-bound, only the diffusible portion, which is almost entirely in the ionic state, can be physiologically active. Indeed, the tissue fluids have approximately the same ionic calcium concentration as does the blood plasma, and there is a state of equilibrium between the two. Cooperman (752), therefore, analyzed the plasma samples not only for total calcium by the usually employed Clark-Collip modification of the Kramer-Tisdall method but, in addition, for ionizable calcium by the use of the McLean-Hastings nomogram. Cooperman compared the values of total calcium and ionizable calcium before and at the end of a night's sleep. Seven men served as subjects in this series; each showed a slightly lower serum calcium at the end of 5 to 7 hours of sleep, with the mean values 10.11 mg per cent before and 9.87 after. As a control test, each subject was required to spend one or more nights in bed awake. The decrease in serum calcium was small under these conditions, but, in general, 1.5 to 2 hours after going to bed, asleep or awake, at night or in the daytime, the drop in serum calcium was greatest. The ionizable calcium never showed a decrease but, on the contrary, appeared to be somewhat raised under every one of the foregoing conditions.

In the animal tests made by Cooperman (752) an exact criterion of sleep was lacking, but dogs were blindfolded and trained to lie quietly on a mattress for long periods of time under conditions that were conducive to sleep. In some tests the dogs were exercised on a treadmill, operating at a slow speed, for 30 to 60 minutes in order to encourage relaxation afterward. In ten trials on five dogs, the effects of 1.5 to 2 hours of rest after mild exercise were a small decrease in total serum calcium and no change in calcium-ion concentration. Without the preliminary exercise the total serum-calcium changes in thirteen trials showed less consistent changes, but again there was no effect on ionizable calcium. When the animals rested 5 to 6 hours, there was, as in the human subjects, a definite decrease in total serum calcium and an increase in ionizable calcium. It appears, then, that rest in the horizontal position leads to an increase rather than a decrease of the physiologically significant serum-calcium concentration, and all considerations based on a postulated decrease are left without factual support.

But what is the meaning of this increase? Is it of significance in understanding the nature and cause of sleep? Not at all, as can be seen from an examination of the serum-protein figures also obtained by Cooperman. There was practically always a marked drop in serum protein in resting men and dogs, under the conditions studied. The drop could be due to the entrance of tissue fluids into the blood vessels. Direct determinations of plasma volume by the Congo red method confirmed this supposition for both the human subjects and the dogs. For example, in one subject the initial plasma volume was 2,625 ml and whole blood volume, 4,874 ml. Two hours of rest, part of it asleep, resulted in a plasma volume of 2,977 ml and whole blood volume, 5,595 ml, or an increase of nearly 15 per cent. The earlier report (1473) was that the blood is diluted during sleep, with the only constituent showing a rise—the chloride ion which is known to be found in higher concentration in tissue fluids than in the plasma. The changes in serum calcium can thus be explained simply as a passive mechanical consequence of the entrance of tissue fluid into the blood vessels during rest or sleep, this fluid containing about the same amount of free calcium but much less bound calcium because of its lower protein content.

As suggested, many data on blood constituents are meaningless in themselves unless one knows how the blood volume was affected under the conditions that prevailed during, or resulted from, the experiment. Blood volume, however, is not an easy figure to obtain accurately. In the first place, one must distinguish between total blood volume and circulating blood volume. The spleen is a known reservoir not only for red blood cells but also for plasma. Yet, removing the spleen does not solve the problem. As shown by Roberts and Crandall (3370), one can inject large amounts of isotonic salt solution or blood into the circulation of normal or splenectomized animals without affecting the blood-volume figures. There is evidence that the portal system is capable of storing large quantities of blood in such a manner that it is not available for dilution with the dye. Furthermore, as pointed out by Waterfield (4126), and also as found by us, the dye method is not satisfactory for determining spontaneous variations in blood volume because most dyes diffuse into the lymph spaces. It should also be remembered that many so-called sleep studies were made on animals or persons "put to sleep" by means of hypnotic drugs, some of which by themselves produce changes in blood volume. Adolph and Gerbasi (22) have shown that sodium amytal led to an increase in blood volume, while ethyl urethane had the opposite effect.

That posture has an influence on the composition and volume of blood in man was demonstrated by Thomson and co-workers (3932) by the use of the dye method. Lying down for 20 to 30 minutes resulted in a decrease in the red-blood-cell count from 4.8 to 4.3 million, in serum protein from 8.1 per cent to 6.9, in hematocrit from 43.6 per cent to 40.3, and in plasma volume an increase from 2,315 to 2,605 ml. The opposite changes occurred on passing from the lying to the standing position for an equal length of time. There was also a greater difference in the packed-cell volumes of blood samples taken from the foot, while standing and on lying down, than of blood samples drawn from the arm under similar conditions. The corresponding pairs of values were 49.3 and 44.7 per cent for blood from the foot, and 47.8 and 44.5 per cent for blood from the arm. Similar relations between posture and blood volume, as well as plasma proteins, were reported by other investigators (3155, 3312, 3757, 3955).

Thus, on standing, there is a passage of fluid from the blood vessels due to increased filtration pressure, and this passing-out of fluid is greater in the leg because of the effect of gravity. That filtration pressure is operative was known to Cohnheim in 1867 and has been studied since then by other investigators, among them Rowe (3457), who created a venous stasis in the arm by a manometer cuff inflated to produce a pressure somewhere between the systolic and diastolic arterial pressures of the subject. Using twelve subjects, and applying various pressures up to 120 mm Hg for 1 to 20 minutes, Rowe produced an increased concentration of serum protein proportional to the magnitude and duration of outside pressure. The non-protein elements underwent no change in concentration, showing that they could pass out of the circulating blood as a part of the filtrate.

Waterfield (4126) used the CO method on eight subjects. The blood volume was lower in the erect than in the recumbent position, the plasma volume decreasing 15 per cent and the cell volume 4 per cent. He also confirmed the earlier findings of a leakage of fluid into the legs in the upright position (4127). The volume of the leg increased by 60–120 ml on standing for 40 minutes, and this change was of the order of magnitude that was to be expected from the blood-volume changes. Youmans and associates (4298) studied the effect of posture on the serum-protein concentration and colloid osmotic pressure of the blood from the foot, from the same viewpoint. There was a marked increase (27 per cent) in serum protein and a still more marked rise (43 per cent) in colloid osmotic pressure on standing, together with an increase of 4 per cent in the volume of the leg. There was also a greater change in the blood taken from the leg than in that drawn from the arm.

The available data on the red-blood-cell counts, packed-cell volume, and hemoglobin concentration seem to be in accord with the foregoing figures for plasma volume and serum-protein concentration. On ten male subjects parallel determinations were made in our laboratory on serum proteins, red-blood-cell count, hematocrit, and hemoglobin: before going to sleep; 1 to 2 hours, 4 to 5 hours, and 6 to 8 hours after the onset of sleep; as well as 1 hour after getting up in the morning. Together with the decrease in serum protein, there were falls in the other constituents studied, the sharpest drop occurring at the end of 1 to 2 hours of sleep. Thereafter there was either a decreased slope or else a slight rise, and a very steep rise 1 hour after awakening. Here, too, the main effect was apparently that of a change in posture with somewhat of an adjustment later in the night. The most consistent decrease was in the hematocrit readings. Walters (4112) had previously reported significant decreases in erythrocyte count, quantity of hemoglobin, and percentage of red blood cells in healthy men on lying down for 20 to 30 minutes but failed to see any connection between these changes and the increased blood volume as reported by others (642, 3312, 3932, 4127). There have also been reports of a lack of effect of sleep on hemoglobin content of the blood (2649, 3757), and in paroxysmal nocturnal hemoglobinuria the hemolytic factor is either more active, or more of it is activated, in sleep than in wakefulness (790, 3373).

It appears that nearly all the changes in the composition of the blood during sleep are explainable by the effect of alternation of posture. In the upright position, with an increase in capillary filtration pressure, there is an oozing-out of blood plasma devoid of protein. In the horizontal position, with decreased filtration pressure, the fluid can return to the blood vessels and thus increase the blood volume, at the same time diluting the constituents that cannot move freely in and out of the circulatory system.

Chapter 6

The Circulation

It was already known to the ancients that the heart rate is decreased during sleep. Modern observers have added qualifications and refinements, based partly on newer and better methods of study and partly on more adequate control of comparative conditions. The decrease in rate as given by various authors ranges from one or two beats up to a dozen or more per minute, depending on, among other factors, sex and age (370, 618, 1523, 1723, 2176, 3031, 3204, 3677, 3818, 4203). As pointed out by Piéron (3192), the assumption of the horizontal position is of itself sufficient to lower the heart rate. As a mean of 18 determinations on himself, he gave the heart rates for standing as 77.8; sitting, 65.3; and lying, 61.2—or a difference of 16.6 beats as a result of changing from the vertical to the horizontal position. Even when one remains in the same position, the pulse rate shows considerable fluctuations from moment to moment, as was found by Boas and Goldschmidt (387) through the use of their "cardiotachometer." This device is an electric counter and recorder, actuated by the beating heart through electrodes tied to the chest, and supplied with sufficiently long wires to allow the subject to move about freely in an average-size room. With this arrangement, which permitted continuous recording for hours or even days, they have studied the variations in heart rate of several hundred subjects in health and in disease, and under a variety of experimental conditions. In practically every case the minimal heart rate during wakefulness was lower than the maximal during sleep. However, the mean pulse during wakefulness for the same subjects exceeded the sleep pulse by 19 beats (82.6 and 63.7). In general, they reported considerable fluctuations of the heart rate not only during waking hours but also during sleep. Loud noises, movements of the sleeper, and unknown influences (probably internal stimuli) caused the heart-rate curve to have a jagged appearance. Daytime sleep produced much less of a drop in pulse than night sleep, the decrease amounting to only 9 beats per minute. The minimal heart rates, which they considered of greater significance than the mean values during sleep, seemed to be related to age and sex. These minimum rates during sleep were 52.7 for men and 57.7 for women. Furthermore, whereas in the waking figures they could find only three instances of heart rates as low as 45, in sleep 14 out of 103 cases had minimal rates between 45 and 36. The range of the heart rates, as would be expected, was much smaller during sleep than in the waking state, with the corresponding ranges for men, 14 and 50, and for women, 18 and 54. There was a decrease in the range during sleep with advancing age, the male and female ranges amounting to 17 and 25 for individuals under 46, and to 11 and 10 for persons over 66. There was no relationship between heart rates during sleep and meteorological conditions, such as temperature, atmospheric pressure, and humidity. It should be noted that the maximal heart rates were observed most frequently during the first 2 hours of sleep and the minimal during the seventh; this pattern is referred to in the discussion of the several variables that may be used for plotting the depth-of-sleep curve (p. 109).

Electrocardiographic studies during sleep were made by several investigators (1981, 2072, 2210, 4069, 4199). Klewitz (2210), in the general lengthening of the cycle, discerned a greater increase in the duration of the ventricular systole than in that of the auricular, although that is the usual occurrence when the heart is slowed. The difference in heart action was considered by him advantageous for the circulation. Kanner (2072) made observations during prolonged rest and sleep and found no difference between them. In both cases the absolute duration of ventricular systole was decreased, and the electrical systole was shorter than the mechanical one. The time of conduction of the impulse through the bundle of His was prolonged during rest, and, therefore, presumably during sleep. Jenness and Wible (1981) stated that in sleep there was a decrease in the P-R interval but an increase in the mean electrical systole.

The heart rates of children show a smaller sleep-wakefulness difference than do those of adults (188, 626, 3877, 4115). Lange (2363), in a systematic study of heart rates, starting with prematurely born infants through children aged thirteen, noted an inverse relationship between age and the decrease in heart rate during sleep. Furthermore, she found that the occurrence of minimal heart rates during the night's sleep gradually shifted from about 9:00 P.M. in infants to 3:00 A.M. in older children. It will be recalled that in adults minimal heart rates are reached in the seventh hour of sleep.

With the different forms of heart disease Klewitz (2209, 2210) found no regularity in changes during sleep. Hearts with valvular defects in the compensated state behaved like normal hearts. In decompensated hearts the fall in rate during sleep depended on the severity of decompensation. In certain cases the rate might be higher in sleep than during wakefulness. Extrasystoles did not disappear in sleep. Klewitz also noted that organic tachycardia was not affected by sleep, while in nervous tachycardia there was a slowing of the heart in sleep. The findings of Klewitz were confirmed by Boas and Weiss (386, 388) by the use of the cardiotachometer. In exophthalmic goiter these authors saw little reduction in heart rate during sleep; the minimal rates were about 30 beats greater than those of normal persons. Crooks and Murray (788), in a study of hyperthyroid patients, obtained sleeping heart rates of over 80/min in 54 per cent of toxic subjects, but only in 3 per cent of non-toxic ones. Thus, the determination of the heart rate during sleep may be of value as a diagnostic procedure in diseases of the thyroid gland.

According to Sutherland (3877), highly excitable children showed greater differences in heart rates than phlegmatic ones. The nocturnal slowing could be abolished by atropine. The slowing during sleep was also abolished in fever and in active rheumatic carditis. Schlesinger (3567) seemed to agree with Sutherland. From the report of Sutherland that atropine prevented a fall in heart rate during sleep it would appear that vagal influences might be involved in this phenomenon. Samaan (3514) accepted this explanation but added that, besides an increase in vagal tonus, there was a decrease in sympathetic tonus. He found that the dog's denervated heart was slowed but little during sleep, and the slowing that did occur he ascribed to lowered body temperature. Boas and Goldschmidt (387) also discussed the possible effect of body temperature on heart rate, but there was no strict parallelism between the two, and the lowest temperature did not correspond in time with the minimal heart rate. They considered, in addition, as possible causes of the slowing of the heart: the low metabolic rate prevailing during sleep; muscular relaxation; the diminution in the number of afferent impulses from other sources; and a generally lowered reflex excitability, favoring a decrease in acceleratory influences constantly playing on the heart. They also marshalled a great deal of evidence in favor of an increase in vagal tonus, including their observation that a marked sinus arrhythmia appeared whenever the heart rate was considerably slowed in sleep.

Jackson (1933, 1934), in recording the heart rate of one subject for twelve nights, detected an anticipatory cardiac acceleration, beginning about 6 minutes before a movement and increasing rapidly in the 30 seconds just prior to the movement. The change in rate in connection with dreaming is described in Chapter 11.

To summarize, the heart rate is decidedly slowed during sleep, more so during the night than during daytime naps.

The greater portion of the work on the circulation during sleep pertains to arterial pressure. Piéron (3192) enumerated older observations, among them those of Tarchanoff (3906), who, in measuring blood pressure in puppies by the direct method, found it to drop 20–50 mm Hg during sleep. Somewhat smaller decreases in blood pressure of adult dogs during sleep were reported by Kernodle and co-workers (2143, 2144).

The effect of the position of the body on blood pressure was studied by several workers (3192), and some reported a fall in pressure on the assumption of the lying position; others, a rise; and still others, various changes. It seems that the influence of the position of the body on blood pressure is less constant than on the heart rate. Even during sleep, as observed by Landis (2359), the position of the subject has little or no effect on blood pressure.

Brooks and Carrol (525), on 127 patients with high, normal, and low blood pressures, found that the drop in pressure during sleep was proportional to the height of the waking blood pressure. In the normal group, whose systolic pressures varied from 110 to 170 mm, with a mean of 142.5 mm, the mean maximal drop during sleep was 24 mm. Müller and Blume (385, 2913, 2915), on many subjects, aged sixteen to forty-five, observed a surprising uniformity in blood pressure during sleep, although the waking blood pressures fluctuated considerably. In sleeping men the mean systolic blood pressure was 94 mm, a decrease of 26 mm from the mean value in wakefulness; in women, 88 mm, a drop of 21 mm. In men with low blood pressure (under 120 mm) the drop during sleep was 22 mm; with higher blood pressures, it was 31 mm. Similarly, in women with low pressures (less than 116 mm) the decrease in sleep was 17 mm; with higher pressures, 39 mm.

The diastolic pressures do not decrease as much as the systolic (626, 2089, 2359, 2913), resulting in diminished pulse pressures. The figures of Landis (2359) for systolic pressure during wakefulness and sleep were 110 mm and 94 mm, a decrease of 16 mm; for diastolic pressure, 74 mm and 68 mm, a drop of only 6 mm, and therefore a change in pulse pressure from 36 mm to 26 mm. In certain cases the diastolic pressure remained entirely unchanged or might even rise a little.

The fall in blood pressure in infants and children during sleep is smaller than in adults (626, 2913, 4027), commensurate with lower waking pressure. As in adults, the decrease is mainly in systolic pressure, diastolic pressure remaining unchanged (188).

In this connection, Boas and Goldschmidt (387) found no relationship between the mean systolic blood pressures and heart rates, but in both men and women the lower the mean (presumably waking) diastolic blood pressure, the smaller was the minimal heart rate during sleep. In men with a mean diastolic pressure of 74 mm, the minimal sleeping heart rate was below 45, but, when the diastolic pressure was 84 mm, the minimal heart rate during sleep was above 61; in women the corresponding pairs of figures were 71 mm and under 50, and 81 mm and over 66. Since there is not a great difference between the diastolic pressure figures in wakefulness and in sleep, the foregoing relationship seems to indicate, as suggested by the authors, that the longer diastole of the slower heart permits a more complete emptying of the arterial tree between heart beats and so determines a lower diastolic arterial pressure.

Many observers hold that the magnitude of the blood pressure drop is in some way connected with the depth of sleep, but there is no agreement on when the lowest point in blood pressure is reached during the night. The older data of Brush and Fayerweather (551) placed the minimum blood pressure in the first hour of the night's sleep. Later studies (525, 2089, 2913) placed it during the second hour. Our data (2176) indicate that the blood pressures 2 hours and 5 hours after the onset of sleep are the same, although the heart is slower after 5 than after 2 hours. Blankenhorn and Campbell (370) found a complete parallelism between the blood pressure and heart rate during sleep, both reaching their minima during the fourth hour. Capecchi (626) located the minimal blood pressure somewhere between 2 and 4 hours after the beginning of the night's sleep, with the minimal heart rate later in the night. It can be stated, as a summing-up of available information, that the lowest blood pressure is more likely to occur in the first half of the night and that it precedes, rather than coincides with, the lowest heart rate during sleep.

According to Brooks and Carrol (525), once the maximum drop in blood pressure had taken place, no similar fall occurred, if the subject was awakened and allowed to fall asleep once more, no matter how deep the subsequent sleep seemed to be. When they kept their subjects in bed all night, but did not allow them to sleep, the fall in blood pressure was less pronounced. On the other hand, Grollman (1523) reported that the blood pressure was the same at a certain hour of the night, whether the subject was awake or asleep. Grollman also stated that, on awakening, the blood pressure did not rise, although the heart rate did, whereas Landis (2359) saw a rapid rise in blood pressure on sudden awakening and a more gradual rise on spontaneous awakening. Blankenhorn and Campbell (370) also noted a rise in blood pressure prior to and after natural awakening at the end of a night's sleep.

That more profound variations in blood pressure during sleep might normally occur was pointed out by MacWilliam (2611, 2612), who called attention to the statistics of incidence of hemorrhages in the brain and lungs, attacks of angina pectoris, and sudden death. All of them frequently occur during sleep in the early hours after midnight. The statistics are not in conformity with the low blood pressures prevailing during sleep, and MacWilliam showed that, on the contrary, very high blood pressures and heart rates might develop as a result of disturbances of sleep by reflex excitations, dreams, and nightmares. In some cases an initial blood pressure of 130 mm would be driven up to 200 mm, a higher pressure, indeed, than might be produced in the same individual, while he was awake, as a result of moderate exercise or excitement. It should be pointed out that, whereas other workers measured the blood pressure during sleep, MacWilliam did so after rousing the subject.

High blood pressure present during wakefulness is affected variously by sleep, depending on the nature of the hypertension. In general, the fall is greater than normal, around 50 mm, usually bringing the systolic pressure to a level corresponding to the daytime value of healthy persons. In patients with transitory hypertension the sleep pressures are always high and that, in the opinion of Müller (2913), indicates that the hypertension is due to an increased excitability of the vasomotor center. He reported several cases of patients with normal blood pressures during the waking hours and high pressures when asleep. Such a condition he called latent hypertension.

Katsch and Pansdorf (2089) stated that in essential hypertension there is a very marked drop in blood pressure during sleep but not in other types of hypertension. Wiechmann and Bamberger (4202, 4203), in discussing the marked drop in blood pressure occasioned by sleep in persons suffering from functional hypertension, emphasized the curative effect of sleep, particularly since the drop in pressure in such persons is the same during daytime naps as in night sleep. The more they sleep, the more they spare their circulation. Campbell and Blankenhorn (618) described some patients whose high blood pressures were or were not reduced in sleep, and so did Müller (2915), who also reported that barbital had no effect on blood pressure during sleep. Wiechmann and Bamberger (4203), using the same dose, 0.5 gm, observed a much greater fall in pressure than in natural sleep, although the heart rate was not affected. Mayo (2725) had some success in reducing the blood pressure in paroxysmal hypertension by the administration of phenobarbital.

Heilig and Hoff (1681) found that a dose of epinephrin, which produced a marked rise in blood pressure in waking subjects, had no effect in the same subjects during sleep.

Müller (2913) thought that the fall in blood pressure during sleep was due to a decreased vasomotor tone, with the slowing of the heart of secondary importance. Blankenhorn and Campbell (370), on the contrary, considered the low heart rate as the chief cause of the fall in blood pressure. It will be recalled that they obtained a complete parallelism between the two, but others found that the minimal heart rate was reached much later than the lowest blood pressure. Stevenson and co-authors (3818), somewhat like Müller, held that there is a periodic fatigue of the sympathetic center concerned in the maintenance of vascular tone. Ustvedt (4027) also referred to the slackening of the blood-vessel tone as the probable cause of the low blood pressure during sleep. Whatever the cause, the fall in blood pressure is probably independent of the low heart rate. Whether or not it is due to fatigue of the vasomotor center is a pertinent question, as, from Mosso's time on, cerebral anemia has been frequently put forward as the possible cause of sleep.

As related by Piéron (3192), the earlier observations on brain volume pointed to a cerebral anemia during sleep. In 1866 Hammond noted a depression of the fontanels in infants while they were asleep. It was further reported that in persons with skull fractures the escape of cerebrospinal fluid was either decreased or stopped during sleep. Mosso, however, made the first laboratory studies in that direction by observing two subjects with skull openings which permitted a simultaneous recording of plethysmographic curves of the brain and forearm. Sleep produced a decrease in brain volume and an increase in that of the forearm; awakening, the opposite effect. Stimuli during sleep, even when the subjects did not awaken, led to a short-lasting rise in brain volume and forearm vasoconstriction. This finding seemed to fit the then firmly held belief that the circulation of the brain is regulated entirely indirectly, through constriction or dilatation of blood vessels elsewhere, either in limbs or in the splanchnic region. Tarchanoff (3906) observed a blanching of the surface blood vessels of the exposed brain of puppies when they fell asleep. Howell (1846) studied the forearm plethysmogram and obtained results that agreed with those of Mosso: an increase in volume during sleep, a transitory vasoconstriction as a result of stimulation, and a sustained shrinking in volume on awakening. About this time the first discordant note was heard, when Czerny (808) reported that in a child with a cranial defect, whom he observed by the method of Mosso, there was a cerebral hyperemia, instead of anemia, during sleep. Thereafter all contributions to the subject seemed to confirm Czerny's rather than Mosso's findings (519, 3031, 3135, 3136, 3677, 3818, 4090). Indeed, as Shepard (3677) pointed out, some of Mosso's own records showed an increase in brain volume at the onset of sleep. Shepard made observations with tambours applied to the scalp over the trephine hole in the skull and over the intact skull as a control. He never observed a fall in brain volume at the onset of sleep. There was always a sustained and marked increase in brain volume, a fall in blood pressure, and no constant change in volume of hand or foot. This combination of changes held for all positions of his two subjects, whether sleep came on gradually, quickly, or with a series of interruptions. Stimuli during sleep led to a fall in brain volume, or a slight rise, then a fall, as was later also observed by Peiper on two children (3135, 3136). Shepard decided that the increase in brain volume during sleep could not be due to venous congestion and reached the conclusion that the brain vessels relax on going to sleep and constrict on awakening. Stevenson and co-authors (3818), using the same method, referred to intracranial pressure rather than volume; but, whenever the brain volume increased, there was also an increase in pressure of the intracranial contents, resulting in an upstroke of the recording tambour, or piston-recorder, lever. They tested, in addition, the effects of morphine and caffeine on brain volume. The former, a depressant, caused an increase in brain volume; the latter, a stimulant, led to a fall. Vujic (4090) observed a rise in cerebrospinal fluid pressure at the onset of sleep and a sharp fall on awakening, and he interpreted his findings as favoring a cerebral hyperemia.

We observed two middle-aged men with trephined skulls, to which we fitted cups connected with recording tambours. In 12 records out of 14 on the first subject, and in 8 out of 10 on the second, there was a definite rise in the intracranial pressure and volume on falling asleep. In no case was there a decrease at the onset of sleep. When the subjects remained awake, there were no changes. On awakening there was a fall in every instance in both subjects, except for the presence of Traube-Hering-like fluctuations on 2 occasions in the first subject, and on 3 in the second. On the other hand, such fluctuations were the rule rather than the exception during sleep, appearing in every one of the sleep records where an increase in intracranial contents was registered. The frequency of these waves varied between 2.5 and 1/min, and the amplitude seemed to increase as the sleep became deeper. Similar waves were described by others (3677, 3818, 4090).

Uhlenbruck (4001), by the plethysmographic method, studied vascular reaction to warmth, cold, pressure, and pain stimuli, and they all led to a decrease in the volume of the extremities. Sleep produced vasodilatation; and awakening, like stimulation, vasoconstriction in the limb, confirming the findings of Howell (1846). However, the notion that the brain volume is regulated indirectly is no longer warranted, for, as was shown by Forbes and Wolff (1237, 4265), the regulation is in part, at least, by cerebral vasomotor nerves.

In the plethysmographic curves published by Howell (1846), there were distinct waves of 60 to 90 minutes' duration, suggesting a short-term cycle that is also in evidence with respect to other sleep concomitants, especially the EEG. In this connection, Ackner and Pampiglione (8) noted fluctuations in the finger volume curves, in association with "spontaneous" EEG changes. They also reported (3087) that early vasomotor responses to repetitive auditory stimuli were alike in most subjects, but later ones showed considerable variability.

Gibbs and co-workers (1427), in measuring the cerebral circulation in man by means of a thermoelectric blood-flow recorder inserted in the jugular vein, saw no significant changes in blood flow from the brain when the subjects fell asleep or when they awakened. However, Kety and his group (2148, 2649), by the use of the N_2O technique, obtained statistically significant increases in cerebral blood flow during sleep—from 59 ml/min to 65 ml/min for each 100 gm of brain tissue. These findings should, once and for all, eliminate the consideration of cerebral anemia (45, 2908) as the direct or indirect cause of sleep.

Chapter 7

Respiration

There is general agreement that sleep leads to changes in the character and rate of respiratory movements, but there are wide differences in reports on the magnitude and direction of these changes. As breathing can be observed by mere inspection, the lack of consistency in the many findings on this variable suggests a complexity of influences or a great lability of the respiratory regulation. Aristotle is credited with noting that, whereas in the waking state inspiration is active and of short duration and expiration passive and slow, the reverse is often true in sleep. Mosso (2906), and recently Oswald (3068), confirmed Aristotle's observation, but Gujer (1555), by the use of a "pneumotachograph," found that in sleep the duration of expiration was lengthened, often amounting to 1.45 that of inspiration, compared to 1.2 during rest without sleep. In his comprehensive monograph on respiration during sleep, Magnussen (2623), employing a mask-and-valve arrangement, in addition to a pneumograph, determined that either type of inspiration-expiration ratio occurred in sleep. However, Magnussen's sleep pneumograms showed no post-expiratory pause. This was also the finding of Cathala and Guillard (663), but Gujer (1555) and Oswald (3068) did record post-expiratory pauses in sleep in human subjects, as did Volkind in dogs (4083).

Mosso (2906) also reported a predominance of thoracic over abdominal breathing during sleep or an inversion of the respiratory movement pattern of wakefulness. Shepard (3677) made a similar observation and came to consider the increase in chest breathing as the most characteristic respiratory change occurring with the onset of sleep. In our laboratory, in nine healthy adults (3287), the amplitudes of the thoracic and abdominal movements, as recorded on a kymograph, were measured and the ratio between the two (T:A) used to indicate the relative changes brought on by sleep. The thoracic excursion was increased in 13 experiments, decreased in 10, and remained unchanged in 7, but in not one experiment was the T:A ratio reversed during sleep. Magnussen (2623) merely noted a dissociation between the two movements during sleep, the abdominal excursion preceding the thoracic one.

For our subjects (3287), as far as could be determined, neither time of day, nor age, nor sex had any influence on the nature of the changes that occurred during drowsiness and sleep. The respiratory rate while lying down and awake varied in different subjects from 8 to 25/min, with a mean of 18. In sleep, in 5 of the 30 experiments the rate was definitely slowed, in 12 there was no change, and in 13 the rate was increased. In 18 tests there was a return to approximately the original rate on awakening. The waking rate varied in the same individual in successive experiments, as did the type of change in drowsiness and after awakening. It was not possible to correlate these variations in the same individual with any other recognizable factor. No wonder other investigators reported an increase (2623) or a decrease (663, 3041, 4083) in the rate of respiration during sleep. Respiratory rates varied with the depth of sleep (2770), with minimal values recorded between 3:00 A.M. and 6:00 A.M. (663).

The lack of agreement on the changes in the rate of respiration with the advent of sleep (1978, 2623, 3287) is due, in part, to a conspicuous irregularity of respiratory movements. In 16 out of our 30 experiments (3287), the irregularity applied to both thoracic and abdominal movements. No subjective or objective phenomena were observed which would account for the changes in the character of respiration, and in successive tests on the same subject the irregularities were not always the same. As a rule, if the respiration was regular in the beginning of the experiment, it became quite irregular during drowsiness, assuming a regular sequence again in sound sleep. In many cases the irregularities were synchronous in both the abdominal and the thoracic movements, but in a few experiments marked periodicity appeared in one of these two types of respiratory movements without being apparent in the other. Usually the irregularity took the form of a considerable shortening of the amplitude of the excursions as compared to normal, lasting for two or three respiratory cycles. In a few experiments, however, there was, instead, at varying intervals, a deep inspiration. In about half of the experiments the variations in amplitude of whatever type were distributed evenly enough to be designated as periodic. That respiration during sleep is likely, at times, to be so periodic as to resemble the Cheyne-Stokes type had been reported by Broadbent (510) and Mosso (2906) in 1877–78, and has since been confirmed by many investigators (38, 39, 1978, 3287, 3376).

Another respiratory phenomenon associated with sleep is snoring, defined by Robin (3377) as "sounds made by vibrations in the soft palate and posterior faucial pillars during sleep." Snoring occurs in both sexes and all ages, but is commoner in older persons, whose palate muscles have a lowered tonus. A dorsal position and an open mouth are factors favoring snoring. Among "organic" causes of snoring are nasal obstructions and edematous changes in pharynx and larynx (1923). Tsukamoto and co-authors (3989), by auditory testing, found that the sleep of non-snorers was deeper than that of snorers.

Schwartz and Fischgold (3623) noted that their sleeping subjects stopped snoring after the EEG indicated an episode of dreaming, suggesting a temporary increase in the tonus of the soft palate. Berger (302), on the other hand, recorded a decrease in the tonus of the extrinsic laryngeal muscles during dreaming.

Snoring is harmless to the sleeper, but can be very annoying to others who may be awake at the time, or have been aroused by the loud noises. Local treatments of snoring comprise surgical amputation or resection of the uvula (1685, 3377), and the injection of sclerosing agents into the soft palate (1131, 3849), both of which methods have been found ineffective. Devices for discouraging the dorsal position of the body and splints for keeping the sleeper's mouth closed (439, 1131, 3377) abound; some three hundred snoring-curtailing inventions have been registered in the U.S. Patent Office (1131). Among general anti-snoring measures proposed are avoidance of food and alcohol intake before retiring (439) and auto-suggestion (1844).

Harrison and co-workers (1653) recorded the respiratory movements of patients who complained of dyspnea at the onset of sleep. Such individuals often showed periodic respiration of the Cheyne-Stokes type during sleep, with an augmented duration of apnea and a gradually increasing depth of the hyperpnea phase, until the dyspnea aroused the subject. The authors concluded that this paroxysmal dyspnea was due to overventilation by reflex stimulation from congested lungs and from the depression of respiration caused by sleep, and not to changes in the composition of the blood.

Although there are differences in the findings concerning the rate and depth of respiration during sleep, all observers noted a decrease in the ventilation of the lungs. Depending upon whether the figures apply to total or only to alveolar ventilation, the reported decreases amounted, variously, to 50 per cent (4215), 20 to 38 per cent (546, 3041, 3376, 4074), or only 5 to 15 per cent (2623).

There is a somewhat greater concordance in reports on respiration in infants and children during sleep, some emphasizing regularity (4094), others a slowing (546, 4079, 4084), though irregularities have also been mentioned (3138, 4026, 4084), the latter including Cheyne-Stokes breathing in newborn infants (4096). A striking regular periodicity of respiration in infants of about 50 minutes' duration was discovered by Denisova and Figurin (914). Respiration was alternately retarded and accelerated, and during the latter phase there were associated facial, head, limb, and body movements, as well as an increased heart rate.

Magnussen (2623) also discovered a somewhat longer respiration cycle in adult sleepers. The alternation consisted of periods of 38 to 52 minutes of regular respiratory movements, preceded and followed by stretches of irregular movements lasting 40 to 60 minutes. There were five distinct cycles in a respiration record of 8 hours and 16 minutes of sleep, giving a mean periodicity of about

100 minutes. A similar cycle of recurring respiratory acceleration has been shown to be associated with the incidence of dreaming (p. 94).

The oxygen intake and CO_2 output have been investigated by several workers, spurred on, no doubt, by the celebrated report made by Pettenkofer and Voit to the Academy of Sciences of Munich in 1866. They declared that during sleep the oxygen intake was more than doubled, while the CO_2 output was markedly decreased. Voit himself found that these conclusions, based on two experiments, were due to faulty calculations, and eleven experiments that he and Pettenkofer subsequently performed indicated that sleep produced a decrease in the oxygen intake. In spite of that, the report became the basis of a hypothesis that there is an active "intramolecular" storage of oxygen during sleep and that sleep is a necessity for that reason. It has since been shown that there is a decrease in oxygen consumption during sleep, amounting to 10 per cent, according to Magnussen (2623), and to over 20 per cent, as reported by Robin and associates (3376). The brain, to be sure, uses as much oxygen in sleep as in wakefulness (2148) but does not store it.

The alveolar partial pressure of oxygen (3376), the oxygen content of arterial blood (2148), and the degree of oxyhemoglobin saturation (352, 353, 4082) show a small decrease during sleep, but not the 6 to 8 per cent reported by Doust and Schneider (970, 971) for the difference between wakefulness and sleep. Mills (2828) challenged the validity of the oxymetric determinations on which the anoxic relation to sleep was based. On the other hand, investigators generally agreed that the partial pressure or percentage of CO_2 in alveolar air, as well as the CO_2 tension in blood, rises during sleep (242, 353, 745, 1075, 1653, 1659, 2269, 3041, 3252, 3288, 3294, 3297, 3374, 3844), though Mills (2828) observed no increase in CO_2 tension in the course of an afternoon nap. Main (2635) noted an increase in alveolar CO_2 pressure in his subjects when they merely changed from the standing to the lying position. Bass and Herr (242), sampling the air several times during each night, found that the maximum values were reached during the first and second hours of sleep. In one case the percentage of CO_2 rose from 6.02 to 6.55 (corresponding to partial pressures of 41.2 and 44.8 mm Hg) 45 minutes after the onset of sleep. Generally, after the first hour there was an irregular downward tendency. Østergaard (3041) noted that the increase of 3–6 mm Hg in the CO_2 tension during sleep was smaller than the 8–9 mm increase in anesthesia. Birchfield and co-workers (352) found that narcoleptic patients, while awake, tended to yield values for the blood gases similar to those of normal persons during sleep.

The responsiveness to increases in CO_2 partial pressures in alveolar air is definitely lowered in sleep (283, 3375). Bass and Herr (242) ascribed the high CO_2 figures to a decrease in the irritability of the respiratory center, and this view was supported by others (283, 353, 1075, 3041, 3288, 3374, 4082). Robin and associates (3375, 3376) related the depressed sensitivity of the respiratory center to a decrease in the number of afferent impulses reaching the center during sleep and, like Wuth (4282), concluded that the hypoxic theory of sleep was untenable. Fink (1170, 1171), commenting on the difficulty of producing overventilatory apnea in the waking state, surmised that "cerebral activity associated with wakefulness is a component of the normal respiratory drive."

Reed and Kellogg (3288) tested the responsiveness to graded CO_2 mixtures containing sufficient oxygen to prevent anoxia at sea level and at an altitude of 14,250 feet. In spite of the changed response curve at the high altitude in wakefulness, the effect of sleep was the same at both altitudes. Different results were obtained by Fleisch (1203), who studied four young adult subjects by the pneumotachographic method under an atmospheric pressure of 330 mm Hg, which corresponds to an altitude of 21,000 feet. In the waking state there was, under these conditions, an increase in the respiratory rate from the normal 18.8 to 22.0/min, with an increase in tidal air from 425 to 578 ml. The minute ventilation was 12.45 liters, instead of the normal 7.75. Sleep resulted in a depression of respiration; and a remarkably prompt one, as it became manifest in 2 to 4 seconds after the onset of sleep. This depression disappeared just as promptly when the subject awakened, demonstrating how rapidly changes in the irritability of the respiratory center can be produced by sleep and wakefulness, under the abnormal pressure conditions prevailing in this experiment.

Krausse (2269) considered it established that there is a relationship between body motility and CO_2 in alveolar air, lowest motility corresponding to highest CO_2 partial pressure. He deemed it necessary to have curves for both of these concomitants before the quality of the sleep of a particular patient could be correctly evaluated. As mentioned in connection with ESR (p. 21), Regelsberger (3299) drew a curve of sleep based on the variation in the partial pressures of CO_2 in alveolar air, but he did not consider it a "depth-of-sleep" curve. Although Regelsberger's interpretation of earlier CO_2 findings (3296) pertained to dissociation between brain and body sleep, his curves bring out oscillations in a sleep variable of 65 to 120 minutes' duration.

The outstanding respiratory feature in sleep is the decreased irritability of the respiratory center, which accounts for the near-unanimity in the findings concerning changes in alveolar air and blood gases. The diversity of, and contradiction in, data on rate, depth, and character of respiratory movements are probably due to the multiplicity of external and internal influences and to the timing of the samplings. The demonstration of a 50-minute cycle in respiratory activity of infants (914), and the somewhat longer periodicity in adults (2623), as well as the alveolar CO_2 curves (3299), together with similar periodicities described in preceding and following chapters, point to the existence of a short-term rest-activity cycle which is the basis of the sleep-wakefulness alternation.

Chapter 8

Digestion, Metabolism, Body Temperature, and Excretion

In general, digestion is not affected in either direction by sleep. This was the considered view of the ancients, and little has been done within recent times to challenge it. However, with respect to particular secretory and motor phenomena, especially gastric function, there is no universal agreement among investigators.

No measurable salivary secretion by the parotid gland in man has been noted during sleep, and the activity of submaxillary and sublingual glands is lower than in restful wakefulness (3584). Grossman and Brickman (1533) compared the pH of human saliva in the daytime and at night, in wakefulness and in sleep. The saliva of subjects who remained awake and active for as long as 24 hours at a time showed the same pH value, 6.7, at night as during the day. Those who slept at night had to be awakened and asked to expectorate. The pH of saliva during sleep was 6.3 as against 6.7 for the waking state.

Concerning gastric motility, Carlson (638), in infants and adults, found that hunger contractions were at least as frequent and strong during sleep as in the waking state. In dogs the contractions were more vigorous and regular when the animals were asleep. Human subjects in the course of a five-day fast had their gastric motility recorded continuously. During sleep the contractions were more frequent than in wakefulness, occupying almost half of the total sleeping time. Wada (4092) also recorded hunger contractions of the stomach as well as bodily movements in one subject during sleep. She noted that stirring was often synchronous with powerful contractions of the stomach. Hellebrandt and associates (1693) reported an increase in gastric motility in sleep. However, in three patients with pyloric stenosis Daniélopolu and Carniol (820) observed a complete cessation of gastric contractions with the onset of sleep and a return to their usual height on awakening. Veit (4044) made electrogastrographic studies by inserting two leads into the stomach through the esophagus or through a duodenal fistula. He differentiated autonomous (intrinsic) peristalsis, with a period of 18 to 25 seconds, hardly affected by atropine, from vagal peristalsis, with a period of 60 to 90 seconds, extinguishable by atropine. The autonomous peristalsis went on in the empty stomach, but in the one woman observed it decreased markedly during sleep, proportionally to the latter's depth, and was promptly resumed upon, or slightly prior to, awakening. McGlade (2753) recorded a series of 20 to 50 foot movements (in three out of twenty-five sleepers), occurring 3 hours after the onset of sleep, and only when certain foods had been eaten. The foot movements were synchronous with openings of the pyloric sphincter.

The secretory function of the stomach is not decreased by sleep, according to the older finding of Friedenwald (1293). Luckhardt and Johnston (2572) and Johnston and Washeim (2007) obtained a rise in gastric acidity, even as their subjects prepared to go to bed, but the acidity was further increased with the onset of sleep and seemed to be proportional to the depth of sleep. The volume of juice usually decreased, and for the same hour of the night it was only half as large when the subject was asleep as when he remained awake. On the other hand, Henning and Norpoth (1701), on the basis of hourly determinations of acidity during sleep, concluded that most normal stomachs stopped secreting during sleep and that only in patients with gastric ulcers was there a continuous high acid secretion. This finding was confirmed by Banche (197). Chalfen (669) reported a decreased gastric secretion during sleep and an increase on awakening. In seven cases out of nine (670) there was no secretion at all from 3:00 a.m. to 5:00 a.m. Conversely, Jores (2020) put the maximum gastric secretion at 4:00 a.m. Winkelstein (4240) made bihourly aspirations of the gastric contents without waking his patients. Free hydrochloric acid was absent or low in normal subjects, but both the secretion and the acidity of the juice showed a marked increase during sleep in patients with duodenal ulcers. Hellebrandt and associates (1693) obtained different results. Their eleven subjects showed a much higher gastric acidity during night sleep than during the day. The mean highest gastric-juice acidities for the group were 58.8 arbitrary units for free acid and 73.8 for acidity in sleep as against 43.8 and 57.8 in the daytime. On the other hand, Reichsman and associates (3305), testing twenty-eight healthy young males, found "no correlations between states of sleeping and waking with HCl secretory rates, natural or histamine-histalog induced." Vandorfy (4035) reported lower figures for the volume of gastric contents of fifty subjects in sleep than in the waking state. Komarov (2233, 2234) also noted a decrease in the secretory activity of stomach, duodenum, and liver, with a lower enzyme content, during sleep.

The secretion of bile, as collected from a fistula in man, is lower at night, with a minimum between 1:00 a.m. and 5.00 a.m., according to Forsgren (1246), who found the same to be true for rabbits which are more active at night than in the daytime. Holmquist (1821), working on hedgehogs, some of which were killed while awake and others when asleep, reported that the bile capillaries were constricted and that there was a decreased number of secretory granules in the acini cells of the pancreas when the animals were killed in the sleeping condition.

The intestinal movements do not seem to be changed in sleep. They are not detectable in sleep if absent in the waking state and vice versa. Niles (3012) listened over the intestines of sleeping persons and found that the peristaltic activity continued unabated. The same conclusion was made by Hines (1776), on studying the motility of a single intestinal loop in a man with a congenital umbilical hernia, as well as by Alvarez (50), who recorded intestinal activity of a patient by a balloon passed into the intestine through a jejunal fistula. Helm and associates (1697), by the balloon method, recorded a clear-cut diminution of intestinal motility in twelve out of sixteen fasting subjects tested. In exteriorized loops of dogs' small intestine, motor activity was not affected by sleep (217, 966).

Peristaltic and haustral movements have been seen in serial X-ray pictures of the colon during sleep (1696), but the human sigmoid colon was quiescent in sleep and became active on awakening (3410).

Basal heat production is usually further decreased during sleep concomitantly with muscular relaxation and low body temperature. Delcourt and Mayer (884), determining BMRs in five subjects, awake and during a short sleep, obtained decreases in three, no change in one, and a slight rise in the fifth. They also found that the dorsal decubitus position commonly imposed on patients for the purpose of measuring their oxygen consumption did not invariably yield lowest values. In some individuals a lower BMR prevailed when they lay on one side, semiflexed, or even curled up. One subject had a smaller BMR when comfortably settled in a deep-cushioned chair than while lying flat on his back. Benedict (291) stated that there is a distinct tendency to a lower metabolic level during sleep. If the level is already very low in the waking state, it probably indicates a more complete than usual muscular relaxation, and it may not be changed in sleep. This was also shown by Necheles and Loo (2978, 2979), who compared the effect of sleep on Occidentals and Orientals. The latter had a much lower rate of heat production than the former. The Chinese seem to be able to relax as much during the waking state as Westerners do when they sleep. Mason and Benedict (2705) similarly studied seven South Indian women but obtained a mean decrease of 9.8 per cent in metabolism during sleep. In two Western women sleep produced a similar lowering of metabolism.

Griffith and associates (1517) did not notice any decrease in oxygen consumption when their two subjects dozed off during a 10-minute basal metabolism test, but, of course, the persons studied were not deeply asleep. Ravaud (3280) obtained a decrease in metabolism in sleep and proposed that the standard procedure for BMR determinations be revised and patients tested under the effect of a hypnotic drug. Several authors (813, 1266, 3624) suggested that only in "nervous" patients did sleep produce a marked decrease in oxygen consumption and that this sleep effect could be put to diagnostic use.

Robin and associates (3376) noted a decrease in oxygen consumption of about 22 per cent in normal subjects during sleep, but Kreider and Iampietro (2274), only about one-half that much. On the other hand, Grollman (1523) found no difference in oxygen consumption between sleep and wakefulness during the hours usually given to sleep. While awakening caused the heart rate to increase, it had no effect on the oxygen intake. Significantly, no change in oxygen consumed by the brain of normal young men resulted from sleep (2148).

Wang and Kern (4115) made many BMR determinations on twelve children between 2:00 A.M. and 4:00 A.M., when they were asleep, and between 8:00 A.M. and 10:00 A.M., after awakening. In every case the heat production was lower during sleep than after awakening, the difference amounting, on the average, to 15 per cent. Williams (4220), studying four children when asleep and after they woke up, obtained in the latter case a mean increase in oxygen consumption of 9 per cent. De Bruin (546), on twenty-two children, also observed a decrease in metabolism with the onset of sleep.

There is a close relationship between weight loss, due to evaporation of water from the skin and lungs, and the metabolic rate, and, as one would expect, the loss in weight is lower during sleep than in the waking condition. Miles (2818), weighing himself on forty nights prior to going to bed and again on getting up in the morning, found that he was losing about 39 gm per hour. The loss on different nights was proportional to the duration of sleep, and he concluded that the longer sleep led to greater restlessness which was probably responsible for the greater loss of weight. However, Freeman (1272) could not confirm Miles's finding. His ten subjects lost about as much weight per hour between midnight and 3:00 A.M. as between 3:00 A.M. and 7:00 A.M.

Burckard and co-workers (571) measured the BMRs of pigeons. During the night, when they were presumably asleep, their oxygen consumption diminished by 15 per cent. This change the authors ascribed to darkness and therefore a decrease in centripetal impulses to the brain, as well as to muscular relaxation. When in three pigeons the brachial plexuses were sectioned, thus considerably suppressing muscle tonus, the nocturnal decrease in heat production persisted but amounted to only 1 to 3 per cent of the daytime rate.

Among the endocrine glands, sometimes spoken of as regulators of metabolism, the hypophysis was reported by Zondek and Bier (4331) to contain a hormone-like bromine compound related to the function of sleep. These authors examined the pituitary glands of 150 species of animals and found most of the bromine in the anterior lobe, some in the pars intermedia. While other organs contained only 1–2 mg per cent, the hypophysis held 15–30 mg per cent. In man (4332) the diencephalic region contains 1.6–1.8 mg per cent, whereas the rest of the brain (samples from cerebrum, cerebellum, and medulla), only 0.5–0.8 mg per cent. The human hypophysis, weighing 0.5–0.75 gm, contains 40–80 gamma of bromine, but the quantity decreases with age so that after the age of seventy-five only a trace of bromine can be found in the gland. Zondek and Bier (4330) called attention to the fact that all hypophyseal hormones heretofore isolated by others were found to be bromine-free. Their alleged hormone "tetra-brom-desiodo-thyroxin," which they likened to thyroxin with the iodine replaced by bromine, accounted for 60 to 65 per cent of all the bromine in the hypophysis and was found by them to produce a sleeplike depression in dogs.

Zondek and Bier (4332) also noted a decrease in the bromine concentration of the dog's hypophysis as a result of narcosis lasting 2 to 3 days (from 15–30 mg per cent to 5–7). Finally, they (4330) reported an increase in blood bromine during sleep and a decrease among patients suffering from manic-depressive psychoses.

Werner (4172) published figures on bromine in the blood of rabbits anesthetized with morphine. In each of eight experiments, two rabbits were used, one narcotized and another as a control. In the morphine-treated animals the blood contained 0.3–1.5 mg per cent bromine, with a mean of 1.0 mg; the blood of the controls, 0.65–1.1 mg and a mean of 0.8 mg. The author concluded that there was more bromine in the blood of the anesthetized animals, although in three of the eight experiments the blood of the control animal had a much higher bromine content than that of the morphine animal, and, as seen above, the range of figures for the anesthetized rabbits exceeded the control range at either end. In addition, the mean values given by Werner fall within the normal range for animal and human blood placed by Neufeld (2988) as between 0.4 and 1.5 mg per cent. Werner also found that the hypophyses of anesthetized dogs contained less bromine than those of control animals (17 as against 23 mg per cent). These results appear more consistent than the blood figures and are the only ones that can be interpreted as a confirmation of Zondek and Bier's discovery. Moruzzi (2891) distinguished between total bromine and non-precipitable bromine in the blood, with a decrease in both during sleep, but the decrease was much more marked in the non-precipitable fraction. These findings are the reverse of those of Zondek and Bier, who reported an increased bromine content in the blood in sleep.

Serbescu and Buttu (3655) could not confirm the findings of Zondek and Bier as regards the hypophysis, in which they found no bromine at all. Zondek and Bier's results have also been criticized by others (1825, 2988).

The adrenalin content of the adrenal glands is decreased during sleep, according to Holmquist (1822), who worked on hedgehogs, animals nocturnal in their habits. He employed both the Folin-Cannon-Denis colorimetric method and the Elliot blood-pressure method for his assays. By the chemical method, the gland was found to contain 3.22 mg in the waking state and 1.56 mg during sleep. The corresponding values by the blood-pressure method were 1.56 mg and 0.66 mg (all figures are mg adrenalin per gm of adrenal gland). Holmquist concluded that there is a close relationship between sleep and the adrenalin content of the adrenal glands.

The effect of sleep on body temperature has long been a topic for debate. It is not that anyone doubts that the body temperature falls during the night, but the fall can conceivably be due to rest in the horizontal position and muscular relaxation. In addition, the fact that one's temperature begins to decrease long before bedtime, and follows its usual 24-hour course even if one stays awake the whole night, has been interpreted as showing that sleep is not directly responsible for the low night temperature. Observations made by Piéron (3192) on several subjects by discontinuous readings and continuous registration led him to conclude that neither the onset of sleep nor awakening had any direct effect on body temperature, provided the subject lay quietly in bed. However, Pembrey and Nicol (3141) held that sleep, as well as rest, was a factor in the nightly temperature drop. In our laboratory the effects of the position of the body and of sleep on the rectal temperature were measured by means of a Leeds and Northrup continuously recording electrical resistance thermometer (2194). The record showed rectal temperature with an accuracy of 0.02° F. Four subjects underwent a number of tests, following one or another of three procedures: (*a*) lying down for about two hours; (*b*) lying down for one hour, then standing up, without leaning against anything, for one hour or more; and (*c*) procedure *b* reversed. The subjects were not told to relax on lying down, but, unless instructed to keep awake, they frequently fell asleep. They were watched directly, and it was thus possible to note when they dozed off and awakened. The time chosen was midafternoon, when the temperature curve has its plateau and shows only minor spontaneous oscillations. Tracings of typical temperature curves are shown in Figure 8.1. Lying down led to a fall in body temperature in a majority of tests, but in some cases there was no change, or even a rise. The mean decrease in temperature was 0.19° F. The tendency to a temperature fall became more accentuated with the onset of sleep, even though here too the temperature remained stationary or rose in a few cases. The mean fall after about one hour of sleep was 0.27° F. Upon awakening, there was a slight tendency to a continued drop in temperature, with the mean drop 0.03° F. for about one-half hour. On lying down after standing up for an hour, there was a fall in temperature in all tests, and it was more marked than on lying down without such a preliminary tiring procedure, the mean fall equaling 0.90° F. Likewise, the opposite procedure led to an unvarying rise in temperature, with a mean of 0.4° F. It appears that the assumption of the horizontal position induces a decrease in body temperature, particularly when the individual experiences muscular fatigue and is inclined to relax—a finding confirmed by Renbourn and Taylor (3314). After the onset of sleep there may or may not be a new decrease in temperature, depending on the time of the day and probably on the degree of muscular relaxation attained in the waking state. For the same reasons awakening may result in a rise, no change, or a fall in temperature.

We then studied the body-temperature curve during night sleep by the same method (2193). There were considerable differences in the rectal temperature curves of a subject for successive nights, both at the time of going to bed and during sleep, the range varying from 0.5° F. to more than 1° F. for a particular hour on different nights (Fig. 8.2). Among the personal characteristics

THE EFFECT OF LYING AWAKE, SLEEPING, AND STANDING UPON RECTAL TEMPERATURE IN MAN

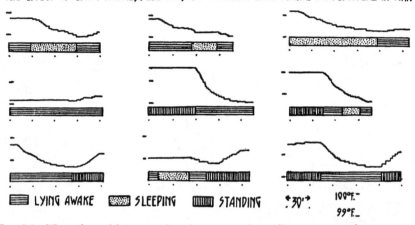

▤ LYING AWAKE   ▦ SLEEPING   ▥ STANDING   •⁑30'⁑•   100°F.⁻
99°F.⁻

Fig. 8.1—The effect of lying awake, sleeping, and standing upon rectal temperature of man, recorded by an electrical resistance thermometer. Dashes to the left of each record indicate 100° and 99° F., respectively; dots underneath the records mark 30-minute periods of time.

of the composite body-temperature curve of a given subject were: the mean nocturnal temperature level and range; the drop from the time of going to bed to the lowest reading of the night; and the difference between the temperature at the time of going to bed and that prevailing at the time of getting up. The last comparison almost always showed that the morning temperature was lower than the evening one by as much as 0.5° F., and this may explain what to many appears a paradoxical phenomenon, namely, a poorer performance (lower efficiency) immediately on getting up than before retiring at night (p. 152).

There was no direct connection between body temperature and frequency of movement during sleep. Generally speaking, there were fewer movements during the downward course of the temperature curve than during its upward swing.

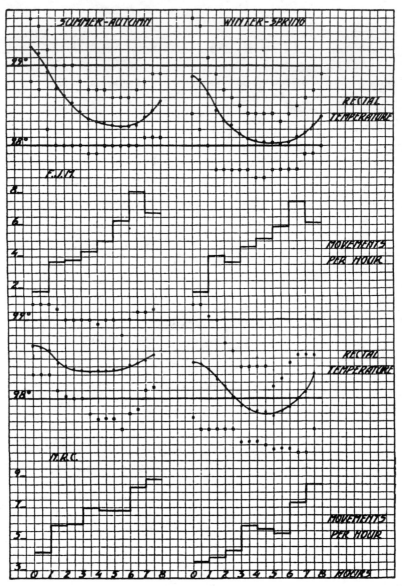

FIG. 8.2—Body temperature and motility during sleep of two subjects for the summer-autumn and winter-spring seasons. The upper four curves are based on data obtained on M (20 nights and 13 nights), and the lower four, on C (14 nights and 27 nights). The temperature curves are drawn through the mean values at the end of successive half-hour periods after going to bed. The dots above and below each temperature curve represent the range of temperature variability—the maximum and minimum temperatures for the particular half-hours during the several nights and not the highest and lowest individual nocturnal temperature records. The body-temperature level—the mean of all the points in the mean temperature curve—was 98.52° in summer-autumn and 98.28° in winter-spring for M, and correspondingly 98.45° and 98.06° for C. The only temperature values com-

We obtained well-defined but different changes in the body-temperature curves as a result of taking alcohol or caffeine prior to going to bed (2943). Alcohol, in doses of 60–75 ml diluted with 4 parts of water, caused a distinct decrease in rectal temperature, compared to normal, during the first half of the night, but during the second half the alcohol curve ran consistently above the normal sleep temperature curve (Fig. 8.3). Normal nights were interspersed

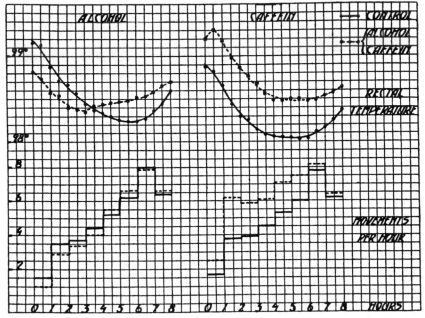

Fig. 8.3—The effect of alcohol (300 and 375 ml in 19 per cent solution) and caffeine (260 and 390 mg) on body temperature and motility during sleep of subject M, plotted as in Fig. 8.2. Curves were based on 10 alcohol nights, interspersed with 12 control nights, and 12 each of caffeine and control nights. The two control body-temperature curves are markedly different because the alcohol series was run in the autumn and the caffeine one in the winter (see Fig. 8.2).

with alcohol nights, and the subjects were given equal volumes of water as a control. On alcohol nights the motility, like the temperature, was below the control during the first half and above it during the second half. Caffeine in

---

mon to both halves of the year, for each subject, were the maximal temperatures at the time of going to bed and shortly thereafter; the minimal temperatures for the corresponding half-hours varied widely.

Under each body-temperature curve is plotted the motility for the season, based on the mean number of movements during successive hours of going to bed. The mean total number of movements per night was 40.1 in summer-autumn and 39.1 in winter-spring for M, and 53.7 and 44.5 for C.

doses of 260–390 mg produced a consistent and marked rise both in temperature and in motility (Fig. 8.3). The caffeine and the control temperature curves were practically parallel to each other, except that during the first half-hour or so after going to bed the rectal temperature under the influence of caffeine rose a little before it assumed its downward course. The motility appeared to be lower when the body temperature was below normal, as in the first half of the night following alcohol, and higher when the body temperature was above normal, as in the second half of the night after alcohol and during the whole night after caffeine. Smaller doses of caffeine, 130 mg, had no effect on body temperature or on motility.

Kreider and associates (2272–75) studied the effects of food intake and varying environmental temperatures on the body temperature of groups of military personnel. Rectal temperature was decreased by over 1° C. during a night's sleep, but the toe temperature dropped from 33° to 11° C. Skin temperature elsewhere showed much smaller decreases than did the rectal one, except at subfreezing environmental temperatures. In the first hour of sleep there was even a tendency for the skin temperature to rise (138, 2273). Somewhat different results were reported by Kirk (2164), who made a series of measurements of the temperature of the sole of the foot by a mercury thermometer protected by a piece of felt strapped to the foot with adhesive tape. In normal persons the sole temperature rose even before sleep set in, reached its maximum at the time sleep was deepest, then fell slowly, at first, and steeply at the time of awakening. In old and feeble people there was, on the contrary, a fall in sole temperature on falling asleep. In schizophrenic patients with catatonia the temperature rise at the onset of sleep was exceptionally great, apparently as a result of a low daytime temperature of the feet.

Piéron (3192) discussed a number of papers dealing with cerebral temperature during sleep but came to the conclusion that, with the instrument available for the purpose, it was impossible to affirm with certitude that sleep had an effect on cerebral temperature. In our laboratory Serota (3658) made a study of the cortical and subcortical temperatures of the cat during sleep by means of implanted thermocouples. The twenty-six cats studied behaved in a normal manner after the operation—walked around in their cages, ate, slept—while connected to a galvanometer by long wires. Needles were inserted into the cortex (suprasylvian, lateral, or splenial gyrus) and hypothalamus. Readings were made every 3 minutes during the various periods of observation, shifting from one thermoneedle to another. The animals were judged to be asleep when they lay down, curled up, and maintained the characteristic sleeping posture for 20 minutes, with a respiratory rate of less than 20/min and a failure to respond to sounds that usually provoked an "investigatory" reflex. The hypothalamus was found to be consistently warmer than the cortex, the difference varying from 0.1° to 0.5° C. Activity, particularly if following excitement, raised the cerebral temperature, both cortical and hypothalamic; rest led to a drop in temperature. During drowsiness, the temperature curves became irregularly rhythmical, with the duration of the waves about six minutes and the amplitude about 0.1° C. These temperature oscillations were different from the wavelike fluctuations in the human brain volume, observed during the onset of sleep (p. 47). Definite sleep resulted in a fall in temperature, greater in the hypothalamus than in the cortex, the gradient between the two narrowing down from 0.5° to 0.3° C. or less. On awakening, the series of events was reversed, the rise in temperature usually manifesting itself first in the hypothalamus. The more marked fall in the temperature of the hypothalamus was not due to its greater distance from the surface, for other regions, such as Ammon's horn or the tail of the caudate nucleus, at a comparable depth, did not mirror it. The temperature did not drop in every case of sleep. Out of 119 sleep curves, 88 showed a fall in temperature; 18, a rise; and 13, no change. When the temperature did not decrease in the hypothalamus, it likewise did not drop elsewhere, showing that there were common interfering causes. Control experiments showed that changes in the circulation were not responsible for the temperature rises and falls but that the latter reflected variations in metabolic activity of the different parts of the brain. Frequently during sleep the hypothalamic temperature began to rise, reaching a maximum in 3 to 12 minutes, when the animal would suddenly stir and change its position. After the cat settled in the new position, the hypothalamic temperature would drop. Serota concluded from his experiments that the hypothalamus, as judged by its temperature changes, was less active during sleep than in wakefulness.

Kosmarskaia and Purin (2247) also recorded the brain temperature of cats, put to sleep by "barbamil" (60 mg/kg). The brain temperature dropped nearly 2° C. in 4 hours, several times the decrease noted by Serota. Furthermore, in the next 4 hours, the brain temperature rose 4° C., ending up with a 2° hyperthermia. The rectal temperature showed similar oscillations. Evidently the state of these cats had no relation to physiological sleep.

Most of the temperature changes occurring during sleep may be due to muscular relaxation, vasomotor adjustments following the assumption of the horizontal position, and, above all, the 24-hour body-temperature curve, which, in return, depends for its establishment and maintenance upon the regular alternation of sleep and wakefulness (p. 138). Quite apart from the general temperature variations are the observations of Serota on changes in regional brain temperature during sleep, which, together with other studies, should enable one to decide whether the center located at the base of the brain is concerned with the production of sleep or of wakefulness.

Piéron (3192) summed up what was known fifty years ago about urinary secretion by saying that it is diminished at night, concomitantly with the decrease in blood pressure and blood flow, and listing as contributory causes the horizontal position, darkness, physical and mental rest, and, finally, sleep itself as a most complete form of rest. Bouchard (424) found urine secreted during sleep to be less toxic than that secreted in wakefulness. "Sleep" urines were also convulsive in their effects, whereas "waking state" urines were narcotizing. On these findings, Bouchard (425) based his "toxic" theory of sleep.

Brunton (550), in a review dealing with the acid output of the kidney and the so-called alkaline tide, listed a number of possible contributory factors which may mask, in one direction or another, the effects of sleep itself, among them variations in food intake, digestive and endocrine tides, posture and muscular relaxation, sweat excretion, quiet, and inhibitory influences from higher centers. It is clear that without a control of these factors one may attribute certain changes to sleep when they are only indirectly due to it. It should be emphasized that there are certain 24-hour rhythms—such as that of body temperature—which, even though in the long run dependent on the alternation of sleep and wakefulness, may persist when one stays awake one or more nights and thus lead to erroneous interpretation of the control tests themselves.

On the volume of urine, Piéron (3192) gave figures reported by sixteen authors on the night secretion of urine compared to day secretion. Of these, eleven found a diminution of urine formation at night, and five an increase; the mean volume per hour was 68 ml for the day and 56 for the night. However, the horizontal position of itself led to an increase in the flow of urine. This fact, confirmed by Bazett and associates (267), may mean that the decrease in the volume of urine secreted during sleep is sufficient to overcome the opposite effect resulting from lying down. Simpson (3713), on the other hand, demonstrated that there was a relation between body temperature and urinary excretion of water. His five subjects were given 100 to 200 ml of water every hour, and urine was collected hourly, even during the night when the subjects had to be briefly awakened for the purpose. There was a negative water balance during the day and retention of water at night. The parallelism between the curves for water excretion and body temperature is quite striking, a sharp drop in urine formation corresponding to the rather abrupt descent of the temperature curve from its daytime plateau. Luederitz (2573) confirmed this relationship, but considered the body temperature as governed by the urinary excretory variation.

The renal plasma flow was found to be uniform in sleep and wakefulness, but between midnight and 4:00 A.M., during "deepest sleep," there was a significant fall in glomerular filtration (3720). However, in congestive heart failure patients, with persistent peripheral edema, glomerular filtration was increased in sleep (191).

There is fairly general agreement that a greater amount of acid products, as determined by titration, is excreted during sleep (619, 2176, 2177, 3713). The pH of urine during sleep is lowered and Endres (1074) explained it as due to the diminished irritability of the respiratory center and a greater CO_2 content and acidity of the blood. Kroetz (2285) and Simpson (3715) also reported a drop in the pH of the urine during sleep. Kaye (2094), while confirming the findings of others that during the night the pH of the urine is lower than in the daytime, denied that this is due to sleep and therefore to lessened ventilation of the lungs and a higher CO_2 tension in the blood. His subject remained awake and engaged in laboratory work, and the nocturnal acidity of the urine appeared just the same, with the lowest pH value, 5.3, at 7:00 A.M. and a high point, 7.1, at 1:00 P.M. Kaye ascribed the nighttime high acidity to a starvation effect.

The excretion of chlorides is decreased during sleep (267, 2176, 3715), as related by Piéron. Bazett and associates (267) observed an alkaline, as well as a chloride, tide on awakening in the morning, even when no food was taken and the subject remained in bed.

Norn (3024), experimenting on himself, ate regularly at 8:00 A.M., 4:00 P.M., and midnight, and slept from 2:30 A.M. to 8:00 A.M. He excreted less water, half as much sodium and chloride, and two-thirds as much potassium during sleep as during the waking state. Inversion of the routine inverted the excretory curve. The onset of sleep was necessary for the "sleep" type of kidney activity to set in. There was no decrease in plasma potassium during sleep, so the lesser excretion of potassium must have been due to another cause. The respiratory depression occurring in sleep could not be wholly responsible for the decrease in sodium and potassium excretion, according to Longson and Mills (2558). Thomas (3924) found that the horizontal position of the body affected the Na:K ratio in the urine.

Leathes (2390) noted a decrease in creatinine and uric acid during the night hours. Campbell and Webster confirmed this finding (619), but others (2176, 3713) detected no change in creatinine excretion in sleep.

Fontès and Yovanovitch (1232) determined the effect of sleep on the elimination of nitrogenous compounds on three young male subjects receiving a standardized diet every 12 hours, a total of 1,150 Cal per meal. The excretion of total nitrogen, urea, and amino acids was decreased by 10 to 15 per cent, but the ammonia excretion was doubled during sleep. Campbell and Webster (619) obtained similar values: a decrease for total nitrogen, urea, and amino acids but an increase in the excretion of ammonia during sleep.

As Simpson ascribed the low urine volume to body temperature, and Kaye the increased urine acidity to fasting, Fontès and Yovanovitch (1233) related the low nitrogen excretion to darkness. Sleep by itself had a slight lowering effect on excretion of nitrogen, but, by staying awake in the dark and sleeping in the presence of light, and a variety of other combinations, it was possible to place the major responsibility for the low nitrogen excretion on darkness.

Another controversial topic is the effect of sleep on the urinary output of phosphates. Again, Piéron's tabulation showed that, out of eleven authors, seven reported an increase in phosphate excretion during the night, and four, a decrease. Campbell and Webster (619, 620) obtained an increased excretion of phosphates during sleep, whether their subject slept in the daytime or at night. I was able to confirm their findings, including the effect of a reversed routine of sleep and wakefulness (2176). Instead of dividing the 24-hour period into two 12-hour portions, I allocated 16 hours to "wakefulness" and 8 hours to "sleep" urine. In another study (2177) I secured a still stricter separation of the two portions, as I had for a subject a person who was carrying out a long-term metabolism experiment on himself and separated the urine he collected during his waking period from that excreted during sleep. The amount of phosphate he excreted per hour during sleep was 15 to 29 per cent higher than that excreted during his waking hours.

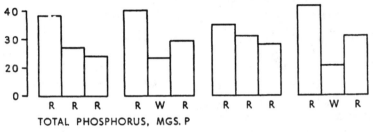

TOTAL PHOSPHORUS, MGS. P

Fig. 8.4—The rate of urinary excretion of total phosphorus by Subject II, during four 6-hour periods of testing (6:00 A.M. to noon). *R*, 2-hour period of rest; *W*, 2-hour period of walking.

Campbell and Webster (619) explained the phosphate tide at night as due to the increased acidity of the urine, "not connected with muscle or nerve metabolism in particular." I, on the contrary, thought that muscular relaxation during sleep might be responsible for the increased excretion of phosphate. Earlier Fiske (1201) noted that there was a gradually decreasing phosphate excretion during the morning hours, followed by an increase in the afternoon. He explained it by assuming "an active retention of phosphate, which later in the day is 'released.'" I confirmed Fiske in the matter of the phosphate excretion during the day and proceeded to test the "retention" idea by asking four subjects to remain in bed awake, without breakfast, from 6:00 A.M. until noon. Three two-hour samples of urine were collected and analyzed for phosphates. A descending curve was obtained in each case. On another day the same subjects were asked to stay in bed during the first and third two-hour periods, but to take a brisk walk (8 miles) during the middle period. In five out of six pairs of tests the phosphate excretion during the walk was much lower than in the same two-hour period of rest on the control days, and correspondingly more was excreted during the period following the walk (Fig. 8.4). The total excreted during the 6 hours was about the same on the two days. It appears that the phosphate metabolized, which under the condition of rest would be delivered to the blood and thus excreted in the urine (since the urinary excretion of phosphates has been shown to reflect their concentration in the blood), was retained by the tissues (muscles?) during activity and released during ensuing rest.

Simpson (3716), who was the only one to report that the phosphate excretion is lowered during sleep, repeated my daytime experiments with slight modifications. Instead of the sequence lying, walking, lying, he employed two other sequences: (*a*) lying, standing, lying, and (*b*) standing, walking, standing. In the first sequence his results were the same as mine; concerning the second he stated that "the results are not clear cut and are difficult to explain." This discrepancy is not surprising. In the first sequence, where standing replaced walking, the individual got tired from standing and undoubtedly relaxed when he lay down. It will be recalled that we (2194) obtained a marked drop in body temperature in persons who lay down after standing up for one hour (p. 58). In Simpson's second sequence—standing, walking, standing—the subjects could not relax after the exercise; hence the indefinite results. Simpson's conclusion was that posture rather than relaxation is the deciding factor. In the vertical position the phosphate excretion is low; in the horizontal position, high. This conclusion, of course, does not explain the variation in phosphate excretion during the day, with the subject fasting, or Simpson's finding that sleep leads to a decrease in phosphate excretion. That muscular relaxation is responsible for the increase in phosphate excretion while lying down awake and during sleep seems to be a valid inference, and most of the changes in the excretion of urine can be traced to one or another of the sleep concomitants or external conditions: horizontal posture, relaxation, low temperature, fasting and darkness.

Part 2

Course of Events during the Sleep Phase

Chapter 9

The Onset of Sleep

Whereas it is easy to distinguish between the conditions of alertness, or being wide-awake, and definite sleep, the passage from one to the other involves a succession of intermediate states, part wakefulness and part sleep in varying proportions—what is designated in Italian as *dormiveglia,* or sleep-waking. Subjectively, there is a feeling of general lassitude, lagging attention, and loss of interest in the surroundings, and from past experience one associates this state with the approach of sleep. Many everyday words are used to designate this condition, among others "sleepiness," "drowsiness," "languor," "inertness," "heaviness of eyelids," and "sluggishness," and I intend to use these terms more or less interchangeably. One word, as common as the others, that I propose to reserve for special use, is "somnolence," and the reason is that in the clinical literature this term often designates a pathological condition—sometimes excessive sleepiness, sometimes hypersomnia, the latter referring to a greater than normal ratio of sleeping to waking hours.

There seems to be no single word in English that can be called the equivalent of the German *Einschlafen,* the French *endormissement,* or the Italian *addormentamento.* "The onset of sleep," "falling asleep," and "going to sleep" are fair equivalents of the foregoing words. Less commonly used words are "dormition" and "hypnagogic state." Critchley (783, 784) employed the terms "predormitum" and "post-dormitum" to describe the process of going to sleep and waking up, and credited W. R. Gowers with coining the word "sleepening" as the opposite of awakening.

Aside from the influence of usual bedtime—discussed under periodicity—fatigue and lack of stimulation, or monotony, favor a feeling of drowsiness which ordinarily precedes the onset of sleep. One expression of this feeling is the paroxysmal respiratory movement of yawning. Barbizet (216) described the yawn as "halfway between a reflex and an expressive movement," lasting 4 to 7 seconds, and often accompanied by stretching. Transient cardiac acceleration and digital vasoconstriction are associated with yawning (1755), which may be an indirect vasomotor adjustment furthering the circulation in the lungs and brain (1006). Conditions of fatigue (3137) which lead to yawning in one person ordinarily apply to others who may witness the yawning—hence the imitative aspect of the act (2875). Lesions in the CNS cause pathological yawning (216, 2482, 2722), and experimentally yawning has been induced in the monkey by stimulating the midbrain or the region of the caudate nucleus and stria terminalis (3243). Lewy (2482) held that yawning, like stretching, might serve to restore the tonus of the muscles involved, but Barbizet (216) saw no particular physiological function for this physical manifestation of drowsiness. Under conditions of monotony, subjects usually relax (61, 2140, 2141, 2568), and their performance deteriorates. Conditioned reflexes in human subjects (2251, 4088) and animals (2887) show longer latencies, decrease in magnitude, and eventually cease.

The behavior of the eyes is often indicative of drowsiness (2392). The closure of the eyelids, especially if it is not intentional, is a sure sign of approaching sleep. But, with the eyelids still open, a peculiar "beady" and dull expression of the eyes is suggestive of sleepiness. Indeed, sleep may set in while the eyes are still open, according to Miles (2815–17), who studied the eye movements in drowsiness by photographically recording this activity. While awake and looking over the visual field, a person's eyes execute rapid saccadic movements in various directions, with "fixation" of the eyes at the end of each movement. The test consisted of shifting the gaze from one luminous dot to another, 40° away in the horizontal plane. In the alert state it took about 0.10 second to rotate the eyes through such an angle, but in extreme drowsiness the time might be as long as 0.16–0.25 second. The fixation was unsteady, resulting in a wavering of the eye to the extent of 1°–2°, or about ten times as great as the normal waking inaccuracy of fixation. Corrective movements usually executed at the end of a long saccadic sweep either were absent in sleepiness or were so exaggerated as to increase the inaccuracy. Long, normally continuous movements might be broken up into short jerks. As the sleepiness became overpowering, not only did the eye movements become slowed but a pendular rolling type of movement replaced the horizontal. According to Miles, the eye muscles continued their activity after vision had stopped, but even before that point was reached the sleepy person was often aware of his condition through the development of diplopia, or inability to fixate a point with both eyes, in spite of an extreme effort to do so.

The findings of Miles were confirmed in our laboratory (2204). Further, a similar impairment of oculomotor performance was produced by small amounts of alcohol, eliciting experimentally the diplopia often associated with alcoholic intoxication. Amphetamine had no effect on oculomotor performance of subjects who were wide awake but led to improvement of the impaired performance in drowsiness.

Magnussen (2621–25) emphasized a sudden rise in foot temperature, along with a gradual decrease in rectal temperature, as an indication of the approach of sleep, or a sign of a "vegetative preparedness for sleep." We (2203) repeated and extended Magnussen's observations by recording the skin temperatures in several locations: toes, soles, and legs, as well as fingers, palms, and forearms. Our results, while confirming Magnussen's findings regarding the feet, did not support his implication of a decrease in sympathetic activity to explain the vasodilation in the feet. Our data showed that, in general, skin temperature fluctuations were greatest in the toes, intermediate in the soles, and least in the calves. The same differential applied to the corresponding skin areas in the upper extremities, but the absolute changes were smaller. Following a meal, if there was a rise in oral temperature, there was a concomitant increase in toe- and finger-skin temperatures. Muscular relaxation, when it led to a lowering of the body temperature, was usually accompanied by a drop in finger temperature and a simultaneous rise in toe temperature. In the pre-sleep hours of the evening there was thus a combination of two influences to raise toe-skin temperature: meal and muscular relaxation. It therefore seemed that the feet, especially the toes, exhibited vasomotor changes that were not characteristic of the skin as a whole, not even of the skin of the extremities, and changes in foot temperature could not be looked upon as variations in general sympathetic activity.

Burch and Greiner (570) considered GSRs to specific stimuli to be measures of performance reflecting alertness. At one portion of the descending curve of specific GSRs, representing drowsiness or very light sleep, there was a "paradoxical spike of over-response," not shown in the curve for non-specific GSRs. The significance of that spike is not clear. Another paradoxical phenomenon was reported by Pavlov and Voskressensky (3131), whose dog, on falling asleep, lost his secretory conditioned reflexes, while preserving the motor ones. At a later stage, he regained the first and lost the second, before finally losing both. Mishchenko (2840, 2841), by the conditioned reflex method, studied differentiation of light and sound stimuli in relation to the onset of sleep in six healthy young men. There were a number of stages between sleep and wakefulness, but the whole period could be divided into two portions: cataleptic and narcotic. In the cataleptic interval conditioned reflexes were present, with inhibition concentrated primarily in the cortex, and cataleptic phenomena appeared first in the hands, then eyes, and later became general. In the narcotic period conditioned reflex activity and reactions to stimuli disappeared, inhibition attacked the subcortical area also, and the cataleptic phenomena were abolished in the order of their appearance and were replaced by relaxation. In this scheme, relaxation, instead of preceding sleep, developed only after a certain depth of sleep had been reached.

As previously mentioned (p. 14), Chauchard (682–85) observed a simultaneous parallel rise in the chronaxies of cortical and peripheral neurones during the period of drowsiness. At the onset of sleep the peripheral chronaxie fell abruptly to its low constitutional value, whereas the central chronaxie continued to rise beyond its high constitutional value. Thus, isochronism is preserved during drowsiness, but heterochronism and loss of "peripheral subordination" are ushered in with the onset of sleep.

The actual passage from wakefulness to sleep is accompanied by a number of changes, some of which were mentioned under the concomitants of sleep. There is a fall in muscle tonus, as seen from a progressive diminution of muscle action potentials (2718) and a decrease in the knee jerk (2552). There is a slowing of the heart rate (387, 3204), a lowering of the blood pressure (545, 3204), a wavy plethysmographic curve (3880), occasionally a paradoxical increase in cardiac reflexes (3746). The insensible perspiration, as measured by the rate of weight loss, increases during the onset of sleep, paralleling the fall in rectal temperature (861, 862).

Kreidl and Herz (2276) saw no differences from the normal in the manner in which blind and deaf people fell asleep. Claparède (708) interpreted this finding as proof that external stimulation or lack of it plays a less decisive part in the onset of sleep than is commonly believed. It is hard to understand why Kreidl and Herz chose to study the effect of blindness and deafness, sensory deficiencies which are deliberately sought by a person who wishes to sleep.

Among the phenomena that characterize the passage from wakefulness to sleep is the well-known "floating" feeling, frequently ending in a "fall" or "start," which may bring the person back to complete wakefulness. Roger (3390) described these muscular contractions as occurring singly or in groups of muscles, in the arm, leg, sometimes the whole body. They usually do not interfere with sleep during the rest of the night. They are more frequent in adults than in children, occur in people who are "nervous," and under circumstances that increase nervousness, fatigue, or agreeable and disagreeable emotional states.

De Lisi (2537) stated that the hypnic myoclonias appear in man and domestic animals, like dogs and cats, 1 to 5 minutes after the beginning of sleep, become extended and intensified during the next 5 minutes, and then subside. They are present in infants and adults of either sex and may appear in any part of the musculature. They may be so widespread as to take on the character of generalized clonic convulsions. To distinguish these phenomena from pathological syndromes, de Lisi called them "physiological hypnic myoclonias."

Pintus and Falqui (3206) investigated the neural mechanism of these dormitional starts. They employed eighteen kittens, one to two months of age, and produced in them various lesions. The myoclonia is not a purely muscular phenomenon, as section of the nerves to the muscles abolished it. When the spinal cord was cut, the myoclonia disappeared below the section. Destruction of the anterior suprasylvian and anterior ectosylvian convolutions abolished the myoclonia contralaterally. However, lesions in other cortical areas, as well as in the mesencephalon, corpus striatum, thalamus, and cerebellum, were without effect. It is clear that these myoclonias are of cortical origin and depend on corticospinal anatomical continuity. What they signify no one has ventured to explain, but Oswald (3067) noted that these jerks "sometimes appeared as a part of the arousal response to a faint but significant external stimulus," as shown by small K-complexes in the EEG. There is no evidence that they are epileptic phenomena (105).

In the "floating" or "drifting off" EEGs of Davis and associates (840, 841), the passage from their stage A to stage B did not occur simultaneously in all parts of the brain. A shift of the focus of maximum activity from the parieto-occipital region to the frontal one with the onset of sleep was also reported by Brazier (463). On the other hand, Darrow and associates (826) noted an increase of the frontal-motor EEG parallelism during the onset of sleep. As the sleep became deeper, this was likely to be replaced by a motor-parietal parallelism.

The Davis group (840) instructed two subjects to signal whenever they felt that they had just "drifted off." One subject did so 20 times, the other 9 times, before falling asleep. The mean duration of the depression of the alpha pattern in four successive groups of five signals for the first subject increased from 2.9 to 13.5 seconds; and in three successive groups of three signals for the second subject, from 6.2 to 22.7 seconds. The authors concluded that "it makes quite meaningless any question as to the exact moment at which a person falls asleep."

The relation between muscular relaxation and the brain-potential pattern at the onset of sleep was determined in our laboratory (366). The subject was asked to hold a light spool between two fingers as he was falling asleep, while his brain potentials were being recorded. At a certain stage of the onset of sleep his muscles relaxed, and the spool dropped from between his fingers. The subject was also asked to report whether he was sufficiently conscious to be aware of having dropped the spool. The spool usually dropped between 0.5 and 25 seconds after the alpha pattern disappeared. When the spool fell 0.5–1.5 (mean 1.1) seconds after the disappearance of the alpha pattern, the subject reported having been aware of it; but when the delay amounted to 6.5–25.0 (mean 14) seconds, the subject was deeply enough asleep not to report dropping the spool. Thus, it would seem that muscle tonus diminishes very soon after the alpha pattern is lost, but the level of consciousness is lowered more slowly. Another possible interpretation is that shortly after the disappearance of the alpha pattern the sleep (or dozing) is so light that the event of the dropping of the spool produces a definite tactile sensation, whereas several seconds later no sensation results from the same kind of stimulus.

Oswald (3068) subjected six volunteers to sound stimuli at lower limits of audibility, at intervals of a few seconds, to which they had to respond by signaling. "The most striking finding, in these situations where the subjects' task was to exercise a high degree of alertness, was the insistent tendency for the EEG to take on the appearance of sleep," coming and going at intervals as short as 3 seconds. Also when subjects were asked to move rhythmically to music, EEG signs of sleep appeared, even though the movements to music continued.

A characteristic (3.5–6/sec EEG pattern, running for about 4 seconds, appears in infants and small children at the onset of sleep. The pattern was first described by Smith (3738) and named "drowsy" waves. In normal children these waves tend to disappear from the age of three years on (460, 811, 1221, 2126, 2981), but a similar EEG pattern may be seen in older children and adults in association with cortical disturbances. Gibbs and Lorimer (1422) described a 30–40/sec EEG pattern appearing in the frontal and to a lesser extent in the parietal and temporal regions during drowsiness in patients with personality disorders. Henriksen and co-authors (1702) reported a case of a thalamic syndrome, in which "EEG studies reveal that although bilaterally symmetrical rhythmic activity may be present when the patient is awake, during drowsiness and deeper sleep a marked asymmetry often appears, with early disappearance of alpha activity and reduction or abolition of spindles on the side involved."

Hodes and co-workers (1797) found that changes in electrical activity during drowsiness of monkeys appeared in subcortical structures, such as the caudate nucleus, earlier than in the cortex, suggesting that the subcortical masses were driving the cortex.

Verzeano and Negishi (4053), studying the electrical activity of several neighboring neurones in the cortex and thalamus of cats, noted that, in the transition from wakefulness to sleep, an enhanced excitatory process developed along the pathways of propagation, but an enhanced inhibitory process developed in the immediate vicinity of the neurones during the passage of the propagating activity.

Concerning the development of sleep, Miller (2823) observed a gradual rise in the threshold of electrical shocks necessary to produce a sensation of pain, as her subjects were going to sleep. Bartlett (233, 234), by the use of an audiometer, established the variations in the auditory thresholds during the onset of sleep. There was a gradual and considerable rise in the threshold intensities, but there were no typical curves. Each individual had his own curve of going to sleep. Entirely different results were obtained in our laboratory (2942, 2944) on dogs and human beings, among the latter, children and adults, mentally normal or feeble-minded. The stimulus used to test auditory irritability was a sound emitted by a magnetic loud-speaker into which was fed a current from an ordinary 110-volt A.C. street circuit, passed through a rheostat. By this means it was possible to vary the intensity of the sound from a hardly audible hum to a very loud blast, and the voltage necessary to produce an audible sound was used to designate the value of the threshold stimulus. An attempt was made to determine whether or not there was a relationship between the time that had elapsed after the "beginning" of sleep and the irritability to auditory stimuli—in other words, the curve of the onset of sleep. In the observations on dogs, the animal was placed in a stand, and a wide band of ticking passed underneath its belly as a sort of sling. The sling was loose enough not to be in contact with the animal when the latter was standing, but, if the dog relaxed his leg muscles, he was supported in the sling. The dogs were taught to remain quietly in the stand, and the observer in the adjoining room watched them through a peep-hole. It was not difficult to detect the development of the drowsy state in such animals, or to tell when they were asleep, by the manner in which they responded to sounds. The human subjects were tested while lying on a couch.

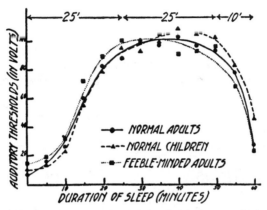

Fig. 9.1—Superimposed curves of auditory threshold changes during the first hour of sleep in three groups of subjects. For the normal adults the plotted values are the means of 996 determinations on eight subjects; for the children, on 571 determinations on eight subjects; and for the feeble-minded, on 668 determinations on seven subjects. The intensity of the sound was plotted as the voltage fed into a loud-speaker.

They were instructed to report when they heard a sound, if awake, or when aroused by it, if asleep. Those children and adults who could follow instructions were asked to hold a piece of paper between thumb and forefinger as they were going to sleep. When the paper dropped, the observer counted that time as "the beginning of the onset" of sleep, and the hearing of the subject was tested a definite length of time thereafter. The waking threshold was, of course, determined for every animal or subject at the start of each session and was found to be fairly constant. The curves of the onset of sleep were strikingly similar for the different subjects and the dogs. They were all roughly S-shaped, showing first a positive and then a negative acceleration. The maximum threshold values were reached 30 to 35 minutes after the arbitrarily set zero time (Fig. 9.1) and were usually followed by a plateau and a downward turn to lighter sleep. There thus appears to be no moment at which sleep may be said to have been reached, but rather a period during which the irritability, as the reciprocal of the threshold sound, gradually falls from its usual waking level.

Another approach to the "time of establishment" of sleep is through the period of "settling down." Motility records show that the sleeper has moved for a certain time after going to bed and then remained quiescent for a fairly long interval of time. Presumably, when the stirring is over for the first time, the subject is asleep. Johnson (1997, 1999) gave the following mean figures for "going to sleep after going to bed"—time in minutes, range in parentheses: unselected college men, 13 (8–23); kindergarten children, 36 (24–64); middle-aged men, 15 (9–25); their wives, 13 (10–17). The figures for the children were obtained by Garvey (1363), and both he and Johnson emphasized the fact that children became quiet much less promptly on going to bed than adults. Page (3075) found 23 minutes to be the mean delay in the cessation of movement after going to bed, using five normal subjects. Kotlyarevsky (2251), in children, noted that unconditioned responses were abolished in 15 to 30 minutes during the onset of sleep. Mayorov and Sandomirsky (2732) reported that "choleric" and "phlegmatic" personality types went to sleep slowly, whereas "sanguine" individuals fell asleep quickly.

It will be recalled (p. 52) that Fleisch reported that under conditions of low atmospheric pressure it took a person only 2 to 4 seconds to fall asleep. Raboutet and co-workers (3254), analyzing sleep EEGs of navigators, found that lower atmospheric pressures favored the onset of sleep, and higher pressures had the opposite effect.

Seasonal influences on the time required to fall asleep have been reported for monkeys (3727) and for children taking afternoon naps (3159). In our laboratory (2200), an attempt was made to determine, for a group of people, of both sexes and of different ages, the ease or difficulty of going to sleep on the basis of a large number of reports that could be treated statistically. It had been our intention to have several grades of ease or difficulty of going to sleep recorded by the subjects. However, this recording was to be done on getting up in the morning, and we soon found that, whereas it was a simple matter for the individual to recall that he had difficulty in falling asleep, it was hard for him to decide whether he went to sleep in the usual fashion or more promptly. So the subject was given two choices for marking his sleep record—that he went to sleep "with ease" or "with difficulty." The individual's tendency to fall asleep was expressed as the percentage of the total number of nights on which he went to sleep with ease. The group, made up of healthy subjects, tended to go to sleep with ease, and the percentage for the group as a whole was around 90, with a range of 63 to 100. As would be expected, the state of the individual at the time of going to bed had some influence on the ease of going to sleep. In the hyperactive state (wide-awake, excited, worried) this percentage was lowest; in the hypoactive state (very tired, sleepy, depressed), the highest; and in the neutral state (moderately tired, indifferent), in between. But the differences were not always statistically reliable, some subjects going to sleep with ease on all nights, irrespective of the state they were in. The subjects went to sleep more easily if they took no naps in the daytime, but again there were numerous individual variations, and the difference was not significant. Nor did the condition of the gastrointestinal tract—the number and type of bowel movements—have any effect on going to sleep with ease. Thus, there was a great diversity among subjects in this respect, although, in general, most subjects had no difficulty in falling asleep.

The time required to fall asleep after going to bed furnishes no information concerning the rapidity with which one passes from a state of wakefulness to one of sleep. It will be recalled, from data on EEG (840) and on the change in auditory threshold (2942, 2944), that the transition is gradual. Magnussen (2622, 2623), by his double system of recording respiration, convinced himself that the transition is practically instantaneous, requiring only a fraction of a second. Drohocki (990) also noted a momentary cessation of breathing, at the beginning of an expiration, though his time estimate ran from 2 to 20 seconds. Both of these investigators observed a repeated reversal of sleep and wakefulness, prior to the setting in of continuous sleep, and their observations are in accord with Oswald's report of a regular alternation of the two states every few seconds (3068). Lawson (2384) also found that the onset of sleep, as judged by the stopping of blinking, occurred in 1 to 2 seconds. It is possible to reconcile the conflicting findings by assuming that the fraction of time occupied by wakefulness gradually decreases, as that given over to sleep increases, till at the end of several minutes one has passed from 100 per cent wakefulness to 100 per cent sleep.

Sturt (3861) tried to determine her judgment of elapsed time during the state of dormition. When sleepy, she started a stop watch and stopped it in what she estimated was 5 minutes. When she was very sleepy, with visual imagery predominating, the actual time elapsed was 3:54; when fairly sleepy (verbal imagery prevailing), it was 4:33; when she was telling herself a story, although sleepy, 4:45. In all cases, however, she stopped too soon. She did not indicate whether, when she was wide-awake, she could estimate 5 minutes' time with greater accuracy than when sleepy.

From the psychological viewpoint, the transition period is characterized by hypnagogic manifestations which, according to Slight (3725), "are intimately linked up and often blended with the so-called conscious thoughts of the moment and are easily accessible for introspection." Several authors, on the basis of self-observations and reports of others, described the successive introspective stages in the transition from wakefulness to sleep (79, 80, 358, 783, 784, 1304, 1305, 1917, 1983, 2345, 2504, 2535, 2723, 2847, 3272, 3418, 3961). The three stages described by Vihvelin (4061) are representative: (a) a progressive narrowing of the field of consciousness, as a quantitative change in psychological processes;

(b) a stage of "pure" hypnagogic hallucinations, as a qualitative change in psychological processes; and (c) a vacillation between wakefulness and sleep, when hypnagogic hallucinations are confused with dreams. Ardis and McKellar (114) pointed out the similarities between hypnagogic hallucinations and the subjective effects of mescaline which would suggest a common principle. Under mescaline, however, the hypnagogic experience of "falling" does not occur and auditory hallucinations are rare.

It is clear that neither physiologically nor psychologically is it possible to say that an individual is fully asleep at a particular moment. Starting with sleepiness or drowsiness, when the person, though fully awake, has a disinclination to activity and a desire for sleep—and going through the phase of preparing for, or yielding to, sleep, followed by a period of part wakefulness and part sleep—one arrives at a stage when the person or animal can be said to be definitely asleep. But definite sleep is not a level value to be ascended from at the moment of awakening. As will be seen, a wavelike alternation of a deeper and a lighter sleep, with characteristic modifications, runs through the entire period of sleep.

Chapter 10

Motility during Sleep

From the discussion of the position of the body during sleep it is clear that the sleeper does not lie completely still during the entire sleep period. At first, motility was merely taken for granted, but with the development of automatic recording equipment, this topic has assumed a very prominent place among the characteristics of sleep investigated. Some writers went to the point of defining that elusive value which is called "quality of sleep" in terms of how often a person moved during the night (2344).

The impetus to these studies unquestionably came from the work of Szymanski (3897–99). But, even prior to that, Maclay (2607), taking up "proper and improper methods of sleeping," noted that a sleeper could, without awakening, turn over and place his face in a new zone, throw his arms above his head, put his hand to his face, rub his nose and face, or throw the covers from around his neck.

Szymanski's device, equally applicable to animal cages as to beds of human beings, consisted essentially of a string carried over pulleys from a suspended cage, or from a bedspring, to a recording lever. The principle is that of a seismograph. It has been modified in minor ways, using pneumatic or electrical transmission instead of mechanical, but the principle is the same—to let the cage or bed record its displacements due to movements of the animal or person. The sensitivity of the apparatus can be made so great that respiration and pulse will appear in the records. In most cases, the device is constructed in such a way as to record movements which a person spontaneously executes during sleep.

The motility records, usually referred to by German writers as *Aktogramme,* showed Szymanski that some animals had several alternating periods of motility and inactivity during the 24 hours of day and night, while others, among them the human adult, had only one of each. He designated the first kind as polyphasic; the second, as monophasic. Although Szymanski's nomenclature has been adopted by others, it should be discarded, as each alternation involves phases of rest and motility, or phases of greater and lesser motility. More appropriate terms would be polycyclic and monocyclic, and these will hereafter be used.

A comprehensive study of normal human adult subjects was made by Johnson and associates (1996, 1997, 1999, 2003, 2004), who collected a large number of motility records from ninety persons and treated them statistically. Their system of tabulation consisted of counting a 5-minute period, in which a movement occurred, as one of motility. The first 15,000 measurements, made on eleven subjects, gave a mean of 11.5 minutes between movements. The mean duration of rest periods was found to be a stable personal characteristic. Their values for typical representatives of groups of healthy sleepers were as follows (all figures in minutes and ranges in parentheses): unselected college men, 12.8 (7.3–21.5); middle-aged men, 9.0 (6.3–12.5); their wives, 10.5 (7.5–14.4). During a night's sleep of about 8 hours there would be, on the average, 38, 53, and 46 movements, respectively, for the three groups. Johnson's system of counting out 5 minutes in which a movement took place led to some unexpected conclusions. Thus, he stated (1996) that their "most typical subject, if he stays in bed 8 hours, spends about one hour and 20 minutes of that time in stirring every 5 minutes or oftener." Likewise, in another paper, Johnson (1997) reported, for adults of middle age, that "it is not unusual for a person to take nearly as much rest on most nights of 6.5 hours as in the average night of 9.5 hours." Naturally, the system of calling 5 minutes a period of motility, if a movement occurred in it, is responsible for the foregoing statements. If he had used 1- or 2-minute intervals, his subjects would have been found to have moved during a smaller percentage of all the periods, i.e., would have spent less time in movement.

The Johnson group did not detect any constant distribution of the movements in the course of a typical night's sleep. After analyzing the results obtained on eleven subjects, they decided (2002) that the distribution of movements was a personal characteristic of the sleeper, "some subjects tending to rest more during the first half of the night; others during the last half; others during the middle."

In a survey of the results, Johnson (1999) published some curves showing striking wavelike variations in the frequency with which the sleepers stirred in successive 5-minute periods. For the night, one could discern a dozen or more small oscillations, but in several curves there were five well-defined waves, suggesting the 85- to 90-minute cycles in EEG and other variables independently "discovered" by others, and discussed in the next chapter.

On the basis of the actograms obtained, Szymanski (3900) divided adult sleepers into three classes: (*a*) subjects showing absolute rest for about 3 hours after the onset of sleep, followed by 3 or 4 periods of relative rest alternating with absolute rest; (*b*) those whose rest was absolute throughout the night; and (*c*) those who had 5 to 7 periods of relative rest during the night's sleep.

No other workers reported subjects belonging to Szymanski's second class, but we tested one apparently normal individual, who could, on being challenged to prove it to us in the laboratory, spend the night in bed practically without any movement. However, he refused to act as a subject more than twice, as he was not well rested in the morning. Szymanski's third class is close to Johnson's subjects with five waves of motility for the night.

It would appear that the average normal sleeper spends a good deal of time in stirring or changing positions. When does he rest, and how much time does he spend in "not moving"? To answer these questions, we had constructed the apparatus shown and explained in Figure 10.1 (2181, 2193). The motility

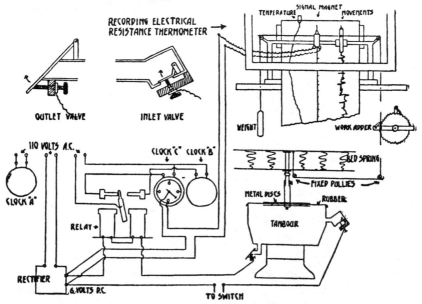

Fig. 10.1—A diagram of the apparatus for determining and for recording motility and rectal temperature during sleep.

The opening of the inlet or outlet valve of the tambour (details shown in upper left-hand corner of diagram) by the movement of the bedspring breaks and keeps open a 6-volt D.C. circuit through a relay, causing the 110-volt A.C. current to start clock *C*, simultaneously interrupting the flow of the current through clock *B*. The time run up by clock *C* or the time lost by clock *B* in comparison with clock *A* is the total time spent in motility by the sleeper during the night's sleep.

The use of the electric clock system for determining the total time spent in motility, as well as of a signal magnet for repeatedly recording successive accumulations of 15 seconds of motility, and the operation of the work-adder in summing up the magnitudes of the individual movements are described in the text.

The rectal temperature curve is recorded by a pen attached to the string of an electrical resistance thermometer, the connection from the thermometer to the sleeper, as well as the construction of the thermometer, omitted from the diagram.

of the sleeper was studied indirectly through the movements of the bedspring which might be either of the vertical multiple-coil type or of the net (hammock) variety. In either case a vertical rod transmitted the movements of the spring to a strong rubber membrane covering a large tambour (30 cm wide and 10 cm high), placed directly on the floor and provided with inlet and outlet valves. A downward movement of the spring, compressing the air, would keep the outlet valve open, and during the upward movement of the spring the inlet valve remained open. When either of these valves was open, an electric circuit through a relay was broken, and this break caused an electric clock, *C*, to start and run until the relay circuit was made again by the cessation of the movement and the closure of the valves. With the clock set at zero (12 o'clock) at the time of going to bed, it was only necessary to read it next morning to find out how much time the sleeper spent in stirring during the night. The inertia of the clock was such that it continued to run for a fraction of a second after the current to it was cut off by the closure of the valves, and thus the amount of time was a trifle more than it should have been. For comparative purposes such a single-clock system would do; but, to get as close as possible to the true time values, we introduced another clock, *B*, which ran continuously, but which was stopped while the valves were open. Using clock *B*, one set it according to a third clock, *A*, which was in no way connected with the apparatus and was therefore uninfluenced by the movements of the bedspring; the time lost by clock *B* compared to clock *A* should have been the time spent in motility. With no inertia in the motors of the clocks, the figures obtained by the use of clocks *B* and *C* should have been the same; but, just as clock *C* furnished figures that were too high, the figures derived from clock *B* were too low. We calibrated the clocks by introducing a signal magnet into the circuit and recording the duration of the movements on a rapidly moving kymograph, with the time marked off in seconds. It was then possible to obtain factors by which the figures derived from clocks *B* and *C* were to be multiplied to give the time actually spent in movement. The greater the number of short-lasting movements, the greater was the difference between the figures furnished by the two clocks; and the employment of two clocks, instead of one, could thus be a source of additional information concerning the type of motility that prevailed during the night. When the clocks were used, no registration system of any kind was needed. The apparatus could be placed under the bed in one's own bedroom, and, if so desired, the clock or clocks might be kept in a distant room. The setting and reading of the clocks were the only manipulations required of the observer, and a source of alternating (regulated) current for the clocks was all that had to be provided for the working of the device. For most purposes, however, the double-clock system could be dispensed with, as the figures obtained by means of either clock were satisfactory if comparative rather than absolute values were sought.

To get the distribution of the movements through the night, in addition to the time spent in motility, a slow-moving kymograph could be set up in a distant room, the face of clock C provided with four contact points at the 15-, 30-, 45-, and 60-second marks, and each of these points connected with a source of current, a signal magnet, and the second-hand of the clock. Whenever 15 seconds of movement were run off, the second-hand completed the circuit with one of the contact points, and the signal magnet recorded it on the moving paper. We have used this device in connection with the clock system.

To compare the frequency with which our subjects stirred with the figures reported by others, we also used a mechanical registration system by means of which a Keith-Lucas lever recorded the actual displacements of the bedspring on kymograph paper. The record showed not only the frequency but also the amplitude of the displacements of the bedspring. The sum of all the recorded displacements gave an indication of the extent of motility during the night, but this sum could be obtained only with difficulty and with no accuracy by measuring and adding the individual lever strokes. To get this information with ease and accuracy, we made the string that led from the bedspring to the writing lever operate a Harvard "work-adder," provided with a revolution counter. Setting the counter at a certain figure before going to bed and reading it the next morning, one got the number of revolutions of the work-adder wheel, to a small fraction of a turn, and, knowing the length of one circumference of the wheel, it was easy to determine the sum-total of all the displacements. The work-adder device, the simplest and cheapest of all we have used, requires no energy to operate and should be very useful for comparative studies where the total motility is wanted rather than the distribution of movements.

When recording motility mechanically, we calibrated the writing-lever strokes in terms of the movements that produced them. As pointed out by other workers, it is impossible to tell from the records what the movements were, but in most cases we could distinguish major movements, owing to turning over or shifting of the entire body, from minor ones, produced by a movement of some part of the body.

We have records of a great many subjects of all ages, in most cases made for special purposes, but their normal or control values had certain trends in common. Rather than hours spent in motility, a typical sleeper would show a clock reading of 3 to 5 minutes, representing about 30 seconds of motility per hour; and that in the face of a total of 20 to 60 movements per night, which is well in accord with the figures given by Johnson for his typical sleepers. Our subjects did not "waste" time in moving—they took about 5 to 10 seconds to change from one position to another. Just how long, on occasion, the sleeper might be awake, if at all, before or after a movement we had no means of knowing, but we knew that he was lying quietly, even if awake, for all but 3 to 5 minutes of the time he remained in bed. Aware from our experience that when one is awake during the night one generally stirs a good deal, we felt certain that our subjects were asleep practically all the time they were at rest, and probably part of the time they "wasted" in movement. By comparison, Cathala and Guillard's figures (663, 1550) of a mean of 15 minutes of motility in 7 hours of sleep are entirely too high.

In our study, the ratio of major to minor movements varied from subject to subject, but was usually less than one. In other words, more than half of the movements were found to be minor. What was more significant, and appeared to be a fairly constant relationship, was the greater motility, whether measured by the clock or by mechanical recorder, during the second half of the night as compared to the first (Fig. 10.2; cf. Figs. 8.2 and 8.3), the ratios varying from

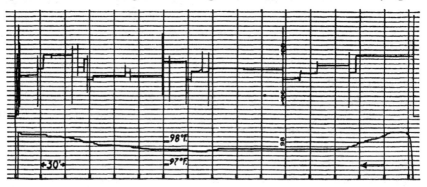

Fig. 10.2—Reduced reproduction of a record of motility during sleep (upper tracing) and of rectal temperature (lower tracing) of subject M. The signal-magnet record was omitted. Arrow indicates the direction of recording.

2:1 to 3:2. Likewise, Laird (2338), by the use of a "somnokinetograph," determined that the average person moves 10 to 12 times per hour, changing his position completely during 4 to 8 of these movements. He suggested (2340) that a gradual increase in movements per hour through the night, termed by him "crescendo sleep," is the normal sleep pattern, thus confirming our findings in this respect. So did Page (3075), on five normal subjects, whose movements for successive 3-hour periods of sleep averaged 12.8, 13.4, and 17.4. Maliniak (2640) employed a pneumatic system of recording her own movements during sleep. A statistical analysis of her figures showed a mean of 4.8 movements per hour, with the first hour least active and the last (sixth) most active. None of these findings are in accord with Johnson's data which indicated that the distribution of movements through the night is a personal characteristic of the sleeper.

Actograms of certain groups of sleepers, such as students (69, 70), pilot trainees (1379), and psychotics (2071), showed no marked deviations from the normal.

A number of conditions were observed to vary with, or affect, motility during sleep. Wada (4092) noted that body movements occurred simultaneously with hunger contractions of the stomach. Griffith (1516), working on college athletes, detected a decrease in the mean rest periods during sleep in the course of the football season, especially after hard and exhausting games. Maliniak (2640) stated that going to bed at an early hour decreased motility and that emotional shocks increased it. Fasting had a calming effect on the first night's sleep, but later on sleep was disturbed by it. Laird and Drexel (2344) studied motility during sleep after light and heavy meals. The former, cornflakes and milk, decreased motility, and the latter increased it. Laird (2339), in eight young men, found a parallelism between urinary bladder-pressure and motility. Greater than usual motility occurred on nights of high urinary output but manifested itself before the development of high bladder-pressure.

Krausse (2269) noted a relationship between the increase in the CO_2 percentage of the alveolar air and the infrequency of movement during sleep. Landis (2360) declared that "there is no correspondence between the frequency or amount of postural activity during the sleep period and the electrical changes of the body," but Titelbaum (3948) found a certain degree of parallelism between the two. Hellmuth and de Veer (1695) studied the influence of the difference between the temperature of the skin and that of the bed on motility in a number of healthy women. Usually there was a difference of 4°–5° C. between the two, but, if it narrowed down to 1° or less, there was an increase in motility. Jackson (1933, 1934) detected an anticipatory cardiac acceleration beginning about 6 minutes before a body movement and increasing rapidly just prior to the movement. In three out of twenty-five subjects McGlade (2753) recorded peculiar leg twitchings during sleep and found them synchronized with the relaxation of the pyloric sphincter.

Meyers and co-workers (2797), in a clinical study of a variety of hypnotics, reported no change in the pattern of sleep motility from these drugs, except in patients with congestive heart failure, in whom motility was increased.

The effect of coffee on motility was investigated by Stanley and Tescher (3780, 3781). The mean number of movements per hour of seven healthy men was 11.4. Taking hot water before going to bed reduced this number to 8.4, but coffee reduced it even more, to 8.1. A feature which made the control or "normal" motility figures unsatisfactory was that, instead of interspersing the "no-drink," water, and coffee nights, Stanley and Tescher ran a whole series of nights with each one. We (2943) avoided this arrangement when we studied the effects of alcohol and caffeine. Taking 300–375 ml of 19 per cent ethyl alcohol about an hour before going to bed, as compared to drinking an equal volume of water on other nights, had no effect on the total motility for the night but materially affected the distribution of the movements. The sleeper was quieter than usual during the first half of the night but more restless during the second. It will be recalled that the body temperature was lower than normal when the motility was lower, and vice versa. This relationship between the general temperature level and the incidence of motility is shown in Figure 8.3, where the effect of 260–400 mg of caffeine is also plotted. Unlike alcohol, caffeine raised the temperature level and motility rate throughout the night. Alcohol and caffeine are taken up here, rather than with the drugs, because they are materials commonly consumed, although it must be admitted that the doses were larger than one would usually ingest. The alcohol, roughly equivalent to two quarts of beer or a quart of light wine, was sufficient to create in most subjects a feeling of intoxication by the time they went to bed. The caffeine administered would be found in 3 cups of strong coffee. Needless to say, the subjects had no difficulty in falling asleep after alcohol but almost always after caffeine. As a control for caffeine, which was taken in capsule form, we had similar capsules filled with lactose, and both the caffeine and lactose capsules were dipped in sugar so that they tasted sweet. The subjects were told that they were given either all caffeine (400 mg), all lactose, or varying proportions of the two. In addition to objective data, they had to record on the following morning their subjective judgment on what they had taken, and how much. The "guesses" for caffeine were correct in about half of the cases, but in the other half they tended to be too high rather than too low.

In infants under ten days of age, Szymanski (3898) recorded from 5 to 6 activity periods occurring evenly by night and day. Irwin (1914, 1915), also observing neonates, found spontaneous motility 6 times greater in wakefulness than in sleep, and this motility increased markedly toward the end of the interfeeding period. Wagner (4094) prepared a catalogue of movements seen in newborn infants in relation to the depth of sleep (p. 9). Wolff (4266) found that the incidence of startle and of other types of movement during sleep in the newborn depended upon whether the sleep was "regular" or "irregular."

It will be recalled that Denisova and Figurin (914) established a 50-minute cycle of alternately slow and fast breathing during sleep in infants. When respiration was accelerated, there appeared a number of accessory phenomena, such as increased heart rate and movements of the body, hands, head, and eyelids. Micturition was also likely to occur during the hyperkinetic phase of the cycle. In our laboratory (150) a similar 50- to 60-minute periodicity of rest and activity was noted in infants. Kliorin (2212), in infants one to nine months of age, noted that periods of immobility tended to be longer (up to 30-40 minutes) the older the infant.

Sleep motility of hospitalized children two and a half to twelve and a half years old was studied by Karger (2080, 2081). During the first hour of sleep pronounced movements were executed, but not so during the remainder of the night. Karger also found that a child's sleep motility was related to his temperament. Lazy and bored children moved little; intelligent and lively ones showed more activity. After sleep had been interrupted, there usually followed a greater motility than was to be expected for that time of night.

Giddings (1434), by means of a "hypnograph," measured motility during sleep in twenty-eight children, nine to fourteen years of age, over a period of 364 nights, giving him a total of 4,717,440 "child-minutes" of sleep. Using the minute as the unit of motility time, instead of 5 minutes as Johnson did, he plotted the number of "active minutes" against each of the hours of the night. Except for the first hour, in which the large number of active minutes was due to the children's still being awake, there was a rise in motility with each successive hour. Girls were found to be sounder sleepers than boys. By the use of a "chronomotometer" Giddings (1438) determined the total time spent in motility by school children, nine to fourteen years of age, during 9 hours of sleep. The time amounted to less than 5 minutes—quite in accord with our findings with respect to sleep of adults (2181, 2193).

Garvey (1363), studying motility during the night sleep, found that his subjects, children two to five years old, moved once every 7.5 minutes on the average. He noted that, although they moved more frequently than adults, children remained still for an hour or more at a time, which adults seldom do.

Garvey (1364) also analyzed the distribution of sleep motility in twenty-two children of nursery-school age in an accumulation of 3,339 nights of sleep. There were distinct oscillations in curves of motility, with a wave length of 60 to 70 minutes. As Garvey put it, "the consistency of these fluctuations from one curve to another, both in number (and hence in mean length) and in variability of length, shows that they tend to be periodic for all the children. . . ." Gaul (1374), using time-lapse photography to record changes in position of a six-year-old boy, noted no distinct cycle of sleep motility—only that the subject moved more often during the second part of the night than during the first. Andreev (71) found that enuretics slept more quietly than did normal children.

A number of external and internal conditions may influence sleep motility in children. Karger (2081) noted that activity just before retiring, or listening to fairy tales, resulted in disturbed sleep. Putting a child accustomed to sleep alone in a room with other children increased his activity during sleep. Curiously enough, sleep was very quiet in fever. Renshaw and co-workers (3319, 3320) found that certain types of moving pictures led to disturbed sleep and increased motility in children six to eighteen years of age. Other moving pictures had a sedative effect. Ingesting 260–400 mg of caffeine between 6:00 P.M. and 9:00 P.M. had as great an effect in increasing motility as certain motion pictures. Giddings (1434), however, obtained no greater effect on sleep motility in children from drinking a beverage containing 200 mg of caffeine than from taking an equal quantity of orange juice. Eating a large amount of food at the evening meal markedly increased motility, but hot or cold baths had no effect. Nor did an hour of study or exercise before going to bed (1435). Emotional states (fear, worry, disappointment, or pleasant anticipation) interfered with quiet sleep (1437).

A lesser motility during daytime naps compared to night sleep was revealed by the results of Marquis (2689) obtained on infants under one year of age. Such infants, in general, moved more frequently than older children and adults but showed less variation from day to day. Boynton and Goodenough (437) reported an average of one change of posture in 25 minutes during naps of a mean length of 79 minutes in twenty-six nursery-school children. Wang (4114) noted that kindergarten children spent over twice as much time in motility during the naps in the summer than in the winter.

De Toni (3956) studied movements of the eyes during sleep in 214 children, three to twelve years of age. The movements were either observed through illuminated eyelids, or, if the latter were not transparent enough, by lifting them. Sleep had to be light for the movements to appear. In the majority of children the eyeballs moved from side to side, in a pendular fashion, 4 to 6 times per minute.

Efimov and Demidov (1043), by applying electrodes to the eyelids of dogs, were able to record the rate of blinking. There was a marked decrease in blinking during sleep. However, Lawson (2384), on the basis of direct observation, noted a complete abolition of blinking with the onset of sleep. Andreev and Ivanov (68, 73), using an electrical recording system, confirmed the existence of slow pendular movements of the eyes during sleep, but maintained that they were related to its onset and termination. In our laboratory (149) slow eye movements were found to be associated not only with the onset of sleep but also with overt body movements during sleep. In addition, binocularly synchronous, jerky movements of the eyes appeared periodically in clusters and seemed to accompany certain types of dreaming (Chapter 11).

The general topic of bodily and eye motility will also be discussed in connection with the depth and duration of sleep, but the material presented in this chapter proves that no normal person sleeps "like a log." On the contrary, he changes positions of the body many times during one night's sleep, though "wasting" no more than 3 to 5 minutes of rest in doing so. One is certainly not justified in judging the quality of sleep entirely or mainly on the basis of how many movements per hour or per night the sleeper made. Although an individual has his own range of motility, that range is wide enough to permit a considerable variation, without his even suspecting it. As shown in a survey (2200), many subjects moved 50 per cent more during certain seasons than they did during others and did not know it. Also, if a certain procedure is found to cut the total time of movement from 5 down to 4 minutes, it cannot be said to improve the quality of sleep or to make it less restless (or more restful), because fewer changes in position, as after alcohol, are not a desirable modification of the normal sleep pattern. Extreme increases or decreases in motility are definitely deleterious, but the definition of "extreme" will vary from person to person and, probably in the same individual, from time to time.

As Johnson and co-workers (2003) have shown by their motion-picture studies, each sleeper has his own repertoire of favorite positions, some mirror images of each other; he alternately, though not in any order, assumes these acceptable positions. Alcohol that temporarily benumbs one's sensations causes a decrease in the frequency of movement, but the resulting discomfort increases motility during the latter part of the night. If the intoxication is too deep to lighten in the course of the night, one wakes up with a "charley horse," a sensation of stiffness and discomfort. Likewise, temporary paralysis may result when a person for one reason or another does not change his position often enough and happens to lie in such a way as to produce a continuous pressure on certain nerves.

By themselves, the motility findings merely suggest that a normal person is not entirely oblivious to the feeling of discomfort from lying too long in one position, even in sleep. However, the cyclical occurrence of activity during sleep, starting with the 50- to 60-minute periodicity in the infant (150, 914), and passing through a 60- to 70-minute one in the preschool child (1364) to the 85- to 90-minute cycle in the adult (902, 1999), points to a hitherto unrecognized time dimension in sleep, not related to a gastric hunger periodicity nor to the alternation of night and day.

Chapter 11

Dreaming

Until about ten years ago, practically all the information on dreaming was derived from the subjective experiences and reports of the dreamers. The latter decided whether or not they had dreamed, and, if they had, related the contents of their dreams. With respect to other events during sleep, one could use objective facts as a check upon the subjective impressions of the sleeper. When a person reported that he had been tossing and turning throughout the night, he could be confronted with his motility records which showed that, out of 7 hours and 45 minutes he spent in bed, he "tossed" for exactly 4 minutes and 12 seconds. As for dreams, the facts themselves are subjective. Their detection, recall, and description depend upon the introspection, memory, and, perhaps, vividness of the imagination of the sleeper. That is why the study of dreams is an ancient lore, and, whereas astrology had long ago given way to astronomy, concerning dream knowledge and understanding moderns were not much further advanced than the ancients. In fact, astrology, fortune-telling, crystal-gazing, and dream interpretation are often practiced today by the same individual.

Older data on dreaming had been gained by the intensive method, involving the recording of many successive dreams by a person, who dreamed frequently, had become intellectually curious about the process, and was temperamentally fit for this type of diary-keeping; or by the extensive method, entailing essentially the application of the questionnaire technique and statistics to the dreaming experience of large groups of people. The information obtained by these two methods is still valid, provided one substitutes "recalled having dreamed" for "dreaming"—something which is inherent in the subjective nature of the report, but was often overlooked. What was needed, however, was a method of objectively recording incidence and duration of dreaming, without, if possible, disrupting the continuity of sleep.

In our laboratory we literally stumbled on an objective method of studying dreaming while exploring eye motility in adults, after we found that in infants eye movements persisted for a time when all discernible body motility ceased (150). Instead of direct inspection, as was done for infant eye movements, those of adult sleepers were recorded indirectly, to insure undisturbed sleep in the dark. By leads from two skin spots straddling the eye to an EEG machine, located in an adjacent room, it was possible to register potential differences whenever the eye moved in its socket. The many investigators who have used this method (260, 472, 515, 1935, 2281, 2282, 2423, 2910, 3238, 3669) generally agree that variations in the corneo-retinal potentials, rather than muscle

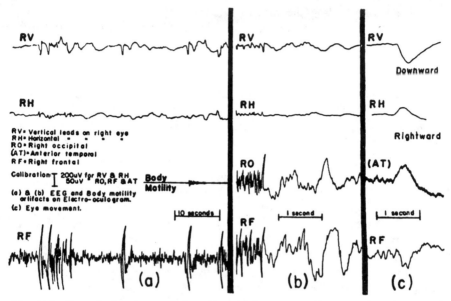

Fig. 11.1—Records showing typical artifacts and an eye movement on an electro-oculogram. Parts (*a*) and (*b*), EEG and body movement artifacts on right vertical (RV) and right horizontal (RH) electro-oculograms; part (*c*), a voluntary movement of the right eye in an oblique direction, with the eyes closed. EEG leads: right occipital (RO), right frontal (RF), and anterior temporal (AT).

action currents, are recorded by this method, but, in any case, it is a faithful indicator of the rotation of the eyeball involved in a movement. By this technique, pendular, often bilaterally asymmetrical, slow eye movements (SEMs), each completed in 3 to 4 seconds, were found to be related to general body motility. In addition, jerky rapid eye movements (REMs) (Fig. 11.1), executed in only a fraction of a second and binocularly symmetrical, tended to occur in clusters for 5 to 60 minutes several times during a single night's sleep (148, 149). In order to correlate the REMs with other concomitants, simultaneous recordings were made of changes in the sleepers' EEG, pulse, and respiration. It was soon apparent that the REMs were associated with a typical low-voltage EEG pattern and statistically significant increases in the heart and respiratory rates (about 10 per cent and 20 per cent, respectively), though occasionally the pulse was slowed. These changes suggested some sort of emotional disturbance, such as might be caused by dreaming. To test this supposition, sleepers were aroused and interrogated during, or shortly after the termination of, REMs, and they almost invariably reported having dreamed. If awakened in the absence of REMs, or when questioned after a night of undisturbed sleep, they seldom recalled dreaming.

As is usually the case, the finding of an association of eye movements with dreaming was not altogether new. Indeed in 1892, Ladd (2320), a professor of mental and moral philosophy at Yale University, through pure introspection, was able to distinguish between the fixed positions of his eyes in deep, presumably dreamless sleep, and their motility during dreaming, cautiously stating that he was "inclined also to believe that, in somewhat vivid visual dreams, the eyeballs move gently in their sockets, taking various positions. . . ." Ladd surmised that "in a dream we probably focus our eyes somewhat as we should do in making the same observation when awake." It is strange that neither Ladd himself nor those who read of his speculations undertook to observe the face of a sleeping person long enough to notice the relatively frequent series of eye movements. Many years thereafter, Jacobson, having noted that eye movements occurred during visual recollection (1935), also observed them during dreaming. In his own words (1937), "When a person dreams . . . most often his eyes are active. Watch the sleeper whose eyes move under his closed lids. . . . Awaken him . . . you are likely to find . . . that he had seen something in a dream." In our subjects, only after the REMs were recorded indirectly were they observed by direct inspection of the sleeper, when his closed eyelids were illuminated by a weak light. Gradual increase in the intensity of the light shining on the eyelids permitted even the taking of motion pictures of the REMs.

Concerning the brain-potential concomitant, it may be stated that dreaming occurs preponderately in stage 1 EEG (p. 26), and then only when it is ascending from stage 2 EEG (901). In the initial stage 1 EEG, descending from the frank wakefulness alpha EEG, there is no dreaming, and REMs are regularly absent. So-called hypnagogic hallucinations are not accepted as "real" and thus are distinguished from dreaming. Furthermore, although the record of the initial stage 1 EEG does not differ from those of the recurring emergent stage 1 EEGs, the auditory thresholds during the latter are greatly elevated. In ten subjects tested, the threshold intensity of a tone of 1,000/second, sounded for 10 seconds and measured by the voltage fed into a loud-speaker, varied from 0.1–0.4 v in the initial stage 1 EEG, but was up to 1.0–1.8 v in emergent stage 1 EEG. By some classifications, a typical stage 1 EEG would be considered as indicative of drowsiness, rather than sleep, or of a transitional state—

between wakefulness and sleep. That may perhaps apply to the initial stage 1 EEG, but the emergent ones are connected not only with behaviorally definite sleep, but also with fairly deep sleep, when judged by auditory thresholds.

Attempts to connect a particular EEG stage of sleep with dreaming are also not entirely recent. In the first edition of this book I suggested that perhaps the EEG method would furnish patterns characteristic of dreaming, but up to that time there was only the statement of the Loomis group that dreaming might be associated with their sleep state *B* (2560). Later, when it was decided by them that "real sleep" might not come on until state *C* (841), dreaming was said to occur in the latter sleep state. In addition, in our laboratory (366), when subjects were awakened during different EEG stages and questioned about dreaming, it was established that the presence of delta waves in the EEG was associated with dreamless sleep. Teplitz (3915) reported that dreaming might occur in connection with any EEG pattern. Among the pre-REM-EEG findings, there are also the isolated statement made by El-Maziny (1071), in a review article, that dreams are associated with a burst of alpha waves in the second stage of the transition from wakefulness to sleep, thus placing their incidence in the initial stage 1 EEG; and a notation on an EEG tracing in a figure in a paper by O'Connor (3038), reading: "spindle" (dream?).

Of the two principal concomitants of dreaming, emergent stage 1 EEG is more significant, as dreaming may occur without REMs. It seems that the presence of REMs is connected with the "eventfulness" of the dream story. If, as one thought, REMs represented scanning movements of the eyes as they followed lively happenings in the dream, relatively "uneventful" dreams would require little or no scanning. An analysis of 105 dream situations, of which 58 related to eventful and 47 to uneventful dreams, showed that the former entailed many more REMs than the latter (904). It is also in keeping with the supposition of scanning that vertical REMs, though much less common than horizontal ones, when they did occur, were associated with looking up and down during the dream, such as watching a blimp dropping leaflets. The amount of ocular activity was also related to the involvement of the dreamer himself in the dream drama. Active dreaming, in which sleeper was actor and spectator, entailed more eye and hand motility than did passive dreaming, in which the sleeper was only a spectator.

General body motility was lessened during REMs, but occasional gross body movements did occur. To test the possibility that such movements might mark the end of one dream episode and the beginning of another, transcriptions of 46 dream narratives of related, continuously progressing events were compared with 31 dream narratives containing two or more distinct and apparently unconnected events. In 46 continuous dreams there were 32 without any body movements, while out of 31 fragmented ones, 21 were accompanied by considerable body motility (904).

Facial movements and occasional vocalization occurred during REMs. Recordings of muscle potentials indicated that isolated movements of the wrist were made with greater frequency during dreaming than at other times, and that there was a relation between such movements and the content of the reported dream. For example, the right hand, left hand, and a foot executed movements in the order named, and the subject, when awakened immediately thereafter, reported that he lifted a bucket with his right hand, supported it with his left, and then started to walk away. Wolpert (4268), who made these observations, also reported that gross body movements, in addition to indicating a transition from one dream story to another, were at times, like the isolated limb movements, appropriate to the dream content. However, there were marked individual differences among the subjects with respect to the frequency with which gross body movements or those of individual extremities accompanied dreaming.

The usual failure of the sleeper to translate his hallucinatory dream activity into overt action may be related to the functional conduction blocks associated with sleep. After Hyde and Gellhorn (1885) produced deafferentation in cats, under dial-urethane anesthesia, by ligation of appropriate dorsal roots of the spinal cord, "even maximal cortical stimulation never induced the degree of tension nor the amplitude in control conditions." The positive Babinski sign in sleep and the observations of Gibbs and Gibbs (1419) that grand mal EEG patterns appearing during sleep do not lead to overt convulsive seizures also point to a functional conduction block.

A representative night's sleep, as revealed by composite data from thirty-three subjects (twenty-six men, seven women) ranging in age from eighteen to sixty-one years (mostly twenty to thirty), and comprising 71 nights, showed a regular succession of 4 or 5 cycles of EEG variations (Fig. 11.2). The length of the cycles was 70 to 90 minutes, with the amplitude greatest in the first cycle and progressively diminishing for the remainder of the night (901). In some subjects stage 4 EEG was present only in the first cycle (or first and second); and in the first upswing the emergent stage 1 EEG appeared only for a few minutes, or was absent altogether. The succeeding cycles were more alike, involving a descent only to stage 2 EEG (or 3), and a much longer stretch of stage 1 EEG, usually 20 to 30 minutes. REMs were generally coextensive with stage 1 EEG, and, because of the brevity of the first emergent stage 1 EEG, both it and the REMs could be missed if recording were done intermittently instead of continuously. For this reason, earlier reports placed the first REM period at about 3 hours after the onset of sleep (149). Also, when the incidence of REMs in four subjects (12 to 16 nights for each) was plotted, it was noticed that two of the subjects showed a marked regularity of pattern from night to night, whereas the other two were less regular (Fig. 11.3). There was a certain consistency, however, in the records of every subject with respect to both incidence and duration of REMs. One sleeper was unique in that REMs never appeared in the first upswing of the EEG, which also never emerged above stage 2.

The continuous recording of EEG variations and incidence of REMs furnished data for the pattern of a typical night's sleep, but it was the intentional awakenings of the subjects during, after, and in between REM periods that

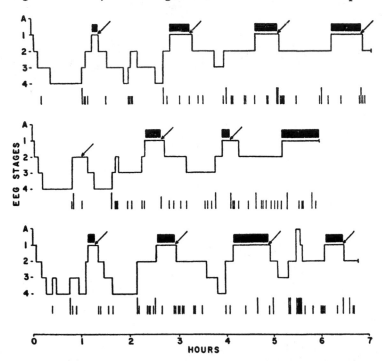

Fig. 11.2—Continuous plotting of EEG patterns for three representative nights. The thick bars above the EEG lines indicate periods of REMs coinciding with emergent stage 1 EEGs. The longer vertical lines at the bottom of each record indicate major body movements (changes in position); the shorter ones, minor movements. The arrows mark the successive EEG pattern cycles (901).

made it possible to apply this method to the elucidation of the nature of the dreaming process. Did the artificial interruptions of the continuity of sleep affect the course of events? They probably tended to shorten the interval between successive REM periods. One subject, in 13 nights of undisturbed sleep, had a mean REM cycle of 110 minutes, but in another 11 nights, with repeated awakenings, REMs recurred, on the average, every 70 minutes. When the subjects were aroused during REMs, the latter, as a rule, did not recur immediately upon the re-onset of sleep, especially if the sleepers were fully awakened and had to describe a dream experience. Awakenings during ocular quiescence did not affect the time of the beginning of the next REM period (901).

The general character of the cyclical variations in EEG pattern during a night's sleep was confirmed by many investigators who employed the REM-EEG method (109, 302, 303, 876, 1254, 1479, 1669, 2069, 2277, 2756, 3190, 3559, 3623, 3840, 3985, 4075, 4197, 4198, 4268, 4269), though not by all (663, 1550). Of course, as data were accumulated, individual peculiarities and deviations from the general rule were reported. Kamiya (2069), in an analysis

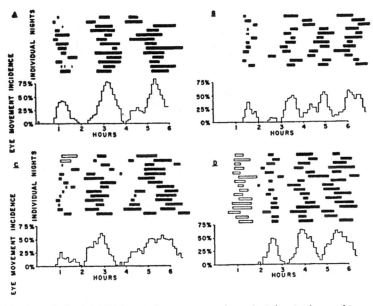

Fig. 11.3—Regularity of REM periods over a number of nights in four subjects (A–D). Each bar represents a single REM period; each row of bars, a single night. The open bars in the diagrams for subjects C and D indicate an absence of REMs, with the peak of the first EEG cycle represented by stage 2 EEG. Composite histograms of REM incidence for the several nights' sleep of each subject, placed under the series of bars, show the greater regularity of REM cycling in subjects A and D than in subjects B and C (901).

of the records of nearly 300 nights of sleep of thirty subjects, noted that, in some cases, the general body motility level during REMs was not much lower than in the periods before and after. However, many REM periods began and ended with a gross body movement. Dream recall was more frequent when the REMs were accompanied by a large increase in the heart rate than when the pulse acceleration was small. Furthermore, many reports of dreaming were elicited from subjects awakened during stages 2, 3, and even 4 EEG, and there seemed to be a marked individual variation in that respect. Kamiya challenged the separation of SEMs and REMs, stating that "SEMs often build up in magnitude and speed . . . into REMs. Also SEMs do not cease upon the onset of REMs. On the contrary the REM period is really a period of heightened SEM as well as REM."

Recall of dreaming was not universally associated with stage 1 EEG; and even less so with REMs. Out of 191 awakenings of nine sleepers during REMs, 152 reports of dreaming were elicited, and out of 160 awakenings of the same subjects in non-REM periods, only 11 recalls of dreaming were obtained (902). Foulkes (1254), however, while getting reports of mental activity in 88 per cent of awakenings during REMs, also noted recalls of such activity in 74 per cent of awakenings in non-REM periods. Foulkes observed that "reports obtained in periods of REM activity showed more organismic involvement in affective, visual, and muscular dimensions than non-REM reports. REM period reports showed less correspondence to waking life of the subject than did reports from spindle and delta sleep. The relatively frequent occurrence of thinking and memory processes in spindle and delta sleep was an especially striking result." Thus, although one depends upon the sleeper's statements in tabulating the data, the decision of whether "dreaming" or "thinking" took place must sometimes be made by the experimenter, on the basis of the structure and content of the report. Similarly, when a subject, definitely asleep by behavioral and instrumental criteria, reports, upon being awakened, that he had not been asleep (1479), his declaration cannot be taken at face value. The same, of course, applies to the statements of many subjects that they never or seldom dream. More properly, they are persons who do not recollect having dreamed, as it may be considered as established that all normal children beyond a certain age and all normal adults dream every night.

The earlier observational and statistical data will be discussed alongside those obtained by the objective REM-EEG method, and agreements and contradictions in the results evaluated. Many historical accounts (415, 416, 2744) and reviews (125, 126, 420, 931, 1166, 1177, 1316, 1488, 1571, 1575, 1657, 1827, 1994, 2102, 2128, 2433, 2491, 2643, 2790, 2801, 2922, 2929–31, 2934, 3001, 3058, 3263, 3334, 3351, 3728, 3865, 4041, 4243, 4245, 4273, 4275) contain no original findings, though replete with discussions.

The frequency of dreaming, expressed as the percentage of nights after which dreaming is recalled, determined by the questionnaire method, and classified by age, sex, and occupation (75, 700, 730, 1604, 2200, 2643, 2807, 2808) is only of academic interest, except that it brings out differences between "re-callers" and "non-recallers." Goodenough and associates (1479) found that "eye movement periods occurred as frequently for nondreamers as for dreamers," but there were significant differences between the two groups in the EEG patterns that prevailed during REMs. In non-dreamers the EEGs were indicative of somewhat shallower sleep. When sleep was interrupted, positive reports of dreaming were made more often by dreamers than by non-dreamers, both during REMs (93 per cent compared to 46 per cent) and in periods free from REMs (53 per cent compared to 17 per cent). Similar results were obtained by Antrobus (109), who also found that the REMs collectively ran for 105 minutes per night (23.7 per cent) for recallers and 82 minutes (18.9 per cent) for non-recallers, with the 23-minute difference statistically significant. The inability of many persons to recall having dreamed, after getting up in the morning, is not surprising, for the memory traces of dreaming are evanescent, as shown by Wolpert and Trosman (4269). Recall of dreaming was best when their subjects were awakened during REMs; it was poorer the longer the interval after the cessation of the REMs. Thus, detailed recall was elicited in 46 out of 54 awakenings during REMs; only fragmented recall in 9 out of 11 within 5 minutes after REMs stopped; and there was complete forgetfulness in 25 out of 26 cases after 10 or more minutes of stage 2 EEG, following stage 1 EEG and REMs. Furthermore, details of dream content were reported more fully when sleep was interrupted while a gross body movement occurred during an REM period.

The incidence of dreaming in the course of a night's sleep is placed by some writers at the beginning and end of sleep (317, 349, 3470), by others only early (1234), or only late (3315), or even continuously (1852), or "every minute of the night" (3561). Bentley (297), who determined that dreaming occurred mainly after the second hour of sleep, came closest to the findings made by the REM-EEG method.

It was generally held that dreaming occurs only in shallow sleep and that deep sleep is dreamless (2933, 3230). Opinions were also expressed that certain dreams are associated with deep sleep (3273), or that dreaming takes place in every stage of sleep (921, 3366, 3915), but recall of dreaming is limited to awakenings from light sleep. Mayorov (2730) drew a depth-of-sleep curve with several evenly spaced shallowings related to dreaming, except that he also placed dreaming at the beginning of the night's sleep, which does not conform to the data obtained by the REM-EEG technique.

That time is greatly compressed during dreaming is a notion that was probably sparked by the famous dream of Maury, who was awakened when a piece of board fell on his neck and later told of a long succession of dream events that led up to his being guillotined. The veracity of this account was challenged by Clavière (719) in 1897, but this did not prevent later writers from suggesting that dreams occurred in a very short time (4110, 4274), down to a few minutes (644, 1568, 1604, 1765), even a few seconds (396, 1611, 2173, 2414, 2718). All the guesses fell far short of the mark. Using the REM-EEG method, dreamers were asked to give a subjective estimate of the duration of the dream episode. In order not to impose too great a task on the subjects, they were told that they would be aroused either 5 or 15 minutes after the beginning of the REMs. Five subjects thus tested gave correct estimates in 45 out of 51 trials, after 5 minutes of REMs, and in 47 cases out of 60, after 15 minutes of REMs (902). When the sleepers were awakened at the end of an REM period that lasted 30 to 60 minutes, the dream narratives were no longer than those told after 15 minutes of REMs (904). In a group of 45 awakenings, dream narratives after 10 to 20 minutes of REMs were as short as those usually reported after 4 to 5 minutes of REMs. In 37 out of these 45 cases a gross body movement was made during the REM period, suggesting that the dream episode was perhaps "fragmented" and that only the terminal fragment had been recalled. Thus, events in a dream seem to run their course at a rate comparable to a real experience of the same time.

Dream contents have been studied in connection with the setting, events, and type of activity recalled, with respect to sex and personality of the dreamer. The dreamer is often aware of the fact that he is asleep and dreaming (534, 2857). The elements that enter into the dream events were analyzed by Hall (1605–11), on the basis of 10,000 dream narratives. Other reports pertain to story (297, 1048, 1049, 1315, 3273, 3366, 4119) or the personality of the dreamer (318, 1053, 2650, 2762, 3590). Still others deal with falling (1638, 1646), flying (3569), levitation (1808, 1838–40), eating (1618), laughter (1538), anxiety (1645), speech (1918), sense of time (1526), hearing atonal sounds (3194), absurdity (676), and sex differences in topics dreamed about (895, 1878, 3905). The Isakower phenomenon—images of amorphous whitish masses—and the "dream screen" have also been the topics of dream research (1361, 1680, 2470–74, 3483). None of these reported contents has the freshness and immediacy of the accounts obtained by the REM-EEG method, especially when narratives of a series of dreams occurring during one night are compared with each other for relatedness or homology of content. Dream stories elicited by Dement and Wolpert (903) from eight subjects for thirty-eight nights showed a common theme running through only seven single-night dream sequences. However, common elements were often incorporated in contiguous dream episodes, occasionally in three; or there might be one item in the first and second, another in the second and third, and still another in all three. This relatedness of dream plots, when present, may be (*a*) the natural pattern, (*b*) augmented by the "unfulfillment" of the dream, resulting from the necessary awakening, (*c*) diminished by the disruption of the continuity and homogeneity created by the awakening, or (*d*) actually initiated by the effect the recital of the dream content had upon successive interruptions of sleep. Further, Trosman and associates (3985) noted the presence of specific common elements in dreams in sequence, with a positive interrelationship among spatial expanse, excitation, activity, interpersonal involvement, and elaboration, and a negative interrelationship among plausibility and a number of other dimensions.

The majority of dream events are visual in character, and the question of seeing objects in color has been answered in the negative (3360), or as a restriction to exciting red hues and calming blue ones (3909), through distinct vision in all natural colors for a fraction of the population, from time to time (606, 2216, 2534, 2808), more often by women than by men (1609), and by neurotics compared to control subjects (3905). From letters received from persons who read about the non-universality of dreaming in color, it is clear that those who deal with colors in their everyday activities (painters, fashion designers) usually dream in colors. One dreams as one thinks.

Several reports have dealt with the dreams of blind persons (369, 396, 925, 1891, 2156, 4185). The dream imagery of the congenitally blind, and of those who lost their sight before the age of five years, is mainly auditory, with some other modalities also present. Schumann (3610–13), who followed the dream of the blind through "rites, myths, legends, fairy tales and folklore," likened the dreams of the blind to the dreams of isolated individuals living in Spitzbergen during the polar season of darkness. Berger and co-workers (303), using the REM-EEG method, found that three persons with lifelong blindness had no REMs during sleep, whereas two subjects, blind ten and three years, respectively, who still had visual imagery, did have REMs. This finding is another indication of the scanning nature of REMs.

Deaf persons used sign language for communication in their dreams, but reported the visual scenes as brilliantly colored (2769). As with the blind, the peculiarities of the dreams are less marked in individuals who became deaf at or after the age of five years.

The age at which dreaming is evident in human beings has been variously given as less than 12 (1860), 13 (1099), 17 (3002), 28 (1536), 36 (368) and 45 months (4231). The question has been asked whether children, old enough to speak, recollect or invent the dream stories they tell (1159). In reviews of the literature (897, 923) the contents of children's dreams are shown to be related to age, giving expression first to anxiety and later to aggression. Delange and associates (876) recorded REMs in children four years old but did not try to determine their association with dreaming. Nor did they mention any concurrent cardiac acceleration. It is probable that the combination of REMs, stage 1 EEG, and an increase in heart rate will establish the age at which dreaming begins.

Barad and co-authors (201) collected dream accounts from residents of a home for the aged and noted that "the majority of dreams reported revealed that the subjects conceived of themselves as diminished in resources and consequently weak, relatively helpless, and vulnerable."

There are enough observations on animals to indicate that some of them, particularly the dog, dream during sleep. Krieger and co-workers (2279) observed spontaneous eye movements in monkeys in sleep and anesthesia, and Weitzmann (4157) recorded an LVFA EEG in monkeys in association with REMs, which totaled 89 minutes in 8 hours (16 per cent) of natural sleep, a fraction comparable to that found in human sleep. Whether the cortical activation sleep of the cat first described by Dement (899) is connected with dreaming (1505) is doubtful, for Jouvet's corresponding "paradoxical phase" (p. 212) is generally accompanied by a decrease in the heart rate. The combination of REM, LVFA EEG, and cardiac acceleration should be achieved in animals, as in children, before dreaming may be said to occur.

Several investigators studied dreaming and dream contents in a variety of pathological states. Saul and associates (3528) reported a greater hostility in the dreams of hypertensives than in those of normotensives. Feeble-minded children and adults had rather simple dreams, which they were inclined to forget (896, 4107). Dreams of schizophrenics did not deviate from normal (2074, 3016); the only unusual feature, as noted by Dement (898), was a tendency to report dreaming of "isolated objects apparently hanging in space, with no movement." A narcoleptic, studied by Vogel (4075), began to dream immediately after falling asleep. Pierce and associates (3190), in enuretic boys, found that the first bed-wetting occurred at the time when the initial dreaming period was to be expected, thus representing a dream substitute (p. 284).

Brain damage is often followed by a cessation of dreaming, particularly if it also interferes with, or abolishes, vision (1461, 1869, 3005). Pre-frontal leucotomy entails a cessation of dreaming, lasting from a few months to two years (3099, 3181, 3562).

That dreams may be of diagnostic and therapeutic significance was recognized by Hildebrandt in 1881, antedating Freud (1289) and others (18, 202, 237, 363, 1288, 1561, 1895, 2583, 3449, 3608) in this respect. The manner in which the patient may modify his account of a dream between the time he first recalled it and his visit to the psychoanalyst was tested by Whitman and co-workers (4197), who utilized the REM-EEG technique for that purpose. Two patients, awakened once or twice per night during a dreaming period, reported the dream contents to an experimenter and in a subsequent interview to their psychiatrist. It was established that certain dreams were told the experimenter and not the psychiatrist, but there were also dreams that were "recalled" for the psychiatrist but not reported to the laboratory observer. Finally, there were major changes and deletions in the delayed retelling of particular dreams. Dreams containing an element which the dreamer expected to bring forth a negative response from the analyst were not retold. By comparing the immediate report with the delayed one, valuable diagnostic information was obtained.

Dream contents have been reported to be affected by events in the individual's life (178), in some cases, happenings during the preceding day—"day residue" (2551, 4117)—even by activities that were interrupted and left uncompleted (397). For those who accept mental telepathy, there are anecdotal stories of dreams affected by the day impressions of other persons (817). On more solid grounds are the effects of subliminal perception, the incorporation of elements of indirectly seen pictures into visual dreams, first described by Poetzl (3219), and confirmed by Fisher and others (1192–96, 2571, 2637, 3679). The incorporation of conscious wishes into the dream events has also been noted (1265, 1360). Stoyva (3840) was able to obtain dream accounts from subjects awakened during REM and stage 1 EEG, "that clearly were in accordance with the dreams suggested by the experimenter during hypnosis." Among unexpected findings by Stoyva were (*a*) a reduction in REM time on experimental nights as compared to nights when no posthypnotic dream suggestion had been operating, and (*b*) a tendency of some subjects to dream on the suggested topic in every dream of the night. Schiff and co-workers (3559), by suggesting during hypnosis a dream-topic requiring much scanning activity, succeeded in obtaining more REMs than when they suggested that the subject look at a still object. They also noticed that the EEG in posthypnotic dreaming was closer to the waking EEG than that of spontaneous dreaming.

Concerning the immediate cause of dreaming, opinions have been expressed that external stimuli are (275) or are not able (3925) to initiate dreaming, but the regularity of repetitive occurrence of dreaming as demonstrated by the REM-EEG method indicates that no external stimulus is needed to start a dreaming episode, though there is a great deal of material accumulated to show that external stimuli may affect the events in a dream (275, 2086, 3925). In our laboratory (904), the effects of external stimuli during REMs were studied in twelve subjects. If the stimulus itself did not arouse the sleeper, he was awakened one minute later. A pure tone of 1,000 cycles/sec, of subliminal intensity, produced an incorporation of the sound into the dream story in only 3 out of 35 trials. Shining a light from a 100-watt lamp into the subject's face never led to awakening, but subsequent arousal revealed a "light" event in the recalled dream in 7 out of 30 instances. A most effective stimulus in that respect was a spray from a hypodermic needle, or simply large drops of cold water falling on the exposed skin of the sleeper. On thirty-three occasions when the spray did not awaken the subjects, falling water was reported in fourteen dream narratives; and on fifteen others that did lead to arousal, the water element was incorporated in six. During ocular quiescence, application of these stimuli initiated no REMs or reports of dreaming upon subsequent arousal. One special stimulus—an electric bell sounded to awaken the subjects—found its way into the dream report in 20 out of 204 routine applications, most commonly as the ringing of a doorbell or telephone. Lengthening the interval between the introduction of the external stimulus and the interruption of sleep furnished information on the course of time in dreaming. "In each of 10 instances, where the stimulus was incorporated and the subsequent interval was precisely timed, the amount of dream action in the interval between the modifying stimulus and the awakening did not vary far from the amount of action that would have been expected to take place during an identical time in reality."

The possibility of internal stimuli causing or affecting the dream contents has been mentioned by several authors (1838–40, 2753, 3484). The effect of thirst, developed by withholding liquid intake for 24 hours, was tested by Dement and Wolpert (904). In none of the fifteen dream narratives obtained from three subjects was there a direct reference to thirst, but in five of them there were elements indirectly related to drinks.

Hormonal imbalance may have an effect on the character of dreams. Finley (1172) reported that a patient experienced pleasant dreams during a 10-day period when she was given pituitary material daily, but in a similar period of adrenal extract administration her dreams were unpleasant. Another account (2771) referred to a patient who had been repeatedly dreaming during her menstrual periods that she was insane, but with menopause these dreams stopped. The effects of drugs were studied by Whitman and associates (4198), using the REM-EEG method to obtain dream narratives from ten volunteer subjects in forty nights of testing. Imipramine led to a decrease in the number of dreams and to an increase in the expression of hostility in the dream narrative. Prochlorperazine produced a greater expression of heterosexuality, and phenobarbital, of homosexuality, in dreams.

The REM-EEG method yielded a number of findings that were not expected from previous studies. The cardiac and respiratory acceleration, as well as the stage 1 EEG, that accompanied REMs indicated a shallowing of sleep and increased body motility. Actually just the opposite happened. Indeed, Georg Mann of the Office of Public Relations of the University of Chicago, in preparing a press release on the research on dreaming, compared the dreamer to a spectator in a theater: fidgeting in his seat before the curtain goes up; then sitting quietly, often "spellbound" by the action, as he follows with his eyes the movements of the actors on the stage; then, after the curtain falls, beginning to stir again. Another unanticipated finding was made by Hawkins and associates (1669), who noted a rise in ESR during dreaming. Perhaps the most striking unexpected observation was the increase in dreaming during the sleep that followed a period of prolonged wakefulness, a sleep that was thought to be very deep. Sleep deprivation, of course, also means a lack of opportunity to dream, and the occasional dream-like behavior of sleep-deprived individuals (p. 221) could possibly be an effort to "catch up" on dreaming. To test the need for dreaming, Dement (900), by arousing sleepers, cut short dreaming episodes as soon as they could be definitely recognized, thus curtailing the time usually spent in dreaming by an estimated 65 to 75 per cent. In eight young male subjects, a total of forty undisturbed nights of sleep showed a mean of about 20 per cent of dreaming (82 minutes of dreaming for a little over 7 hours of sleep). These were designated by Dement as base-line nights. After 3 to 7 consecutive nights of dream curtailment—necessitating, incidentally, night after night, a markedly progressive increase of 40 per cent to over 300 per cent in the number of experimental awakenings—five subjects dreamed a mean of 112 minutes, or 27 per cent of the total mean sleep time, during the first "recovery" night. Increased dreaming, though less marked, was also present in succeeding "recovery" nights. That sleep interruption as such was not responsible for the increase in dreaming time was demonstrated by awakening six of the subjects during non-dreaming periods, but otherwise duplicating exactly, for each subject, the number and distribution of awakenings he underwent during the dream-curtailment nights. No increase in dreaming was evident during the sham "recovery" nights. It should be added that anxiety, irritability, and an increase in appetite were produced in the experimental subjects when their dreaming was curtailed but not when they were aroused during dreamless stretches of sleep. Dement tentatively interpreted his striking findings "as indicating that a certain amount of dreaming each night is a necessity. It is as though a pressure to dream builds up with the accruing dream deficit during successive dream-deprivation nights—a pressure which is first evident in the increasing frequency of attempts to dream and then, during the recovery period, in the marked increase in total dream time and percentage of dream time."

Some of the views and opinions concerning the nature of dreaming are philosophical, even metaphysical (125, 305, 539, 583, 1001, 1338, 1450, 1841, 1842, 2130, 2158, 2603, 2638, 2639, 3692, 3693, 3696, 4076, 4267), and are not susceptible of translation into biological terms. A surprising number of writers compared the dream action to psychotic behavior, starting with Radestock (3257), who in 1879 quoted Kant as stating that "the lunatic is a wakeful dreamer," and Schopenhauer as observing that "a dream is a short-lasting psychosis, and a psychosis is a long-lasting dream," and followed by others, perhaps developing this notion on their own (52, 300, 349, 1126, 2088, 3581, 3770). Dreaming has also been compared to narcissistic regression (2311, 3316, 4237), and children's dreams to the behavior of savage peoples (2763). The interaction of the conscious and unconscious, operating during sleep, as developed by Hartmann (1656), has also been held responsible for dream processes (2905, 3950, 4010). Freud's idea (1289) that the dream is the protector of sleep has its adherents (1217, 2968) and opponents (520, 2905), with further notions that the dream can be both a protector and a disturber of sleep (1217), or neither (4011). Brody (520) advanced the view that the dream regulates sleep, and Ullman (4007–14), that dreaming protects the sleeper from external danger. There are also theories based on cellular and organ fatigue and similar hypothetical changes (419, 798, 885, 2553, 2731), hypnosis (4139) and inhibition (3126)—the last-mentioned advanced by Pavlov who, disregarding his own theory that sleep is a generalized cortical inhibition, explained dreaming by declaring that when one part of the cortex is inhibited, another part gets into a reversed state of excitation (p. 346).

Granted that dreaming is a hallucinatory experience, it nevertheless possesses the elements of analysis and integration that characterize the levels of waking consciousness (1007, 2801), but the performance is poorer and the memory of events shorter (1333, 3657). To those who insist that because dreams occur they must serve a particular purpose, it may be pointed out that not all processes have a teleological explanation. Vomiting, for instance, when it is elicited by some irritating matter in the stomach, serves a good purpose in evacuating the stomach and removing the irritant. The same vomiting act, when resulting from motion sickness, serves no physiological purpose. The explanation of the latter type of vomiting is that the vestibular centers in the medulla were unduly excited from the unusual motion of the body, and this excitation has spread to the neighboring vomiting center. This explanation is correct, but it is not teleological. Dreaming may be considered a crude type of cortical activity associated with a recurrent appearance of stage 1 EEG in the course of a night's sleep. Because this is an emergent stage 1 EEG, rising from a lower level of cortical function, it is less effective in furthering analysis, integration, and recall than the initial stage 1 EEG. As such, dreaming need not have a special function (4016) and may be quite meaningless (2298). The effects of dream curtailment, discovered by Dement (900), may be due to interference with an acquired habit. When one develops a craving for sweets—no vital nutritional necessity—and the supply is temporarily cut off, one may resent the curtailment and may overindulge, for a time, when the supply is restored.

The age at which dreaming first occurs during sleep is synchronous with the appearance of thinking in the waking state. Dreaming is nothing more than the consequence of repetitive cortical activation or "paradoxical phase" of the periodic variation in sleep EEG patterns. A sketch of the probable phylogenetic and ontogenetic development of this phase of sleep into dreaming constitutes a part of the evolutionary theory of sleep and wakefulness, presented in the last chapter of this book.

Chapter 12

The Depth of Sleep

The depth of sleep is usually expressed in terms of the magnitude of a variable that a particular investigator has been studying. It so happens that the fluctuations of the several concomitants of sleep do not run synchronously in the course of a night's sleep, and the curves of the depth of sleep vary with the concomitant measured.

The oldest depth-of-sleep curve was published one hundred years ago by Kohlschütter (2228) who charted it by plotting the figures for the intensities of sounds required to awaken the sleeper at different hours of the night. Kohlschütter found a tremendous increase in the auditory threshold by the end of the first hour of sleep and nearly as precipitous a drop to a low value by the end of the third hour, then a gradual, but insignificant, decrease for the remainder of the night. This curve, often referred to as "classical," found its way into many textbooks, one writer copying it from another. It remained for Swan (3886) to show the meaninglessness of the curve by analyzing its construction. It appears that, out of 74 observations distributed over 16 successive half-hourly intervals of several nights' sleep, 33, or 45 per cent, were rejected by Kohlschütter as "unsatisfactory." They were so designated because, if included, they would give the depth-of-sleep curve a jagged appearance, and Kohlschütter decided, a priori, that the curve must be smooth. Michelson (2804) obtained a curve whose peak was similar to Kohlschütter's, but the descending part was not so steep, not so close to the baseline, and had several undulations. Depth-of-sleep curves of Moenninghoff and Piesbergen (2855), also based on auditory thresholds, of Czerny (808), who used faradic shocks, and Lambranzi (2352), who employed both auditory and visual stimuli, differed from those of Kohlschütter and of Michelson in that each showed a secondary peak, not as high as the first one, about two hours prior to awakening. The common feature of all these curves was the very deep sleep during the first hour or two and the relatively shallow sleep in the hours that followed.

Endres and von Frey (1077, 1079, 1081), using the bristle method of the latter, studied the irritability to touch and pain stimuli during sleep in seven subjects. Each subject had his own characteristic curve, but in general the depth-of-sleep curves resembled the classical ones, as the threshold value of the tactile stimulus rose to 100 times, and that of pain 8 to 40 times, the pre-sleep levels soon after the onset of sleep. The investigators then developed the concept of the "amount" of sleep (*Schlafmenge*) as the product of the depth of sleep and time—in other words, the area between the depth-of-sleep curve and the axis of the abscissae. The area for the first two hours of sleep was greater than that for the remainder of the night, and that fact is responsible for the idea, as old as the oldest sleep curves, that one gets the greatest "beneficial" effects from the first two hours of sleep.

Among the variables followed through the night's sleep was the heart rate studied by Boas and Goldschmidt (387), who presented a tabulation of the time of occurrence of minimum heart rates during sleep. While the minima for some of the fifty-one men and fifty-two women studied were found in every hour of sleep, the mode for each sex was in the seventh hour. The composite curves for the two groups showed the minimum heart rate for the men to be near the end of the seventh hour; for the women, during the sixth hour. Conversely, the mean maximum heart rate occurred 2 hours and 55 minutes after the onset of sleep, but the incidence of the maxima was even closer to the onset of sleep: out of 102 persons, 28 had their highest heart rate during the first and 27 in the second hour of sleep. And these are the hours when, according to the classical depth-of-sleep curves, sleep is deepest. Further, considering how easily the heart rate is affected by almost any activity of the organism, as well as by external and internal stimuli, one cannot lightly disregard the entirely objectively established heart-rate minima during sleep. The striking similarity between the heart-rate curves and the ESR curve may be more than accidental (Fig. 12.1). Some process (or processes) tending to decrease the ESR and increase the heart rate may be at its lowest at the junction of the third and last quarter of the night's sleep.

Katsch and Pansdorf (2089) looked upon the fall in blood pressure as an indication of the depth of sleep, and they found a maximal fall two hours after the onset of sleep. Blankenhorn and Campbell (370, 618) located the minimum pressure during the fourth hour of sleep. More striking was the recording of blood pressure by Brush and Fayerweather (551), which showed a distinct first wave about 1½ hours in duration. The plethysmographic records of Howell (1846) revealed several wavelike oscillations 1–1½ hours apart. According to Capecchi (626), the lowest pressure is reached 2–4 hours after the beginning of sleep; the lowest heart rate a little later; and the body temperature trough still later. One may summarize the somewhat conflicting findings by saying that the lowest arterial pressure is attained some time during the first half of the night, while the lowest heart rate occurs during the second half.

Magnussen (2623), as previously mentioned (p. 50), discerned five periods of variations in the respiratory movements in the course of a night's sleep—a periodicity of about 90 minutes. Bass and Herr (242) suggested that the partial pressure of CO_2 in the alveolar air be accepted as an index of the depth of sleep, thus placing it in the first hour after the onset of sleep. Regelsberger (3297) invented an apparatus that automatically analyzed and continuously recorded the CO_2 concentration of the alveolar air for long periods of time and used it for measuring changes in sleep. Simultaneously determining variations in ESR, Regelsberger, it will be recalled (p. 21), obtained parallel changes in the two variables, with intervals of 1 to 2 hours between crests of succeeding waves. Richter (3337), after studying the sleep of sixteen subjects, decided that the rise in the ESR level was a better indication of the depth of sleep than the auditory

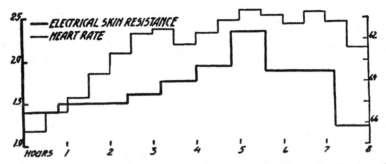

Fig. 12.1—Concomitant changes in ESR and heart rate during a night's sleep. *Thick line:* variation in the mean ESR level for successive tenths of a night's sleep, expressed as ratios of the ESR level prevailing at the time of going to sleep and based on determinations made on eight subjects during 34 nights; *thin line:* mean heart rates for successive half-hourly periods of a night's sleep, based on data in Figures 37 and 38 of Boas and Goldschmidt (387). The highest mean ESR level and the lowest mean heart rate are reached in the third quarter of the night's sleep.

threshold method, but Landis (2360), from figures obtained on one subject, concluded that the ESR level was not an indication of the depth of sleep. Titelbaum (3948) located the highest ESR in the latter part of the night, when sleep, as judged by other criteria, is certainly not deepest. A suggestion of some waves can also be seen in the ESR record of Figure 12.1, though, as a composite curve, it hides variations occurring in individual night records. Rutenfranz and coworkers (3482) detected a resemblance between their ESR curves and Czerny's bimodal depth-of-sleep curve. Levy and co-authors (2467) noted that periods of arousal were marked by sharp drops and slow recovery of the ESR in their subjects, and that finding points up the increase in ESR seen by Hawkins and associates (1669) during dreaming.

Johnson (1999), in recording the frequency with which sleepers stirred during a night's sleep, discerned, as previously indicated, five well-defined oscillations, with a mean duration of about $1\frac{1}{2}$ hours. Suckling and associates (3863) found a good moment-to-moment correlation between motility and depth of sleep, as well as between heart rate and depth of sleep. On the other hand, minimal heart rates and maximal motility occur during the second half of the night's sleep. In our laboratory we tested the relationship between the depth of sleep and the proximity of the testing to a preceding movement in terms of time. The depth of sleep was determined by the apparatus described in connection with establishing the curve of the onset of sleep (p. 76). The results (2944) were based on some three hundred tests on six subjects. The frequency of movement and the intensity of the threshold sound varied considerably in the different subjects. Each of these variables seemed to be characteristic for a given sleeper and were not as such related. Thus, the most quiet sleeper, on the average, required the least intensity of sound to awaken him. However, for each sleeper there was a relationship between the magnitude of the stimulus and the length of the period of immobility immediately preceding the test. The ascending portion of the curve was S-shaped, resembling the curve for the onset of sleep (Fig. 9.1) obtained by the same method. The curve reached its height in 15 to 20 minutes, instead of 25 to 35 minutes as at the onset of sleep, then turned downward. It should be remembered that this is a composite curve and applies to time after a movement at any hour of the night. That means that the depth of sleep would be very small at 1:00 A.M., if tested 5 minutes after a movement, and might be very great at 6:00 A.M., if 15 to 20 minutes had elapsed since the subject stirred. Statistically, considering that the subjects moved more frequently later in the night, there were not as many chances to test a sleeper, 15 to 20 minutes after he moved, at 6:00 A.M., as there were at 1:00 A.M.; but, when he did remain quiet for a longer time, his sleep was progressively deeper up to, on the average, 15 to 20 minutes. Beyond that the sleep became lighter again, probably to lead to a new movement. Unfortunately, it was impossible to determine the depth of sleep in relation to the incidence of the next movement because the subject was awakened or semi-awakened by the test itself. But again, statistically, the movements were likely to be separated by 5 minutes at one time and by 30 at another, and the results were in accord with that expectation.

Wagner (4094), using pain, tactile, olfactory, and auditory stimuli to determine the depth of sleep in 197 newborn infants, was able to list seven stages of depth in terms of duration and extent of responses made by the infants at each stage. In the waking state the infants were generally active, moved parts of the body as well as mouth, eyes open. In light sleep these movements continued; eyes were closed, but eyelid movements were present. In deeper sleep the infants were quiet, with an occasional eyelid, mouth, or body movement. In succeeding stages the eyelid and mouth movements were totally absent, while body movements continued; all movements stopped, but breathing was irregular; in deepest sleep, no movements, breathing regular. Gentry and Aldrich (1395), using Wagner's system of grading the depth of sleep, studied the "rooting reflex"—the ability of an infant, whose cheek has been touched lightly, to turn its head toward the side of stimulation and open its mouth, presumably to receive the nipple. The rooting reflex was weaker the deeper the sleep, to the point of complete disappearance. Wagner (4096) also established that during an afternoon interfeeding period newborn infants were likely to sleep deeply for 17 to 22 minutes. This figure is close to that obtained by Reynard and Dockeray (3325), as well as the mean duration of complete quiescence seen in older infants (150). Furthermore, the complete rest-activity cycle in these older infants is 50 to 60 minutes, comparing well with the 50-minute respiratory cycle reported for infants by Denisova and Figurin (914).

De Toni (3956) considered sleep to have reached its greatest depth in children when the pendular eyeball movements had decreased from 8–10/min right after the onset of sleep (also just before awakening) to only 1/min. Garvey (1364), studying the distribution of motility in twenty-two children of nursery-school age, distinguished waves of motility of 60 to 70 minutes' duration—longer than the infants' 50- to 60-minute sleep cycle, but shorter than the 85- to 90-minute sleep cycle of adults.

EEG data reveal a definite cycling, as discussed at length in Chapter 11. Several cycles can be discerned in the figures published by Brooks and associates (524), and an even sharper delineation can be seen in the plotting of the changing EEG by Hoffman and associates (1810), though it was apparently unnoticed by the authors. In a record of one night's sleep of 420 minutes' duration, there were five waves of 75 to 105 minutes in length, or a mean of 84 minutes. Reichert and Woehlisch (3304) presented a night's EEG record, with an initial cycle of about 3 hours and succeeding cycles shallower and shorter. In our laboratory (149) we also placed the first dreaming episode after about 3 hours of sleep, till continuous recording revealed the missed emergent stage 1 EEG about $1\frac{1}{2}$ hours after the onset of sleep. In any case, the 85- to 90-minute EEG periodicity (901), though entailing successive dreaming activity, is essentially a depth-of-sleep oscillation. However, during dreaming, sleep is neither as shallow as the EEG would indicate, nor as deep as Jouvet's "paradoxical phase" of sleep in cats (2033). It must be remembered that the latter is accompanied by a slowing of the heart, whereas, during dreaming, the heart rate is increased. The EEG cycling is fundamentally the same in man and cat, and, to complete the analogy, in young kittens the cycle length is 20 to 30 minutes and in adult cats, 30 to 45 minutes.

Another example of the 85-minute periodicity may be found in the reports of Ohlmeyer and co-workers (3045, 3046) on the recurrence of penile erections, with a mean duration of 25 minutes, during sleep, as recorded automatically in seven healthy subjects, twenty to forty years old, with eight to thirty-four observations per subject. The authors referred to the 85-minute cycle as the "biological hour"—corresponding to the "short rhythm" of Regelsberger (3299).

Among the deviations from the normal, sleep has been reported to be very deep in patients suffering from migraine (1352), cachexia (2574), enuresis (3852), and acne (3879), but light, as judged by the EEG patterns, in neurasthenics (2703).

Several authors dealt with the inadequacies of depth-of-sleep determinations based on single variables, and others suggested methods of their own, or reviewed the general field of the depth of sleep (582, 598, 1459, 1565, 2080, 2441, 2921, 3023, 3195, 3506, 3614, 3798, 3799, 3995, 4145, 4168, 4173–75, 4250–61, 4317, 4335).

In considering the many depth-of-sleep curves published since 1862, one is struck by the consistently sharp increase in sleep depth during the first hour or two. The explanation is not far to seek. The four or five oscillations that appear and reappear for several variables—motility, circulation, respiration, ESR, EEG —are approximately 1½ hours in length. The initial waves are strictly superimposed upon each other, producing a sharp peak, but the succeeding ones are often slightly out of phase and tend to cancel each other. Therefore, composite curves tend to become shallower and more blurred. That was true of our data on the relation between the depth of sleep and the time elapsed from a preceding body movement (1994), as well as the successive REM-EEG variations during a single night's sleep (901). Therefore, instead of a composite depth-of-sleep curve, based upon many nights of sleep, for one or more subjects, one should draw a representative curve of a night's sleep, such as shown in Figure 11.2. But here one finds, as pointed out in the beginning of this chapter, that by selecting one or another variable one can show that sleep is deepest in the early, middle, or late part of the night. What does stand out in many individual curves, and tends to be obscured in the composite ones, is the existence of a basic rest-activity cycle, 50 to 60 minutes long in infants, longer in children, still longer in adults, and that a representative night's sleep of about 8 hours is likely to be made up of five such cycles (Fig. 11.2). The implications of this short-term periodicity are further discussed in the last chapter of this book.

Chapter 13

Duration of Sleep

The time spent in sleep, or, considering the periods of various degrees of drowsiness at the onset and termination of sleep, the time between going to bed at night and getting up in the morning, is one of the easiest characteristics of sleep to study. It has been thoroughly investigated, and considerable statistical data are available, particularly with respect to the sleep of infants and children. The figures were gathered either by the questionnaire method from parents or by direct observations made in institutions, where a number of children could be studied under comparable, though admittedly not always ideal, conditions.

In general, the figures show a gradual, somewhat irregular, decrease in the duration of sleep with age, but there is a difference between estimates or proposed norms and actual observational figures (2566).

A newborn infant is said to sleep for 22 hours out of 24 (2665, 2743, 3867), or 20–22 hours (1004, 4004), or 19–20 hours (558, 789). A publication of the Children's Bureau, U.S. Department of Health, Education, and Welfare (89), issued in 1955 and reprinted as late as 1961, informs parents that for "the first week or two a baby may be awake only about 2 hours out of the 24." Factual data tell a different story. Gesell and Amatruda (1411), for one newborn infant observed for 15 days, and Parmelee (3095), for another watched for 7 days, obtained mean total durations of sleep per 24 hours of 14 and 17.8 hours, respectively. More telling are the figures given by Parmelee and co-workers (3096) for seventy-five full-term neonates, for the first three days of life, of which the mean was only 16.6 hours, though for individual infants it ranged from 10.5 to 23 hours. These investigators also established the mean longest unbroken sleep for the group—4.4 hours, again with a tremendous range of 2.1 to 10 hours. Unfortunately, there is little information on the maximum duration of wakefulness in neonates (3095).

Concerning young infants under six months of age, the total duration of sleep is given by Dukes (1004) as 18 to 20 hours, by the Children's Bureau's anonymous author (89) as 15 to 17 hours, and by others (558, 1465, 3053) as 13 to 15 hours.

These figures are close to the values obtained by us (2196) in a study of nineteen infants, reared under family home conditions, rather than institutional care. Table 13.1 shows the data obtained from protocols kept by the infants' mothers on specially designed forms and from continuous actograms, both of which were collected daily. The period covered was 24 weeks (from the 3d to the 26th, inclusive) during which the infants remained lying in their cribs, except when lifted to be fed and cared for, and thus furnished information concerning the motility which could be translated into intervals of wakefulness and sleep. As an infant might at times be awake and quiescent, the figures for sleep were, if anything, slightly higher than the true figures, but certainly not lower. As can be seen from Table 13.1, each infant had its own range and mode of total hours of sleep, the percentage of sleep time ranging from 49 to 68 per cent or from just under 12 to over 16 hours out of the 24. For the group as a whole, the mean total number of hours of sleep decreased from 14.8 for the first 4-week period to 13.9 for the last, or about 1 hour (Table 15.1). Our findings are in agreement with earlier reports (3170, 3928, 4124) which pointed out that infants varied markedly in the duration of "quality" of their sleep, depending upon personality, state of health, and conditions under which the infants were reared.

From birth on there is an uneven division between night and day with respect to the hours of sleep (1411), the infants sleeping about two-thirds of the time from 8:00 P.M. to 8:00 A.M., and only one-half of the "daytime" 12 hours. This night-day disparity increases as the infant gets older, and by the age of three months there is usually an unbroken period of about 10 hours of sleep at night, and a gradually decreasing time spent in short naps in the daytime (p. 133). In the second six months of the infant's life, the decrease in the total duration of sleep is due mainly to the shrinking of the daytime sleep to one morning and one afternoon nap, the duration of the unbroken night sleep remaining practically unchanged.

During the second year the child learns to walk, and his field of activity is thus widened. He is also able to remain awake longer, and one of the two naps, usually the morning one, is given up. The total duration of sleep fluctuates between 13 and 14 hours; the afternoon nap separates two periods of wakefulness of 5 to 5.5 hours each. From this age until the child begins to attend school his night sleep remains unchanged, and the nap is gradually decreased to one hour, then given up altogether. In some cases the nap is refused at the age of two and a half years, as found by Flemming (1210); in other cases, depending upon child and parent, the child will continue to take and enjoy his afternoon nap until the age of seven, or even beyond. The decrease in the amount of sleep from 13 to 14 hours in the second year to 12 at the end of the fifth is due mainly to the shortening and later abandonment of the afternoon nap, according to Foster (1252), who analyzed records kept by mothers of 1,000 children less than eight years of age. The total hours of sleep for the three- to five-year-olds, as given by different authors, run

TABLE 13.1

FREQUENCY DISTRIBUTION OF TOTAL HOURS OF SLEEP PER 24 HOURS, FOR 19 INFANTS, DURING THE PERIOD OF OBSERVATION (WEEKS 3–26) AND THE VARIATION IN THE MEAN DURATION OF SLEEP OF INDIVIDUAL INFANTS FOR THE WHOLE 24 WEEKS

Hours of Sleep per 24 Hrs.	Infants																			Total
	6M	1M	7F	8M	5F	2M	4F	9M	10M	6F	3F	8F	4M	2F	7M	3M	9F	10F	5M	
7– 7.99	2																			2
8– 8.99	8		1	2																13
9– 9.99	11	5	4	4	1				1	1	1									27
10–10.99	26	17	5	11	6	1	2	2	3	3	1									76
11–11.99	34	22	9	13	9	12	4	3	8	10	9	1		2		3	2	1		142
12–12.99	57	27	33	40	33	29	21	7	13	18	14	8	6	10	6	6	5	2	1	336
13–13.99	25	27	55	51	55	34	41	19	40	31	23	31	11	19	19	31	12	13	3	540
14–14.99	1	16	29	34	27	47	39	30	27	35	51	45	34	40	39	18	24	23	15	574
15–15.99	4	11	9	8	20	26	37	16	37	33	35	42	44	43	36	34	37	32	44	548
16–16.99		3	7	1	8	14	19	10	14	10	25	14	26	32	37	26	26	25	51	348
17–17.99			1	3	3	4	5	4	8	9	7	5	7	12	20	27	10	19	38	182
18–18.99			2		1	1			2	5	1		1	8	5	16	7	5	5	59
19–19.99									1	2	1			2	1		1	4	2	14
20–20.99																1				1
Individual means of hours of sleep	11.76	12.72	13.20	13.20	13.68	14.16	14.40	14.40	14.40	14.40	14.64	14.88	15.36	15.36	15.60	15.60	15.60	15.60	16.32	
Per cent of time spent in sleep	49	53	55	55	57	59	60	60	60	60	61	62	64	64	65	65	65	65	68	

from 14 to 15 (265, 1004), through 11 to 12½ (924, 1210, 1691, 3281, 3326). Flemming (1210) considered the fifth year a very critical one in the life of the child, with sleep difficulties more prevalent than before or after, and requiring very good management in the passage from two shorter periods of wakefulness to a single long one, when the nap is given up.

Reynolds (3326) reported that the amount of sleep taken by a preschool child varied considerably from day to day, but there was a fairly constant mean over several weeks. However, there was no consistency in the variations of different children, and at no time did her group of seventy-seven children between the ages of one and a half and six years behave like a unit in the periodic changes in the duration of sleep. What a child lost one day he would make up the next, and vice versa, thus maintaining a sleep balance over a longer period of time.

According to White (4189), preschool children with higher intelligence quotients sleep less than children who are not so bright. Shinn (3682) compared the day and night sleep of 30 nursery-school children at Vassar College with that of 135 children of the same ages in Honolulu. The Vassar children slept less, but their mental age was higher, and the author thought that this relatively higher intelligence might have been the cause of the shorter sleep. A negative correlation between mental age and total sleep was also found by Wagner (4097). These results may indicate that greater mental development and superior intelligence cause the young child to move forward in lengthening its period of daytime wakefulness.

Ilg (1896) traced the decrease in the number of naps in infants and children, from 4 to 5 at the age of four weeks; 3 at the age of sixteen weeks; and one long forenoon nap and an unstable afternoon one at the age of forty weeks. The single nap after the noon meal at fifteen to eighteen months may be difficult to attain at twenty-one months, and the nap may become a real problem at two and a half years of age. At the age of four to five and a half years the majority of children may take a "play nap"—a period of lying down by parent's request, without actually falling asleep. The duration of the single afternoon nap is given as 1–1.5 hours (674, 3631), and the onset time seems to be seasonally affected, especially in children who take longer to fall asleep (3159). In general, children are slower in going to sleep and sleep less as they get older (812).

Some adults reacquire the afternoon nap routine, if at home or under conditions permitting them to take time out of their daily activities. One or two hours of sleep enables such individuals to stay up longer in the evening than they could otherwise. The refreshing effect of a half-hour "catnap" at the end of the working day, before or after the evening meal, is in a different category: the influence is psychological rather than physiological, as discussed in Chapter 36 (p. 365).

From the data on the duration of sleep of American and British primary-school children, six to thirteen years of age (60, 1004, 3053, 3281, 3918), it is evident that there is a decrease from 11 to 13 hours at the lowest age to 8.5–10.5 at the highest. There appears to be no correlation between the length of sleep and success in school work. From a study on over five thousand Japanese children (1670), it appears that they sleep less than do Western children (1691), the mean duration of 10 hours at the age of six decreasing to 8.5 hours at thirteen.

There seem to be no sex differences in the duration of sleep in children under eight years of age (1253), but in older ones the reports are varied both with respect to length and regularity (1106, 1670, 3281).

In an investigation of mental and physical traits of one thousand gifted children, Terman (3917) found that they slept longer on the average than unselected children. The differences in minutes for seven successive ages (from seven to fourteen years) were 23, 16, 25, 35, 27, 50, 44. These figures are in disagreement with the finding that superior school work is not related to duration of sleep (3918), but Hayashi (1670), with his large series, obtained the same relationship. It will be recalled that, among very young children, superior intelligence seemed to be associated with shorter sleep, and Terman's own figures show no differential in favor of brighter children until they have reached the age of seven. It is possible that superior mental ability in younger children permits them to remain awake longer, whereas the increased mental activity of older gifted children produces greater fatigue and, therefore, greater need for recuperation at the end of a waking period.

The time of going to bed has also been the object of statistical analysis. Foster (1252) declared that the shortening of the night's sleep, as the child gets older, is done at the expense of going to bed later rather than a change in the hours of getting up. The time taken to fall asleep—about 20 minutes—is approximately the same for all ages. Wittstock (4247) also traced the gradual postponing of the hour of retiring for the night with age. The hours of going to bed advanced from 8:00 P.M. for children five to eight years old to 9:00–10:00 P.M. for older children and adolescents (60, 2758). The relative constancy of the hour of arising is probably connected with school attendance which starts at about the same time of the day for children of different ages. The increase in the percentage of children who do not awaken spontaneously would indicate that they are not getting as much sleep as they might, were they not awakened. This percentage, according to Terman and Hocking (3918), fluctuates about 20 until the age of eleven, then begins to mount, reaching 48 at age eighteen. The authors' explanation of the progressively greater failure of adolescents to awaken spontaneously is that at that time they change from a vesperal to a matinal type of sleeper, although they admit that it may be due to their having to do more homework in the evening than do younger children.

For youths between thirteen and twenty-one, figures for the duration of sleep (75, 1004, 1670, 3053, 3918) run from 8.75 to 7 hours, approaching the mean value for the general adult population.

Statistical data on the duration of sleep in adults point to a fair constancy for a group, a variability from person to person, and in the same individual from night to night (428, 615, 728, 1372). The mean is usually given as 8 hours, women sleeping longer than men (232, 615), except for data obtained in an institution for the insane, where the opposite was the case (2319).

Caffeine in small doses (65–130 mg) did not impair the "quality" of sleep (1817) but larger quantities did. The duration of sleep was also decreased by larger amounts, with the mean figures, in hours: control nights, 7.52; 65–130 mg caffeine, 7.47; 200–260 mg, 7.30; 325–390 mg, 6.59. The effect of caffeine did not depend on age, sex, or previous caffeine habits of the individual.

We (2200) have analyzed the duration-of-sleep figures obtained from twenty-five subjects covering several thousands of nights. The number of hours slept per night averaged almost exactly 7.5 for the group as a whole. But that number of hours is less informative than the ranges of the individual means which were as low as a little over 6 hours for some subjects and well over 9 for others. Those who regularly used an alarm clock did not predominantly fall into the short-hour fraction but seemed to be distributed among the others. Allowing each subject a 2-hour period within which he usually went to bed, we determined the mean duration of sleep when the subjects retired for the night earlier or later than usual. As would be expected, in the former case the mean length of the night's sleep increased to a little over 8 hours; in the latter, it dropped below 7. Furthermore, individual mean differences varied from a few minutes to over 3 hours. The same conclusion was reached from analyzing the figures for the duration of sleep with respect to the mode of awakening, whether the latter was spontaneous or artificial (by alarm clock, by outside noises, or by being called). About 60 per cent of the awakenings were spontaneous for the group as a whole, but there were subjects who nearly always, others who frequently, and still others who rarely, used an alarm clock. Here, too, the means show that artificial awakening shortened sleep, cutting it down to 7.2 hours from 7.8, the latter prevailing when awakening was spontaneous. The group as a whole slept 35 minutes more if permitted to awaken spontaneously than when sleep was artificially terminated. But for some subjects the duration of sleep was nearly the same, indicating that they would awaken at a certain time, whether they set the alarm clock or not; for others the time was shortened by over two hours, suggesting that they used artificial means of awakening only when they went to bed late, or else habitually "underslept" during work days and made up for it by sleeping later on rest days, or by going to bed very early on certain nights. There were three subjects who slept about one hour more when they used an alarm clock than when their sleep was terminated spontaneously. All three were habitual alarm-clock users and ordinarily went to bed early as they apparently needed a great deal of sleep. In short, the effects of both variations in the hour of going to bed and in the mode of awakening indicate that what is true of a group, and can be expected or predicted, does not apply to an individual member of that group. There is no more a "normal" duration of sleep, for either children or adults, than there is a normal heart rate, or height, or weight. Comparisons with composite values may tell an individual whether his particular figure is close to or far removed from the mean, but in most cases attempts to reach that mean are either impossible, unnecessary, or both.

Special conditions, activities, or occupations seem to be related to the duration of sleep. A survey of the sleep habits of "509 men of distinction" (2331) and of "1000 leaders in science, art, industry, and politics" (456) yielded modes of 8 hours per night, though about 2 per cent at each extreme slept 5 and 10 hours, respectively. Hersey (1718) thought that a person's mood underwent wave-like oscillations, a cycle lasting 4 to 6 weeks and varying somewhat with age, temperament, intelligence, and marital status. He considered, among other factors, the possible influence of sleep. The duration of sleep for a group of twelve unskilled workers was the same, whether they were at the peak or at the bottom of the "mood wave." It thus appeared that duration of sleep could not be considered as a valid cause of regular variations in affective tone. Different results were obtained by Barry and Bousfield (232, 428), who reported a definite positive correlation between the feeling of well-being, or euphoria, and the length of the previous night's sleep in 413 undergraduates. Those who slept from 8 to 8.75 hours felt better than those who slept less than 8 hours, and considerably more so than the students who slept less than 6 hours. On the other hand, sleeping over 9 hours seemed to be less beneficial. Women who slept longer than men reported a significantly higher euphoria.

Sheldon (3676) worked out a scale for body structure and temperament, with three theoretical types, although the majority of individuals have a mixture of temperaments, with one or more predominating. Of the extreme types, the viscerotonic, represented by the fat boy of the *Pickwick Papers,* likes to sleep, sleeps well and long, preferring to retire early and get up late. The cerebrotonic type, with "the lean and hungry look," is a poor sleeper, is most alert late at night, hates to go to bed as well as to get up, and is often "worthless" in the early part of the day. The somatotonic, or athletic, type requires little sleep, likes to get up early, and feels good in the morning.

Concerning special conditions, Williams (4222) noted an increase of 20 minutes to one hour in the duration of sleep at altitudes over 10,000 feet. Graveline and associates (1506) found that a subject continuously submerged in water for 7 days required only about two hours of sleep per 24 hours. Submersion in water for 10 hours each day did not seem to affect the duration of sleep (1508).

To test the recuperative effects of different durations of sleep, Weygandt (4183) carried out a series of tests on himself, each of a half-hour's duration, involving some arithmetical performances and learning by heart. The tests were made before going to bed, after varying periods of sleep during the night, and again in the morning. In all cases sleep produced improvement in performance, but for the addition tests one hour of sleep was as good as several, while for memorization 5 hours of sleep were needed to make his performance as good as it usually was in the morning. Weygandt concluded that the recuperative power of sleep lay in the first few hours and that the morning period of relatively light sleep was of slight value. The opposite conclusion was reached by Fortune (1250), who used an ergograph to measure the amount of work he could do with the index finger of his right hand. Likewise Moore and co-workers (2876) reported a definite relationship between the number of hours slept and muscular efficiency on the following day. They analyzed the data collected in 1,500 tests on twenty-six women whose sleeping hours varied from 6 to 9. The longer the subjects slept, the better was their muscular performance. Vitenzon (4068) noted that 2 to 6 hours of sleep, instead of the customary 7 to 8, deleteriously affected "visual trace reactions" of human subjects.

Tuberculosis patients were found to sleep 8 to 8.5 hours (293), but hospitalized individuals usually sleep longer than they do at home (3474). Acne was said to be associated with longer than usual sleep (3879), but this finding has not been confirmed (729). Gans (1352, 1356) successfully treated migraine by putting his patients on a "sleep diet" of no more than 7.5 hours per night. Puech and associates (3247) studied a child with hydrocephalic anencephaly, who slept well from 10:00 P.M. to 8:00 A.M. and, at the age of five years, did not take daytime naps. That child, however, recognized members of her family, could laugh, and had an almost normal EEG. She differed therefore from the typical anencephalic behavior pattern (p. 23).

To summarize the findings on the duration of sleep, the gradual decrease in the total hours of sleep per 24 hours can be expressed as an increased ability to remain awake, parallel with anatomical maturation and physiological development. The relative wakefulness capacity of the individual is increased fourfold, as the young infant has to "pay" with two hours of sleep for each hour of wakefulness, whereas in the adult corresponding payment amounts to only half an hour. The absolute capacity for remaining awake increases from a few minutes at birth to 15 to 17 hours in the adult—the "natural" maximum in a sleep-wakefulness rhythm of 24 hours. The extension of this absolute maximum under artificial routines of living is discussed in Chapter 18.

Chapter 14

Awakening

In many respects the process of awakening is the reverse of the onset of sleep, except that in non-spontaneous termination of sleep the passage to the waking state is sudden rather than gradual. Such a sudden waking is likely to produce a feeling of bewilderment in the subject, with a certain disorientation of behavior, as described long ago by Gudden (1547). It is well known that a person may be aroused by an alarm clock and fall asleep again after silencing the alarm. What is not so well known is that every normal person probably awakens several times during a single night. Some would call these interruptions of sleep semi-awakenings, but in all situations spontaneous passage from sleep to wakefulness involves several stages of *dormiveglia:* it is just as hard to say that the sleeping person has awakened at a certain moment as it is to determine the exact time of falling asleep. That one can be awakened during the night and not remember it has probably been the experience of everyone. The person aroused may be asked a question—for instance, to give a certain friend's telephone number, which he does correctly—and is then permitted to fall asleep once more. Next morning he is found to have forgotten the incident but, if reminded about it, may recall it. It has also been pointed out that to turn over while lying close to the edge of the bed, without falling out, requires some control of one's movements, while in a state of, at least, semi-awakening. Very young children, accustomed to sleeping in a crib with protected sides, often fall out of a flat bed during their sleep when first changed from the former to the latter.

To determine the incidence of spontaneous awakenings during the night, our subjects were instructed to press a key, activating a signal magnet, whenever they were sufficiently awake to recall the instruction. Aside from awakenings that inadvertently went unrecorded, not all that were recorded were remembered on getting up in the morning (2193). One subject pressed the key 101 times in the course of 20 nights; only 16 of these overt awakenings occurred during the first half of the night's sleep. There was a correlation between the frequency of awakenings and the incidence of body movements, and a lightening of sleep. In general, toward the end of the night, sleep is considerably lighter, movements and awakenings more frequent than in earlier sleep. There is a gradual increase in the number of afferent impulses: from a distended bladder; perhaps from a contracting empty stomach; also probably from the muscles, as suggested by the rise in body temperature. All these factors tend to produce more frequent lightening of sleep to the point of semi-awakening and, aided by noises and daylight, finally bring the sleeper to the point of actual awakening. Even then, some people, if they find the hour too early, can go back to sleep, but others have difficulty in reverting to sleep under such conditions and usually give up after a few fruitless attempts. In this respect, also, awakening resembles going to sleep, which is easy for some and difficult for others.

A detailed description of gradual awakening, including hypnopompic phenomena, obtained by introspection, was given by Grotjahn (1535, 1537), who, shortly after getting up, recorded the effect of external and internal stimuli on himself as the state of sleep gave way to that of wakefulness. De Lisi (2537) found that, on the motor side, awakening is characterized by tonic activity, such as stretching, whereas the onset of sleep is accompanied by myoclonus. Otto (3072) considered stretching and yawning on awakening as indications of the completeness of the preceding night's rest. Both are indulged in by children and adults who enjoy normal sleep. Max (2719), who studied action potentials from the arm and hand muscles of deaf-mutes at the onset of sleep, made similar observations during awakening. Whether sudden or gradual, awakening was almost always accompanied by overt movements which were superimposed upon, and masked, the basic muscular changes. In twenty records, where no visible movements were seen during awakening, there was an increase in the magnitude of the muscle potentials, reaching maximum values right after awakening. Subsequent muscular relaxation would cause the muscle potentials to decrease but not to the level prevailing before awakening. The mean potential in fifty-two cases of after-sleep relaxation was 1.35 microv, compared to a mean of 0.76 microv before awakening. Grollman (1523) studied blood pressure, cardiac output, pulse, and oxygen consumption during awakening. Of these, only the heart rate was definitely accelerated at the termination of sleep. Boas and Goldschmidt (387) obtained a few cardiotachometric records at the time of awakening. Some subjects showed a sharp increase at the time of overt waking-up; in others there was a gradual rise in heart rate for several minutes prior to awakening.

The speed with which one can pass from sleep to wakefulness under special conditions was shown by the results of Fleisch (1203), previously referred to in connection with the quickness of falling asleep, when the atmospheric pressure was decreased to about 330 mm Hg. This change, as indicated by a sudden increase in respiratory activity, could be accomplished in 4 seconds or less.

The paucity of papers describing the process of awakening, as contrasted with the onset of sleep, is very easily explained. It is a relatively simple matter to sit up for an hour or so while the subject is falling asleep, but the time of awakening is so uncertain that very few investigators have made any observations on it, except when awakening occurred at the end of a short nap or when it was automatically taken care of by a system of continuous recording. Some work has been done on performance after awakening, by comparing the scores obtained late at night with those early in the morning. This research formed a part of studies of 24-hour variations in performance, discussed in Chapter 16. In general, a person's performance is worse after getting up in the morning than before going to bed, paradoxical though such a finding may appear. Omwake (3055) submitted five subjects to three tests before they retired for the night, and after they had had 2, 4, 6, or 8 hours of sleep, respectively. The tests measured the swaying of the body in the standing position; hand steadiness, as judged by the ability to hold a stylus in a hole without touching the edges; and checking off numbers from a given list. All these tests showed a marked deterioration after 2 hours of sleep, as compared to the scores obtained before going to bed, and a gradual improvement, as the period of sleep was lengthened, but even after 8 hours of sleep the performance was not up to the pre-sleep level. Evidently, immediately after getting up, irrespective of the hour, one is not at one's best.

The feeling of having rested well during the night, handled on a statistical basis (2200), appeared to be a matter of an even chance for a group as a whole, i.e., the number of mornings when the subjects reported that they felt "well rested" fluctuated around 50 per cent of the total. For individual subjects the percentage varied from 0 to 100. Thus, certain subjects habitually woke up feeling well rested, others hardly ever. This phenomenon may be related to the character of the person's 24-hour curve of temperature and performance (p. 151).

A particular type of performance after awakening that engaged the attention of psychologists is the capacity for recalling learned material. Lay (2385) tested the ability of eleven young subjects to memorize, and to recall 12 or 24 hours later, "nonsense" words. Some learned these words by heart quicker in the morning, others in the evening. But irrespective of the ease or difficulty with which the words were memorized, the material learned in the evening was retained better than that learned in the morning. Similar results were obtained by Ploog (3218). Newman (2995) found that sleep following learning led to better retention of "non-essential" material—the equivalent of nonsense syllables—but not of meaningful material. Gibb (1417) extended the intervals after learning nonsense syllables to 48, 72, and 96 hours, and obtained like results. Jenkins and Dallenbach (1976) had two subjects learn nonsense syllables by heart, and tested their retention of the learned material 1, 2, 4, or 8 hours later. With the data obtained as a control, they had the same subjects memorize similar material at night, between 11:30 P.M. and 1:00 A.M., let them go to sleep, and aroused them 1, 2, 4, or 8 hours after the onset of sleep. The amount retained was always greater following sleep than after a corresponding period of wakefulness, with the added difference that, whereas in the waking state the curve of retention had the familiar form of a continued decline, scarcely more was forgotten after 8 hours of sleep than after 2. The authors concluded that "forgetting is not so much a matter of decay of old impressions and associations as it is a matter of the interference, inhibition, or obliteration of old by new." Dahl (810) modified the technique by adding figures to the syllables and testing recognition of the learned material, when it was mixed with new material in a test list. Recognition was better after 6 to 8 hours of sleep than after an equal period of wakefulness, but with 1- or 2-hour intervals it was the other way around. Thus Dahl's results are only in partial agreement with those of Jenkins and Dallenbach, who obtained better retention after every period of sleep tested. A still different retention curve could be drawn from the data on two subjects reported by Van Ormer (4038, 4039). His subjects showed the same retention after one hour of sleep as after one hour of wakefulness. From then on, however, the curves of retention of nonsense syllables followed those of Jenkins and Dallenbach for a while, i.e., the curve went down in the waking state but remained horizontal in sleep. After 8 hours of sleep, retention was better than after 8 hours of wakefulness. Worchel and Marks (4278) had two subjects learn nonsense syllables late at night, with or without a preliminary period of 1.5 hours of sleep. Learning ability was impaired by the short sleep, but relearning the syllables after a night's sleep was unaffected by either of the two learning routines. Finally, Graves (1507), experimenting on herself, found learning just before going to bed at night favored retention, provided the latter was tested 72, 96, or 144 hours afterward, but not when the interval was 24 or 48 hours. There is thus a good deal of variety in the results, probably because of differences in subjects and procedures, but, in general, it appears that going to bed immediately after memorizing suitable material favors retention, as against remaining awake for some time thereafter.

"Sleep-learning" or acquiring new knowledge while asleep has been the topic of science fiction as well as laboratory investigations. Leshan (101, 2439) was able to abolish the nail-biting habits of eight out of twenty boys who were admonished to do so 16,200 times in 54 nights of their sojourn at a summer camp. Hoyt (1847) used a variety of procedures in presenting ten Chinese words and their English equivalents to sleeping subjects. Comparing the time it took to learn these equivalents following a night's sleep, Hoyt concluded that learning did not occur during sleep. Others (1255, 2443) reported success. Perhaps the most extensive study of sleep-learning was made by Simon and Emmons (1073, 3706–8) on twenty-one subjects, who were given ninety-six questions and answers at 5-minute intervals throughout the night's sleep, while their sleep EEGs were monitored. The percentage of items recalled correctly on awakening the next morning decreased as the percentage of alpha frequencies decreased, and shortly after the alpha pattern disappeared the item recall stopped. The authors concluded that learning during sleep was "impractical and probably impossible." They reached somewhat similar conclusions from a critical analysis of ten other sleep-learning studies (3708), including those of Leshan (2439) and Hoyt (1847).

Does one know how long one slept and, if so, with what accuracy can one tell time when awakened? What are the cues that determine one's time sense? Vaschide (4040) tested thirty-three persons who thought they could wake up at a certain time. Those with superior education made an error of 25 minutes on the average; persons with a rudimentary schooling, 13 minutes; uneducated ones, 7 minutes. It may mean that the less educated a person is, the more dependent he becomes on natural cues, disregarded by others. An individual who has access to, and can tell time from, a timepiece will be less likely to watch the shadows than one who cannot determine the time of day from an instrument. Boring and Boring (414) studied the time sense during sleep in four subjects. Their time sense was found to be poor, each tending to name an hour later than the actual one, when aroused during the night. There was no improvement with practice. The errors tended to be greater when sleep was deepest. The subject who dropped off into deep sleep almost at once made maximal errors during the first hour of sleep; the other three, whose sleep deepened gradually, made their biggest errors during the third hour. The most useful cues were the feeling of fatigue or restedness and later in the night sensations from bladder and digestive tract. A memory of dreaming or occurrence of periods of wakefulness was usually indicative of a late hour.

A somewhat different procedure, more like Vaschide's, was employed by Frobenius (1301, 1302), who fixed a certain time for each of his five subjects to awaken during the night. The tests made on 250 nights revealed that the subjects were able to wake up within 5 minutes of the time set for them. That remarkable feat of time-telling probably exceeds the ability of most people to tell time during the waking hours. Brush (552), who regularly slept about 8 hours, was able to awaken at a chosen time in the morning by subvocally repeating 10 times when he went to bed: "Wake me up at x o'clock." The actual time of awakening was closer to the time set than to the habitual time of waking up in the morning. Bladder sensations did not seem to matter, except that, when marked, they led to awakening at an earlier hour than set.

Omwake and Loranz (3056) determined the ability of twenty college girls to wake up at a specified time and found that some subjects possessed such a special ability, whereas others did not. The most successful were also the most confident ones. In about half of the cases the good subjects awakened within

30 minutes of the appointed time, but some came closer than that, and a few woke up exactly on time. Out of one hundred students questioned, only eleven believed that they could awaken at an assigned hour (1059).

The ability of many persons not so much to wake up at a deliberately set time (3039) as to awaken spontaneously at almost the same hour every morning is related to the establishment and maintenance of a 24-hour rhythm, discussed in Chapter 15.

To summarize, awakening—the reverse of falling asleep—is usually gradual when spontaneous, but can be fairly sudden when brought about by powerful external or internal stimuli. Awakening is a characteristic of sleep, distinguishing it from such sleep-like states as coma or anesthesia. Immediately after awakening, a person can be just as drowsy as before going to sleep, and his performance is often paradoxically poorer than at night before going to bed. Partial or even complete awakenings occur several times during the night and are not usually remembered; they become more frequent toward the end of the customary period of sleep; finally, because of increasing difficulty in lapsing back into sleep, they culminate in overt termination of sleep, or "awakening" in the everyday meaning of this word.

Part 3

Periodicity

Chapter 15

The 24-Hour Sleep-Wakefulness and
Body-Temperature Rhythms

Periodicity is a common phenomenon in nature, expressing itself in the seasons of the year, the phases of the moon, the day and night of the rotation of the earth, the twice-daily ebb and flow of the tide. Some or all of these external changes affect the activity of organisms, ontogenetically and perhaps phylogenetically, giving rise to a variety of biological periodicities, superimposed on the intrinsic endocrine, digestive, rest-activity, and other physiological fluctuations (113, 141, 143, 299, 536, 647, 995, 1574, 1581, 1594, 1687, 1688, 2186, 3306, 3747). The courses, rounds, or series of repetitive or recurring phenomena, events, conditions, or states have been variously, and often interchangeably, designated as rhythms, cycles, or periods.

For the purposes of this discussion, the term rhythm will be used to designate a regularly recurring quantitative change in some particular variable biological process, irrespective of whether or not it takes place in a cell, tissue, structure, organism, or population. Two conditions are necessary to make such a recurring change into a rhythm: (*a*) it must be extrinsic in origin, depending upon a regular change in the environment, such as light or temperature, usually associated with terrestrial or cosmic periodicity, developing in each biological system de novo; and (*b*) when fully established, it must persist for some time, even when the environmental changes are absent. Except that the regulating mechanism need not be nervous, a rhythm may be likened to a conditioned response, which is also individually acquired and depends on an extrinsic reinforcement for its establishment, yet will persist for a shorter or longer time in the absence of such reinforcement. The term cycle, on the other hand, will apply to repetitive series of events or to successive changes of state, either qualitative or quantitative in nature, and its distinctive feature is the order of occurrence, rather than duration. Cycles are intrinsic in origin and have to run their course to be completed. They may be influenced by internal and external conditions, which may affect them quantitatively, but seldom qualitatively. A good example is the cardiac cycle which may be affected—in duration and magnitude of change—by drugs, nerve impulses, or temperature variations, but which is intrinsic in origin and development. A third type of biological recurrence, which, like the rhythm, is extrinsic in origin, but is so directly dependent on environmental changes that it shows no persistence of variations when the external conditions are made uniform, will be referred to as causal, synchronous, associated, or coupled periodicity. The regularity or irregularity of periodicity is a function of the external variation with which it is coupled (3543, 4166).

As an example of a rhythm, one may refer to the behavior of the hermit crab (*Clibanarius misanthropus Rino*), at Arcachon on the shore of the Atlantic Ocean, which is positively phototactic at neap tide, when the layer of water is thin, and negatively phototactic at spring tide, when, with the layer of water thick, it need not protect itself (1812). Brought into an aquarium, half-light and half-dark, it shows a definite 14-day rhythm, retreating into the dark portion of the tank during neap tide, then moving into the light part during spring tide. The development and persistence of this bi-weekly rhythm is certainly not a matter of "natural" organization, for the same crab, living on the shores of the Mediterranean Sea, where there are no tides, is always positively phototactic. External conditions rather than an innate hereditary mechanism must be responsible for the establishment of the fortnightly rhythm in the hermit crab. And yet many investigators hold that biological rhythms are inherited (1632) or, at least, endogenous, rather than exogenous in character (144, 2027), or partly one and partly the other (142, 144). In addition to the obvious 24-hour day-night periodicity, a 24-hour 50-minute lunar day rhythm has been discerned in the spontaneous activity of the rat (537). A similar double timing of pigment dispersion and oxygen consumption of the fiddler crab led Brown (535) to postulate the existence of a mechanism "which can perceive some kind of physical force in the environment hitherto not known to affect living organisms." That the moon is believed to have an influence on animal and human behavior is shown by the reference to insanity as "lunacy."

The terms applied to biological variations related to the 24-hour alternation of night and day include the Greek-derived nyctohemeral, diel, and diurnal. The term circadian was coined by Halberg (1584) to designate a periodicity of about 24 hours, in part individually acquired, but inborn, in the main. The term "diurnal" is often taken as the opposite of "nocturnal," and the lack of a word in English to comprise both night and day makes it desirable, to avoid any misunderstanding, to use the somewhat awkward number-word combination of "24-hour" period.

The alternation of sleep and wakefulness in man is a good example of the multiplicity of factors concerned in recurring phenomena. In the newborn infant, there is the operation of the 50- to 60-minute basic rest-activity cycle

(150), but it soon becomes coupled with the 3- to 4-hour gastric cycle and the daily astronomical and social periodicity, eventually becoming a 24-hour rhythm. Aside from the general effect of gastric motility (3335, 3336, 3912), 3-hour and 4-hour feeding schedules will lead to a marked increase in activity of neonates toward the end of the particular interfeeding periods (2690, 2878). On a "self-demand" feeding schedule (3717), the interfeeding periods were longer at night than in the daytime, with means in a study of 4 infants (2690) 3.61 and 2.86 hours, respectively, tending—incidentally—to be an integer of the basic rest-activity cycle.

As previously pointed out (p. 115), from birth on there is a disparity between the total hours of sleep during the two halves of the 24-hour period. Table 15.1 shows that the mean duration of sleep, between 8:00 P.M. and 8:00 A.M., for a group of infants under our observation (2196), was 8.5 hours during the third week of life. Night sleep time gradually rose to and then surpassed 10 hours during the twelfth week and thereafter remained remarkably constant to the end of the twenty-sixth week. An entirely different variation was found in the mean total duration of sleep for the 8:00 A.M. to 8:00 P.M. interval which even in the third week was not quite 6.5 hours, or two hours under the duration of the night sleep. The total length of the day sleep decreased slowly and continuously until it was a little over 3.5 hours in the twenty-sixth week. For the first half of the period of observation (weeks 3 to 14) the decrease in the day sleep almost exactly balanced the increase in the night sleep, but thereafter the decreasing values for the day sleep completely accounted for the progressive falling-off in the total duration of sleep per 24 hours.

The constantly increasing influence of acculturation and the resulting disparity between the day and night sleep-wakefulness demarcations are shown in the 6 curves of Figure 15.1. The day-night asymmetry already present in the first 4-week period (weeks 3 to 6) becomes more pronounced in the following 5 periods. The night portions of the curves (8:00 P.M. to 8:00 A.M.) are well established during the third 4-week period. However, in all 6 periods the incidence of sleep is greatest for the hours of 1:00 A.M. to 3:00 A.M.; the fractions of time spent in sleep during these two hours, for the 6 periods are, successively, 0.795, 0.895, 0.955, 0.970, 0.965, and 0.985. The day halves of the curves show two characteristic features. One is that the lowest incidence of sleep is not in the middle of the day, but toward its end, corresponding to the evening meal hours. For the first 3 periods the hours with the least sleep were 6:00 P.M. to 8:00 P.M., and for the last 3, 5:00 P.M. to 7:00 P.M.; the corresponding 6 values of diminishing sleep fractions were 0.460, 0.395, 0.295, 0.245, 0.225, and 0.190. The other feature is the establishment of regular daytime nap periods of 10:00 A.M. to noon, and 2:00 P.M. to 4:00 P.M. A suggestion of these naps can be seen in the curves for the third and fourth periods (weeks 11 to 18), but they are definitely marked-out in the last two periods (weeks 19 to 26).

In analyzing our findings, Gifford (1442) divided the first 6 months of the infant's life into two fairly equal parts. In the first trimester, when the decreasing daytime sleep hours were balanced by the increase in the duration of night sleep—the total sleep time remaining unchanged—the infant passes from "an undifferentiated phase" to an "evidence of ego functioning, the capacity for delaying immediate instinctual satisfaction, and a primitive awareness of time and external reality." In the second trimester, when the day sleep time continues to decrease, while the night sleep time remains unchanged, there is a "beginning of object relations." The infant acquires an occipital EEG pattern (p. 27), smiles, and "shows a rapid advance in perceptual integration . . . associated with increased awareness of his surroundings and with the capacity for visual communication between himself and his mother."

One girl infant's adjustment to the community 24-hour pattern was so striking as to merit special description. She was a first child, and her parents were suffi-

TABLE 15.1

PROGRESSIVE CHANGES IN THE GROUP MEAN DURATION OF
INFANTS' SLEEP FROM THE THIRD TO THE
TWENTY-SIXTH WEEK OF LIFE

Week	Number of Infants	Duration of Sleep in Hours		
		Total per 24 Hours	"Day" Half 8:00 A.M.– 8:00 P.M.	"Night" Half 8:00 P.M.– 8:00 A.M.
3	10	14.86	6.36	8.50
4	14	14.77	6.44	8.33
5	15	14.70	6.28	8.42
6	16	14.46	6.04	8.42
7	16	14.35	5.66	8.69
8	16	14.52	5.48	9.04
9	19	14.70	5.47	9.23
10	19	14.95	5.39	9.56
11	19	14.82	5.18	9.64
12	19	15.01	4.96	10.05
13	19	14.90	4.86	10.04
14	19	14.92	4.91	10.01
15	19	14.65	4.64	10.01
16	18	14.55	4.43	10.12
17	18	14.46	4.33	10.13
18	18	14.41	4.34	10.07
19	18	14.19	4.24	9.95
20	18	14.24	4.22	10.02
21	18	14.04	4.02	10.02
22	18	13.98	3.95	10.03
23	18	14.10	4.06	10.04
24	18	13.91	3.86	10.05
25	17	13.88	3.82	10.06
26	16	13.69	3.61	10.08

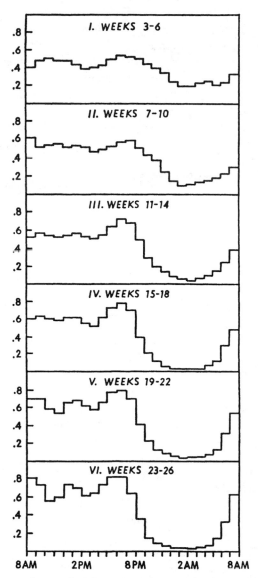

Fig. 15.1—The mean sleep-wakefulness partition in each of six successive 4-week periods of observation of a group of infants (2196). The 24 hour-marks, from 8:00 A.M., shown at the bottom of the lowermost section, apply to all sections. The height of the line at each hourly division represents the mean fraction of the hour during which the group was awake. The area below each composite demarcation line is the total fraction of wakefulness for the entire 24 hours of each 4-week period. Conversely, the areas above the composite demarcation lines are the corresponding sleep fractions. The mean total hours of sleep for the six periods were, successively, 14.70, 14.63, 14.91, 14.52, 14.11, and 13.90 hours. For weekly values see Table 15.1.

ciently indulgent to permit her to set her own sleep-wakefulness and feeding schedule. The top and bottom of Figure 15.2, in which the progress of this infant is shown, do not differ from any other infant's chart. They show an initial haphazard distribution of sleep and feedings and a terminal adjustment to an uninterrupted 10-hour sleep during the night (8:00 P.M. to 6:00 A.M.), with short naps and feedings during the intervening hours. But there the similarities end. The infant began her adjustment with a possibly lunar 25-hour periodicity. This periodicity is evident from the successive displacement to the right of the clusters of daily feedings, the white spaces of wakefulness, and the bands of "long" sleeps, which all together give the impression of a milky way running diagonally across. From the fourth to the middle of the seventh week a whole 24 hours was thus gained, and the milky way begins its second spiral. (It is best to envisage the chart as the side-surface of a cylinder, with a circumference of 24 hours, slit along the midnight line and laid flat. With a slight distortion, the lines would form a continuous time-line, as the end of one day is the beginning of the next.) The second turn of the milky way is whiter, due to a partial consolidation of the sleep and wakefulness fractions, and also slightly steeper, because of the shortening of the period from 25 hours to a mean of 24.86 hours during the 4-week interval between the middle of the seventh week and the middle of the eleventh. The mean total duration of sleep up to this point is slightly over 63 per cent of the time, which is quite in agreement with the corresponding figures for other infants. The third spiral of the milky way has a much greater slope than the first two, requiring 7 weeks (to the middle of the eighteenth week) to gain 24 hours, and the mean period is lowered to 24.5 hours. The mean total duration of sleep during the 7 weeks in question is down to 61 per cent of the time. From the middle of the eighteenth to the end of the twenty-first week, the consolidated long sleep hours, as well as the much widened light space, appear stationary, indicating that the periodicity is now down to the astronomically correct 24 hours. However, the adjustment to the community pattern is imperfect, as the long sleep starts at midnight or later. A secondary adjustment, involving a temporary shortening of the period to 23.86 hours, causing a leftward displacement of the night sleep to the 8:00 P.M. to 6:00 A.M. interval, occurred during weeks 22–24, and the last 2 weeks of observation again show a 24-hour periodicity, with adjustment—both astronomical and social—complete. The mean total duration of sleep from the middle of the eighteenth week fluctuated about 57 per cent of the time, which is again in accord with the data for other infants. How many other infants would manifest a similar non-24-hour periodicity prior to complete 24-hour adjustment, if their parents were as indulgent as those of this infant girl, is hard to say, but we noted a suggestion of spirals in the chart of another infant, who enjoyed a complete self-demand schedule of feedings. However, the charts for practically all of the other infants show a rather definite, though not always

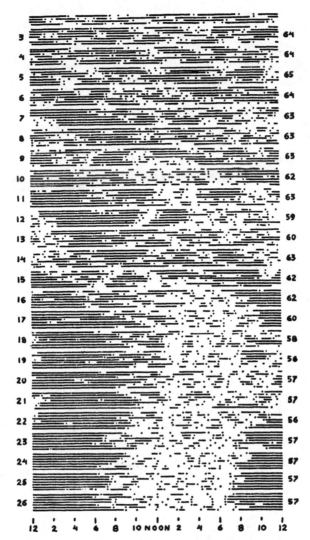

Fig. 15.2—The incidence of sleep, wakefulness, and feeding in Infant 4F, from the 11th to the 182d day of life (2196). Each line represents a 24-hour calendar day. The lines are sleep periods, measured to the nearest 5 minutes; the breaks in the lines, wakefulness; the dots, feedings. Each group of seven lines is separated from adjacent groups by a double space. The weeks are indicated on the left; percentages of time spent in sleep during the successive weeks, on the right; time, in 2-hourly intervals, at the bottom.

sharp, consolidation of the night sleep at the conventional hours by the twelfth to fourteenth week of life.

Lange (2363) published figures on day-night sleep-wakefulness distribution, from a complete lack of differentiation in premature neonates through age groups of 5 to 8 months, 11 to 21 months, and 4 to 13 years, confirming our findings on the establishment of the 24-hour sleep-wakefulness rhythm in human beings.

That there is a 24-hour variation in body temperature was known for a long time. Piéron (3192) gave 1842 as the date of the first systematic study by Gierse. Baerensprung (176) in 1851, in addition to self-observation, followed the temperatures of individuals of different ages, from infants to adults, and noted a coincidence of maxima and minima for both body temperatures and heart rates. Others (1889, 1890, 1987, 2195, 2655, 3043) observed the influence of muscular activity and food intake. The effects of sleep on body temperature were already considered (p. 58), but rest in bed for several days did not abolish the 24-hour curve (2786, 4272). The earlier view (1229, 1412) that the body-temperature changes were due to variations in the irritability of the regulating center was shown to be untenable (962). The endocrine system (1921) and "unknown" factors (528, 2024) were added to muscular activity, food intake, and sleep, as determinants of the 24-hour temperature rhythm.

The first systematic studies of the development of the body-temperature rhythm in human beings were made in 1904 by Jundell (2051) and in 1908 by Gofferjé (1465). Jundell's data are presented in Table 15.2, together with data we (2206) collected some 30 years later. Our observations were made on neonates at the Chicago Lying-in Hospital and on older infants and children at the Bobs Roberts Memorial Hospital. The newborn were entirely normal, and the older ones were in the hospital for observation or for the correction of nutritional disorders, were not "sick," and did not have fever. Their rectal temperature was determined every two hours, except that between midnight and 8:00 A.M. only one reading was made—at 4:00 A.M. The immediate environmental temperature was read off from a thermometer attached to the child's bed. The periods of sleep and wakefulness, of feeding, and activity were also noted.

From four to ten children of each of the following age groups were observed for about 10 days: newborn, older ones up to 6 months, 7 to 12 months, 13 to 24 months, 25 months to 6 years, and 7 to 13 years. For each subject we determined the daily temperature mean range (MR) and then the range of the mean of the composite curve for the period (RM). We also noted the variations in the individual mean 24-hour temperature ranges and constructed composite curves for the different age groups. The room-temperature data were handled in the same manner as those for the body temperature. In addition, we looked for the relative constancy of high and low temperature values with respect to their magnitude and hours of occurrence. This constancy, or lack of it, could be determined for the individual or age group by obtaining the ratio of MR to RM, which was high when the high and low temperature points were reached at different hours on different days, and approached 1.00 as the 24-hour temperature curves became more superimposable.

TABLE 15.2

THE RATIO OF THE MEAN 24-HOUR TEMPERATURE RANGE (MR) IN A GIVEN AGE GROUP
TO THE RANGE OF THE MEAN (RM) OR COMPOSITE 24-HOUR BODY-
TEMPERATURE CURVE FOR THAT AGE GROUP

(Degrees in Centigrade)

Age Group	Number of Sub-jects	Variation in Individual 24-Hour Tem-perature Ranges	Group Mean 24-Hour Tempera-ture Range (MR)	The Mean 24-Hour Body-Temperature Curve for the Age Group			MR/RM
				High	Low	Range (RM)	
Based on Our Data (2206)							
Newborn..........	10	0.35–0.74°	0.62°	36.95°	36.68°	0.27°	2.30
1–5 months........	5	0.62–1.02	0.80	37.28	36.72	0.56	1.43
7–11 months.......	6	0.74–1.15	0.98	37.38	36.56	0.82	1.20
14–22 months......	6	1.18–1.80	1.67	37.51	35.95	1.56	1.07
3–6 years.........	4	1.39–1.86	1.56	37.50	36.15	1.35	1.16
7–13 years........	4	1.10–1.82	1.44	37.73	36.36	1.37	1.05
Based on Data of Jundell (2051)							
Newborn..........	18	0.17–0.53°	0.38°	36.86°	36.76°	0.10°	3.80
Newborn..........	15	0.23–0.63	0.44	36.87	36.72	0.15	2.93
Newborn..........	14	0.17–0.67	0.39	36.96	36.70	0.26	1.50
Under 6 months....	54	0.32–1.50	0.69	37.33	36.81	0.52	1.33
2–5 years.........	3	0.94–1.43	1.22	37.47	36.37	1.10	1.11
19–22 years........	5	0.85–1.23	1.06	37.24	36.24	1.00	1.06

In Table 15.2 it can be seen that there is a parallelism between the two sets of body-temperature figures, but that ours are uniformly higher than Jundell's. This discrepancy may be due to the fact that our 24-hour curves were based on 10 observations daily, whereas his were based on only 6. In a general way, the group mean of the 24-hour temperature range increases with age, but during the second year of life there appears rather abruptly a marked increase in the magnitude of that temperature range, which is now almost doubled in value and definitely exceeds that of older children and adults. This increased range involves a very low minimal temperature, as only in this age group does it fall below 36° C. It will further be noted that the MR:RM ratios are high at first (also higher for our subjects than for Jundell's, and probably for the reason stated above), but come close to 1.00 before the children reach the age of two years, indicating a more complete 24-hour regularity.

In sections 1–4*A* of Figure 15.3 are shown the successive daily temperature curves as well as the composite curves for a neonate, an infant of three and a half months, a fifteen-month-old child, and one nine years of age. We selected the three-and-a-half-month-old infant as the one that had the highest 24-hour temperature range in its age group, and the fifteen-month-old child as the one with the lowest in that category. We thus obtained 24-hour temperature ranges of about the same magnitude (1.02° and 1.18°, respectively), although the means of 24-hour ranges for the two groups were 0.8° and 1.67°. Yet the successive daily temperature curves of the older child can be superimposed upon each other more easily than those of the younger (secs. 2 and 3 of Fig. 15.3).

That living for a time in a world run on a 24-hour schedule is in itself insufficient for the establishment of a pronounced 24-hour temperature rhythm can be seen from sections 5 and 5*A* of Figure 15.3, in which the body-temperature variations of a twelve-month-old hydrocephalic child are plotted. No regular temperature variation is evident in section 5, and the mean 24-hour range is only 0.46°, or in the category of the newborn. Section 5*A* shows a slight tendency for the room temperature to be higher in the daytime than at night, and the same is true of the composite body-temperature curve. Furthermore, the 24-hour body-temperature curve may be lost even after it has been presumably well established, as appears from section 6, which represents the variations in body temperature in a child of nine years who had developed a brain tumor and had been unconscious for about a year. Here, too, one finds a mean 24-hour body-temperature range of only 0.58°, with a suggestion of 24-hour regularity (sec. 6*A* of Fig. 15.3). That child had to be fed artificially and was usually given three meals between 8:00 A.M. and 6:00 P.M. When the feedings were spaced equally, every 8 hours, the slight 24-hour regularity was lost, as is shown in sections 7 and 7*A,* and the MR:RM ratio increased from 1.53 to 2.66, although the mean daily temperature range remained unchanged (0.6°). Usually the temperature of this child fluctuated between 37° and 38°, but from time to time it would go through periods of hyperthermia with much greater temperature fluctuations. The temperatures for two such periods are plotted in section 8, from which it can be seen that, with some delay and irregularity, the body temperature seems to vary with the room temperature.

Our results demonstrated that, while there may be a 24-hour fluctuation in body temperature even in young infants, the 24-hour temperature rhythm, in the sense of a regularly recurring and superimposable variation, first appears during the second year of a child's life. A gradual approach to that state can be discerned during the first year in that the 24-hour variation increases in magnitude practically from birth on. The full establishment of the body-temperature curve can be placed in the second year of life because of the sudden

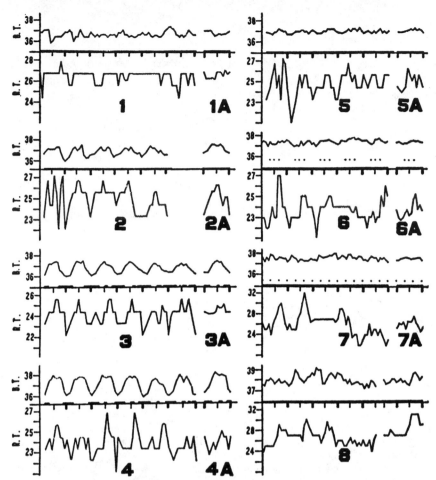

FIG. 15.3—Ontogenesis of the 24-hour body-temperature rhythm. In all sections body temperature (B.T.) is plotted above and room temperature (R.T.) below the horizontal line. Temperature figures are in degrees C., and the scale is the same in all sections, except for room temperatures in sections 7, 7A, and 8, where it is half that scale. Time is indicated on the horizontal line in 12-hour intervals—a thick mark for midnight, and a thin one for noon. In sections 3, 3A, 4, and 4A, the thin portions of the horizontal lines refer to periods of wakefulness. Section 1A is plotted from the means of values used for section 1, and the same applies to the other A sections.

Sections 1 and 1A: normal newborn infant, first six days of life.

Sections 2 and 2A: normal infant, three and a half months old—a suggestion of regularity in the 24-hour body-temperature curves.

Sections 3 and 3A: normal child, fifteen months old. The body-temperature ranges are about the same as in section 2, but the regularity is more marked.

Sections 4 and 4A: normal child, nine years of age. Note nicks in daytime body-temperature plateaus, coinciding with naps.

Sections 5 and 5A: infant, twelve months old, with hydrocephalus.

Sections 6 and 6A: child, nine years old, with brain tumor and hydrocephalus, unconscious for one year. There is a suggestion of higher body temperatures following feedings (indicated by dots above the horizontal line). MR:RM = 1.53.

Sections 7 and 7A: the same child as in section 6, but feeding routine changed—the three daily feedings are separated by equal time intervals. Suggestion of regularity in body-temperature curve is lost. MR:RM = 2.66.

Section 8: the same child as in sections 6 and 7, during two of the occasional periods of hyperthermia.

marked increase in the 24-hour body-temperature range and the approach of the MR:RM ratio to 1.00. Learning to walk, with its resulting widening of the sphere of the child's activity, is probably the outstanding influence during that time. It is in this year that the mean minimal temperature is below 36° C., suggesting that the almost incessant waking-hour activity of children under two years of age leads to greater fatigue and more complete muscular relaxation.

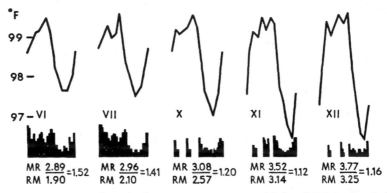

Fig. 15.4—Composite 24-hour body-temperature curves of infant MM in the sixth, seventh, tenth, eleventh, and twelfth months of life. Both the mean daily temperature range (MR) and the range of the composite five-day temperature curve (RM) increased as the infant grew older; at the same time the MR value approached the RM, showing a greater superimposability of the daily curves and a smaller MR:RM ratio. The maxima of all five composite temperature curves are about the same, with the greater 24-hour temperature ranges due to progressively lower minima.

The shaded areas under the five body-temperature curves represent hourly variations in motility, recorded by the device described in Chapter 10. During the sixth and seventh months the infant remained in his crib all the time, but his motility was much lower during the night sleep than in the daytime naps, as shown by the two slight dips in the motility chart. Distinct dips in the plateaus of the last two body-temperature curves correspond to the two daytime naps.

The establishment of the 24-hour body-temperature curve in an individual infant was followed by Mullin (2941), who obtained MR:RM ratios of 2.5–3.0 during the first five months of the infant's life. From the sixth month on, the ratio began to decrease rapidly. It can be seen in Figure 15.4 that, as ranges of the 5 composite 24-hour body-temperature curves increased, the MR:RM ratios decreased. The maximum body temperatures were not changed, and the increase in range was due mainly to a lowering of the minimal temperature during the night, from a little over 97.5° F., in the sixth and seventh months, to below 96.4°, in the eleventh and twelfth. During the last three months of the first year the infant gradually became more active and crawled around a great deal when taken out of his crib. At the age of eleven to twelve months this infant reached a stage in the establishment of a regular body-temperature rhythm usually attained several months later.

On the other hand, mere staying in bed does not necessarily abolish a previously established 24-hour body-temperature rhythm. We were able to follow the oral temperature changes of a young man who had been in bed for sixteen months following an attack of acute anterior poliomyelitis. This patient had complete and total paralysis of all muscles of both upper extremities and partial paralysis of the other muscles. On the basis of 4 weeks' observations, with oral temperatures taken bi-hourly from 8:00 A.M. to 10:00 P.M., that patient showed a perfectly normal body-temperature curve. His lowest temperature figure was always at 8:00 A.M., with a mean of 97.6° F. The biggest change was from 8:00 A.M. to 10:00 A.M., after which a fairly good plateau was maintained for the rest of the day, with a peak at 4:00 P.M. (98.8°). Thereafter the temperature began to fall slightly, and at 10:00 P.M. it was 98.4°. The patient followed a normal routine with respect to sleep and wakefulness as one could predict from his body-temperature figures.

Additional observations were made on seven institutionalized feeble-minded patients, six children and one adult. An attempt was made to study children of very low mental development, classified as idiots or near that level, spending their entire time in bed, so that their motility as well as temperature could be recorded over the 24-hour period. Rectal temperature was taken every two hours by nurses of the institution, and motility readings, by the "work-adder" method, were made every hour by orderlies who also wrote down on the record sheet whether the patients were asleep or awake and, if awake, whether they were lying quietly or were active. The six children could be divided into two groups: (*a*) children who were not particularly active in the daytime, though they slept well at night; and (*b*) children who showed a very good 24-hour variation of observed, as well as recorded, motility. Table 15.3 shows their daily body-temperature ranges, with the means. The ratios of the latter (MR) to the range of the mean, or composite, 24-hour temperature curve for the period of observation (RM) appear to be high for the first group and put it developmentally—by reference to Table 15.2—into the class of infants under six months of age. As the mental age of two children was close to one year, while that of the third was over two years, it indicates that a 24-hour variation in muscular activity, in addition to cerebral development, is necessary for the establishment of a good 24-hour temperature curve. This condition was met by the second group. Their MR:RM temperature ratios would put them among infants between six months and one year of age, and their mental ages corresponded to this temperature classification. Here a well-developed 24-hour rhythm of activity seemed to be the deciding factor. The 24-hour temperature and motility curves of two children, one from each group, are shown in Figure 15.5. It will be noted that the rise of the body temperature of St in the morning precedes, and the fall in the evening follows, the increase and decrease, respectively, of the child's motor activity. This was also true of the other two children in this group, Sh and Si, and is indicative of a lack of immediate dependence of temperature on motility, which characterizes an established body-temperature curve. From Fa's records it can be seen that there is no parallelism whatsoever between the motility and the temperature curves, and that, also, applied to Wh and Ma.

Patient Ha was in a class by herself, as she was twenty-nine years old and showed a very poor 24-hour motility rhythm. However, her MR:RM ratio was the lowest of all and put her, from the temperature standpoint, among older

TABLE 15.3

THE RATIO OF THE MEAN 24-HOUR BODY-TEMPERATURE RANGE OF EACH OF SEVEN IDIOTS (MR)
TO THE RANGE OF THE MEAN OR COMPOSITE 24-HOUR BODY-TEMPERATURE
CURVE OF THE SAME INDIVIDUAL (RM)

(Degrees in Fahrenheit)

SUBJECT	CHRON-OLOGI-CAL AGE IN YEARS	MEN-TAL AGE IN MONTHS	24-HOUR ACTIVITY VARIA-TION	NUM-BER OF DAYS OF OBSER-VATION	VARIATION IN 24-HOUR BODY-TEM-PERATURE RANGE	MEAN OF 24-HOUR RANGE (MR)	MEAN 24-HOUR BODY-TEMPERATURE CURVE			MR/RM
							High	Low	Range (RM)	
Fa (female)....	12	13	Poor	14	0.2–1.6°	0.7°	98.3°	98.1°	0.2°	3.50
Wh (female)....	11½	28	Poor	9	0.3–2.2	1.0	98.3	97.8	0.5	2.00
Ma (male).....	11	11	Absent	15	1.2–3.0	1.8	98.9	97.8	1.1	1.63
St (female).....	10	11	Good	11	0.8–3.2	1.9	98.9	97.5	1.4	1.36
Sh (female)....	7	11	Good	15	0.6–2.4	1.6	98.9	97.7	1.2	1.33
Si (male).......	13	10	Good	19	1.0–3.0	1.7	99.0	97.7	1.3	1.31
Ha (female)....	29	13	Poor	14	0.3–1.6	1.0	98.6	97.7	0.9	1.11

children, even though her mental age was thirteen months. Whether we were dealing with the effects of a certain feeding and sleeping routine that had been repeatedly imposed on Ha for twenty-nine years is hard to say.

Concerning the mentality, motility, and general behavior data on the six children, they may be said to confirm the results previously reported by us (2206), and point to the individual establishment of the 24-hour body-temperature curve. This curve is conditioned by mental and physical development, routine performance of certain tasks, and an asymmetry with respect to food intake and sleep.

Even a uniformity in hours of sleep and schedule of meals and activity does not insure a completely repetitive 24-hour body-temperature curve in human beings. The occurrences of everyday life are likely to influence the temperature through excitement, resulting in temporary emotional hyperthermia or "psychogenic fever" (51, 512, 1135, 2185, 3313, 4188). Renbourn and Taylor (3314), in thirty-two subjects, found that the rectal temperature was not always higher than the oral one, and that values for rectal temperatures at distances of 5.5, 13, and 21 cm from the anus did not show any orderly gradient in different individuals. Mellette and associates (2768) noted a sex difference in the incidence of maxima and minima of the rectal temperature curves. Peak temperatures in women occurred two hours later and troughs over one hour earlier than in men, resulting in a greater temperature drop per hour, though the total decrease was smaller for women. By taking temperature readings for several days, one usually succeeds in obtaining a smooth 24-hour curve, but such a composite curve does

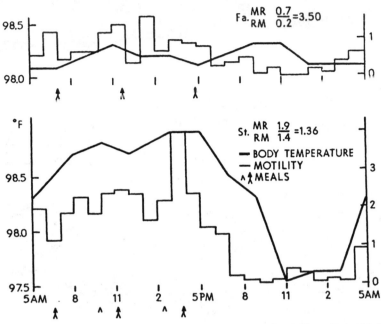

Fig. 15.5—The 24-hour variations in body temperature and motility of two high-grade idiots with infantile cerebral palsy (Table 15.3). *Upper records:* no well-defined body-temperature curve; motility slightly higher in the daytime than at night. *Lower records:* marked 24-hour body-temperature and motility variations; patient usually asleep between 6:00 P.M. and 5:00 A.M. and very active in the daytime, particularly in the afternoon.

not reveal the magnitude of the day-to-day variations in temperature for the same hour. Over 18,000 temperature readings we have accumulated (2202) permitted us to determine the time of incidence and the constancy of the maxima and minima, as well as the degree of dispersion or concentration of the values pertaining to particular phases of the various temperature rhythms. In the several parts of Figure 15.6 are histograms, arranged horizontally, for the frequency with which certain temperature readings occurred at different hours in individual subjects. The ranges of readings for almost any hour often exceeded the range of the mean 24-hour body-temperature curve. Yet, distinct modes can usually be discerned in frequency distribution curves, formed by the right-side ends of the histograms. The 6:00 A.M. temperatures of parts *A* and *B*, pertaining to one person, show at once the least dispersion and greatest resemblance to the conventional probability curves. Although the mean maxima of both curves are at 2:00 P.M. and minima at 2:00 A.M., many 2:00 P.M. temperatures are lower than some 2:00 A.M. values. On the contrary, parts *C* and *D*, also of one individual, show a much greater concentration of temperature values for every hour of the day and night. In *C* all the temperatures taken from 11:00 A.M. to 7:00 P.M. were higher than all the temperatures from 11:00 P.M. to 6:00 A.M. The maxima of both *C* and *D* are at 3:00 P.M., while the minima occur at 3:00

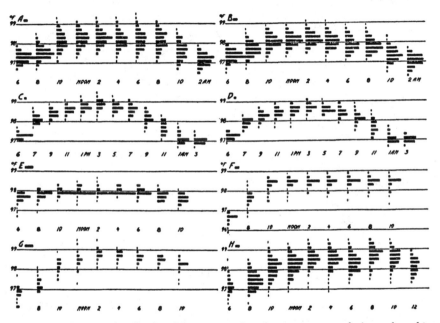

FIG. 15.6—Frequency distribution histograms of oral temperatures of six male subjects for the different hours of the day and night. The vertical temperature scale is the same for all eight parts of the figure. The succession of hours is not a time scale, but only reference points to the groups of horizontal bars above them. The length of each horizontal bar corresponds to the number of times particular temperature values occurred, with the bar next to each letter representing 20 readings.

A: 3192 temperature readings, 10 per 24 hours, for subject K during three summers, mid-May to mid-October; *B:* 3352 temperature readings for the same subject during four winters, October to March; *C:* 3254 temperature readings, 12 per 24 hours, for subject R during three summers, June to August; *D:* 3236 temperature readings for the same subject during four winters, December to February; *E:* 656 temperature readings, 9 per day, for subject F, from March to May of one year; *F:* 1019 temperature readings, 9 per day, for subject H, from February to August of one year; *G:* 357 temperature readings, 9 per day, for subject M, from February to April of one year; *H:* 2962 temperature readings, 10 per day, for subject L, for one year.

A.M., giving a 12-hour separation of the two, as in parts *A* and *B*. Frequency distribution curves of the incidence of the maxima and minima, not reproduced, also resembled probability curves, with a greater dispersion of the hours of individual daily maxima than of the daily minima. This difference results in a smoother crest and a sharper trough of the 24-hour curves. Part *G* resembles parts *A* to *D*, even though it is confined to the waking hours and is based on a rather small number of days. The mean maximum is 98.81°, occurring at 2:00 P.M., and the rise is somewhat steeper than the fall.

A different type of curve is shown in part *H*. This person's temperature modes were all the same from noon to 4:00 P.M., although the 2:00 P.M. mean was the highest, but the maximum daily temperature was reached only at 8:00 P.M. The minimum was at 4:00 A.M. (not shown in the figure), with the maximum-minimum interval about 8 hours. In these four individuals 24-hour temperature minima occurred at about the same time, during sleep, while the maxima were reached either in the afternoon or in the evening, but were constant for the particular person.

A third type of curve is seen in parts *E* and *F*. Instead of a peak, there is a plateau, which is quite distinct in *E,* and almost extreme in *F*. In *E* the morning rise was small, and the modes were the same, 98.0°, from 8:00 A.M. to 8:00 P.M. The mean temperatures did not vary more than 0.02° from noon to 4:00 P.M. In *F* the rise was sharper from 6:00 A.M. to 10:00 A.M., but thereafter the mode was the same, 98.6° F., till 10:00 P.M. From noon to 8:00 P.M., the mean temperatures did not vary by more than 0.07° F. This was the only subject whose temperature was the hypothetical 98.6° F. in about 40 per cent of all the readings made between 10:00 A.M. and 10:00 P.M.

To summarize, the development and maintenance of 24-hour sleep-wakefulness and body-temperature rhythms stem from being born into, and living in, a family and community run according to alternations of light and darkness, resulting from the period of rotation of the earth around its axis.

Chapter 16

24-Hour Variation in Activity and Performance

The adaptation of man and higher animals in their activity and rest to the alternation of day and night is well known, but the absence of such a day-and-night rhythm in lower animals, and in the young of higher ones, was brought to light by Szymanski (3897–99), who obtained activity records, or actograms, of a wide variety of animals (p. 81). Szymanski found that periods of activity and rest alternated in all the species observed, but, with respect to coincidence or non-coincidence of the activity rhythms with the 24-hour succession of day and night, he divided the animals into two classes, which are referred to here as monocyclic and polycyclic. Albino rats are polycyclic, with 10, or 12 to 16 (4141) periods of activity in 24 hours. Dancing mice have 9 such cycles; white mice, 16; and gray mice, 19.

Szymanski classified canary birds with adult human beings as monocyclic creatures which have a highly developed sense of sight and therefore take one unbroken rest period during the darkness of the night. Polycyclic animals, on the other hand, receive their information about external happenings mainly through their tactile and olfactory senses. There is, then, during growth and development a gradual transition from the tactile and gustatory perception of the polycyclic human nursling to the optical predominance seen in the monocyclic child.

An animal may be polycyclic and still be influenced to some extent by the alternations of day and night. Rats are predominantly "night" animals, though not monocyclic. Galamini (1337) studied the habits of several white rats. They would wake up about 4:00 P.M., eat, move around a great deal until midnight, sleep for 3 to 4 hours, get up and remain active until 8:00 A.M., when they would sleep for 8 hours, resuming their activity at 4:00 P.M. Their body temperature was also dicyclic: first maximum at 10:00 to 11:00 P.M.; first minimum at 4:00 A.M.; second maximum at 7:00 A.M.; second minimum at 1:00 to 5:00 P.M. The British short-tailed vole (field mouse), Microtus, was observed by Davis (837) to have a short 2- to 4-hour rhythm of feeding activity and a longer 24-hour activity cycle, with its peak following sunset, and a higher mean activity during the night than in the daytime. Herring and Brody (1717) found the peak of metabolic activity of the rat to be before midnight and the trough before noon, the difference in oxygen consumption from maximum to minimum amounting to 25 to 30 per cent. The horse, as observed by Steinhart (3798), has its longest period of sleep between 1:00 and 5:00 A.M., and, when kept in the stable, its longest waking period from 3:00 to 8:00 P.M. Among the six hundred horses he studied, some had as few as 3, others as many as 16, periods of sleep, not equally distributed. The mean number of sleep periods was 9, with 4 of these in the lying position. The horse hardly ever lies down for more than an hour and is rarely asleep in any position for more than 3 hours at a time. The free activity of sheep and pigs, from 6:00 A.M. to 6:00 P.M., amounted to 78 per cent and 88 per cent, respectively, of their 24-hour totals (801).

Wald and Jackson (4101) noted that rats increased their running activity several times, if deprived of food or water. They concluded that "high running is not, therefore, a reliable sign of well being. . . . When healthy, intact animals are most completely provided with their needs, they run minimally." Mice have also been shown to increase their activity prior to feeding, presumably from hunger (7). Rabbits, under laboratory conditions, with continuous access to food, were most active at night (2195). When food was available only for 6 hours in the daytime, the animals quickly adapted themselves to this feeding routine, and their activity became rather monocyclic, increasing sharply in the morning, prior to feeding time. Thus, activity of polycyclic animals can be affected both by the amount and hours of availability of food.

The total motility was found to be about 6 hours out of 24 for the non-hibernating hedgehog (1719), as well as for the rabbit (2195). In the human subject one can compare night and day motility only when the subject is bed-ridden or is kept in bed for some special purpose. The feeble-minded children described in the preceding chapter showed that a good 24-hour activity variation was associated with a well-established body-temperature curve. Page (3075) recorded the motility of five normal adults for a mean of 17 days and 10 nights each. The "day" motility was recorded in the morning only, from 8:00 to 11:00 A.M., and the night (sleep) motility, from 9:00 P.M. to 6:00 A.M. The mean rest periods for the group were over 6 minutes in the daytime and over 11 minutes during sleep at night. On the other hand, the mean number of movements per hour was 7.86 for the day period and 4.63 for the night. We obtained motility records on two normal individuals who spent several 48-hour periods in bed. Daytime (waking) motility was found to be 6 times as great as night (sleep) motility for each subject. Although there was no consistency in the hour-to-hour fluctuations in motility during the waking hours, the night motility pattern was preserved. In each case there was greater motility during the second half of the night than during the first.

That the individual's capacity for doing mental or physical work is not the same throughout the waking period has been known for a long time. Many attempts have been made to detect such variations in different tests. Lombard (2552) found that the greatest knee-jerk was obtained in the morning, right after breakfast, and that from then on there was a falling-off in the height of the response till bedtime. Dresslar (979) determined the time required to tap a telegraph key 300 times, running six tests daily at 2-hour intervals, from 8:00 A.M. to 6:00 P.M. Speed of performance was lowest at 8:00 A.M., improved gradually up to 4:00 P.M., and fell off a little at 6:00 P.M. Dresslar did not study performance in the evening, but Bergström (306) measured muscular efficiency from 7:00 A.M. to 10:00 P.M. and obtained a rather smooth curve of performance, with minima early in the morning and late at night and a maximum at 2:00 P.M. However, other tests made by Bergström led him to conclude that "there is no general type of daily rhythm." Marsh (2691), in a variety of tests involving muscular activity, reported the type of performance curve obtained by Dresslar and by Bergström, but he also had conflicting results which he ascribed to interfering factors. Hollingworth (1818) found that performance in more strictly motor tests showed a well-defined curve, whereas in "mental" tests there was a gradual decrease in efficiency from early in the morning to the end of the waking period. He concluded that there was no evidence of "organic rhythms or diurnal factors" in the performance of the tests. Gates (1372, 1373), studying the efficiency curve of 165 college students, observed an improvement up to noon, a falling-off after lunch, a new climb to a midafternoon maximum, then a downward tendency until the end of the school day. Freeman and Hovland (1274), in a review of the literature on this topic, prepared a table of contributions on variation in sensory, motor, and mental performance. They divided the performance curves into four classes: (*a*) a continuous rise in performance through the whole period of observation; (*b*) a continuous fall; (*c*) a morning rise and an afternoon fall; and (*d*) the reverse of *c*. All the curves we have obtained fit into class *c*, namely, a peak in the middle of the waking period.

Considering the possible interrelationship between performance and muscular tonus and between the latter and body temperature, we (2182) studied the speed and accuracy with which various manipulations could be carried out, employing a number of tests that could be easily repeated several times during the waking period. At first we used only such tests as could be performed on the subject by himself, at home, immediately after waking up in the morning and just before going to bed. The tests were made five times daily: immediately upon getting up, one hour later, just before the noon meal, just before the evening meal, and just before going to bed. Each of the six subjects performed one or more tests at a time, for 20 days or more, and the mean figures for the speed and accuracy of performance at different times of the day were determined. One subject was made to go through a number of tests ten times daily for 20 days, as a check upon the shape of the curves based on figures obtained from the five-tests-a-day series. In many cases there was a continued improvement in performance with the repetition of a test, but this improvement did not influence the relationship of the mean values for the different times of the day. To compare the efficiency of performance in the several tasks done during the day, the first value for speed or accuracy was considered as unity, and the reciprocals of the ratios of the later values to the first one were used as indices of performance at other times of the day. The tasks were selected from a wide list of standard tests, all involving muscular activity, either as movement or as steadiness. There were no problems to solve, and, except for multiplication, the individual tests required little or no mental activity on the part of the subject.

The six tests requiring no special apparatus were: (*a*) dealing a pack of cards into four hands, face of cards downward (156 cards); (*b*) sorting the same pack of cards, face upward, according to the denomination; (*c*) drawing a line between the double lines of a five-pointed star seen as reflected by a mirror, without touching either of the double lines—"mirror drawing"; (*d*) copying a text of five-letter nonsense syllables, 400 letters in all; (*e*) transcribing a text of 400 letters into a code that had been previously learned; (*f*) multiplying an eight-digit number by another eight-digit number on paper, three multiplications to a test. In all these tests performance was based on the time it took to accomplish a given task (measured by a stop-watch), and in the last four tests on the number of errors made. More cerebral activity was obviously involved in tests *d–f* than in *a–c*. A test for steadiness was (*g*) the ability to hold a metal stylus in one of several holes, of varying diameter, in a metal plate, without touching the edges of the hole. Any contact between the stylus and the plate closed an electric circuit which actuated a counter. Scoring was based on the number of contacts made in three one-minute trials separated from each other by one minute of rest. Another test for steadiness was (*h*) the ability to stand upright, with eyes closed. The inevitable swaying of the body in the course of one minute was recorded (2400). As a rule, two or more tests were run at the same sitting at the end of which the body temperature was measured by means of a clinical thermometer held in the mouth for 5 minutes.

There was an agreement in the results obtained on the same test in different subjects. The curves of both speed and accuracy of performance showed a well-marked rhythm, with minima early in the morning and late at night and a maximum in the middle of the day. In most cases where five tests were made daily, the mean figures for the noon tests were slightly higher than for the 6:00 P.M. tests, the actual maximum probably lying in between but closer to the noon hour. The composite body-temperature curve was somewhat higher at 6:00 P.M. than at noon, with the highest temperature attained later than the hour corresponding to the maximum of performance. Otherwise the temperature curve was quite parallel to that of performance. Of the remaining three daily trials, the performance immediately upon getting up was usually but not always inferior to that obtained just before going to bed, an observation made by previous workers. The second morning trial, one hour after the first, yielded results almost always higher than those obtained late in the evening. For illustrative purposes the mean figures for speed and accuracy of performance for 20 days in one subject, from 7:00 A.M. to 11:00 P.M., with ten tests daily instead of five, are given in Figure 16.1. It can be seen that in this subject the curve of

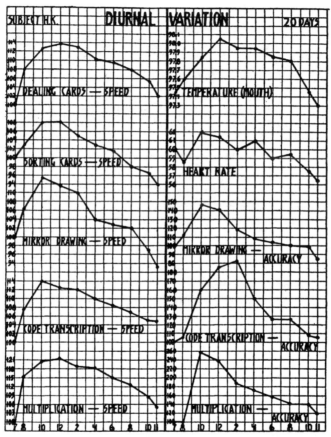

FIG. 16.1—Variation in speed and accuracy of performance, expressed as reciprocals of the ratios of the time it took to perform a task and the number of errors made to the time and errors made in the first series of tests at 7:00 A.M., at which hour the speed and accuracy of performance were taken to be 100. One subject, 10 trials per day, means for 20 days. The actual mean figures for the 7:00 A.M. trials were: dealing cards, 45.5 seconds; sorting cards, 96.5 seconds; mirror drawing, 17.1 seconds, 8.4 errors; code transcription, 291 seconds, 1.28 errors; multiplication, 283 seconds, 4.9 errors. Mouth temperature, in degrees F., and heart rate, in beats per minute, are given in actual figures and not as reciprocals of basal values.

performance reached its maximum rather early in the day, but the same was true of his body-temperature curve. The swaying (ataxia) tests, as well as hand steadiness, showed a similar parallelism between the body-temperature curves and those of performance. In Figure 16.2 body temperature and hand steadiness, the latter expressed as the reciprocal of the number of contacts the stylus made with the edges of the opening, were plotted for two subjects on the basis of 20 days' trials. As no observations were made between noon and 6:00 P.M., it was impossible to say just when the best performance occurred, but in one subject it was probably closer to noon, while in the other it was nearer 6:00 P.M.

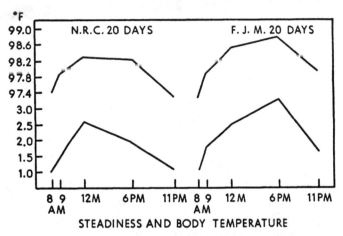

STEADINESS AND BODY TEMPERATURE

Fig. 16.2—Variation in hand steadiness, expressed as reciprocals of the ratios of the numbers of contacts made in three 1-minute tests to the number of contacts made at the 8:00 A.M. trials, at which time the steadiness was taken to be 1. Two subjects, five trials per day, means for 20 days. *Upper curves:* body temperature, in degrees F., in terms of actual figures, and not as reciprocals of basal values; *lower curves:* hand steadiness, with mean numbers of contacts at the 8:00 A.M. trials equaling 27.6 for subject C, and 21.9 for subject M.

The subject with the early peak of steadiness had a correspondingly early temperature maximum, and the subject with the late peak of steadiness had a late temperature crest. Omwake (3055) also found that hand steadiness and the ability to stand upright with least swaying were better in the afternoon than early in the morning, but she, like all the other workers in this field, did not determine the variations in body temperature at the various testing periods.

Because of the definite relation of the speed and accuracy of carrying out certain tasks to body temperature, we later (2205) investigated the possible relation of body temperature to performances which were purely sensorimotor and sensory-mental-motor—simple reaction time (RT) and choice RT. The tests were made on six subjects at various times of the day: at 9:00 A.M. and 11:00 A.M., and at 1:00, 3:00, 5:00, 7:00, and 9:00 P.M. A complete test consisted of twenty trials each for (*a*) simple RT to white light; (*b*) simple RT to sound of a telegraph key; (*c*) choice RT to green light but not to red; (*d*) choice RT to sound of a bell but not to that of a telegraph key. The apparatus used was a Hipp chronoscope measuring RT in milliseconds. There was for a time a gradual improvement in RT scores, but this improvement was not related to the influence of body temperature, which manifested itself at different levels of achievement.

The results obtained in this study yielded a curve showing a progressive decrease in RT during the morning and early afternoon and a rise in the late

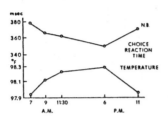

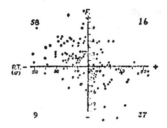

FIG. 16.3—Variation in RT to visual stimuli, with choice, and oral temperature for subject B, based on means for 12 to 23 trials for the different hours of the day, each trial comprising 20 RTs. *Upper curve:* RT in milliseconds; *lower curve:* temperature in degrees F.

FIG. 16.4—Relationship between changes in body temperature and changes in visual RT for subject T, based on 120 pairs of observations, usually separated by 2 or 3 hours. Body-temperature changes are plotted along the ordinates, and RT changes along the abscissae. In the majority of pairs of observations a change in body temperature in one direction was accompanied by a change in RT in the opposite direction, 95 (58 + 37) showing such a relationship, against 25 (16 + 9) in which body temperature and RT varied in the same direction.

afternoon and evening. That this variation in RT frequently was related to the body-temperature curve can be seen in the sample curve for one of the subjects, giving the temperature and visual choice RT (Fig. 16.3). The ability to respond promptly appears to be best in the middle of the day, when the temperature is highest, and poorest in the morning and late evening, when the body temperature is lowest.

A fairly good relationship between body temperature and RT was observed regardless of the time of day, indicating that there is probably no RT curve independent of the temperature. On the contrary, it would appear that RT was always connected with the body temperature, which, whenever it changed, was accompanied by a change in the opposite direction in RT. The relationship between temperature and RT was brought out by the data which were obtained by averaging together the RTs for tests made when the temperatures were the same, regardless of time of day. This inverse relationship was true of both simple and choice RTs.

Further analysis of the temperature and RT relationship was made by comparing pairs of successive tests made on the same day. The paired tests for each subject were divided into groups on the basis of whether the oral temperature in the second tests was higher or lower than in the first. The corresponding changes in RT from the first test to the second were then examined for the number of increases, decreases, and no differences within each temperature-change division. The evidence indicates an inverse relationship between RT and body-temperature changes. There were more than three times as many cases of RT changes in the opposite direction to that of temperature as there were cases of their moving in the same direction (Fig. 16.4).

The foregoing data were based on spontaneous, or naturally occurring, changes in body temperature. The same association of temperature with RT could be demonstrated by changing the body posture in the manner described on page 58. If, after standing for one hour, one assumed a horizontal position for another hour, the oral temperature would fall. In fourteen experiments on five subjects that procedure resulted in the following changes, with the ranges for the five subjects given in parentheses: oral temperature, $-0.64°$ F. ($-0.45°$ to $-0.90°$); simple visual RT (all time values are in msec), $+30$ ($+6$ to $+51$); simple auditory RT, $+30$ (-7 to $+72$); choice visual RT, $+27$ ($+9$ to $+61$); choice auditory RT, $+30$ ($+1$ to $+49$). Several experiments in which the subject first lay down, then stood up, resulted in a rise in body temperature and an accompanying decrease in RT.

While some of the tests studied could be designated as neuromuscular, others, even though they had a motor component, are often referred to as "mental" tests. Bills (342–44) made an exhaustive study of separate responses (equivalent to RTs) in such tasks as color-naming, adding digit pairs, naming opposites, code substitution, and other repetitive performances. They all showed decrements in speed and accuracy with continued activity, but the decrements were much smaller than one obtained in "physical" tasks. Furthermore, even though the subject tried to maintain a certain pace, the performance was not continuous but interspersed with short pauses, occurring at the rate of about three per minute. Bills called these pauses "blocks" and defined them as interruptions of activity of a duration equal to, or exceeding, twice the mean time required for a response. Prolonged performance tended to increase the frequency and duration of the blocks; but, if the normal (not followed by block) RTs were computed, hardly any decrement would be found in their values. The extra blocking, according to Bills, "gives the worker enough rests to compensate for the fatigue which would otherwise develop." Errors tended to occur with blocks, either just before or just following a blocking pause. Thus, a block represented at the same time a lowered reactive capacity and a rest which raised that reactive capacity. The block permitted the subject to continue his performance for a long time without a marked decrement in RT proper, but with longer and more frequent blocks as evidence of some fatigue. One would expect to find no variation in RT, even though greater fatigability later in the day might tend to increase blocking. To test this hypothesis, we constructed a modified Bills apparatus, by employing an electric counter whose hand traveled around a dial divided into one hundred sectors. Every time the circuit was made, the hand jumped one division of the dial. We placed a disk on the shaft operating the hand of the counter and pasted one hundred strips of colored paper over the sectors of the disk, six different colors, never the same color in adjacent spaces, and in no definite order of succession. The procedure consisted of the subject naming a color and at the same time pressing a key which brought on the next strip, when the color-naming and key-pressing were repeated, for 5 minutes. The subject was thus setting his own pace, which he was to make as fast as he could. Each closure of the key was marked on a kymograph by means of a signal magnet; a second signal magnet marked the time, and a third was used by the observer to mark corrected and uncorrected errors in naming the colors. Corrected errors manifested themselves in the lengthening of the RT. The tests were made nine times daily, at 2-hour intervals, from 7:30 A.M. to 11:30 P.M. Although there were some changes in performance from minute to minute even during the short periods of the tests, the findings presented here were for the entire 5-minute tests. The gross RT was determined by dividing the total time (5 minutes) by the number of signal-magnet marks made by the subject during that time. The net RT was measured in a like manner, but only after excluding all blocks, or, by definition, RTs over twice as great as the mean RT. By this separation of the short from the long pauses, one obtained the total number of blocks, the collective blocking time, and the mean duration of the blocks. The results obtained on three subjects, on the basis of 9 full days per subject, showed that the highest body temperature and lowest gross RT were reached, on the average, at 3:30 P.M. The net RT, which could be expected to remain unchanged, was also lowest when the body temperature was highest. The number of blocks per minute, somewhat more irregular than the RTs, showed its lowest value in the afternoon tests, and highest in the evening, with the morning in between. The mean length of the blocks was also lowest in the afternoon tests, and the same was true of the errors, corrected and uncorrected.

In interpreting the results in the light of Bills's findings, i.e., considering the number and particularly the duration of the blocks as indices of mental fatigue, one must infer that there is a 24-hour variation in the state of the nervous system which determines the degree of mental fatigability at different hours of the waking period. Highest body temperature, best performance rate, and, now, lowest fatigability are all reached almost synchronously in the afternoon. Both morning and night hours show the opposite characteristics, but, in general, the temperature is lower, performance worse, and fatigability greater immediately upon getting up in the morning than they are at night just before going to bed. That, of course, does not mean that one does not benefit by the night's sleep. As will be seen later, failure to sleep during the night will be reflected in performance during the following day. What it does mean is that right after getting up in the morning the body temperature is likely to be lower than before going to bed, with the body-temperature curve for the night often asymmetrical.

An opportunity to follow color-naming performance "around the clock" presented itself when, in a study made at the Naval Medical Research Institute (2197), nine young male subjects adhered to a rotating schedule of duty, in

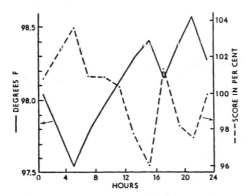

FIG. 16.5—Variations in group mean oral temperatures, taken at different hours of night and day, and concomitant variations in the group mean time required to name series of 600 colors, the latter expressed as percentage of total group mean scores for the period of observation, with 100 per cent equaling 312 seconds. *Solid line:* oral temperature; *broken line:* color-naming score.

practice on large surface vessels of the U.S. Navy. The subjects had 24 hours of duty in each of 5 successive 96-hour periods, averaging 6 hours per day, but distributed in a rotating manner, with five 4-hour shifts between 8:00 P.M. and 4:00 P.M., and two 2-hour intervals between 4:00 and 8:00 P.M., when the watches were "dogged." There were 12 to 14 hours of freedom from "standing watch," permitting long continuous periods of sleep at different hours on successive days. The composite body temperature shown in Fig. 16.5 is not a continuous 24-hour curve, but is made up of sections obtained during watches in different parts of the 96-hour cycle. The subjects were awake and active, except during the 4:00 P.M. to 8:00 P.M. period, when, aside from brief testing, they were free to relax. That they did so is revealed by the notch, between 3:00 P.M. and 9:00 P.M., in the otherwise unbroken rise of 1° F. in the composite group body-temperature means. Variations in the mean group time of 312 seconds required to name 600 colors were plotted in terms of percentage deviations from the group mean, to equalize the values of the scores of individual subjects. As can be seen, the time required for color-naming varied inversely with the body temperature, the correlation coefficient between these two variates equaling —0.8874, statistically highly significant (P <0.01).

Continuous day-and-night oculomotor performance was measured in eighteen subjects, kept awake for 24 hours (2204). By a modified American Optical Company Ophthalmograph, photographic recordings were made of binocular fixation, lateral scanning eye swings, and blinking rate. Poorest oculomotor performance occurred in the early morning hours coinciding with greatest drowsiness, but lagged behind the incidence of lowest body temperature. However, without intervening sleep, there was a spontaneous improvement in oculomotor performance later in the morning and in the afternoon when the drowsiness abated. Likewise, as shown in Fig. 22.1, the feelings of fatigue of a group of fifteen subjects manifested 24-hour fluctuations during 98 hours of continuous sleep deprivation (2957).

Speed and accuracy of performance may be slightly better or poorer on getting up in the morning than before going to bed at night, but they are low in either case, the peak or plateau appearing in between. These findings are not in agreement with the older notions concerning the removal of accumulated metabolic waste products or the "recharging of the battery" during sleep, which would call for the best performance early in the day, followed by a gradual deterioration. That activity itself may lead to improved performance was shown by Noll (3019), who tested the mental efficiency of a group of students before and after a 3-hour examination. The majority of the subjects did better at the end than at the beginning of the examination. A drop in performance in the early afternoon (1372, 2416, 3481), leading to double peaks in the efficiency curve, may be related to a "let-down" experienced after heavy noontime meals.

The ability to guess the time of the day, as well as to judge the passage of time, has also been related to the 24-hour rhythm (1054), or more directly to the changes in body temperature (1260, 1261, 1787). The excitability of the cerebral cortex, as judged by conditioned salivary responses of a child, showed a rise from 7:00 to 11:00 A.M., a plateau till 7:00 P.M., and a downward turn thereafter (3724). Rather indefinite data have been reported for the variation of the ESR (1139, 3295, 3593). For the alpha pattern in man, Bjerner (360) obtained a good 24-hour curve, with the lowest frequency, in four out of five subjects kept awake all night, at 4:00 to 6:00 A.M.

Grabfield and associates (1497, 2694) tested the 24-hour variation in sensitivity to faradic current in three subjects. The daytime values fluctuated, but, between 8:30 P.M. and 8:30 A.M., either when the subjects remained awake or when they were awakened to be tested, lowest sensitivity was at 4:00 A.M. Jores and Frees (2029) tested the sensitivity of the teeth to painful stimulation by faradic shocks in twenty normal subjects. Of these, seventeen were tested from 8:00 A.M. to 8:00 P.M., and the remaining three from 8:00 P.M. to 6:00 A.M. There was a gradual increase in sensitivity during the day, reaching its highest point (lowest threshold) at 6:00 P.M., when it started to decrease, reaching its lowest level after midnight. Though Schumacher and associates (3609) reported that pain thresholds were uniform throughout a 24-hour period of enforced wakefulness, we (2201) were able to confirm the findings of Jores and Frees for the 6-hour period of 6:00 A.M. to noon. In twenty-two series of tests on two subjects, there was a direct relationship between the rise in body temperature and increased sensitivity to painful stimulation of the skin by a tetanizing faradic current. Furthermore, when relaxing in the sitting position for one hour led to a fall in a subject's body temperature, there was a corresponding decrease in sensitivity to pain, whereas subsequent standing up for one hour, if it resulted in a rise in the body temperature, was associated with an increased sensitivity.

Bogoslovsky (393, 394) investigated the variability in sensitivity of the dark-adapted eye to electric current in four female subjects. From 9:00 A.M. on, the sensitivity rose until 12:30 P.M., then gradually and irregularly fell to a minimum at midnight. This variability was confirmed with respect to sensitivity of the eye to light (4049). Kris (2281) noted a 24-hour variation in the periorbitally measured eye potential level, with the value immediately upon getting up only about one-half of the day's peak.

Mice were found to be more susceptible to audiogenic convulsions at night, when their body temperature was high, than in the daytime, when their temperature was low (1586).

The frequency of humming sounds varied, for eighteen subjects, from a mean of 218 early in the morning to 241 at noon and 212 at night (3466), suggesting a relation to the sleep-wakefulness rhythm.

That temperature had an effect on the rate of biological processes has been known for a long time. By means of the Van't Hoff-Arrhenius equation, it is possible to calculate the critical thermal increment, or the temperature characteristic, designated by the Greek letter μ, which stands for calories per gram mol of activating energy of the reacting system. These values for 360 different biological processes were listed by Crozier (794). The graph he published reveals a multimodal frequency of occurrence of certain μ values. Clear modes are exhibited at 8, 11, 12, 16, 18, 20, 22, 24, and 32 thousand calories. Stier (3822) found a μ value of 23,500 cal. for the frequency of the activity cycle of the 2-day-old mouse. Our data on performance in relation to body temperature did not always give the same μ value for a certain task for different subjects, but, in general, simpler tasks gave low μ values, and more complicated acts, higher values. The speed of sorting playing cards yielded μ values of 23,000 cal., while the speed of code transcription, mirror-drawing, and multiplication gave values of 40,000 to 50,000 cal. For visual choice RT of subject T, the μ value was 46,980 cal. Hoagland (1787) determined the μ value of the rate of counting to 60 by one subject, who took 52.0 seconds to do it at a body temperature of 97.4° F., and only 37.5 seconds at 103.0° F. It was 24,000 cal.

Treating the heart-rate figures by the same equation, we obtained a μ value of 29,400 cal., comparable to the values reported by others for the same activity. The μ values for the performance speed and RTs were definitely higher than those listed by Crozier for comparatively simple biological processes. It may be added that μ values for the alpha pattern of the brain oscillogram, as determined by Hoagland (1788–90) and Jasper and Andrews (1963) over the enormous range of temperatures obtainable in patients with diathermy hyperpyrexia, were only 8,000–16,000 cal. A μ value of about 8,000 cal. was also found for the frequency of the cat's EEG for a body temperature range of 28°–37° C. (2227). It appears that the chemical reactions that govern the EEG pattern are different from those involved in higher mental activity.

There is a definite difference in the degree of mentation required of the subject for simple RT and RT with choice. In the former, alertness is all that is needed; but in the latter, where the individual is to respond to one type of signal and not to another, analysis and judgment are the added requirements, reflected in the longer time, roughly 0.1 second. It is significant that the effect of temperature is more marked on RT with choice than on simple RT. Subjectively, the individual tested could allow his mind to wander when his simple RT was measured, just getting ready to respond when he received the preliminary warning of the imminence of stimulation, but he had to be "on his toes" throughout the period of testing of his RT with choice, if he wished to avoid incorrect responses and reprimands from the observer. The effect of body temperature on RT with choice is a definite suggestion of variation in mental work with body temperature.

Assuming that the effect of body temperature indicates that one is dealing with a chemical phenomenon, there are two possible interpretations of the relationship between temperature and RT: either (*a*) mental processes represent chemical reactions in themselves or (*b*) the speed of thinking depends upon the level of metabolic activity of the cells of the cerebral cortex, and, by raising the latter through an increase in body temperature, one indirectly speeds up the thought process.

Whatever their correct explanation, the results show an unmistakable connection between body temperature and speed and accuracy of responding and performing—what is usually designated as efficiency. This relation of performance to temperature gives the 24-hour body-temperature curve a new significance. It was seen in Figure 8.2 that each of the two subjects reached his minimal body temperature during sleep at a different time. Quite by accident, Figure 16.2 shows the daytime temperatures of the same two subjects in relation to their hand steadiness. One subject had his temperature peak earlier in the day than the other and also reached his minimal temperature earlier during sleep.

There are two distinct types of body-temperature and efficiency curves, with the peak reached early in the waking period in one and later in the other. In addition, there are intermediate gradations between the two extremes. Lay (2385) long ago reported that some persons learned better in the morning, others in the evening. There are advantages and disadvantages in being a morning or an evening person (3072, 3346, 4247). Evening persons are likely to want to remain awake late at night when everyone goes to bed, and in turn they are inefficient during the early working hours of the day. Léopold-Lévi (2435) developed this idea further by dividing humanity into four groups: (*a*) those who go to bed late and get up early; (*b*) those who go to bed early and get up late; (*c*) those who go to bed early and get up early; and (*d*) those who go to bed late and get up late. He accounted for the existence of these four classes on the basis of the predominance of one or another division of the visceral nervous system and also certain endocrine influences. Sheldon (3676), as noted (p. 120), developed a scheme for body structure and temperament, both of which appear to be related to going to bed and getting up at certain hours.

The existence of distinct "morning" and "evening" types is also an everyday observation, among students particularly, some preferring to study late at night and sleep late in the morning, while others like to go to bed early and study early in the morning. As we were able to establish in some subjects, "morning" people have their temperature peaks early in the day, shortly before or shortly after noon, and the opposite, of course, applies to "evening" people. Three of the four different performance curves listed by Freeman and Hovland (1274) can be explained on this basis: ascending performance curves were probably obtained on "evening" subjects; descending on "morning" subjects; curves with a peak or plateau in the afternoon on intermediary types. This occurrence was particularly likely since many tests were made on a few subjects and during "office" hours, from 9:00 A.M. to 5:00 P.M.

To summarize, most of the curves of performance can be brought into line with the known 24-hour body-temperature curves, allowing for individual skewing of the curves toward an earlier or later, rather than a midafternoon, peak. For each individual there probably exists a drowsiness temperature level, above which it is easy to remain awake and below which it is progressively harder to do so. The results of studies made on persons kept awake for a long time, to be discussed later, will serve to complete the evidence and lead toward a better understanding of the body temperature as an index of the 24-hour sleep-wakefulness rhythm, in both its establishment and its persistence.

Chapter 17

24-Hour Variation in Visceral Activity

A great number of studies on the variation of visceral activities have been made entirely apart from any connection with the physiology of sleep. Jores (2022, 2024, 2025) reviewed and summarized these contributions, using figures from the different original articles. Some measurements were made only during daytime hours, others embraced the waking period of 15 to 16 hours, and still others extended over the entire 24 hours.

No regular curves of 24-hour variations in erythrocyte counts have been established (2020, 2371, 3687), except in anemia, in which Jores (2024) observed a maximum count at 5:00 P.M. and a minimum at 7:00 A.M. However, hemoglobin and hematocrit values were found by Renbourn (3312) to be highest at 7:00 A.M., with a precipitous decrease in the morning and afternoon, and a low at night. For the erythrocyte sedimentation rate, a 24-hour variation has been affirmed (2030, 4303) and denied (3312). Conflicting reports have also been made on the existence of a 24-hour variation in the counts of leucocytes (538, 2024, 3674) and lymphocytes (1070, 3674), but there is a general agreement on the variations in eosinophils (p. 169).

For plasma proteins, Renbourn (3312) noted no changes during the day and evening, but "a significant fall after 10:00 p.m., independent of bed rest, with a suggestion of a rise commencing about 2:30 a.m." A 24-hour variation has also been reported for the fibrinolytic activity of the plasma (557), as well as for its content of cholinesterase (3473), cholesterol (4311), glutathione (4310), and ethyl alcohol (2066).

Cullen and Earle (799) followed the pH of the blood in ten normal individuals from early in the morning until late at night. There was a rise in pH, individual increases for the day varying from 0.01 to 0.07 pH. The onset of sleep (p. 33) leads to a decrease in the pH of the blood during the night.

Forsgren (1244) could discern some changes in the non-protein nitrogen of the blood plasma, which he related to the 24-hour rhythmicity in liver function. Holmquist (1823), in determining total serum calcium in five young men and in fifteen rabbits, found the maximum values in human serum during the night (and sleep) and in rabbit serum during the day (and rest). Maximum total calcium values corresponded to minimal adrenalin concentration in the blood and to lowest body temperature. This finding is in disagreement with the findings of other investigators, that the serum calcium is lower during sleep than during the waking state (p. 35). Ehrström (1052) reported no uniformity with respect to 24-hour variation of the serum-calcium concentration: of a total of 100 patients, in 20 the morning serum-calcium values were the lowest of the 24-hour period, in 30 the highest, and in the remaining 50 somewhere in between. Plasma magnesium concentration was found to be highest at night (3472) and that of iron (1620, 2714), in the morning.

Heart-rate variations have been followed by several investigators (387, 1108, 1766, 2772, 2781, 3231, 3945). In a comprehensive study of the ontogenetic development of the 24-hour periodicity, Lange and co-workers (1690, 2363) established (*a*) a shift in the incidence of the minimal heart rates from 9:00 P.M. in infants to 3:00 A.M. in children, and (*b*) a gradual widening of the 24-hour range (with the mean value in each case considered 100) from 96 to 104 in neonates to 84 to 118 in children four to thirteen years of age. The parallelism between the heart-rate and body-temperature curves is striking, though Boas and Goldschmidt (387) failed to detect it (p. 42). A change in 8 to 11 (3904) or 10 to 20 (2202) beats per minute corresponded to one of 1° F. (2202), but, as shown in the next chapter (p. 182), the clear-cut 24-hour heart-rate variation is not a rhythm but a simple coupled periodicity related to alternation of rest and activity.

Brooks and Carrol (525) obtained lower arterial blood-pressure values in subjects during the night, even when they were kept awake. Subjects who slept during the night had a lower blood pressure in the morning, 3 hours after awakening, than during the evening, and there was a gradual rise in the course of the day. Mueller and Brown (2937), from data pertaining to hourly blood-pressure determinations on 87 persons—26 with normal, and 61 with elevated, pressures—placed the maximum blood pressure at 6:00–7:00 P.M., and minimum at 3:00–4:00 A.M., for both groups of subjects. Similar maxima and minima were reported for venous blood pressure (2286, 2772), minute volume of the heart (2286), and rewarming time for extremities (1766).

Among the few scattered data on the 24-hour variation in respiration are the maximal vital capacity (2286) and ventilation of the lungs (4074) in man in the afternoon, and the minimal after midnight, and the 20 to 25 per cent decrease in the respiratory rate of monkeys during the night (3555).

Concerning 24-hour variations in the activities of the digestive system, low pH values of human saliva (1533), as previously mentioned (p. 53), were obtained during the night. Henning and Norpoth (1701) reported a high gastric acidity in the morning hours, but Hellebrandt and associates (1693), on the

contrary, found the highest gastric-juice acidity during the night hours devoted to sleep. Gastric motility was also greater at night. The secretion of pep-
sinogen, as judged by the rate of excretion of uropepsin, shows a distinct 24-
hour curve (1413), which is absent in patients with Addison's disease, suggesting that the adrenocortical hormone influences gastric secretory activity. Forsgren (1242) noted a reciprocal relationship between the secretory and glycogenic functions of the liver, the highest secretion of bile occurring in the daytime, when the glycogenic activity is lowest. Josephson and Larsson (2032)
collected bile from a fistula in a patient. Maximal secretion occurred between
11:00 A.M. and 1:00 P.M., and minimal at 5:00–7:00 A.M., differing from the
bimodal curve of Dastre (831), with maxima at 9:00 A.M. and 9:00–11:00 P.M.
Hamar (1614) determined the amount of glucose resorbed from the lumen
of the isolated jejunum of the rat. At 9:00–10:00 A.M., 30 to 40 per cent was
absorbed, but this rate rose to 70 to 80 per cent at 6:00–7:00 P.M.

Holmgren (1819) determined the 24-hour variation in fat content of the
intestinal wall, lungs, and liver, and in the appearance of the acinal cells of the
pancreas of large white rats, killed at 2-hour intervals through the 24-hour
period. Histologically and chemically, the highest fat content of the intestinal
wall was found at night (2:00 A.M.), the lowest in the daytime (2:00 P.M.).
The gastrointestinal contents varied in the same sense. When the rats were fed
in the afternoon (after a 24-hour fast) or at night, the fat infiltration of the
intestine was greater after the night feeding than after the day feeding. This
difference led Holmgren to conclude that not purely alimentary factors but
rather greater absorption determined the higher fat content of the abdominal
wall at night. The zymogen granules in the pancreatic cells also fluctuated.
When the intestinal wall was rich in fat, there were few zymogen granules
present, and vice versa. Liver fat showed the same variation as intestinal-wall
fat, but the glycogen content of the liver was variable, with the lowest concentration most often at 10:00 P.M.

There is a great deal of repetition and confusion in the numerous reports on
the glycogenic function of the liver, particularly since comparisons are often
drawn between monocyclic man, active mainly in the daytime, or largely dicyclic rats, most active during the night, and polycyclic rabbits. Holmquist
(1820) analyzed the livers of rats for glycogen simultaneously with a histological examination of these organs. The glycogen content of the liver varied
in a bimodal fashion over the 24-hour period, with maxima at 2:00 P.M. and
2:00 A.M., and minima between. Like Galamini (1337), he found the body
temperature of the rat to show two peaks, with the lowest temperatures when
the glycogen content of the liver was highest. Holmquist (1821) also examined
the livers of hedgehogs, killed at night, when they were active, or in the daytime, when they were asleep. Livers of animals killed during their waking
period had a small amount of glycogen, but their bile capillaries were dilated,

and the acinal cells of their pancreases contained a large number of zymogen granules; the reverse was true when the animals were killed during sleep. Aagren and co-workers (1) also described cyclic changes in the glycogen content of the liver in rabbits, rats, and mice. Independently of food intake, glycogen accumulated in the liver at night and gradually disappeared during the day. The glycogen content of the liver was found to be highest in the early afternoon and lowest early in the morning in guinea pigs (3162) and chickens (1061). Jores (2021) detected a bimodal curve in the bilirubin content of the blood in monocyclic man, with peaks at noon and midnight, and lowest values at 8:00 A.M. and 8:00 P.M. He considered this bimodality, as well as variations in uribilinogen excretion in the urine, as evidence of a 24-hour rhythm in hepatic function.

Forsgren (1245-48) saw a connection between liver activity and water retention. During its assimilatory phase the liver takes up water as it lays up glycogen; it gives up water, forms urea, and produces bile during the secretory phase. In man the assimilatory phase is at night; the secretory, in the daytime. Higgins and co-workers (1763) determined the changes in gross weight of the rat liver, as well as its water, glycogen, protein, and fat contents, for a 2-day period following a single feeding. A group of rats which fasted for 22 hours was given an ample meal, and small numbers were killed thereafter at 2-hour intervals. The curve of changes in the weight of the liver was found to be bimodal, the first mode occurring at 5:00-7:00 P.M. and the second between 11:00 P.M. and 1:00 A.M. The water, glycogen, and protein contents followed the curve for the total weight changes, but the fat did not, with its curve very nearly a horizontal line. During the second day changes in weight of the liver were absent, except that at 3:00 P.M. there was a transitory increase in weight, mainly due to the retention of water. The same authors (1764) later reported that the 24-hour variation in liver weight and composition was due to the rats' feeding habits. When they controlled the food intake, so that the animals ate as much in the daytime as they did at night, the 24-hour variations largely disappeared.

There is a similar diversity in the reports pertaining to 24-hour variations in the blood-sugar level and sugar tolerance in normal and diabetic individuals. Hatlehol (1661) noted that in young diabetics the blood sugar, instead of going down continuously during fasting, might show a low value in the evening and a higher value the following morning. According to Hatlehol, the cause of the "paradoxical" rise in blood sugar during the night was not muscular inactivity; nor was blood sugar affected by changing the meal hours. Maximum blood-sugar values in diabetics, treated (3654) or untreated (1929) with insulin, were attained in the morning, and minimal values in late afternoon or evening, but in some patients there was a sharp increase in blood sugar between midnight and 3:00-5:00 A.M. (2362). In healthy subjects Jores (2020) found blood sugar to be highest at 4:00 A.M. and lowest at 3:00-4:00 P.M.

Sugar tolerance was reported by Harding and co-authors (1630) to be lower in the afternoon (4:00 P.M.) than in the morning. Möllerström (2853), however, stated that in diabetes the tolerance is higher in the afternoon (noon to 3:00 P.M.) than either in the morning or in the evening. He came to this conclusion by observing the effects of meals on the blood-sugar curve. The same meal had different effects on blood sugar depending on the hour of the day; and, at the time of greatest tolerance (or least sensitivity), there was a tendency to a spontaneous decrease in blood sugar, so that after a meal the blood sugar sometimes fell to a level lower than the fasting value. Krasnjanskij (2263) detected several waves in the 24-hour blood-sugar curve, with a rise after each meal. Hussels (1879) noted variations in alimentary hyperglycemia at different hours of the day, related to which one of three constitutional types the normal subject belonged.

Allcroft (44) found that the blood-sugar level of the lactating cow showed 24-hour variations, whereas that of dry cows did not. Pitts (3210) related the blood-sugar variations in the rat to its feeding habits.

Dobreff and Saprjanoff (954) analyzed the cerebrospinal fluid of five subjects every 3 hours for 24 hours. The sugar concentration was highest at 8:00 A.M., and lowest at 2:00 P.M., with respective values 55–72 and 40–47 mg per cent. The chloride value was greatest at 5:00–8:00 P.M. (870–970 mg per cent) and least from 8:00 A.M. to noon (700–860 mg per cent). The leucocyte count showed no distinct variation.

Euler and Holmquist (1111) studied the 24-hour variation in the adrenalin content of the blood, as well as the adrenal glands, in hedgehogs and rabbits. The former had a higher adrenalin concentration during the night than in the daytime; the latter showed two maxima, between 4:00 and 10:00 A.M., and between 4:00 and 10:00 P.M. In man, the adrenalin content of the blood plasma, followed from 6:00 A.M. to 6:00 P.M., showed peaks at 8:00–9:00 A.M. and 2:00 P.M., perhaps related to food intake.

It is evident that many of the 24-hour changes in the composition of the blood, in liver content and activity, and in metabolic processes are connected with the feeding routine and, therefore, indirectly with the mode of existence. Some variations may be more definitely related to the alternation of sleep and wakefulness, with a predominance of assimilatory and catabolic processes, respectively.

A 24-hour variation in kidney activity is absent in infants at birth but begins to manifest itself at the age of four to six weeks by a smaller volume of urine voided at night than in the daytime (328). The nocturnal olyguria has been reported by many investigators (194, 282, 1406, 2017, 2028, 2788, 2789, 3024, 3713, 3720, 4074). Gerritzen (1405–08) measured the diuretic effect of drinking a given amount of water or 0.7 per cent NaCl solution every hour, with food at regular hours or also taken every hour. The effect was least at night and greatest in the afternoon or evening. Papper and Rosenbaum (3090), who obtained similar results, ascribed them to an increased secretion of antidiuretic hormone and a decreased excretion of sodium salts. The same explanation was offered by Dell and Kayser (890), who noted an increase in water diuresis when subjects were kept in the dark. Sirota and co-workers (3720), by various "clearance" procedures, established that the renal blood flow was constant throughout the 24 hours, and so was glomerular filtration, except for a "slight but significant fall" between midnight and 4:00 A.M. However, there was a considerable increase in tubular reabsorption of water, which accounted for the decrease in urine flow.

A decrease in the pH of the urine and a greater excretion of acid at night has also been a common observation (620, 2176, 2177, 2831, 3555, 3713). Kaye (2094) held that starvation rather than sleep was responsible for the high acidity of urine secreted at night. Chloride, sodium, and potassium ions seem to follow the 24-hour water-excretion curve, except for a marked rise in chloride excretion in the morning (282, 2832, 3024, 3713, 3714, 3779). Gerritzen (1406) regarded the chloride excretion as part of the 24-hour hepatic rhythm. Mills and Stanbury (2832) noted that the characteristic 24-hour curves of excretion of sodium, potassium, and chloride persisted "in subjects continuously active, or continuously recumbent, for 24 and once for 48 hours, with or without sleep, fasting or taking small meals, etc." Stanbury and Thomson (3779), from their study of electrolyte excretion, concluded that "changes in glomerular filtration may help, but changes in tubular function were mainly responsible for cyclic changes in electrolyte excretion."

Total nitrogen excretion is highest at 8:00–10:00 A.M. and lowest at night (619, 732, 1232, 4074). The excretion of uric acid is also low at night (3713), but the opposite is true of ammonia (619, 1232).

The 24-hour kidney excretory rhythm may be affected by "life situation," "altered behavior" (3591), sojourn in the Arctic during the continuous summer daylight (2545), as well as by pathological insufficiency (2777). In addition to the 24-hour rhythm, Menzel and co-workers (2774, 2776–80) discerned 12-, 8-, and 6-hour periodicities, even 7-, 23-, and 25-hour rhythms, by a system they called "period analysis." A parallelism between body temperature, and electrolyte and ketosteroid excretion has been reported (955, 2788), and the administration of cortisone was followed by a virtual abolition of the 24-hour kidney rhythm. The effect of large amounts of exogenous adrenocortical hormone does not prove that the kidney rhythm is normally dependent on endogenous adrenocortical control (3407).

The urinary excretion of phosphates was discussed at some length in dealing with concomitants of sleep (p. 65). That more phosphate is excreted in the afternoon than in the morning was established by several investigators (511, 732, 1201). This disparity applied to subjects in their fourteenth and sixteenth

days of fasting (2177). We followed the phosphate excretion in a number of
subjects, for several days each, under normal eating conditions, during fasts of
several days' duration, and with exactly the same meals taken every 12 hours.
In all cases the urine was collected for successive 4-hour periods, 4 of these
during the waking hours and 2 during sleep, necessitating an artificial awakening of the subjects once during the night. In the first series the subjects chose
their diets, and the number of meals was either 3 or 2, but the qualitative and
quantitative composition of each subject's meals was kept constant. Sample
curves of phosphate excretion for two of the six subjects who followed this routine are shown in Figure 17.1. There seems to be a fairly consistent 24-hour variation in phosphate excretion, with the 7:00–11:00 A.M. period usually showing the

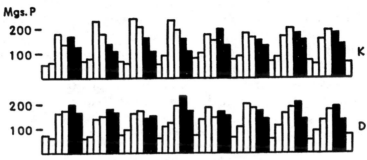

Fig. 17.1—Urinary excretion of phosphates by two subjects, in successive 4-hour periods,
on a customary eating and sleeping routine. Hours of wakefulness (white columns):
7:00 A.M.–11:00 P.M.; hours of sleep (black columns): 11:00 P.M.–7:00 A.M. The amount
of phosphates excreted during the second half of the sleep period was nearly always smaller
than that excreted during the first half; the lowest amount of phosphates was usually
excreted during the 4-hour period after getting up in the morning.

smallest excretion, and the greatest phosphate excretion occurring variously
during the 3:00–7:00 P.M., 7:00–11:00 P.M., and 11:00 P.M.–3:00 A.M. periods.
The difference between the two graphs is probably due to one subject (D)
eating 3 meals per day, while the other (K) ate only 2, at noon and at 6:00 P.M.,
thus "fasting" between 6:00 P.M. and noon of the following day. The incidence
of food intake seems to be decisive, but in both subjects the excretion of phosphates was greater during the first half of the night than during the second. In
another series three subjects fasted for 3, 4, and 3 days, respectively, with controlled diets before and after. There was a great deal of irregularity in the
several 24-hour curves of phosphate excretion, but there was always more phosphate excreted between 11:00 P.M. and 7:00 A.M., the time devoted to staying
in bed, and almost entirely to sleep, than from 11:00 A.M. to 7:00 P.M., a portion of the waking period. The excretion of phosphate was greater for the
11:00 P.M.–3:00 A.M. period than it was between 3:00 and 7:00 A.M. In a last

series four subjects in six tests, totaling 26 days, ate exactly the same meals every 12 hours, while continuing their ordinary sleep-wakefulness routine. In all cases but one there was a greater or lesser increase in the night excretion over the day, and even the subject who showed no difference on a high protein diet did so on a low. Again, during the majority of nights, the phosphate output during the first half of the night was greater than during the second, while that was not the case for the corresponding two 4-hour periods in the daytime.

It was concluded that the character of the diet and especially the distribution of the meals had an important influence in shaping the 24-hour curve of phosphate excretion. As all meals are usually taken between 7:00 A.M. and 7:00 P.M., the urinary phosphate output is greater between 7:00 P.M. and 7:00 A.M. than during the daytime 12 hours. Eating the same amount of food every 12 hours tends to make the curve bimodal, but there still seems to be more phosphate excreted during sleep than during the corresponding 8 hours of wakefulness. Finally, and most consistently, under either normal and 12-hour eating schedules or during fasting, more phosphate is excreted between 11:00 P.M. and 3:00 A.M. than between 3:00 and 7:00 A.M. It will be recalled that Simpson (3716) ascribed the increase in phosphate excretion during sleep to the assumption of the horizontal position, but that would not explain the inequality between the two halves of the night. Another explanation is that muscular relaxation may be responsible for the release of phosphate, and one would expect the relaxation to be greater during the first half of the night, when the body temperature is falling, than during the second half, when it is rising and when motility is on the increase (2177). Phosphate excretion reflects the phosphate concentration in the blood plasma. If the hypothesis concerning the connection between muscular activity (phasic or tonic) and phosphate retention is warranted, the phosphate-excretion curve may be looked upon as reciprocally portraying a 24-hour muscle-tonus curve.

Bochnik (389) plotted 24-hour curves for 25 variables pertaining to motor, sensory, and vegetative activities. Mitotic cell division in human epidermis proceeds much faster at 9:00–10:00 P.M. than between 5:00 and 10:00 A.M. (751). Similar 24-hour variations have been reported for mitosis in epidermal cells of mice, rats, and hamsters (687, 688, 1598, 1602), but with greater activity in the daytime. Mitosis, like several other variables, seems to be related to the hormonal secretion of the adrenal cortex, as reflected in the eosinophil count, plasma 17-hydroxycorticosteroids, and excretion of urinary ketosteroids. The existence of a 24-hour variation in circulating eosinophils has been abundantly demonstrated for man (959, 1213, 1601, 1792, 2062, 3908, 4065), monkey (2809), and mouse (538, 1586, 1600, 4065). For man, the 24-hour curve of the eosinophil count is almost a mirror image of the body-temperature curve, as shown by figures in the papers of Halberg and associates (1601) and Hobbs and co-workers (1792). Because the eosinophil count may vary from under 50 to over

$1000/mm^3$ in different persons, and in the same person on different days, its variation is usually expressed in relative, rather than absolute, terms. The decrease in the mean eosinophil level of a group of subjects from 6:30 to 8:00 A.M. amounted to 45 to 60 per cent. Halberg and Ulstrom (1599) have found no characteristic morning drop in eosinophil count in infants one to seven months old, but did so in fifteen-month-old infants. In Addison's disease, hypopituitarism, and after bilateral adrenalectomy, the eosinophil rhythm is absent (1590, 1596, 1601), as it is in patients receiving corticosteroids every 3 hours (2062). In blind persons the morning eosinopenia is less marked than in seeing persons (110, 2357, 2468), but hemidecortication (1591) and mental deficiency (1589) do not affect the eosinophil rhythm. In epileptics, seizures seem to coincide with minimal eosinophil counts (1588), suggesting an association of plasma corticoid concentration, or high body temperature, or some other 24-hour variants, with some factor precipitating or favoring the fits.

The spectacular spontaneous morning eosinopenia is more than matched by evoked eosinopenia. Epinephrine administration and stressful situations were followed by all but a disappearance of eosinophils from the circulating blood of mice (3759). After hypophysectomy, the evoked eosinopenia in mice was only about one-half the pre-operative one, but ACTH could still produce a decrease in cell count of 87 per cent. In human subjects, an intravenous injection of 1 mg of adrenalin produced "manifest tremor, tachycardia, substernal tightness, and anxiety," with a drop of the eosinophil count as much as 70 per cent (from 650 to $200/mm^3$) in 4 hours (3934). Nor-epinephrine produced only one-sixth of the eosinopenic effect of epinephrine (1870). Bonvallet and co-workers (410) teased dogs by offering them meat, but snatching it away when the animals tried to grab it. The mean drop in eosinophil count was related to the emotional reaction of the animals. In dogs which did not react, it was 14 per cent (range, 0–36); in those which reacted moderately, 26 per cent (range, 0–70); and in strongly reacting animals, 59 per cent (range, 25–90). In students during examinations or performance tests (2145, 3934), in athletes engaged in competitive activity (1771, 3318), and in patients under emotional tension (1870), similar eosinopenia was observed. A 24-hour curve of plasma corticosteroid concentration has been found in rats (1553), monkeys (2809), and man (1264, 4000, 4120); in man, even when deprived of sleep (2949). The excretion of ketosteroids by the kidney also shows a variation (1772, 2326, 3201, 3202), with a sharp morning rise and a 24-hour curve—a mirror image of the eosinophil-count curve and parallel to the body-temperature curve (1583).

Porter (3233–35) demonstrated that in cats and monkeys (*a*) there was an increase in electrical activity in the posterior hypothalamus following stress or epinephrine injection; (*b*) electrical stimulation of the tuberal and mammillary areas produced eosinopenia; and (*c*) the destruction of these areas abolished the eosinopenic effects of both epinephrine and stress. Mason (2706) raised the corticosteroid level of the plasma by stimulating the infundibular region of the hypothalamus in monkeys. The 24-hour variation in plasma corticosteroids may well reflect a similar variation in the secretion of ACTH (3158).

To summarize, the only dramatic addition in the field of visceral activity since the first edition of this book has been the proved existence of a hypophyseal-adrenocortical 24-hour periodicity, as revealed in the eosinophil count, plasma corticosteroid concentration, and ketosteroid excretion. There are many visceral activities that show a 24-hour variation. Some are rhythms, others mere coupled periodicities, as can be seen from the ease with which they can be modified, which is the principal topic of the next chapter.

Chapter 18

Modifiability of the 24-Hour Periodicities

Attempts to modify 24-hour periodicities in animals and man may be divided into three categories: (*a*) the effects of changes in environmental conditions—such as illumination and temperature—and of feeding and activity routines on the periodicity itself; (*b*) a shift in phase without changing the 24-hour wave length up to the point of complete inversion; and (*c*) the establishment of non–24-hour periodicities (1581, 1583, 2022, 2186, 4165).

In general, continuous darkness has no effect on an established 24-hour rhythm, and continuous light tends to abolish it. The rods and cones of the catfish retina are dark-adapted during the night and light-adapted in the daytime. This alternation was unaffected by continuous darkness, but continuous light caused the rods and cones to be light-adapted (4167). The same type of finding applies to the lizard Anolis, which is green at night and brown in the daytime (3260), the mitosis rhythm in the mouse (636), and activity rhythms of rodents (529, 837, 1515, 2005). Continuous darkness in some cases shortened the 24-hour wave length (607, 2936), whereas continuous light either increased it (607, 1227, 1228, 2006, 2936) or disorganized it (529), when it did not abolish it. Blindfolding abolished the 24-hour blood-sugar and body-temperature variations in rabbits (2019), but enucleation of the eyes made the rhythm longer or shorter in the rat (3342), or made it possible to establish a rhythm coinciding with 24-hour changes in environmental temperature (530). Rodents raised in the dark developed an "arhythmic, or poorly defined diel activity pattern" (607), and reports of well-developed 24-hour rhythms under these conditions (1227, 2005) did not indicate that other environmental 24-hour variations (noise, temperature) had been excluded. Hypophysectomy did not affect the 24-hour rhythm of the catfish retinal elements (4167) but completely abolished the skin-color rhythm in lizards, which became permanently green—their night color (3260). In rodents removal of the hypophysis was reported to result in no effect on the 24-hour activity (2936); an early suppression with later recovery (2466); or first a lowering of the body-temperature level with an eventual abolition of day-night temperature differences (1156).

Lemkuhl (2418, 2419) connected the 24-hour activity cycle of pigeons not only with light and darkness but also with hunger. After extirpation of the cerebrum, the activity of the pigeons was diminished and the normal periodicity changed, but in about 4 months the animals regained their previous reactivity to different light situations and to hunger. Lemkuhl concluded that the mechanism of this rhythmicity was "subcortical," although it was hard to draw analogies between parts of the brain in the pigeon and in mammals.

In three human subjects Mills and co-workers (2834) disrupted the 24-hour urinary rhythm by the administration of potassium salts at 4-hourly intervals for 3 nights. After this disruption the subjects remained awake for 24 hours, consuming small hourly meals. In spite of the constancy of the new conditions, the normal urinary rhythm was promptly restored. Thyroid medication raised the body temperature (2202), and complete sleep deprivation for 3 to 4 days tended to lower the body-temperature level (161, 2271, 2957), without affecting the 24-hour rhythm.

The phase shift in the 24-hour rhythm in animals was usually carried to 180° by a complete inversion of the light-darkness alternation. Galbraith and Simpson (1340), in 1903, produced such a reversal of the 24-hour body-temperature curve in monkeys, but the inverted temperature curve was not so regular as the normal one. The authors also shifted the light-and-darkness changes, instead of completely reversing them (3:00 A.M.–3:00 P.M.), with equally good results. They finally left the monkeys entirely in the dark or had the light shining continuously, and the 24-hour temperature curve gradually disappeared. The monkey is a distinctly "optical" animal by Szymanski's classification and does not preserve its body-temperature rhythm in the dark. Birds, also highly "optical" animals, responded likewise to the reversal of the light-darkness schedule (1767). Practically all other reports pertained to the activity (529, 607, 1227, 1228, 2005) or mitosis (1585, 1587) rhythm of rodents, which could be easily inverted by reversing the hours of illumination, or by changing the external temperature (531) or the feeding schedule (1225), with the latter two conditions not as powerful as the light-darkness reversal. In the monkey it was also possible to invert the 24-hour oxygen-consumption rhythm (3726).

Mosso (2907), in 1887, tried to invert his own body-temperature curve by reversing his living schedule but gave up the attempt after 4 days, as he developed a fever which he ascribed to the change in routine. In 1902 Benedict and Snell (292) were unable to produce such an inversion in the body temperature in a subject who had reversed his sleep and waking routine for 10 days; but this period may not have been sufficient, as seen from the results of Toulouse and Piéron (3959), who demonstrated an inversion of the body-temperature curves in night nurses 5 or 6 weeks after the change from day to night duty was made. Gibson (1432) likewise obtained an inversion of the temperature curve in two subjects who moved from New Haven to Manila, with a time difference between the two places of nearly 12 hours. He suggested that a possible "explanation of Benedict's results is to be found in the depressing effects of environmental conditions, such as darkness, artificial illumination, the unusual absence of noise and external activity and in the habitual and regular reactions of the body to these influences." Results similar to Gibson's were reported by Osborne (3065), following a trip from Melbourne to London. However, Polimanti (3223) reported the case of a pharmacist, who, after living on a reversed routine for 6 years, did not have an inverted body-temperature curve. From the details he supplied, one can see that his subject did not reverse his routine completely. In our laboratory (2202) the 24-hour body-temperature and heart-rate curves were inverted in several subjects. Burckard and Kayser (572) inverted the body-temperature rhythm of a bed-ridden idiot by changing the illumination and feeding schedules. Wittersheim and co-workers (4246) were able to invert the performance curve, though the inverted curve showed greater variability than did the normal one. Halberg and co-authors (1593) inverted the incidence of convulsions in patients, in addition to the body-temperature and eosinophil-count rhythms. Migeon and associates (2810) noted no change in the usual 24-hour variation in plasma corticosteroids and in urinary ketosteroids in night workers, but a reversal of the former was accomplished by Perkoff and associates (3158) on an inverted routine.

A kidney excretion rhythm for potassium, and to a lesser extent for sodium and chloride ions, which persisted after 4 weeks of night work was reported by Mills and Thomas (2829, 2833). Phosphate excretion changed promptly on the reverse schedule, however, indicating that its 24-hour curve was a simple coupled periodicity (p. 132). Luederitz (2573) detected a dependence of the reversal of the body-temperature rhythm upon that of the urinary water-excretion rhythm. Spontaneous inversion in the kidney excretion rhythm has been reported in cirrhosis with ascites (2010), and sleep-wakefulness inversion, in old age (390).

A gradual shift in the body-temperature (585) and other rhythms (1212) has been described by travelers who moved into new time zones. A successful attempt to develop 3 different 24-hour body-temperature curves in the 3 watch-standing sections of the crew of a submarine was made by Utterback and Ludwig (4028) and is discussed in connection with the hygiene of sleep and wakefulness (p. 316).

The older (4074) and more recent (3526) failures to invert the body temperature were undoubtedly due to the expectations of results in 2–3 days. It usually takes a week or two to adjust to a markedly shifted or inverted routine, and reports of prompt changeovers are more surprising than the failures (2019, 3671). Some persons offer greater resistance to a change in phase of their 24-hour rhythms than others, just as there are individual differences in giving up old habits and in acquiring new ones.

It has been possible to develop non–24-hour rhythms in invertebrates (1492–94, 2174, 2183) as well as vertebrates. Although Johnson (2005) and Hemmingsen and Krarup (1698) could not break the 24-hour rhythm in rats by subjecting them to an alternation of 8 hours of light and 8 of darkness, Browman (532) succeeded in doing so by manipulating both light and environmental temperature, and using rats bred for 25 generations in continuous light. It has been possible to develop two activity peaks per 24 hours in rats by changing the ratio of light and darkness (146). Tribukait (3975) could change the activity rhythm of mice by slowly shortening the light-darkness period to 21 hours or lengthening it to 27 hours but not much by going outside this range. When he tried to develop an artificial rhythm of 19 hours, the mice reverted to an apparently endogenous periodicity of 23.5 hours (3974). The only successful attempts to produce a 12-hour rhythm were reported by Shcherbakova (3555) for the monkey and by Savvateev (3530) for the hen.

Efforts to establish a 12-hour rhythm in man have uniformly failed. In our laboratory, we tested this routine on subject S, who slept twice every 24 hours, from 4:00 to 7:00 or 7:30. After 33 days on this routine, the subject reported that he felt fine and did not experience any difficulty in keeping up his schedule. However, he did not acquire a distinct 12-hour body-temperature curve, although his composite 24-hour curve showed a secondary dip at 7:00 P.M., in addition to the primary one at 7:00 A.M. Both of these "lows" were reached 2.5 to 3 hours after going to sleep, but the mean primary minimum (7:00 A.M.) was 96.95° F., whereas the secondary one (7:00 P.M.) was 97.8° F., or nearly 1° higher. Likewise the afternoon maximum was 98.55° F., whereas the night maximum was 98.95° F. It was reached toward midnight, and was identical with the highest body temperature usually attained by this subject at 8:00–10:00 P.M. on a normal 24-hour routine. When one takes into consideration that, according to S's statement, irregularity was one of his few outstanding habits, it becomes clear that a person of regular living habits would be still less likely to acquire a good 12-hour body-temperature curve in a comparable length of time. Mills and Stanbury (2827, 2830) also failed to develop a kidney excretory rhythm of 12 hours, though the total period of observation was only 48 hours and all too short for the purpose. Halberg and co-workers (1593), from data on two subjects, concluded that "two alternations of rest and activity within 24 hours, even if maintained for years, are not associated with 12-hour rhythms, neither in number of eosinophils nor in body temperature."

No more successful were attempts to develop a 48-hour rhythm in our laboratory. K and T, the two subjects of this experiment, slept at the usual time but stayed awake for 39–40 hours instead of the customary 16–17. They observed this schedule for 30 days, or fifteen 48-hour periods. Figure 18.1 shows their oral temperature curves for three successive 10-day, or 5-cycle, periods. There is a striking similarity between the two sets of curves. In all cases the temperature during the evening of the "second" day was considerably lower than at the same time the previous evening. With this low temperature went a state of marked sleepiness, much more intense than that of the night before. However, when one compares the curves for the three successive 10-day periods, one cannot fail to notice a retrograde change. The curves for the first five periods looked more skewed than the others—more like one 48-hour wave, with a kink corresponding to the hours of the first night. The temperature range for the second 24 hours is over twice that of the first. During the second

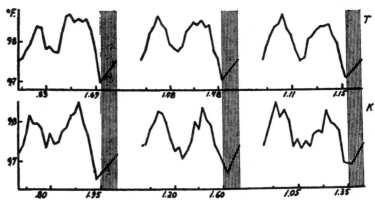

Fig. 18.1—Composite 48-hour mean oral temperature curves of two subjects for three successive 10-day (five 48-hour) periods. Living routine involved 40 hours of unbroken wakefulness and 8 hours of sleep (shaded areas) every other night. Time marks, noon and midnight. The temperature curves became more distinctly bimodal, with the body-temperature ranges for the two 24-hour fractions (shown under the time lines) approaching each other as the routine was continued—a complete failure to establish a single 48-hour body-temperature curve. Compare the similarity of the curves for the two subjects with the marked differences between the corresponding body-temperature curves of the same two subjects on 21-hour and 28-hour routines of living, shown in Figures 18.2 and 18.3.

10-day period the disparity between the two 24-hour sections is smaller, and during the third they are nearly alike. In other words, persistence in that routine gradually drove the subjects back to the 24-hour cycle which they were trying to abolish. It will also be noted that at first the oral temperature went up to a higher level in the second afternoon than it did in the first, but toward the end of the month it was the other way around. It also became progressively harder to stay awake during the first night of each 48-hour interval, and the efficiency during that night was so low as to nullify completely the "time-saving" feature of this routine. It appears that by sleeping at the usual time every other night, the subjects were, figuratively speaking, tearing down one night what had been built up the night before. That is probably why the 48-hour temperature curves looked more and more like two 24-hour curves as time went on. Thus, neither one-half nor twice the usual length of the rhythm is a suitable wave length for an artificial rhythm.

We decided to adopt a new time interval not too far removed from 24 hours to make one too sleepy, or not sleepy enough, at the scheduled bedtime. We chose 21 hours and 28 hours for the sole reason that they gave an 8-day and a 6-day week, respectively, and thus permitted the subjects to work out a weekly schedule that would not be in conflict with their teaching and research. On the 21-hour schedule they went to bed 3 hours earlier every day, and in the course of a week they gained 21 hours, or an extra 21-hour period, making 8 artificial days in the week. On the 6-day week, they went to bed 4 hours later every day, so that in the course of a natural week they lost 24 hours, or a whole day. Again, K and T were the subjects, running each artificial-day routine for 6 weeks, with a "normal" 6-week period in between. Similar as their body-temperature curves were on the 48-hour schedule, they were entirely different on the 21- and 28-hour routines. As shown in Figure 18.2, T had no difficulty in acquiring either a 21 hour or a 28-hour body-temperature rhythm. In each case it took him one week to make the change. K, on the other hand, continued with the 24-hour cycle, in spite of diligently following the prescribed schedules (Fig. 18.3). A noteworthy feature in T's body-temperature curves is the relation between the length of the cycle and the range of the mean or composite temperature curve, (RM): for the 21-hour cycle the RM was 1.21° F.; for the 24-hour cycle, 1.66° F.; and for the 28-hour cycle, 1.75° F. That sleep and wakefulness had some effect on K's body temperature is shown by the differences in the successive daily temperature curves, particularly on the 28-hour routine. When K slept during the night, his 24-hour temperature range was greater, and the curve smoother, than when he was obliged to sleep during the day. The time of going to sleep (incidence of first long period of quiescence) and the motility records were also different for successive "sleeps" on the artificial schedules. Compared to the corresponding figures on the 24-hour routine, the ease of going to sleep was greater, motility during sleep was smaller, and duration of sleep was longer on each of the two artificial cycles when the hour of retiring was at night; the reverse was true for sleep following daytime retiring hours.

It was not necessary to wait for several weeks' records to determine whether a subject was likely to acquire a body-temperature curve corresponding to the artificial cycle. By the use of the MR:RM ratio (p. 139), one could tell how superimposable the temperature figures were when arranged according to the 21- or 28-hour schedules; particularly when dividing the 8 or 6 cycles of the week into two halves—when the sleeping hours fell predominantly during darkness and when they occurred during the hours of light—the two half-weekly composite curves would resemble each other if the new cycle was established and would differ if the subject persisted in his 24-hour rhythm.

With this in mind we had four subjects follow an artificial routine for 2.5 weeks: two—the 21-hour cycle, and two—the 28-hour one. One of these subjects showed a definite swing to the new cycle; the other three, including R, did not. Going on a 28-hour routine, R could not sleep during the day hours and was very sleepy when the schedule called for staying up at night. Even though he undertook to follow the artificial routine for a longer time, he felt

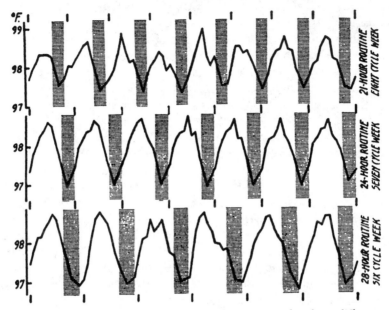

Fig. 18.2—Weekly body-temperature curves of subject T under three different routines of sleep and wakefulness. *Upper curve:* 21-hour routine of 15 hours of wakefulness and 6 hours of sleep; *middle curve:* customary 24-hour routine of 17 hours of wakefulness and 7 hours of sleep; *lower curve:* 28-hour routine of 19 hours of wakefulness and 9 hours of sleep. Shaded areas represent time spent in bed, usually in sleep. Each curve is based on five weeks of following one or another routine of living. Eight, seven, and six well-defined body-temperature waves can be discerned in the three corresponding weekly records, with the minima always in the shaded areas.

obliged to return to the regular 24-hour routine to be able to carry on his laboratory work and studies.

Obvious factors that seemed to interfere with adjustment to a non–24-hour rhythm were, besides light, the greater noise level and higher air temperatures in the daytime. In 1907 Lindhard (2518) produced an inversion of the body-temperature curves of members of his expedition in one week during the winter darkness in Greenland. As an approximation to uniform environmental conditions, a chamber in Mammoth Cave, Kentucky about 60 feet in width and 25 feet in height was secured as living quarters for subjects R and K from

June 4 to July 6, 1938. In that chamber, off the route traversed by conducted parties of tourists, the darkness was absolute when the artificial light used during the waking hours was turned off; the silence was also complete; and the temperature was always 54° F., not varying more than 1° in a year. The only unpleasant factor was the high humidity amounting to almost complete vapor saturation. Beds, a table, chairs, washstand, and platforms for the subjects' motility-recording equipment were provided by the management of the Mammoth Cave Hotel. From the same source came their meals, once or twice

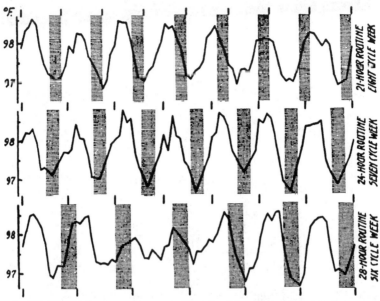

FIG. 18.3—Weekly body-temperature curves of subject K under the three routines of living described in the legend to Figure 18.2. Each weekly record shows seven body-temperature waves, with the minima in the shaded areas on the customary 24-hour routine, but not on the artificial 21- and 28-hour sleep-wakefulness schedules.

daily, to be eaten at once or later, depending on the schedule which was different for each day of the week. Oral temperature was taken every 2 hours during the waking period and 4 hours after retiring, which necessitated the use of an alarm clock. The waking period was of 19 hours' duration; and the period of darkness and staying in bed, usually but not always entirely devoted to sleep, 9 hours. A light breakfast was eaten shortly after getting up, and two larger meals were taken at the end of 7 and 13 hours, respectively, of the waking period. The chilly atmosphere made warm clothes necessary, particularly when sitting down, and was also conducive to frequent strolling through the cave. A large portion of the time was devoted to reading, studying, and working on motility records.

Toward the end of the first week R was completely adapted to the new routine. He had no difficulty in sleeping, was usually quite sleepy at retiring time, and even sleepier at the time of getting up, after 9 hours of sleep. He nearly always had to be awakened at the end of the sleep period, and his motility was about the same during every one of the 6 sleep periods. In Figure 18.4 are shown composite weekly body-temperature curves for the last 3 weeks

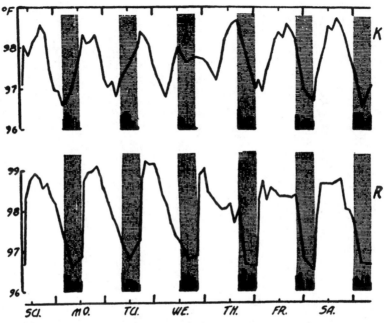

FIG. 18.4—Weekly body-temperature curves of subjects K and R under an artificial routine of 19 hours of wakefulness and 9 hours of sleep. Shaded areas represent time spent in bed; solid black areas show hourly variation in the incidence of 15-minute periods of quiescence: the larger the area, the smaller the motility. Each weekly record was based on the mean temperature values during the last three weeks of a stay in Mammoth Cave. K's weekly record has seven 24-hour curves, as in Figure 18.3, but R adapted himself to the 28-hour schedule, and his temperature record exhibits six waves per week, with the minima always in the shaded areas.

spent in the cave. It can be seen that R had 6 well-defined temperature waves, whereas K's weekly record contains 7 waves. R's temperature was always low at the time of getting up, but within the next hour it rose 1.5°–2° F., which it never did on a normal routine. Furthermore, the daily temperature range, as in T's case, was much higher than normal when the body-temperature rhythm was of 28 hours' duration.

K's behavior, like his body temperature, was entirely different. He could sleep very well when his sleeping hours in the cave coincided, or nearly coincided, with his customary sleeping time and a low temperature level. At other times he either had difficulty in falling asleep, or woke up too early, or both. His motility at such times was naturally greater than normal. Staying in bed for 9 hours, even during the upswing of the body-temperature curve, inevitably resulted in preventing the curve from reaching its usual height, as can be seen from the portion of K's temperature graph for Wednesday afternoon. The period from Tuesday evening to Wednesday noon was one in which the two subjects were in opposite phase with respect to each other's temperature rhythm. At 5:00 P.M. on Tuesday K was usually wide awake, and his temperature was near its maximum. R was then awakening, and his temperature was low. Toward midnight as K's temperature was falling, R's was above 99° F. At 4:00–6:00 A.M. on Wednesday K's temperature was at its lowest, well below 97° F., and he had difficulty in keeping awake. R's temperature was at that time above 98° F., and he was wide awake. Between 6:00 A.M. and noon K's temperature was steadily rising, and he was less and less sleepy. At noon, when his temperature reached 98° F., he was quite awake. During the same 6-hour period R's temperature was falling, and he was getting sleepier, as he usually did toward the end of the period of wakefulness. At noon his temperature was close to 97° F., and he could hardly keep awake. On the other hand, on Saturdays and Sundays the two body-temperature curves were practically parallel to each other. This was repeated week after week during the subjects' stay in the cave.

On leaving the cave, R's temperature curve quickly swung back into the 24-hour rhythm but did not acquire its usual range at once. The mean temperature figures for the first successive 5 weeks showed daily ranges of 1.54°, 1.56°, 1.68°, 1.83°, 1.88° F. During the first week he had difficulty in sleeping on certain nights, when by the 28-hour schedule he should have remained awake. But even during the first week he had a good 24-hour rhythm, and in 3 weeks or so his 24-hour body-temperature range was back to its normal value.

In K's case he could compare the temperature curve during the stay in the cave not only with the normal curves before and after but also with the 21-hour and the 28-hour curves obtained on the corresponding routines at our laboratory in Chicago. K's normal 24-hour (composite weekly) curves had a range of a little over 1.6° F. during the winter months and a little under 1.5° F. during the summer. Compared to these curves, his temperature curves on the 21-hour and the 28-hour regimens in Chicago were somewhat flatter, with both under 1.4° F. in range. In Chicago K's temperature peak was reached at 2:00 P.M., occasionally as early as noon or as late as 4:00 P.M., and that held true for the 21-, 24-, and 28-hour routines. In the cave, however, the maximum shifted very early to 6:00 P.M., where it remained, with a few exceptions, for the rest of his stay underground. K's minimum temperature was usually reached at 2:00–4:00 A.M.; the same applied to the temperature while in the cave, but on both the

21-hour and the 28-hour routines in Chicago the minimum tended to occur earlier—as early as 10:00 P.M. toward the end of each experiment.

It is hard to account for the later maximum of K's body temperature in the cave, or for the earlier minima on the artificial routines in Chicago, except as evidence of the tendency of the 24-hour temperature curve toward some disorganization, in spite of the fact that there was no distinct substitution of 21- and 28-hour curves for the normal 24-hour one.

From the results of these experiments it appears that there is no foundation for assuming that some cosmic forces determine the 24-hour rhythm, aside from "rest, movement, food intake, and sleep" (2022). On the contrary, the rhythm seems to be conditioned by activity of the organism which may adapt itself to the astronomical periodicity of day and night. The revelation that some individuals offer a great resistance to the development of an artificial routine of living does not vitiate the factual demonstration that the establishment of an artificial cycle is possible. Until many more observations of different individuals living on various routines become available, it is impossible to state the causative factors that contribute to the apparent fixity of the 24-hour rhythm. Age has been mentioned as one possible factor. Among the several subjects in this experiment K offered the greatest resistance to change, and he also happened to be the oldest of the group.

An opportunity presented itself for one male and two female subjects to be tested for adjustment to an 18- and a 28-hour routine of living by a sojourn in an outlying section of Tromsö, Norway, located well above the Arctic Circle (69°39′N. lat., 18°58′E. long.) for 9 weeks, from May 21 to July 23, 1951, during which period the sun did not set (2198). Three weeks were allowed for the adjustment to each of the two artificial routines, with two weeks on the normal 24-hour schedule between. In the female subjects there was a disruption of the 24-hour body-temperature rhythm, but there was no change in the 24-hour body-temperature curve of the male subject. The striking feature in all three subjects was the promptness with which the heart rate adjusted itself to both the 18- and 28-hour routines. As can be seen from Figure 18.5, in 72 hours on an 18-hour routine, there are four distinct 18-hour heart-rate curves, but only three 24-hour body-temperature curves, and in 168 hours on a 28-hour routine, there are 6 heart-rate and 7 body-temperature curves. Thus, although under the normal routine of living there is a complete parallelism between the body-temperature and heart-rate 24-hour curves, the former is a true rhythm, resisting a change, once established, whereas the latter is a periodicity coupled with the schedule of meals, activities, and sleep.

Lewis and Lobban (2477–80, 2544) followed the effects of living on a 21-, 22-, and 27-hour routine in several groups of explorers stationed in Spitzbergen during the continuous daylight of the summer. There was a partial adjustment to the artificial routine, more so for body temperature than for urinary excre-

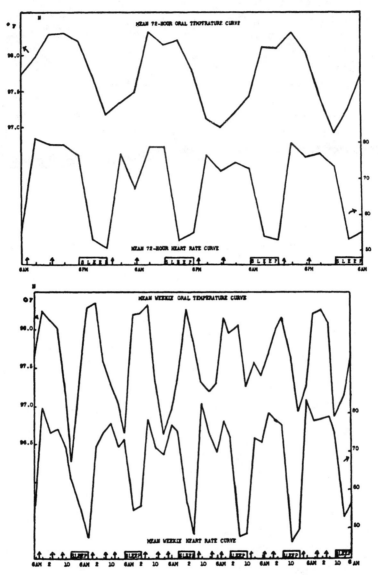

Fig. 18.5—Mean oral-temperature and heart-rate curves of subject K on artificial 18-hour (*upper curve*) and 28-hour (*lower curve*) routines of sleep and wakefulness. Each curve is based on a three-week period of following one or the other routine (seven 3-day or 72-hour periods and three 7-day or 168-hour periods). Hours of sleep are shown in boxes and mealtimes are marked by arrows on base-line.

tion of water, potassium, and chloride ions. The potassium 24-hour excretory rhythm was particularly resistant to change. In a non-Arctic setting, out of eight subjects who lived on a 22-hour schedule for 6 weeks, only one developed a 22-hour urinary rhythm.

Adams and co-workers (13) studied the behavior of two B-52 combat crews confined in a crew-compartment mock-up and tested with a battery of five performance tasks and four psychophysiological measures. Their results indicated that "men are able to work for periods of at least 15 days, using a 4-hour-on and 2-hour-off work-rest schedule continuously without any marked change in performance efficiency or in psychophysiological functioning." No information was given concerning the preservation or modification of the 24-hour rhythm.

From what is known about the establishment, maintenance, and modifiability of the 24-hour alternation of sleep and wakefulness, with associated rhythms and coupled periodicities, this alternation is based on a combination of nervous (probably cortical) and endocrine (probably hypophyseal-adreno-cortical) individually acquired mechanisms. No cosmic or hereditary factor need be invoked, though neither is excluded. An acceptable theory of sleep and wakefulness must account for the adjustment to the 24-hour alternation of night and day, as well as for the modifiability of the 24-hour rhythm after it has been established.

Chapter 19

Meteorological and Seasonal Influences

The 24-hour rhythm of sleep and wakefulness, even when it is well established, is subject to influences of, or at least varies with, other internal or physiological cycles as well as external meteorological and astronomical periodicities of shorter or longer duration.

Among the shorter physiological cycles one may mention the 50–60 minute rest-activity cycle and the 3–4 hour gastric motility cycle in the infant, which are lengthened to 80–90 minutes and 5–6 hours, respectively, in the adult. For longer periodicities, Richter (3341) noted cyclic fluctuations, 4–6 days in duration, of sleep in three psychotic patients; and Gjessing (1455), a 3–4 week alternation of a "reaction phase" in catatonics, when they slept only about 2 hours per night, with an "interval," when their sleep lasted about 7 hours. Hersey (1718), as previously indicated (p. 120), made an extensive, though somewhat obscure, study of moods that affected workingmen's psychic fatigability and efficiency. There were definite "highs" and "lows" in the mood cycle, whose duration varied from 4 to 6 weeks, shorter in younger than in older men, in introverts than in extroverts, in the dull than in the more intelligent, in the submissive than in the aggressive, in the single than in the married. However, the mood cycle did not seem to have any effect on sleep. Conversely, Hersey concluded that the sleep changes could not be held responsible for the highs and lows of the mood cycle.

The menstrual cycle in the human female is accompanied by definite changes in mood in most subjects. We (2200) compared the sleep records of nine young women, comprising 82 menstrual nights and 702 control nights. There were less "ease of going to sleep," greater motility, and longer duration of sleep, as well as a better recall of dreaming, on menstrual compared to normal nights. Of these variables, only the increase in recall of dreaming, which occurred on 65 per cent of the nights during menstruation, instead of the "control" 48 per cent, was of statistical significance.

In observations made by Rubenstein (3465) on the BMR and basal body-temperature variations during the menstrual cycle on sixteen normal women, twenty-one to thirty-nine years of age, he established low points in the early-morning body temperature and BMR (97.73° F., and 52.01 Cal. per hour) at the time of the pre-ovulative vaginal smear; the high points (98.42° F., and 54.46 Cal. per hour) coincided with the premenstrual smear. In other words, at the time of awakening in the morning the body temperature of these subjects was nearly 0.7° F. higher at certain times of the menstrual cycle than at others. That the 24-hour body-temperature rhythm is preserved during the menstrual temperature swings has been demonstrated by taking temperature readings in the evening, as well as early in the morning (2202). An analysis of the readings obtained in two subjects during 34 menstrual cycles revealed an almost complete parallelism between the evening and morning menstrual body-temperature curves, with a range of 99.13°–97.93° F. for the former, and of 98.53°–97.34° F. for the latter. Thus, temperatures taken in the evening, and probably at any other fixed time, are just as satisfactory as basal temperatures for revealing the ovulatory and other phases of the menstrual cycle, and, incidentally, oral temperatures are as indicative as are rectal and vaginal ones.

Meteorological, climatic, and seasonal influences constitute the major external periodicities that may play upon the 24-hour rhythm. Barometric pressure, temperature of the air, direction and force of winds, humidity, rainfall, and proportion of sunshine have all been considered in attempts to discover the effects of environmental conditions on sleep. No correlations were noted between changes in atmospheric pressure and depth and duration of sleep (3064, 3076, 3458). However, in eighteen subjects, with 3,522 nights of sleep, we (2200) detected a slight increase in motility during sleep when the barometric pressure was higher than usual, but the difference was not statistically significant.

Boynton (436) found that extremes of room temperature were unfavorable for the continuity of the afternoon naps of nursery-school children. The optimum room temperature was 50°–60° F. Scott (3631), in a similar study, and Shinn (3682), in records of both day and night sleep of children, could detect but little effect from changes in room temperature when it varied from 68.5° to 82.5° F. Changes in humidity were also without influence on sleep (3064, 3682).

In the records of our subjects (2200) we tried to correlate various sleep characteristics with outdoor temperature, room temperature, humidity, precipitation, and combinations of the foregoing. No definite correlations could be established.

For the longer seasonal periodicities there are several reports which fail to agree with one another. Haas (1565) found sleep to be deeper in the winter than in the summer. According to Hayashi (1670), the Japanese sleep longest in the winter, next longest in the autumn, less in the spring, least in the summer. Erwin (1106), from a study of the sleep of 409 children, concluded that sleep was longer in the fall and winter than in the spring and summer, but Garvey (1363) noted no seasonal differences in children's sleep. Laird (2336) stated that sleep was poorest in the spring, when "calcium metabolism" was at its lowest, and best in the late autumn, which was the high serum-calcium season.

In two subjects (2193) we found the motility and the temperature levels during sleep to be higher in the summer and autumn than in the winter and spring. In a more extensive study of the sleep records of twelve subjects over 1,785 nights, distributed fairly evenly over the four seasons (2200), we detected seasonal variations in several sleep characteristics, some of which, however, were not found to be statistically significant. The percentage of nights on which the subjects went to sleep with ease showed a bimodal curve for the year, the best seasons in this respect were spring and autumn, with percentages of 95 and 93, while the figures for winter and summer were 90 and 87, respectively. Although our subjects appeared to have no difficulty in going to sleep in any season, these small differences are statistically significant. Motility during sleep and recall of dreaming, both with significant seasonal variations, each show a single yearly cycle. Motility was least in the spring and greatest in the autumn. Lowest incidence of recall of dreaming seemed to coincide with the highest motility. The number of hours slept and the feeling of being well rested on getting up in the morning did not show either marked or statistically reliable seasonal differences.

In a long-range study of seasonal variations in the different sleep characteristics, the subjects were two girls, H and E, who were six and a half and four and a half years old, respectively, at the beginning of the period of observation. They were leading normal lives, occupying themselves with the usual pursuits of children of elementary-school age. They slept in separate rooms, under ordinary home conditions, the only "abnormality" being the presence of recording devices under and near their beds. They quickly became accustomed to the presence of the recording instruments and learned to set them and to care for the records very much as adult subjects did under similar conditions. They usually went to bed at 7:30–8:00 P.M. On school days they got up before, or were awakened at, 7:00 A.M.; on other days they were allowed to sleep longer, though they seldom did. The duration of the night sleep was thus about 11 hours. The younger girl continued to take afternoon naps for 2 years. Both children were in good health and had no serious illnesses during the 3-year period of observation. Minor ailments and instrumental imperfections caused the elimination of certain records, and short vacations also led to the loss of a few nights at a time, with the result that the data to be discussed were based on a mean of 290 days per year per child, with no month furnishing less than fifteen satisfactory sleep-motility records. As can be seen from Table 19.1, there was a marked seasonal variation in motility, whether expressed in terms of numbers of the hundredths of work-adder turns per hour or in seconds spent in movement per hour (p. 83). Figure 19.1 for the month-to-month variation in mean hourly motility for the entire period shows that the annual cycle was repeated three times for each of the two children. Of the seasons, summer was characterized by the highest and winter by the lowest motility, with the autumn and spring figures between and of about the same magnitude. The mean air temperatures were usually lowest in January and February and highest in July and

TABLE 19.1

SEASONAL VARIATION IN MOTILITY DURING SLEEP, AS JUDGED BY DIFFERENT CRITERIA, IN TWO GIRLS—H, AGED NINE AND ONE-HALF YEARS, AND E, AGED SEVEN AND ONE-HALF YEARS, AT THE END OF THE PERIOD OF OBSERVATION

Criteria of Motility		Winter (Dec., Jan., Feb.)	Spring (Mar., Apr., May)	Summer (June, July, Aug.)	Autumn (Sept., Oct., Nov.)
Motility measured in hundredths of "work-adder" turns per hour of sleep, means for 1936, 1937, 1938	H	12.7	13.8	20.3	15.0
	E	13.6	17.8	24.0	17.7
Number of seconds spent in movement per hour of sleep, means for 1936, 1937, 1938	H	19.9	20.1	22.6	19.3
	E	22.5	29.6	32.6	29.7
Number of movements per hour of sleep, means for 1938	H	5.75	6.45	5.53	5.47
	E	7.30	6.60	5.94	6.65
"Going-to-sleep" time—number of minutes elapsing prior to the onset of the first period of immobility of 15 minutes or longer, means for 1938	H	24.3	21.5	22.2	24.1
	E	8.7	7.2	8.9	8.1
Percentage of nights in which long period of immobility set in at once after going to bed, means for 1938	H	6	8	0	0
	E	28	39	27	30
Number of quarter-hours of immobility per night of 11 hours, means for 1938	H	22.6	20.6	22.2	22.0
	E	19.1	20.1	20.5	19.5
Number of periods of immobility of one hour or longer per night of 11 hours, means for 1938	H	0.75	0.64	0.78	0.83
	E	0.48	0.70	0.60	0.55

August, and the same was true of motility. There was, in addition, an annual variation in motility levels, 1938 being highest and 1937 lowest, and the ratios for the 3 years about the same for each of the two subjects. The U.S. Weather Bureau data for the 3 years showed no variations in Chicago temperature, atmospheric pressure, or precipitation, which might be related to the variations in motility. The seasonal differences, however, were quite independent of the general motility level, which was consistently higher for E than for H.

Compared to the curve for seasonal variation in motility for our group of twelve subjects, with the highest motility in the autumn and lowest in the spring, the children's curves showed a shift of one season for the maximum and minimum, but the same semiannual separation of the two extremes. As shown in

Figure 8.2 (p. 60), in our earliest study of seasonal variations in motility during sleep, on two adults (2193), motility was found to be higher in summer and autumn than in winter and spring. Thus, in the three separate investigations, lowest motility occurred in (*a*) winter and spring, (*b*) spring, and (*c*) winter, or, in general, during the colder portion of the year.

The time spent in movement, also higher for E than for H, showed less of a seasonal variation, suggesting that the seasonal differences applied more to the extent of the movements than to their incidence. To test this supposition, a detailed study was made not only of the incidence of the individual movements

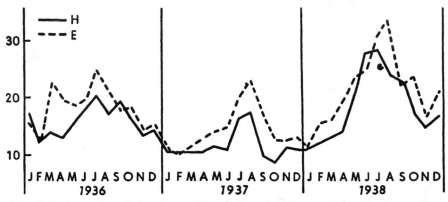

Fig. 19.1—Seasonal variation in motility during sleep in two girls, H, nine and one-half, and E, seven and one-half years old, at the end of the period of observation. Total number of records for the three years for each child: 870. Motility is expressed as the mean number of hundredths of work-adder turns (Fig. 10.1) per hour of sleep for each of 36 successive months. There is a general parallelism between the two curves, with the lowest motility values in the winter and the highest in the summer, and the motility of H usually smaller than that of E (Table 19.1). There is also a variation in the sleep motility of both children for each of the three years: designating the motility level for 1936 as 1.00, the motility levels for 1937 and 1938 are, respectively, 0.74 and 1.19 for H and 0.79 and 1.17 for E.

during sleep, as recorded by a signal magnet in series with the electric-clock circuit, but also of the distribution of periods of immobility of 15 minutes' duration or longer for each of the children for the year 1938. The occurrence of the first such period was taken arbitrarily as the beginning of sleep. As shown in Table 19.1, there was little seasonal variation in the "ease of going to sleep," but the smallest mean figures (21.5 minutes for H and 7.2 minutes for E) prior to the onset of a long period of immobility coresponded to the spring months, in that respect agreeing with the seasonal figures for the twelve subjects referred to above. The percentage of nights on which a long period of immobility set in at once after going to bed was also highest in the spring. The distribution of the rest periods themselves revealed no consistent seasonal variation whatsoever (Fig. 19.2). The curves for each child show a characteristic downward course, to be expected from the usually increasing incidence of movement during the night, but the 4 seasonal curves cross and recross each other repeatedly. The total numbers of periods of immobility per night (Table 19.1) were about the same for all seasons. Again, the individuality of the "rest" pattern manifested itself in each group of 4 seasonal curves. The number of immobility periods was greater for H than for E, and, probably because of H's slower onset of sleep, the greater incidence of periods of immobility occurred, in her case, during the second and third hours of sleep, while E's curves had their highest points during the first and second hours.

Superficially, it appears to be possible to demonstrate the presence or absence of a seasonal variation in motility during sleep by choosing the appropriate criterion. Actually, however, there is no contradiction in these apparently inconsistent

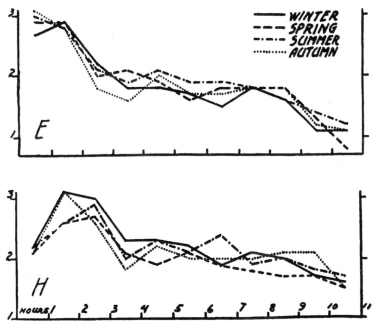

Fig. 19.2—Variation in the mean hourly incidence of periods of immobility during sleep for two girls, H (288 nights) and E (309 nights), based on data gathered during 1938. Immobility is expressed in quarter-hours in which no movement occurred; immobility of 15–29 minutes counted as one, 30–44 minutes as two, 45–59 as three. Winter: December, January, February; spring: March, April, May; summer: June, July, August; autumn: September, October, November. The curves for the four seasons show no consistent variations in either subject, but, on the contrary, indicate a distinct individuality irrespective of season with regard to the total periods of immobility per night, greater for H than for E (Table 19.1), and their distribution through the night's sleep. The maximum immobility was the same for both subjects, and the difference in its hour of incidence was probably related to the earlier onset of sleep in E than in H (Table 19.1).

conclusions. What the figures indicate is a fairly stable individual pattern of motility during sleep, showing the same distribution of movements and immobility periods over the 4 seasons of the year. The time one spends in making the movements and particularly the extent of the movements themselves do show a seasonal variation. During the cold season of the year one's movements during sleep are confined to the warmed-up area of the bed, the outlying "cold regions" discouraging extensive movements. Quite the opposite is the situation during the warm season, when movement is encouraged by the absence of bedcovers and the relief obtained from a complete transfer of the body from a warmer to a cooler portion of the bed surface.

A marked seasonal difference for the duration of sleep was reported for a herd of hamadril monkeys, which slept for about 8.5 hours during the May–July trimester, as against 14.5 hours in the December–February one (3727). It seems that length of daylight and environmental temperatures were the deciding factors.

Seasonal differences in the 24-hour body-temperature curves of two subjects are shown in Figure 15.6 (p. 146). A close look at parts *A* and *C* of that figure, representing summer body temperatures, and parts *B* and *D* for winter data, will reveal that the histograms for the different hours of the day, as well as their modes, were higher in the summer. There were also many more temperature readings above 99° F. in the summer for both subjects. Night temperatures, including the early morning "basal" ones, were the same in both seasons. Adam and Ferres (9), who compared the body temperatures of groups of subjects in the temperate climate of Oxford (64.1° F. dry bulb and 56.3° F. wet bulb) and the humid tropical climate of Singapore (79.9° F. dry bulb and 72.2° F. wet bulb), obtained similar 24-hour body-temperature curves in both places. At Singapore, however, the mean values were 0.43° F. higher for rectal temperatures, and 0.35° F. higher for oral ones, than at Oxford (differences statistically highly significant).

Iampietro and associates (1890) compared the 24-hour body-temperature curves of several subjects at Natick, Massachusetts, Mount Washington, New Hampshire, and Fort Churchill, Canada, and concluded that living in diverse climates had no effect on the 24-hour body-temperature pattern. On the other hand, Lobban (2543) tested natives of Yukon Territory in midsummer and midwinter for differences in the urinary excretion of water and potassium and chloride ions. She found that "in about half the native subjects the diurnal excretory rhythms which we have come to regard as normal in subjects from temperate zones were either absent or were very much reduced in amplitude." Similar findings were made on "white" subjects who had been living in the same arctic environment for some months.

The impression of steamer passengers taking "Midnight Sun" cruises along the coast of North Norway has been that the local inhabitants sleep very little or not at all during the summer, as one sees people at piers of towns at all hours of the day and night. Actually the duration of sleep for a sample of the population of Tromsö, Norway, was only about one hour less in the summer than in the winter. Indeed, the continuous daylight of the summer seems to be less disturbing than the near-continuous darkness of the winter (2199). Kjos (2169) noted far fewer subjective complaints or objective signs of sleep difficulties among 407 school children of Tromsö in April than in January. A group of five men, who, as members of the British North Greenland Expedition of 1952–54, spent two years at a latitude of 77° N., slept, on the average, a little under 8 hours per night, with no marked seasonal trends (2475).

Finally, Winkel and Hamoen (4239) found a seasonal variation in the appearance of a "sleep pattern" in the EEGs of 741 patients examined in one year. The pattern, characterized by (a) flattening of previously normal EEG, dissolution of alpha and appearance of theta and delta waves, and (b) reappearance of alpha after acoustic stimulation, showed up in 2.5 per cent of the patients in the spring, 9.9 per cent in the summer, 6.3 per cent in the autumn, and 6.2 per cent in the winter.

Meteorological and seasonal periodicities, as well as geographic and climatic differences in light-darkness ratios and environmental temperature and humidity, influence mood and behavior and may thus affect sleep indirectly. The fundamental 24-hour sleep-wakefulness rhythm is not changed by these external periodicities.

Part 4

Interference with Sleep and Wakefulness

Chapter 20

Induction of Sleep

Animals and persons can be induced to fall asleep or to change to a state closely resembling sleep by a variety of physical and chemical methods. The simple procedure of rocking the cradle, sometimes accompanied by the singing of a lullaby, has long been a favorite way of inducing sleep in infants. Holding a baby in one's arms, gently restraining its movements, has also stood the test of time as a physical soporific. Although these methods may be frowned upon in modern nursery-room practice, their efficacy has never been denied. In the laboratory Sidis (3691), employing guinea pigs, cats, dogs, and children, produced sleep by limitation of movement, aided at times by a continuous monotonous sound. The puppies Sidis used were from three weeks to three months old. Wrapping a cloth around them, he immobilized them in the dorsal position and kept their eyes closed by placing his fingers on their eyelids. After a few attempts to free themselves, the puppies became quiescent and eventually fell asleep. On repetition of the experiment the animals could be put to sleep with greater ease, until it was no longer necessary to immobilize them. Sidis concluded that sleep was caused by a "diminution in the variability of the volume of sensory impressions."

I repeated these experiments on several puppies, from one week to three months of age but omitted the monotonous sound. I also employed a slightly different method of keeping the puppies quiescent (2178). I simply placed the animal in the dorsal position in the "trough" formed when the forearm was held horizontally close to the body. The puppy's head fitted into the hollow of the hand, and the fingers could be closed (if necessary) around its head or on the eyelids. In this way, the trunk and limbs of the animal were entirely free, and it rarely struggled but rather nestled against the warm body of the observer. After a few minutes in this position, the body and limb musculature could be seen to relax progressively, and a little later the puppy invariably fell asleep. In many cases the onset of sleep was preceded by a yawn or two and by a general trembling or startle movement of the legs, especially of the paws. When respiration was recorded, the breathing could be seen to become regular, in rate and in amplitude, after such a startle movement. Once definitely asleep, a puppy could be manipulated considerably without waking it up. The outstanding feature of its condition was a complete muscular relaxation, particularly of the trunk and head. By dorsiflexing the hand upon the forearm, the puppy's head could be gradually lowered without arousing the animal. The length of time that the puppy remained asleep varied greatly. As a rule, it was only a matter of a few minutes before the animal awakened. Yawning and startle movements frequently accompanied awakening, but the most constant and striking occurrence was an increase in the tonus of the body musculature. Thus, in puppies, immobilization which was conducive to muscular relaxation was alone sufficient to induce sleep.

That monotonous stimulation was not needed was also demonstrated long ago by Coriat (758), who likewise studied the effect of immobilization in animals and of muscular relaxation in man: "The subject was directed to completely relax all his muscles, with the result that when the limbs were elevated they fell by their own weight." His subjects usually fell asleep in about 15 minutes, whether a monotonous sound stimulus (buzzer) was used or not. When the muscles were held tense, no sleep resulted. "Changes from muscular tension to muscular relaxation produced sleep: changes from muscular relaxation to muscular tension induced complete wakefulness in the drowsy subject." I repeated Coriat's observations (2176) and was able to confirm them in every particular. On many occasions I had observed persons who were instructed to "lie quietly" for about 30 minutes prior to having their BMR determined. Even though these measurements were made shortly after getting up in the morning, the subject often fell asleep while waiting for the test. Coriat's findings were also confirmed by Lovell and Morgan (2568), who found that control subjects relaxed as well as one group which was submitted to a recurrent sound stimulus and another group given instructions to relax.

Of significance in this connection is the work of Miller (2823), who studied the reactions of seven subjects to induction shocks sent into the fingers of one hand (p. 76). The shock was of such intensity as to be painful, and it generally resulted in a flexion of the arm at the elbow. Her subjects were trained for months to relax completely during the tests. Compared to control experiments, extreme muscular relaxation led to a reduction of the extent of the flexion, an increase in RT, and a diminution of the apparent intensity or unpleasantness of the stimulus. On many occasions there was no movement in response to the shock. Relaxation frequently resulted in sleep. We (2201) were not only able to decrease the sensitivity to pain in subjects who were sitting down and relaxing for one hour, but correspondingly to increase it by having the relaxed subjects stand up for the next hour (p. 159). There is thus a similarity between the phenomena accompanying the onset of sleep and the condition of muscular relaxation: in both cases there is a raised threshold of excitability.

Though not needed, repetitive light or sound stimuli are conducive to sleep (1367, 3070), at times assisted by autosuggestion (944–47). When frank sleep is not achieved, distinct drowsiness may develop. Kennedy and Travis (2140, 2141) noted a decrease in muscle action potentials, as well as poorer performance, in carrying out monotonous tasks. Drowsiness has also been induced in subjects whose breathing sounds were amplified (2294, 2295); who were submitted to prolonged mild anoxia (3735); were breathing warm air (756); were rotated slowly (1509); or were merely asked to lie down to have their EEGs recorded (2135).

That monotony of surroundings may play a significant part in the production of sleep can be seen from the incidence of sleep during the study of conditioned reflexes, particularly in Pavlov's laboratory, where sound insulation was most complete (3121, 3122, 3124). Pavlov himself definitely connected "internal inhibition" with the onset of sleep, and this led to the development of his theory that sleep is a generalized cortical inhibition (p. 344). Krasnogorski (2264) established a number of "active points" on the skin of the leg in the dog. The tactile stimulation of one or another of these points always preceded feeding, and the animals responded to such stimulation in a characteristic manner. An "inactive point" was also stimulated from time to time, but this was not followed by feeding. Stimulation of the "inactive point" often caused the onset of sleep. Similar findings on man and animals were explained in Pavlovian terms, as negative induction or internal inhibition, by other investigators (335, 1482, 2307, 2430, 3088). Curiously interpreted was the behavior of a dog conditioned by Kupalov (2308), with feeding as the unconditioned stimulus. The dog was allowed to move around, as "some foreign authors attempted to consider the convincing facts of Pavlov as a particular phenomenon, due to the special conditions of technique, by which the animal is placed in a stand, and its freedom of movement is limited." After eating fast 18 times, then slowly another 8 times, the animal, evidently satiated, lay down and fell asleep. This loss of interest in the feeding was considered by Kupalov an irradiation of internal inhibition and a direct cause of the onset of sleep. Similarly interpreted was the ease with which children went to sleep in the evening, while being tested for conditioned responses, as due to greater inhibitability (3673), or irradiation of low excitability (2265).

Rosenthal (3415) has shown that no special conditioning is necessary to produce sleep. He studied the orientation or "investigatory" reflex in puppies and dogs. It is the response of a dog to a certain stimulus, like a sound, produced by the observer, by turning to the direction from which the sound came in order to investigate the situation. Since nothing happens, the dog turns his head back to the normal position. The sound is now again produced, and again the dog "investigates." Repeating this procedure a number of times, one finds that the dog finally refuses to investigate further, having by this time presumably convinced himself that the sound has no special significance. This loss of interest is designated by Pavlov and his school as an inhibition of the investigatory reflex. Rosenthal created such a situation for his dogs, either using special sound stimuli or else letting the setting of the laboratory furnish the dogs with spontaneous occurrences to be investigated. In each case the animals fell asleep after being kept in the room for a while. Such a tendency for dogs to fall asleep when placed in a stand and trained to remain quiet for a certain interval of time is familiar to almost everyone who has had occasion to study basal metabolism, gastric and intestinal motility or secretion, and has usually been ascribed to monotony. The dogs that we (2944) studied (p. 77) had no conditioned reflexes developed in them at any time, and yet they almost always fell asleep when left in a room by themselves.

The notion that internal inhibition always precedes sleep is also challenged by the observations made on a dog during conditioned salivation produced by daily injections of morphine (2180). Such a dog brought into the room where he usually received the injection would begin to secrete saliva, the setting of the laboratory acting as a continuous conditioned stimulus. This went on until the injection of morphine, by producing first stimulation and later depression, terminated the conditioned secretion, and the interval could be made as long as one or two hours. Usually the animals appeared quite alert prior to the administration of morphine, but the dog in question had a tendency to fall asleep while in the laboratory under observation. As drowsiness developed, the conditioned salivary secretion gradually diminished, and with the onset of sleep it would stop entirely. Waking the dog resulted in a full resumption of the salivary flow. The only way to insure a steady uniform conditioned salivation was to keep the dog awake by talking to it or by moving around the room. A typical example of the secretory activity of this dog is shown in Figure 20.1. These results were based on the behavior of one dog, but since then this phenomenon has been seen in several dogs under similar conditions. In all these animals there was no inhibition of the conditioned salivation before the development of drowsiness, but the latter, on the contrary, led to a gradual decrease in salivation. There was a definite proportionality between the two, with no secretion at all during frank sleep. Yet Kamensky (2067) explained a similar return of conditioned reflex activity in a dog after 20–30 minutes of sleep as a restoration of the working capacity of its cerebrum.

A situation similar to that of the dog left alone, when it is specially contrived for observational or experimental purposes, is spoken of as sensory isolation or deprivation. When subjects are deprived of external stimulation for one or more days, they tend to suffer a decrease in intellectual ability (1716, 4333) and in test performance (1716, 3634), though improved learning capacity has also been reported (4050). Hallucinations (326, 1716, 3752, 4182, 4323), anxiety and depression (4323, 4324), and a tendency to sleep (4086, 4087) have been observed in normal persons, and disorganization, in patients with anxiety or obsession (164). Rioch (3359) found that normal cats kept in the dark for 48–72 hours slept, or, at least, were quiescent for 18–20 hours out of 24. Real sensory deprivation as created by Struempell (3854) in his celebrated patient was said to produce an immediate onset of sleep, but Ballet (192), who studied a man with a hysterical loss of gustatory, olfactory, cutaneous and proprioceptive senses, doubted the reality of the "sleep" that could be induced by excluding vision and hearing. Complete deafferentation is probably incompatible with the maintenance of wakefulness, but monotony of stimulation, or an absence of external stimuli, is often sufficient to induce sleep.

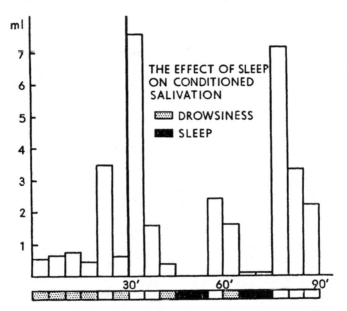

Fig. 20.1—A typical example of the effect of drowsiness and sleep on the rate of conditioned salivary secretion, for successive 5-minute intervals, before and after the injection of morphine, which acted as an unconditioned stimulus (thick vertical line). During the first 20 minutes of conditioned secretion the dog was drowsy (eyes half-closed), and the secretion rate was 0.4–0.7 ml. For the next 5 minutes the dog was kept awake, and the quantity of saliva secreted rose to 3.5 ml. Permitted to become drowsy again, the dog secreted only 0.6 ml in the last 5 minutes prior to the injection of morphine. Post-injection secretion of saliva was 7.6 and 1.6 ml for the first two 5-minute intervals. The dog then became very drowsy, and the 0.4 ml shown for the third 5 minutes was really collected in the first 2 minutes. During the fourth and fifth periods the dog was definitely asleep and snoring, and no saliva came out of the fistula for 13 minutes. The repetition of wakefulness, drowsiness and frank sleep led to the secretion of 2.4, 1.6, 0.1, and 0.1 ml for the sixth to the ninth periods. Aroused again and kept wide-awake, the dog secreted 7.2, 3.3, and 2.2 ml, respectively, for the last three 5-minute intervals.

Entirely different methods of inducing sleep consist of either injecting certain substances into the blood stream, brain ventricles, or brain tissue itself, or of stimulating or destroying certain regions of the brain stem. Among the older observations are those of Litwer (2539, 2540), who made some experiments to test the toxic theory of sleep of Bouchard (424), based on the alleged convulsive action of urine secreted during sleep and the narcotic effect of urine secreted in the waking period. Litwer produced convulsions and death in rabbits by the intravenous injection of concentrated urine (osmotic pressure 2.5 to 7 times that of body fluids), but not with the same urine when diluted; he ascribed the positive results obtained by Bouchard to the concentration of solids in the urine used for injections.

Forsgren (1243, 1247), also experimenting on rabbits, employed aqueous extracts of livers taken from sleeping rabbits. These, when injected subcutaneously into rabbits that were wide awake, rendered them sleepy. He concluded that sleep might be governed by some substance produced in the liver.

Parenteral administration of milk was found to have a sleep-producing effect by Lust (2584). He treated a child who suffered from sleeplessness, which followed an attack of encephalitis, by intramuscular injection of 2 ml of milk. The child slept soundly through the night. Omitting the milk injection next night caused the sleeplessness to return. The child's body temperature was raised by the injections of milk, and other protein-containing materials had an equal sleep-producing effect if they led to a rise in body temperature. An increase in temperature from 37.3° to 37.8° C. was sufficient to induce sleep. Lindig (2519), in general, confirmed Lust's finding that anything that raised the body temperature would lead to sleep.

On the basis of the supposed decrease in the calcium concentration of the blood during anesthesia, and of his own finding of a similar decrease during sleep, Demole (908) considered the possibility of calcium being taken up by the brain as the cause of sleep. To test this hypothesis, he injected (after a preliminary exposure of the brain under ether anesthesia) from 0.25 to 2 mg $CaCl_2$ in 0.025–0.05 ml of water into the region of the gray matter close to the infundibulum and tuber cinereum of a number of cats. The result was sleep, lighter or deeper, lasting from 30 minutes to 3 hours, depending upon the dose of $CaCl_2$ injected. There was also a slowing of the pulse and respiration, narrowing of the pupils, and an appearance of the nictitating membrane. When he injected the salt into other regions of the brain, sleep was not produced. Into two cats he injected KCl, which led to stiffness and convulsions—not to sleep. Demole could abolish the effects of a KCl injection by $CaCl_2$, but not vice versa.

Berggren and Moberg (304) repeated Demole's experiments, also on cats, using $CaCl_2$ and KCl solutions, isotonic with the blood, and controlling their injections by merely inserting the needle or by introducing Ringer's solution.

They obtained sleep with either of the two salts, sometimes from merely inserting the needle, but the effective region delineated by them coincides with that given by Demole. Yoshihara (4292) produced typical sleep in cats and monkeys by injecting doses of CaCl₂, comparable to Demole's, into the tuber cinereum, but not when injecting it elsewhere. He found that his animals would awaken when exposed to cold (—4° C.) but went back to sleep when returned to a warm room.

Cloetta and Fischer (722) also confirmed Demole's results with calcium. They tested, in addition, the effects of injecting salts of other metals. The magnesium ion had a less certain effect and had to be used in larger amounts than calcium. Strontium produced a mixture of inhibitory and excitatory symptoms. The effect of barium was marked stimulation when injected into any part of the brain, which was not true of the other ions. Potassium likewise caused psychic and motor excitement, but only when injected into the infundibular region; its action was of brief duration and could be abolished by calcium. Sodium was without any effect.

Brunelli (548) obtained similar results by injecting various salts into the tuber cinereum of cats: sleep from calcium and magnesium, and excitement from potassium, barium, and strontium. He interpreted his results as corresponding to what one might expect from the effects of these ions on the permeability of cell membranes: a decrease in permeability leading to depression; an increase, to stimulation.

In this connection, Cloetta and co-workers (723) found a slight increase in the calcium and potassium content of the brain during sleep, with the increase greater in the infundibular region than in other parts of the brain. They therefore concluded that the calcium ion participated in the production of sleep, although as previously stated (p. 35), they realized that the calcium taken up by the brain could not account for the amount that supposedly disappeared from the blood. Katzenelbogen (2092) also analyzed the brain and its various regions for calcium. He experimented with cats under the effects of diallylbarbituric acid narcosis. He found as much calcium in the brain of anesthetized animals as in those of controls. There was more calcium in the hypothalamus than in any other region, but here also there was no difference between the control and narcotized animals. While Katzenelbogen's finding suggests that "calcium may play a certain role in the function of the hypothalamic region," it shows that calcium is not a factor in determining the state of the animal (wakefulness or anesthesia). Katzenelbogen (2091) had previously reported that there was a decrease in the calcium content of the blood as well as of the cerebrospinal fluid in cats when under the influence of diallylbarbituric acid for some 18–22 hours. The ratios of the fluid calcium to blood calcium, however, did not permit him to conclude that sleep is associated with marked changes in the permeability of the blood-cerebrospinal-fluid barrier to calcium.

Although Demole did not obtain as typical a sleep picture by intraventricular injection of CaCl₂ as he did by introducing the salt into the hypothalamus, Lafora and Sanz-Ibáñez (2323, 3517) worked out a method that yielded good results in cats. At first they employed the customary suboccipital puncture of the fourth ventricle, and control injections of colored solutions showed that the liquid rapidly diffused through the aqueduct into the third ventricle. Amounts of CaCl₂ varying from 0.5 to 1 ml of a 5 per cent solution, when thus injected, produced sleep in 1–2 minutes. The onset of sleep appeared quite natural and was preceded by yawning, assumption of the horizontal position, and slowing of the respiration. The sleep was exceptionally deep and lasted from 3 to 6 hours. Smaller doses of CaCl₂ led to a lighter and shorter-lasting sleep. In all cases, however, the cats could be aroused by appropriate stimulation and, when allowed to do so, fell asleep again. Because some animals died from cessation of respiration shortly after the injection, the authors improvised a way of reaching the third ventricle directly: they exposed and cut the occipito-atloid ligament and introduced a urethral sound through the fourth ventricle and aqueduct into the third ventricle. They could then obtain the usual sleep effect with half as much CaCl₂ as they had to use previously. Injections of KCl led to excitement lasting an hour or more, followed by a semblance of sleep. Somnifen, luminal, and dial, introduced by the same method, were less efficacious than CaCl₂. Tonkikh (3957) produced sleep in cats by the injection of CaCl₂ into the brain ventricles, but the sleep did not appear "natural."

Marinesco and co-workers (2681–83) performed a variety of experiments on fifty cats, some of which they used more than once. They were among the first to repeat and confirm Demole's observations. In addition to intrahypothalamic and intraventricular injections, they also tried intravenous ones. Choline, introduced intravenously, led at first to agitation, trembling, and muscular hypertonus, but within 30 minutes the cats fell asleep. The sleep reached its greatest depth in 1–1.5 hours and lasted for 3–4 hours. Intravenous injections of KCl had an effect similar to that which followed choline injections, but CaCl₂ produced sleep in 10 minutes. The authors pointed out that both choline and potassium act as parasympathetic stimulants and interpreted their finding to mean that sleep is probably due to an excitation of the "parasympathetic center" in the hypothalamus.

Hess (1740) obtained sleep in cats, with the sympathetic system removed by operation, after an intraventricular injection of ergotamine. The pupils were small during the ergotamine-induced sleep, but they dilated reflexly in response to acoustic and tactile stimuli. The pupils also exhibited the paradoxical response to light which, according to Hess, is characteristic of physiological sleep: there was a momentary widening prior to the narrowing, particularly if the light stimulus was applied at the onset of sleep when the pupils were not yet fully narrowed.

Dikshit (937, 938) studied the effects of intraventricular and intrahypothalamic injections of acetylcholine in cats. Small doses (0.0001–0.0005 mg) of the drug produced a "condition closely resembling sleep" which came on in 10–30 minutes and lasted for 2–3 hours. Control injections of physiological salt solution were ineffective, while pilocarpine caused excitement. He considered these results a confirmation of the view that sleep is a parasympathetic phenomenon. Dikshit also found acetylcholine in the brain, more in the basal nuclei than elsewhere.

Hoffer (1809) injected acetylcholine into human volunteers who thereupon became tired and sleepy, going to sleep hours before their usual bedtime. Hoffer concluded that the effects were due to an increased parasympathetic tone.

Legendre and Piéron (2408–13) reported the discovery of a "hypnotoxin." They could not conveniently extract it from the brain of a dog that had been kept awake for several days, nor were blood transfusions successful. However, 4–6 ml of cerebrospinal fluid, obtained from a dog that had been deprived of sleep and injected into the fourth ventricle of another dog (after withdrawing from the latter an equal volume of fluid), caused the development of marked drowsiness and histological brain changes characteristic of prolonged sleeplessness. "Normal" cerebrospinal fluid, when similarly injected, had no effect.

Ivy and Schnedorf (1926, 3580) repeated Piéron's experiments and obtained depression and sleep in normal dogs, after an injection of 8 ml of cerebrospinal fluid from other dogs that had been kept awake. However, all recipients of cerebrospinal fluid, or of physiological salt solution used as a control, showed a rise in body temperature, averaging 2.6° F., if they were depressed by the injection, which confirmed the earlier findings of Lust (2584) and Lindig (2519).

Kroll (2287) obtained an extract of brain tissue from sleeping rabbits and cats which, when injected intravenously or suboccipitally into waking animals, caused the latter to fall asleep. It did not make any difference how the donor animals were put to sleep (by pernocton, intraventricular injections of $CaCl_2$) : the brain extracts were equally soporific. Extracts of the non-hibernating hamster's brain were without effect, but those made of the hamster's brain during hibernation produced a state of deep sleep, lasting from 2 to 35 days, when injected into cats. The cats' body temperature fell from 1° to 2° C., they behaved like partially poikilothermal animals, and their blood sugar was decreased to about one-half its normal value. Extracts of other organs of the hibernating hamster had no sleep-producing effect. However, Neri and associates (2986, 2987) failed in an attempt to demonstrate the liberation of soporific materials into the blood stream of a sleeping dog. Having established a cross-circulation in two dogs, they induced sleep in one of them by thrusting a needle into the infundibular region. Nothing happened to the second animal while the first one slept. The authors concluded that sleep resulted from purely nervous action and not from hormonal or chemical influences.

Schuetz (3594), by a curious line of reasoning, decided that the antidiuretic principle of the posterior lobe of the hypophysis should "cause, deepen, or prolong natural sleep," and found this to be the case, at least for afternoon naps, in eighteen out of thirty-five subjects tested. Faltz and co-workers (1136) confirmed Schuetz's findings but disagreed with his reasoning.

The induction of physiological sleep, as distinguished from anesthesia, by electrical stimulation of parts of the CNS was pioneered by Hess (1732–51) in 1927. Using specially constructed electrodes, he inserted them from above through openings in the skull into the gray matter surrounding the third ventricle, in a number of cats. Depending on the exact spot stimulated, he produced a variety of effects, such as modification of respiration, swallowing, salivation, glycosuria, micturition, defecation (in the proper position of the body), and ocular changes. When the direct current was passed through certain portions of the periventricular gray, a typical syndrome of drowsiness was produced, and this condition was followed by the onset of sleep. If the floor of the room or cage was kept wet, the cats refused to lie down. Otherwise they retired to a corner, curled up, yawned, and behaved as any normal animal would prior to going to sleep. When finally asleep, the animals could be awakened and then allowed to fall asleep again.

Though Hess's findings were challenged at first (1651, 3270), they have since been abundantly confirmed. The essential elements for successful induction of sleep are a frequency of stimulation of 4–6/sec and a voltage of 2.5–3.5 (33, 34, 1712, 1752, 1875). Higher frequencies or intensities of current reverse the effects and lead to arousal. Whether the stimuli are delivered to the thalamus (33, 34, 1875, 2866), hypothalamus (195, 1631, 1725, 1927, 1928, 2811, 3245, 3807), or both, matters little. Indeed, sleep has been produced by stimulating the occipital cortex of rats (580), and stimulation of the caudate nucleus led to motor inactivation (32), drowsiness (1671), and sleep (3094) in the hands of different investigators. The notion of Hess and others (195, 2865) that sleep is produced by the stimulation of an anteriorly located hypnogenic or trophotropic zone, related to parasympathetic activity, and arousal by that of posteriorly placed dynamogenic or ergotropic zone, connected with sympathetic activity, is not supported by the findings of Parmeggiani (3094) and Favale and associates (1144, 1145): either sleep or arousal may be produced from the stimulation of almost any locus in the brain stem, even peripheral nerves (3225), provided one adheres to the rule concerning voltage, frequency, and perhaps pulse shape and duration. These facts, by themselves, do not rule out the existence of two centers, for, as shown by Nulsen and co-workers (3029), the stimulation of a given spot on the cerebellar cortex will either facilitate or inhibit cortically induced movements of a certain muscle, depending on the frequency of stimulation, and yet facilitation is accomplished via the fastigial nuclei and inhibition via the dentate. There is no such distinct separation of nuclei in the brain stem, and evidence for the duality of sleep-wakefulness control must therefore be based on considerations other than opposite effects elicited from high and low frequencies and intensities of stimulation.

Production of lesions in different parts of the brain—the counterpart of stimulation—has also been used in the induction of sleep. Bremer (473–77) made two cat preparations which have since become standard laboratory material: (*a*) *encéphale isolé* (EI), produced by a transection of the lower part of the medulla, and (*b*) *cerveau isolé* (CI), by cutting the midbrain just behind the origin of the oculomotor nerves. The EI permitted the study of cortical activity under the influence of olfactory, visual, auditory, vestibular, and musculocutaneous impulses, but in the CI the field was narrowed practically entirely to the influence of olfactory and visual impulses. According to Bremer, an EI cat manifested alternations of sleep and wakefulness, with the usual concomitants of each, including appropriate EEG patterns. A CI cat behaved like a sleeping animal, and its condition was ascribed by Bremer to a suppression of the incessant flow of afferent impulses, produced by the midbrain transection. Apparently the olfactory and visual impulses were insufficient to keep the animal awake, and the cerebral cortex was, for practical purposes, deafferented. Hodes (1796) produced an EEG synchronization in cats by reducing proprioceptive inflow through a muscle relaxant (Flaxedil).

More limited injury was done by Marinesco and co-workers (2681–83), who passed a polarizing current through the brain stem of cats. With anelectrotonus they obtained characteristic sleep, resembling calcium effects, in four cases out of nine; with catelectrotonus, sleep was produced in three experiments out of nine, but it was slower in developing and not very definite. The polarization caused detectable lesions, and, whenever sleep was produced, the lesions could later be found in the gray matter around the third ventricle, from the optic chiasm to the mammillary bodies. Specifically, lesions in the thalamus, behind the thalamus, and in the floor of the third ventricle were without effect.

Contrary to the foregoing, Spiegel and Inaba (1899, 3766) made stabbings, under anesthesia, in the inner and outer portions of the periventricular gray and the aqueduct without causing any abnormality in the sleep-wakefulness alternation of rabbits and dogs. On the other hand, injury to the thalamus led to sleep, lasting for weeks in some cases, but the animals could always be aroused by appropriate stimulation.

Ranson (3266–68) found that lesions of the hypothalamus produced drowsiness in cats, whereas faradic stimulation led to excitement. It is now clear that the rate of stimulation was too high to produce sleep. Harrison (1650–52) confirmed Ranson's findings, including the effects of high frequency stimulation. Ranström (3271) also obtained sleepiness in cats by electrolytic destruction of the posterior part of the hypothalamus but noted that, if he used N₂O anesthesia and allowed the animals to recover quickly after the operation, sleep did not set in for several hours. Ranström therefore concluded that the delay in the onset of sleep was due to the action of substances liberated during the necrosis of the destroyed tissue acting on nearby parts of the brain stem. In the meantime, Nauta (2976) reported that in rats extensive bilateral lesions of the hypothalamus in the immediate vicinity of the mammillary bodies were found to produce somnolence, but similar lesions in the region of the hypothalamus rostral to the mammillary bodies were found to produce sleeplessness. Nauta concluded that there is a distinct sleep center as well as a waking center. The sleepless rats did not live long enough to furnish information on the permanence of their waking state. However, Jorda and Manceau (2016, 2644), who induced sleep in guinea pigs by lesions in the mammillary and juxta-mammillary regions, could also induce continuous wakefulness by injury at the level of the preoptic and suprachiasmic zones. The wakeful animals usually died on the third day, but one guinea pig survived for 26 days, constantly active, losing weight, in spite of increased food intake.

Miller and Spiegel (2821) found that lesions in the subthalamus led to sleep in cats, with the thalamus and hypothalamus intact. Schreiner and associates (3592) induced drowsiness in cats by lesions in the intralaminal nuclei of the thalamus. Knott and associates (2223) noted that the drowsiness of cats tended to disappear in a few days, if some hypothalamic tissue was left intact. Collins (742), using monkeys, observed that the effects of unilateral hypothalamic lesions lasted only two days, whereas bilateral lesions were effective for two weeks. Hafer (1578), also working on monkeys, was able to correlate the degree of drowsiness with the amount of hypothalamic damage, as shown by anatomical studies. Several other investigators (57, 171, 2531, 2796, 3592) obtained substantially the same results on cats as on monkeys.

Clinically the hypothalamic region was associated with the sleep function through the studies of sleeping sickness by Mauthner (2717) and Economo (1030–39), and it may be pointed out that, although papers on the effects of brain stem lesions appear periodically (605, 1973, 1984), no one has as yet reported prolonged sleeplessness in man resulting from such lesions.

The induction of sleep for therapeutic purposes, so-called sleep cure or *Dauerschlaf,* has been practiced for many years (375, 1027, 1090, 3548), but is constantly being "rediscovered." The procedure involves the employment of hypnotics and tranquilizers by means of which the patient is kept asleep for 12 to 22 hours each day for one to 4 weeks (72, 162, 504, 1925, 2351, 3052, 3133, 3835), sometimes combined with electroshock (111, 2663), or conditioned reflex training (276, 2660). Many authors (78, 175, 263, 264, 270, 470, 503, 586, 894, 1127, 1370, 1925, 2068, 2142, 2415, 3021, 3255, 3278, 3497, 4146, 4208, 4209) dealt with the general topic of sleep therapy. Others applied themselves to the treatment of particular conditions, mainly nervous and mental diseases (72, 162, 163, 504, 741, 874, 880, 951, 1351, 1894, 1924, 2231, 2700, 2874, 3052, 3082, 3420, 3791, 3792, 4058), with arterial hypertension (310, 2085, 2325, 3519, 3675, 4151) next, and a variety of miscellaneous ailments (311, 1317, 1344, 1443, 2270, 2711, 3171, 3568, 3641, 3850, 4055, 4142–44, 4177). It has even been suggested that the infirmities of old age could be successfully overcome by the sleep cure, as Braines (455) was able to rejuvenate an old dog by this method.

To summarize, two essentially different procedures have been considered in artificially interfering with the sleep-wakefulness alternation. Human beings and animals can be made drowsy, or sleep may be induced, by immobilization leading to muscular relaxation, or by excluding as much as possible the inflow of afferent impulses from the sense organs. In addition to functional deafferentation, there are more drastic procedures of acting chemically, electrically, or mechanically on one or another region at the base of the brain, hypothalamus, thalamus, areas between, or near them. Whether the drowsiness and sleep thus induced involve the activities of a sleep center, a wakefulness center, or two mutually antagonistic centers is discussed in the succeeding chapters.

Chapter 21

Modification of Sleep and Wakefulness

This is the only new chapter, as all the findings to be discussed were made over a decade after the first edition of the book was published. The fundamental discoveries of the part played by the various nuclei spread through the brain stem reticular formation (BSRF) in influencing the depth of sleep and the degree of alertness were reported only in 1949–50 by Moruzzi and Magoun and by Lindsley and associates. Studies of the effects of stimulative and destructive procedures, after these discoveries, were furthered by the use of permanently implanted macro- and microelectrodes and the recording of EEGs and other potential changes in man and animals. From results obtained by the manipulative procedure in the cat, Moruzzi and Magoun (2900) suggested the possibilities that (*a*) "cortical arousal reaction to natural stimuli is mediated by collaterals of afferent pathways to the BSRF, and thence through the ascending reticular activating system (ARAS), rather than by intra-cortical spread following the arrival of afferent impulses at the sensory receiving areas of the cortex," and (*b*) "a background of maintained activity within this ARAS may account for wakefulness, while reduction of its activity either naturally, by barbiturates, or by experimental injury and disease, may respectively precipitate normal sleep, contribute to anesthesia or produce pathological somnolence." Lindsley and associates (2531), in the same animal, observed the following effects of chronic lesions:

> After destruction of the anterior midbrain tegmentum or hypothalamus, sparing sensory connections to thalamus and cortex, the animals usually appeared asleep. Their EEGs exhibited slow waves and spindle bursts. Ordinary stimulation was ineffective, but stronger auditory or nociceptive stimuli evoked motor responses and EEG desynchronization. Arousal was brief, usually not outlasting stimulation. After mesencephalic interruption of the medial and lateral lemnisci and spinothalamic tracts, the animals were not abnormally sleepy and showed waking EEGs. When relaxation or sleep occurred, arousal and EEG activation was readily induced by afferent stimuli and usually persisted for long periods after stimulation. Of these two systems influencing the cortex, that through the tegmen-

tum and hypothalamus thus appears of greater importance in maintaining wakefulness and inducing EEG arousal upon afferent stimulation.

The BSRF, as the name indicates, is a poorly defined collection of gray masses, extending from the medulla to the diencephalon, but the suggestion of Olszewski (3054) that the term BSRF be dropped has not been followed. The BSRF has been the topic of symposia and the title of several reviews, of which probably the most comprehensive are the ones by Segundo (3645), Brodal (517), and Rossi and Zanchetti (3427), the latter containing 682 bibliographical references. The term "system" has also come into use, as the physiological counterpart of the anatomical BSRF, for the interaction of its several parts and its rostral and caudal connections.

The fundamental discoveries of the functions of the BSRF were confirmed, elaborated upon, or discussed from the physiological, psychological, and clinical viewpoints by many investigators (81, 119, 406, 518, 1003, 1219, 1279–85, 1366, 1390, 1826, 1882, 1885, 1904–6, 1909, 1911, 2528, 2533, 2626–32, 2707, 2892–98, 3248, 3271, 3515, 3571, 3646, 3788, 3789, 3919). In addition, it was established that both facilitatory and inhibitory influences can be exerted by the BSRF, caudally as well as rostrally (119, 159, 378, 1713, 1856, 3329), and that these effects can be obtained from the lowermost regions (1854, 1857, 2570, 2627, 2628, 3329). It is therefore proper to speak of a descending reticular activating system (DRAS), in addition to the ARAS. Individual neurones in the BSRF have multiple synaptic connections and exhibit the phenomena of occlusion, inhibition, and facilitation (53, 2605). By physical isolation of the BSRF (409) and by cross-circulation experiments (3249), it was shown that BSRF activity can be affected by the composition of the blood (CO_2, adrenalin), though ordinarily there is an integration of nervous and humoral factors (409, 1854, 3645). The BSRF also probably exerts its influence on cortical activity by extraneural, aside from neural, mechanisms. The neurohumoral mechanisms may be adrenergic (3450, 3645), cholinergic (922, 2555, 3120, 3355–57, 3494), or both (449, 1134).

The hypothalamus innervates the entire hypophysis and can probably influence it by the humoral route also (2904). In turn, pituitary hormones can affect the hypothalamus and thus other parts of the CNS, including the cortex. Sawyer and Kawakami (2095, 3531) noted two EEG phases in the post-coital behavior of the female rabbit: (*a*) sleep spindles, lasting several seconds to 30 minutes, when the animal is drowsy, if not sleeping, and (*b*) "hippocampal hyperactivity," 8/sec high voltage EEG from hippocampus and its connections, with the animal depressed, but moving its jaws and eyelids. This EEG after-reaction can be induced by 5/sec low voltage (0.01–1.0) stimulation of the hypothalamus through implanted electrodes, with EEG spindle phase starting at once, and the hippocampal phase replacing it sooner than after coitus. The after-reaction can also be elicited by the injection of pituitary gonadotropins and other sex steroids, but the latency is greater than after electric stimulation.

Rostral to the BSRF proper is the thalamic reticular formation, separate and independent of specific thalamic relay nuclei (1622), giving rise to the non-specific or diffuse thalamic projection system (DTPS) to the cortex and also in a descending manner to the BSRF (522) and farther caudally (3564). Unlike the specific thalamic projection system (STPS) which produces an arousal reaction in the area of projection on the cortex, the DTPS causes the excitation to spread widely (522), though perhaps more to the frontal areas than to others (3790). The DTPS was investigated by Jasper and associates (1875, 1959–61, 1966), by Morison and Dempsey and co-workers (2880–82), and by others (1286, 2163, 3089, 4111). Though the view is not universally accepted (115, 2757), the DTPS is said to exert an influence on cortical activity secondary only to that of the ARAS. According to Jasper (1960), the DTPS seems "to play a unique role in the regulation of whatever functional significance we may attribute to the alpha rhythm," and perhaps is also related to maintaining a certain level of alertness (1961).

A somewhat different view of the function of DTPS is derived from the production of rhythmically recurrent cortical potentials synchronous with thalamic stimulation at the rate of 8–12/sec, the recruiting responses of Dempsey and Morison (910, 911), also studied by others (31, 122, 521, 1968, 4052). The recruiting responses are distinct from the arousal responses which can be mediated by the DTPS as well as by the ARAS, if the frequency of stimulation is much higher, the two types of responses involving separate systems (121, 3565, 3947). Conversely, recruiting responses can be obtained from structures below the thalamus (112), especially if the voltage is small (3244) and the frequency low (2600, 2630). Recruiting responses can even be obtained in waking animals (112, 1122) but may be more related to sleep spindles than to the alpha pattern (697, 2220, 2221, 2426, 2885). The DTPS differs from the ARAS in not being sensitive to either epinephrine or barbiturates, but mainly in exerting short-lasting effects, perhaps related to attention (1962), as compared to longer-lasting alertness mediated through the ARAS (2528). It seems that there are elements of antagonism, as well as of synergism, in the influence of the ARAS and DTPS on cortical processes.

Hernández-Peón and associates (1708–15) demonstrated the role of the BSRF in simple learning (positive conditioning) and habituation (negative conditioning), as well as attention. Habituation occurs in neonates (500) and in CI preparations (2646), indicating that neither an active cortex nor lower BSRF is needed for the process. Dishabituation, equated with the arousal response (2646, 2647) and attention (1350), is also mediated via the ARAS. Indeed, Sharpless and Jasper (3672) and Schwab and co-workers (3619) showed that a mild EEG arousal response is itself subject to habituation.

The "arrest reaction" (1875, 1960), obtained in waking animals by stimulating the DTPS, may be like the standstill or "still" reaction of Byrne (598), as the animal remains immobile and fails to respond to usual stimuli. Its clinical aspects were studied by Fischgold and Lairy-Bounes (1181, 2348), who noted that in brain-stem lesions one gets an "arrest reaction" if wakefulness is maintained and an "arousal reaction" if hypersomnia prevails. Cortical lesions may abolish the "arrest reaction" even in wakefulness.

That the cerebral cortex is involved in awakening, as well as in the maintenance of wakefulness, was stressed by Bremer and Terzuolo (489–92). The corticofugal influences on the BSRF, producing reverberating circuits, were also emphasized by others (715, 1283, 1710, 1858, 1908, 2542, 2896, 3424, 3648, 4118). Mollica (2861, 2862) was unable to provoke an arousal response in a CI cat by stimulating various cortical areas, but could do so by stimulating the mesencephalic tegmentum. He concluded that the ability of the cortex to "awaken itself" depended upon its connection with bulbopontine reticular structures. On the other hand, Batsel (257) found that CI dogs, which exhibited a continuous pattern of spindles and slow waves in the acute state, if kept alive for several days, began to show EEG patterns of sleep and wakefulness, the wakefulness lasting for several hours at a time. Surgically isolated cortical areas (479, 1706, 2284) exhibit rhythmical activity, though somewhat different from other cortical regions anatomically connected with underlying structures.

The hippocampus may be connected with the BSRF by two routes (15) and has been shown to exert a greater blocking effect on conduction in the BSRF than other cortical areas (16). Electrical stimulation of neocortical points in the rabbit (3330) and BSRF in the cat (3112) elicited LVFA in the neocortex and HVSA in the hippocampus. At the onset of sleep there was a neocortical synchronization and hippocampal desynchronization (3105), and converse, but still reciprocal, EEG changes at awakening (1511, 3105, 3353). During the "paradoxical phase" of sleep (p. 212), when neocortical activity resembled that of wakefulness, the slow hippocampal waves were most pronounced (601, 1503, 2082). Hippocampal stimulation during sleep did not lead to arousal (2538, 4047), though, at times, it was followed by a peculiar "running" reaction, and this behavior led to the conclusion that the hippocampus has an "aspecific" inhibitory action on the BSRF.

In a study of neuronal activity of an EI cat preparation, Verzeano and Negichi (4051, 4053) observed an enhancement of the excitatory process along pathways of propagation in cells of cortex and thalamus in transition from wakefulness to sleep. However, there was an inhibition of activity in neighboring neurones. In cortical areas, neurone activity was increased in some units (3495) and decreased in others (1115, 1849) during arousal. Bremer and Stoupel (486, 487) noted evidences of both facilitation and inhibition in cortically evoked potentials during arousal caused by BSRF stimulation. Evarts and co-workers

(1121) obtained a smaller cortical response to geniculate stimulation in wakefulness than in sleep. Caudate nucleus stimulation at low rates led to depression and sleeplike behavior in CI preparations (777, 4019).

The behavior of the EI preparation was studied by making lesions at different levels of the pons. Although vagal stimulation could abolish spontaneous spindling (2895, 4307), cutting the vagi or suppressing the special senses did not affect the alertness of the EI cats (3388). Bilateral gasserectomy abolished wakefulness (3386, 3387, 3428), except for rare periods (2863). Otherwise intact cats, whose pons was cut electrolytically in front of the trigeminal outflow, showed low voltage EEGs and ocular behavior suggestive of wakefulness (255), but olfactory and visual deafferentation produced a sleep EEG pattern (256). However, LVFA returned after 1–2 days. If rostropontine, instead of midpontine, lesions were made in the animals, HVSA EEG was induced for the entire survival period of up to 6 days. Some small amount of nervous tissue in the upper pons was needed for wakefulness. Midpontine pretrigeminal cats could also be put to sleep by repetitive light stimuli (117, 118, 2645). Other observations on midpontine (254, 2899) and EI (252–54, 757, 2616–18) preparations led to the postulation of the existence of an active hypnogenic mechanism in the caudal part of the brain stem, extending into the medulla. This would mean that there are two sleep systems—one in front and the other behind the wakefulness system.

The pons is also involved in a phase of sleep in the cat which lasts 10–15 minutes and is characterized by a LVFA resembling the EEG of wakefulness, alternating with a 20–30 minute period of HVSA. Dement (899), who first recognized LVFA sleep as real sleep, rather than temporary wakefulness, also noted that it did not differ much in depth, as judged by the auditory threshold, from HVSA sleep, but he called it "activated" sleep because of the EEG pattern of cortical desynchronization or activation. Incidentally, the LVFA sleep is an excellent example of the non-reliability of the EEG pattern as a sole criterion of sleep, let alone the depth of sleep. Jouvet, Michel, and associates (2033–50) published a series of papers on the two phases of sleep, referring to the LVFA as "paradoxical phase" (p.p.), later as "archi-sleep," to distinguish it from the HVSA "neo-sleep," still later "rhombencephalic" sleep, to indicate its origin in a pontine structure. The general findings pertaining to the EEG pattern of LVFA have been abundantly confirmed (295, 1118, 1503, 1625, 1834, 1851, 1883, 1884, 2082, 3425), and in some respects its character and concomitants resemble the emergent stage 1 EEG in man, associated with dreaming activity of the cortex (p. 94). Points of resemblance include (*a*) the waking type EEG; (*b*) their appearance, in natural sleep, only following a period of HVSA sleep; (*c*) the presence of REMs; and (*d*) the increased respiratory rate. LVFA sleep in the cat, however, is accompanied by (*a*) a marked muscular relaxation, especially in the nuchal region, whereas in man snoring is suspended, suggesting an increase in the pharyngeal muscle tonus; (*b*) more significantly, a cardiac slowing, as contrasted with an increase in the heart rate in man; and (*c*) a great rise in auditory threshold, as against a moderate rise in man—by comparison with the threshold during the initial stage 1 EEG. Spindles of 5–8/sec have been recorded in the cat during the LVFA phase, but their presence in man has so far not been established.

Evarts (1118) and Huttenlocher (1883, 1884) noted an inverse influence of sleep in the cat on the spontaneous and evoked discharges of neurone units in the BSRF. The rate of spontaneous discharge was, by and large, higher in HVSA than during quiet wakefulness, and highest in LVFA, whereas evoked discharges were decreased in HVSA sleep and almost entirely absent during LVFA. The latter finding is in line with the high thresholds of arousal in LVFA.

By decortication and lesions in, and transections of, the brain stem of the cat, Jouvet and his group demonstrated that the HVSA requires the presence of an intact cortex, whence it is spread caudally, whereas the LVFA originates in the pons and travels rostrally, probably via the limbic midbrain circuit described by Nauta (2977), bypassing the BSRF on the way to the cortex. It was shown that in the intact cat it was possible to induce a period of LVFA by stimulating certain points in the midbrain or pons, provided this was done during HVSA sleep and the voltage was very low. Furthermore, having done so once, it was impossible to repeat the effect for 15–30 minutes. This refractory interval suggested that the LVFA was due to the liberation of some neurohumoral agent, for whose production and accumulation HVSA, or something associated with it, provided the stimulus. The agent is perhaps of a cholinergic nature, as atropine suppressed the effect and eserine prolonged the LVFA, though not the frequency of the cycle. As the Jouvet group sees it, LVFA depends on some internal mechanism for its run of about one-third of the total sleep time, whereas the neocortically originating HVSA is initiated by external conditions of monotony of stimulation, darkness, and quiet, that lead to the onset of sleep.

No teleological explanation of the alternation of LVFA and HVSA in sleep has been offered, but the time dimensions fit in with the basic rest-activity cycle (p. 88), which is longer in man than in the cat, and longer in adult humans and cats than in infants and kittens. With their cardiac and other concomitants, the two sleep phases will be utilized in the elaboration of the evolutionary theory of wakefulness, sleep, and dreaming presented in the last chapter of this book.

Bonvallet and co-workers (407), in cats and dogs, under Flaxedil, obtained a decrease in activity and an appearance of a slow wave EEG after distending the carotid sinus, and did so by a purely nervous mechanism, independently of the blood-pressure level. Confirmed by Mazzella and co-workers (2735), the carotid sinus effect represented the first example of an afferent inflow that dampened rather than activated the cortex via the reticular formation (887,

888, 1761)—comparable in its uniqueness to the reflex pupilloconstriction by the peripheral action of light. The bearing of the discovery of the carotid sinus effect on the elucidation of the possible cause of idiopathic narcolepsy and cataplexy is discussed in Chapter 23.

To summarize, within the 1949–59 decade, by the tools provided by the EEG machine and implanted electrodes, and through the modification of sleep and wakefulness by lesions and stimulations, gifted investigators made three significant discoveries: (*a*) the existence and functions of the non-specific ARAS and DTPS; (*b*) the LVFA phase of sleep alternating with an HVSA one, as the basis of the short-term rest-activity cycle; and (*c*) the unique role of the carotid sinus in the induction of sleep.

Chapter 22

Deprivation of Sleep

Organ extirpation, as a means of determining its function through the ensuing deficiency symptoms, has long been a recognized method in physiological research. Depriving the organism of a certain activity is the functional counterpart. Fasting and prolonged sleeplessness have been used to study the effects of lack of food and of sleep.

The first experiments on the effects of depriving animals of sleep were performed in 1894 by Manacéine (2642), who found that puppies died when kept awake for 4–6 days (92–143 hours). They showed a marked hypothermia, amounting to 4°–5° C., at the end of the experiment. The red-blood-cell count decreased from 5 to 2 million, but later it increased, due, according to the author, to a thickening of the blood. Necropsies revealed capillary hemorrhages in the cerebral gray matter. Tarozzi (3907) kept three adult dogs awake by walking them when necessary. They died after 9, 13, and 17 days, respectively, with their body temperature down to 35° C. However, they showed no oligocythemia during the test; nor did Tarozzi find any cortical hemorrhages on postmortem examination. A histological study of the nervous system of Tarozzi's dogs by Daddi (809) revealed a diffuse chromatolysis and vacuolization of protoplasm in the cells of the cerebral cortex, particularly in the frontal region. Similar cortical cell changes in sleep-deprived dogs were reported by Agostini (29) and Okazaki (3048), and in guinea pigs by Jorda (2016). A most extensive series of experiments were made by Legendre and Piéron (2401–13, 3191, 3192), who deprived some twenty dogs of sleep for periods varying from 30 to 505 hours, but in no case beyond the point where they showed extreme sleepiness. The animals were always in good physiological condition and ate well. When very sleepy, the dogs became hyperirritable, but by appropriate sensory (auditory) stimulation their conduct could be brought back almost to normal. They showed evidence of muscular hypotonus, manifested by a sinking of the head and bending of the paws, when no attempt was made to keep them awake. There were no significant changes in the composition of the blood, blood pressure, heart rate, respiration, or body temperature. Definitely localized degenerative changes were found in the brains of animals killed at the time when they were very sleepy. These changes consisted of shrinking of the cells, displacement of nuclei, vacuolization of cytoplasm, and disappearance of Nissl granules. They were most marked in the two deep layers of the prefrontal cortical region (giant pyramidal and polymorph cells); less marked in the sigmoid gyrus; and completely absent in the occipital cortex, cerebellum, medulla, and spinal cord. The amount of damage was proportional to the degree of sleepiness. If the animals were permitted to sleep, they were completely restored to normal by one period of sleep, as no cellular changes could then be detected in their brains. The injection of cerebrospinal fluid taken from very sleepy dogs into the fourth ventricle of normal dogs produced sleepiness in the latter. The brains of the hosts showed the same cellular changes as those of the donors. Injection of cerebrospinal fluid from normal animals led to neither sleepiness nor degenerative nerve-cell changes. It was found that the hypnotic properties of the cerebrospinal fluid could be destroyed by keeping it at 65° C. for 5 minutes or by oxygenation. The chemical agent was not dialyzable and could be precipitated by alcohol. Ivy and Schnedorf (1926), as previously mentioned (p. 203), repeated the experiment with the cerebrospinal-fluid transfer from sleepy to wakeful dogs. It will be recalled that, in addition to profound sleep, their animals developed a hyperthermia.

Our work (2178) was confined to observations on twelve puppies, from six weeks to three months of age, with their litter mates serving as controls. As a rule, two puppies from the same litter, as nearly alike in every respect as could be found, were used together, one being kept awake and the other continuing its normal routine. In several cases a daily record was made of their weight, body temperature, heart and respiratory rates, blood sugar, alkaline reserve of the blood, hemoglobin, and red-and-white-blood-cell counts. Each experiment was preceded by a period of preliminary observation, under normal conditions, of about two weeks' duration. The period of experimental insomnia varied from 2 to 7 days. It was easy to keep the animals awake during the first day of the experiment, but on the second and succeeding days it was progressively harder. From our protocols it appeared that it was hardest to keep them awake when they were not walked; easiest when they were walked frequently and when their attention was attracted to something during the rest periods. Thus, bringing in the control litter mate and allowing it to play with the experimental animal often banished drowsiness from the latter completely. But after 3 or 4 days of continued wakefulness, the puppy would lose all interest in its surroundings. Some puppies developed a definite photophobia and attempted to get into dark corners when walked.

Extreme sleepiness manifested itself by a muscular weakness, the animals' front paws flexing anteriorly and giving them the appearance of being "flat-footed." At this point the puppies were allowed to sleep, or both the experimental and the control animals were killed. Those puppies that were permitted to sleep appeared completely recovered the next day, except for two that died without awakening. Some puppies ate and drank well; others refused food when they were very sleepy. There were no appreciable variations in the body temperature of the sleepless puppies, nor were there any important changes in the heart rate, respiratory rate, blood sugar, alkaline reserve of the blood, hemoglobin, or white blood cells. Minor variations were observed, but similar variations were present in the control puppies, although the two did not always run parallel. The only marked change noted was in the red-blood-cell count, which fell appreciably, sometimes more than 25 per cent, in the experimental animals.

The results of a neurological study of the various parts of the CNS were entirely negative. Abnormalities could easily be detected in the preparations from the experimental puppies, but similar abnormalities could be seen in the nerve cells of their normal litter mates.

Deprivation-of-sleep experiments were also carried out on rabbits. Crile (779) kept rabbits awake for 96–118 hours. He observed a slight rise in body temperature and a slowing of the respiration but no change in the reaction of the blood. By histological methods lesions were found in the liver and adrenal gland as well as in the CNS.

Bast and associates (244–48, 2388) kept sixteen rabbits awake by placing them in cylindrical cages, revolving slowly on a horizontal axis. The rabbit had to change its position about 8 times per minute when placed in such a cage, but the total distance covered in 24 hours was less than 1.5 miles. It took from 6 to 31 days for the animals to show extreme sleepiness, heralded by a sudden fall in body temperature, which at times amounted to 4°–5° C., and by a slowing of the pulse and of the respiration. The authors found degenerative changes in the cells of the CNS; but, instead of being confined to certain areas of the cerebral cortex, in the rabbits these changes were limited to the cells of the medulla and the spinal cord (245, 247). The thyroid and adrenal glands also showed degenerative cellular changes.

Stern and associates published several papers (3811–13) pertaining to the "blood-cerebrospinal-fluid barrier," a figurative barrier to the passage of certain substances from the blood into the cerebrospinal fluid. Their work consisted of analyzing the blood and cerebrospinal fluid of dogs that were kept awake for 8 to 14 days, and determining the ratios of the concentrations of certain constituents in each medium. Prolonged wakefulness (3811) led to a marked decrease in the potassium content and a simultaneous rise in the calcium content of the cerebrospinal fluid, causing the K/Ca coefficient in that fluid to fall from a normal value of 2 to less than 1. Sleep brought about a return to the normal K/Ca coefficient. In addition, Stern and associates (3813) found that a positively inotropic effect on the frog heart could be obtained by dog's blood, when diluted no more than 1:100, and by dog's cerebrospinal fluid, in a dilution of not more than 1:10. After 24 hours of wakefulness this inotropic effect was obtainable with 100 times greater dilutions of the two media. However, if insulin (0.1–0.5 units/kg) was administered, wakefulness did not increase the inotropic power of either the blood or the cerebrospinal fluid. The vasoconstrictor power of the two media was also increased by wakefulness but remained unchanged if insulin was given during that period. Stern maintained that introduction of insulin prevented the increased sympathomimetic effect of the blood and cerebrospinal fluid on the heart and blood vessels which usually developed when the dog remained awake for 24 hours. Insulin also increased the permeability coefficient to sugar and potassium, thereby maintaining a normal level of potassium in the cerebrospinal fluid, in spite of a drop of potassium in the blood. Insulin caused an increase in the calcium content both of the blood and of the cerebrospinal fluid.

Demidov and co-workers (905) have studied the effect of a thyroid preparation on the changes produced in the blood and cerebrospinal fluid of the dog after 24 hours of wakefulness. They ran three series of experiments: wakefulness alone, thyroid administration alone, and simultaneous wakefulness and thyroid administration. They determined in each case the non-protein nitrogen, urea, chlorides, bromides, potassium, calcium, and glucose in blood plasma, serum, and cerebrospinal fluid, before and after the experiment. Some constituents were modified in the same direction by sleeplessness and thyroid, others in opposite directions, showing an unequal permeability of the blood-cerebrospinal-fluid barrier to the different constituents of the blood plasma under these conditions. From the stimulating effect of the thyroid preparation on the sympathetic system and of insulin on the parasympathetic, Stern (3812) concluded that the hormones of the thyroid and pancreas had a definite influence on the alternation of sleep and wakefulness. She further surmised (3811) that this influence manifested itself in the changed permeability of the blood-cerebrospinal-fluid barrier, which, in turn, affected the electrolyte composition of the cerebrospinal fluid. Changes in the composition of the fluid led to functional changes in the brain, with sleep as a result. As previously stated (p. 36), Katzenelbogen's studies of the distribution of calcium between the blood and the cerebrospinal fluid gave him calcium coefficients which did not suggest that sleep might be associated with marked changes in the permeability of the blood-cerebrospinal-fluid barrier to calcium.

Bunch and associates (564, 565) compared the learning ability of rats after varying periods of wakefulness (up to 48 hours) with that of well-rested animals, using a multiple-T water maze. Sleep-deprived rats performed 10 to 21 per cent better than the control ones. In another series, Licklider and Bunch (2514) found that rats died after 3 to 14 days of enforced wakefulness, but mainly from fighting with each other. Kept awake for 20 hours out of 24, rats could go on for many weeks, though they also became highly irritable and inclined to fight. During the 4 hours of rest permitted them daily, the rats were inactive for about 3—double that of control rats. They also succumbed sooner to complete sleep deprivation than did rats not subjected to weeks of 20-hour per day enforced wakefulness. As could be expected, sleep-deprived rats (4131, 4161) and kittens and puppies (1150) went to sleep faster, or had shorter "sleep latencies," than did rested animals.

Ukolova (4005) observed a neurotic type of disturbance of salivary conditioned reflexes in dogs deprived of sleep for 48 hours, and Svorad and coworkers (3884, 3885), using rats, were able to induce sleeplessness by developing a conditioned fear of the electric shock reinforcement or by repeated intraperitoneal injections of "psychton" (beta-phenyl-isopropylamine). An experimental neurosis previously developed in rats did not become worse as a result of insomnia induced by the excitant amine. Susceptibility of rats to sound-precipitated convulsions was not affected by a 24-hour sleep deprivation (3666). Feldman (1150) noted a progressive slowing of the EEG in kittens and puppies, together with a decreased reactivity, during 60–84 hours of enforced wakefulness.

Webb and Agnew (4133) noted an inverse relationship between age and resistance to exhaustion in rats maintained on a constantly moving wheel in a study of sleep deprivation. At the age of sixty-three days, young rats were not exhausted even after 216 hours (9 days) on the rotating wheel. But groups of older rats, aged 89, 147, 170, and 220 days, succumbed in 156, 110, 80, and 68 hours, respectively. The greater resistance to sleep deprivation of younger animals is in line with their greater ability to withstand anoxia and profound hypothermia (p. 327).

The first sleep deprivation study on man was made in 1896 by Patrick and Gilbert (3115) who kept three young subjects awake for 90 hours, during which time they submitted themselves to a variety of physiological and psychological tests. The only control was the performance of the subjects on the day after the first sleep period that terminated the prolonged vigil. The experiment was performed only once, but there was a certain consistency in the results obtained on the three subjects. In general, there were decreases in sensory acuity, quickness of reaction, motor speed, and memorizing ability. Two significant observations were visual hallucinations in one subject and a gradual decrease in body temperature, with the preservation, however, of the 24-hour temperature curve. The subjects not only did not lose weight but even gained some. They slept for 12 hours at the end of the experiment and seemed to be completely restored to normal on awakening.

Another 26 years passed before a similar experiment was performed by Robinson and Herrmann (3378)—also once—on 3 men. Their subjects were kept awake for 65 hours. The performance tests comprised steadiness, accuracy of aiming, muscular strength, ability to name letters, and mental arithmetic. The period of sleeplessness was preceded and followed by control periods of observation (11–26 days before and 4–5 days after). The performance scores "were not affected by insomnia in any marked or consistent manner." Robinson and Richardson-Robinson (3379) could likewise detect no difference in the performance ability of a whole class of students who were kept awake for 24 hours, compared to a control group who had the usual amount of sleep. The authors ascribed this lack of an observable effect in the "sleepless" group to an extra amount of effort, which was sufficient to compensate for the deficiency that was probably present.

The results of our experiments, started in 1922, were published only in part (753, 2176, 2400). Altogether we employed some thirty-five subjects, all men but two, and mostly students. The number of individual periods of sleeplessness studied exceeded 60, and the duration was usually 60-odd hours, or staying awake until late in the evening of a third day of sleeplessness. I have remained awake on more than one occasion over 100 hours and, with the aid of benzedrine sulphate, as long as 180 hours.

The original intention was to maintain the routine of living in everything but sleep. The subjects were to undress and go to bed at the usual time but were to keep awake throughout the night. That aim could sometimes be achieved during the first night of continued wakefulness, but was entirely impossible during the second. Indeed, the only way one could remain awake was by engaging in some sort of muscular activity, even if it were no more than talking. Thus, we were studying the effects of loss of sleep as well as those of almost uninterrupted muscular activity.

While there were differences in the subjective experiences of the many sleep-evading persons, there were several features common to most. As indicated above, during the first night the subject did not feel very tired or sleepy. He could read or study or do laboratory work, without much attention from the watcher, but usually felt an attack of drowsiness between 3:00 A.M. and 6:00 A.M. The drowsiness was accompanied by an unpleasant itching of the eyes. Next morning the subject felt well, except for a slight malaise which always appeared on sitting down and resting for any length of time. However, if he occupied himself with his ordinary daily tasks, he was likely to forget having spent a sleepless night. During the second night the individual's condition was entirely different. His eyes not only itched but felt dry, and he could abolish that sensation only by closing his eyes, which made it extremely hard to remain fully awake, even if walking. Reading or study was next to impossible because sitting quietly was conducive to even greater sleepiness. As during the first night, there came a 2–3 hour period in the early hours of the morning when the desire for sleep was almost overpowering. At this time the subject often saw double. Later in the morning the sleepiness diminished once more, and the subject could perform routine laboratory work, as usual. It was not safe for him to sit down, however, without the danger of falling asleep, particularly if he attended lectures. Attempting to take down lecture notes usually resulted in failure. After a few words had been written correctly, his hand would begin to slip, and, instead of writing, there was unintelligible scribbling. A new effort led to only a short-lasting improvement of the writing. At times, even the pencil fell out of the subject's hand; apparently, he could not keep up the very slight pressure of the fingers necessary to hold it. All efforts could be sustained for only a short time. An example of this failure was the repeated inability of the subject to count his own pulse for as long as a minute. After counting to 15 or 20, he invariably lost track of the numbers and would find himself dozing off.

The third night resembled the second, and the fourth day was like the third. For this reason we adopted, as a standard procedure, a waking period of 62–65 hours. At the end of that time the individual was as sleepy as he was likely to be. Those who continued to stay awake experienced the wavelike increase and decrease in sleepiness with the greatest drowsiness at about the same time every night.

Objectively, from the watcher's standpoint, the appearance of the sleepless person seemed quite normal, particularly during the daytime and when he engaged in some form of muscular activity. After the first night, however, the subject had to be supervised very closely, as sitting down, even in the daytime, rendered him extremely sleepy. Thus, he would fall asleep when taking his temperature and when his blood pressure or ESR was being determined; but he usually remained fully awake when performing a test that required his active participation. If permitted to lie down, he would be found asleep in less than a minute. This condition was utilized by us in making repeated alternate measurements of one or another variable, during sleep and wakefulness, within a few minutes' time. Usually the subject would close his eyelids merely to relieve the itching or slightly burning sensation in the eyes, but that only accentuated his tendency to fall asleep. He often pretended (or perhaps that was his intention) to go out into the hall so as to have more room for strolling, but in a minute or so the watcher would find him sitting on the stairway step, fast asleep. When aroused, he often vehemently denied having been asleep and would show resentment at being distrusted. This tendency to hyperirritability and irascibility could be banished by making the subject walk briskly for a few minutes, but it would soon return. Mild-mannered persons became ill-tempered under continued efforts to keep them awake, and in that respect their behavior resembled very closely that of well-trained children who often become quite unmanageable if they stay up past their usual bedtime.

Another feature was the irrationality of action that could be called semi-dreaming, probably what Patrick and Gilbert (3115) referred to as hallucinations. In carrying on his work, the subject often made remarks that clearly did not fit the situation. When questioned, he would report that he was under the impression that he was talking to the watcher on a topic which, as the watcher knew, had not entered into the previous conversation at all. The subject then, as a rule, concluded that he must have been dreaming, although he was definitely awake, from the observer's viewpoint, and even engaged in some activity. It scarcely need be added that the watchers were changed frequently and had plenty of sleep. On rare occasions the subject reported that he had to keep the watcher awake.

The quantitative studies made during prolonged sleeplessness yielded results that could be properly evaluated not only on the basis of the progressive changes that occurred during that particular period but also by comparison with the data gathered on the same subject in the course of control periods before and after. For each subject there was a range of day-to-day variations which had to be exceeded during the sleepless period before any significance could be attached to the figures obtained. It was impossible to make all the different tests on every subject, but some tests were repeated year after year on successive groups of subjects.

In general, there were no deviations from the normal range in the vegetative functions of the subjects: heart rate, blood pressure, body temperature, basal metabolism, appetite, composition of the blood and urine. The red-blood-cell count and hemoglobin percentage were determined in groups of subjects from time to time with variable results. We were particularly interested in this blood constituent because the results on animals indicated a decrease in the number of red blood cells on prolonged lack of sleep. Individual subjects gave consistent results on successive periods of sleeplessness, but for the twenty subjects examined for this variable there was no general tendency toward an oligocythemia. However, at the time of going to bed, the red-blood-cell count and hemoglobin were lower than in the morning of the same day in the majority of cases.

In studying the effect of loss of sleep on the nervous system, we employed only those tests which had been previously reported as demonstrating the effects of fatigue and of depressing drugs. The tests chosen fell into two classes: those in which effort is not a determining factor and those in which it may be one. The first group comprised the knee-jerk, pupillary response to light, cutaneous sensitivity to faradic current and to the Von Frey hairs (touch and pain), visual acuity, EEG, and ESR (3948); the second group consisted of body steadiness (graphic Romberg test), hand steadiness, naming of opposites, naming of colors, mental arithmetic, and RT (visual, auditory, and visual with choice). Of the first group of tests one can only repeat what has been said about the vegetative functions: no consistent variation for the group as a whole, with respect to all the tests but one, namely, sensitivity to pain. By the use of the Von Frey test hairs, we (753) studied six subjects, and, whereas the cutaneous sensitivity to touch remained unchanged, that to pain showed a progressive increase (lower thresholds) during the period of wakefulness in every one of the eleven selected points on the face and hands. During the latter part of the period of abstention from sleep the subject's general behavior and reactivity (including diplopia) were very much like those of persons under the influence of a large dose of alcohol, such as 1 ml/kg. With such doses of alcohol Mullin and Luckhardt (2945) obtained in their subjects a decreased sensitivity to pain, but also no change in sensitivity to touch. Extremely sleepy and drunken individuals may behave alike, but they manifest diametrically opposite changes in their ability to receive nocuous cutaneous stimuli without experiencing pain.

EEG records (365) showed a rapid change of patterns when the subject was repeatedly permitted to fall asleep and awakened shortly thereafter. There was a succession of many regular patterns, which varied in rate from 1 to 14 per second, in addition to a distinct high-frequency beta pattern. Blake (366) described this condition as follows:

> With the subject lying down, delta waves predominated, even while he talked, and disappeared only when he made an extreme effort to concentrate. Muscular tone was so low that a spool was never held more than 15 seconds, even with distinct effort, and usually dropped as soon as placed in his hand. He was never aware of having been asleep and he answered every question that he heard, but it sometimes took a strong auditory stimulus to arouse him to the point of responding.
>
> It seems, therefore, that he did sleep, but was unable to differentiate between it and wakefulness. To check the maximum duration of wakefulness, the subject counted as long as he could. Counting took great concentration and was paralleled by a marked change in potential pattern, from the delta rhythm to a great discharge of beta waves. Even with this effort, he lost consciousness at a count between 3 and 10, and, in about as many seconds, the potentials drifted back to the usual slow waves.

The second group of tests showed, in general, a decreasing performance ability during the period of sleeplessness. Aside from individual variations, there were two other factors complicating and distorting the results: (*a*) the 24-hour variation in performance, or better scores when the persons were wide-awake and their body temperature higher, and (*b*) efforts made by the subjects to perform as well as, or better than, during the control periods. This latter tendency showed up in the color-naming test. A large cardboard on which were pasted colored squares, arranged in random sequence in ten rows of ten squares each, was presented to the subject to be named consecutively. The observer counted the number of mistakes (corrected and left uncorrected) made and the time required for naming the entire one hundred items (about 1 minute). Prolonged sleeplessness had no effect on the score of this test (time and errors). But, if the subjects were required to name several hundred (400–1,200) items, both the time and the number of errors were much greater than with a similarly large number of colored squares under control conditions. The deterioration would set in, as a rule, with the third or fourth hundred. It means that the sleepy individual could make a successful short-lasting effort. This, it will be recalled, was the conclusion also made by Robinson and Richardson-Robinson (3379).

In every subject, we studied the sleep that terminated the long period of sleeplessness. Allowed to sleep as long as they pleased, most subjects slept from 11 to 13 hours. This sleep was deeper than usual, on an hourly basis; there were fewer movements, major and minor, and less time was spent in movement than during control nights. The pattern of motility remained unchanged: there was more motility during the second half of the night's sleep than during the first. It was thought that the recovery sleep was likely to be dreamless, but Dement (900), by employing the REM-EEG method, demonstrated that, on the contrary, dreaming activity was heightened by prolonged wakefulness. That observation was the starting point of his research into the effects of deprivation of dreaming, previously discussed (p. 105).

Reports of other investigators confirm earlier findings. Herz (1720), with himself as subject, performed a test once, remaining awake for 80 hours. No functional deviations from the normal were observed, except an increase in the number of polymorphonuclear neutrophile leucocytes and a decrease in lymphocytes. A group of professors at George Washington University (82) observed two men and four women who went without sleep for two nights and two men who remained awake for three nights, also each subject only once. There was a gradual increase in the leucocyte count to levels definitely above the normal in six out of the eight subjects. Otherwise, the results were negative.

Rakestraw and Whittier (3261) kept eight normal men awake for 48 hours. The subjects were on a uniform diet. The two 24-hour samples of urine from each subject were compared with that collected during the 24 hours preceding the experiment. Blood samples were taken at the beginning, in the middle, and at the end of the 48-hour period of wakefulness. Determinations were made of the urinary total nitrogen, ammonia, chlorides, phosphates, uric acid, and total acidity; the blood was analyzed for sugar, non-protein nitrogen, urea, phenols (both free and conjugated), uric acid, chlorides, alkali reserve, total acid-soluble phosphorus, and lactic acid. The results showed no consistent alteration in the urine components. Likewise keeping the diet constant, Kroetz (2285) studied the urine and blood of two subjects, each kept awake on two occasions for periods varying from 52 to 80 hours. There was no evidence of an increase of acid metabolites in either blood or urine.

Laslett (2373, 2374) found that staying awake for 72 hours led to much poorer performance in various tests than did wakefulness for 50 hours. Miles and Laslett (2819) photographically recorded the eye movements of five college men who remained awake for 66 hours. The general behavior of the eyes was the same as that described by Miles for the onset of sleep (2816), showing how close such subjects were to the sleeping state even when still ostensibly awake. Weiskotten (4148) stayed awake for 62 hours, preceded and followed by a week of control observations. The tests employed involved memory and speed and accuracy of performance. He found that attentiveness and rapidity suffered more than accuracy and that deterioration of performance did not set in until the middle of the second night of wakefulness. Following the same routine, Weiskotten and Ferguson (4149) continued the study of "the effects of fatigue induced through loss of sleep on the learning process," keeping three subjects awake for 66 hours. The results were similar to those obtained by Weiskotten on himself. Emphasizing the fatigue factor in sleeplessness, the authors ascribed the poorer performance to a diminution in attentiveness and in the ability to concentrate.

Katz and Landis (2090) were approached by a young man, twenty-four years old, who offered himself as a subject for an experiment on the effect of abstention from sleep. He was convinced that sleep was only a habit and, as such, could be broken without any ill effects. By arrangement with the authors, he was given a night-watchman's clock, with instructions that he register the time every 10 minutes as proof of his being awake. He remained "awake" for 231 hours, the collective 10–30-minute periods of sleep, as shown by misses on his record, amounting to only 5.25 hours. His weight, pulse rate, blood pressure, and BMR did not change. His speed of typewriting decreased. On the fourth day he had hallucinations. Later he became more and more confused and irrational, did not know where he was, and accused the observers of trying to ruin the experiment. He developed delusions of persecution and became so unmanageable that the experiment had to be discontinued. It is hard to evaluate the results. The subject appeared to have been slightly psychopathic, and it was not known how many naps shorter than 10 minutes he managed to take. But it is clear that a person can remain practically awake for as long as 10 days without any detrimental effect on his physical health.

Warren and Clark (4122) employed Bills's method of "block"-recording (342) in studying the effects of 65 hours of wakefulness on four subjects. The results were largely negative, as were our own by the same technique.

Since 1939 there has been a tremendous amount of research into the effects of sleep deprivation. In the main (161, 713, 1041, 1269, 1323, 1480, 1648, 1666, 1707, 2570, 2641, 2956, 2957, 3997), reports on physiological processes were confirmed, sometimes with additional details. But there were also entirely new findings and differences in the interpretation of old ones. The excretion of 17-ketosteroids was not changed by sleep deprivation (377, 1269, 3999), but the plasma concentrations of 17-hydroxycorticosteroids were significantly decreased by only one sleepless night (2949). Likewise, the electrodermal activity and pupillary response were changed after one night of wakefulness (3588). Burch and Greiner (569) noted a downward trend in the amplitude of the specific GSR to electric shock with continued sleep deprivation. Critical flicker frequency was decreased (1648), and so was the amplitude of visual accommodation (712), after a moderate sleep loss.

Several authors dealt with performance in a variety of tests, sleep deprivation affecting it not at all, or in a downward direction (377, 429, 469, 640, 641, 695, 1020, 3154, 3551, 3663, 4211–14). By analyzing 22,000 self-administered RTs, obtained from five subjects during fifty-two sleep deprivations, Bjerner (360) noted characteristic long RTs or "pauses" in the carrying out of the serial tests which coincided with changes from alpha to slow wave EEGs. These long RTs and pauses tended to occur in the early morning hours, when the alpha frequency was smallest (p. 158). Mitnick and Armington (2846) reported a decrement in alpha pattern during prolonged wakefulness, to the point of almost complete disappearance (129), with a paradoxical alpha—"stimuli that normally produced alpha block were found to elicit alpha rhythm." The stimuli apparently brought the subject back into something resembling normal quiet wakefulness (815, 1469). Rodin and co-workers (3383) found that, after a sleep loss of 58 hours, the alpha pattern could not be sustained for more than 10 seconds. The Walter Reed Medical Center research team (1440, 1441, 4225–27) also associated the decline in alpha activity with the duration of sleep deprivation; and the presence of longer RTs with lapses or "blocks," or "micro-sleep," under conditions of monotony militating against sustained alertness.

That the body temperature retains its 24-hour rhythm, though its mean level may be somewhat decreased in continuous wakefulness, as first described by Patrick and Gilbert (3115), has been confirmed on normal subjects many times and is still being reconfirmed (161, 2271). However, really striking data in that direction were published by Murray and co-workers (2956, 2957) at Walter Reed. In Figure 22.1 are shown mean body temperature changes and variations in self-ratings of fatigue of fifteen subjects, kept awake for 98 hours. The two curves are almost mirror images of each other, and the mean group self-rating of fatigue stops climbing when the temperature stops falling. These findings support the earlier conclusion that after two successive nights of sleep deprivation the subjects are about as sleepy as they are likely to get, except, of course, for the 24-hour rhythmical up-and-downs. In contrast to the decrease in body temperature observed in normal persons during sleep deprivation, the body temperature, as well as the heart rate, of hospitalized chronic schizophrenics was raised by 100 consecutive hours of wakefulness, for which they volunteered as subjects (2237). However, their performance in tests deteriorated progressively and they "remanifested their acute psychotic picture as it had been observed at the time of their admission to the hospital." As mentioned in Chapter 25 (p. 257), the frequency of epileptic attacks was increased during sleep deprivation (320), though no morphological or chemical changes in the blood of epileptics were detected under such conditions (203).

As could be expected, amphetamine (3996) prevented the deterioration in the performance of a variety of psychomotor tests during sleep deprivation. In a visual size-judgment test, prolonged wakefulness caused an overestimation of size (639), much greater than that produced by 200 mg of chlorpromazine, though a placebo had a somewhat greater effect than the tranquilizer. Sleep deprivation was also found to be more effective than chlorpromazine in impairing the score of a continuous performance test (2838).

Among 275 servicemen who had undergone 112 hours of sleep deprivation,

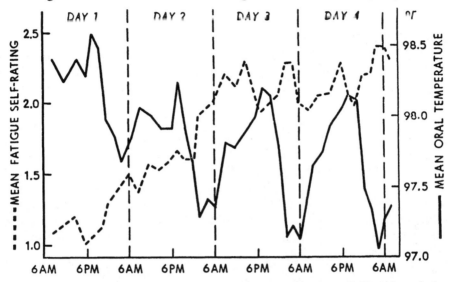

Fig. 22.1—Mean group oral temperatures and fatigue self-ratings of 15 subjects during 98 hours of sleep deprivation, represented in Fig. 1 of Murray and co-workers (2957). Measurements were made 10 times per 24 hours, at 2 to 3 hour intervals. The fatigue self-rating scale consisted of four steps: *1*, not tired; *2*, little tired; *3*, pretty tired; and *4*, dead tired.

Although the group 24-hour oral temperature rhythm was strikingly preserved during the entire period of sleep deprivation, the group mean oral temperature levels for the four successive 24-hour intervals, as determined from 594 original temperature readings kindly supplied by Professor Murray, were 98.16, 97.76, 97.71, and 97.68° F. The drop of 0.39° from the mean temperature level of the first 24 hours to that of the second 24 hours was statistically highly significant, both on the basis of group mean differences and on that of individual subject differences (Ps < 0.001).

The mean group fatigue self-rating levels for the successive 24-hour intervals were 1.21, 1.67, 2.11, and 2.17. The increases in the group fatigue self-rating levels, from the first to the second and from the second to the third 24 hours, 0.47 and 0.44, were statistically highly significant (Ps < 0.001).

Tyler (3996) saw a few instances of behavior resembling symptoms of acute schizophrenia. The EEGs of some of his subjects also appeared like those of psychoneurotic patients. Beginning with Agostini (29), several observers have noted psychotic behavior in intentional and accidental prolonged wakefulness (377, 461, 3180), but even when the symptoms stopped short of psychosis, they indicated profound personality changes, as reported by Seymour (3663) and the Walter Reed group (2888, 2889, 2954, 2955). Using the Rorschach test, Loveland and Singer (2567) were able to predict which subjects would hallucinate during sleep deprivation, and Cappon and Banks (628, 629) noted that "highly nervous and highly neurotic subjects . . . were not able to withstand sleep loss as well as subjects scoring low" in the nervous scale of the Cornell Medical Index. As everyone has his breaking point, sleep deprivation has been exploited for "brain washing" purposes or to extract false confessions from prisoners (1777, 2380, 3032, 3523).

There are several reports dealing with the effect of partial loss of sleep. On five different occasions Smith (3740) deprived herself of some sleep on three successive nights and studied her own performance in a variety of tests. It took her as much as two weeks to reach her pre-experimental level after each period of curtailed sleep. Laird (2328) attempted to determine the effect of the loss of a night's sleep on the performance of five subjects. "Both quantity and quality, especially the latter, are adversely affected by the loss of a night's sleep," was his conclusion. Laird and Wheeler (2346) also described the effect of shortening one's sleep by two hours nightly for a week. Their three subjects had several weeks of practice in mental multiplication of one three-digit number by another, doing fifteen such multiplications per sitting. After a week of short-sleep rations each subject could solve the fifteen problems in less time and with an undiminished accuracy.

Freeman (1271) investigated the effect of curtailed sleep on the performance of two subjects, himself and his wife, for 28 consecutive days. "The amount of sleep was systematically varied to include seven periods each of 4, 6, 8, 10 hours," and a mean duration of sleep of 7 hours per night. The tests were given at 9:00 A.M. and 9:00 P.M. and consisted of measurements of finger oscillation, discrimination reaction, manual pursuit, and memory span, and "the tonus accompaniments were photographically recorded." There was no consistent variation in performance, but the tonus accompaniments of the work were greater after nights when the sleep was short. Subjectively, both Freemans became "cantankerous" and had to forego attendance at all social functions to preserve their reputation for congeniality. In another report Freeman (1272) compared the effects of 4 and 8 hours of sleep on energy expenditure, as measured by muscular tension (technique of tendon deformation) and insensible weight loss. He submitted five subjects to two work-output tests: finger oscillograph and bicycle ergometer.

"When the same subject is changed from 8 to 4 hours of sleeping, the subsequent energy used both during the rest and work tends to be abnormally high."

How long can a person stay awake? The results of sleep deprivation experiments do not furnish information on the absolute wakefulness capacity of man because, as pointed out, after 48–60 hours of wakefulness, the subject's condition and performance are so far below the usual wakeful level that the term "wakefulness" loses its accepted meaning. To determine the maximum span of wakefulness, as a part of an established sleep-wakefulness rhythm, requires a period of adjustment to a cycle longer than 24 hours, and so far no such experiment has been performed. One can only make a guess in that direction, and it would be over 20 hours. The absolute wakefulness capacity of man may become a practical rather than a theoretical matter, if physiological cycling is to be put on a non–24-hour basis in subterranean, undersea, or extraterrestrial operations.

The interpretation of the effects of sleep deprivation varies with the aspect studied and results obtained. Tyler and co-workers (3998) considered their EEG findings "to indicate that the mental effort required either for working a problem or in staying awake during experimental insomnia produces an increase in the rate of the electrical activity of the brain." Malmo and Surwillo (2641) also held that their "data supported the conclusion that sleep deprivation had the effect of increasing the level of activation . . . and not as a drift toward sleep." Ax and Luby (161), however, interpreted the changes in autonomic responses "as evidence for decreased arousal or activation and profound central sympathetic fatigue." Scholander (3588) concluded that the effects on autonomic responses studied by him were "due to a conflict between a wish to stay awake and the successively increasing sleepiness induced by the sleep deprivation and the monotony of the experimental situation." Be that as it may, nearly all attempts to keep animals or human beings awake involve continued muscular activity, and therefore the effects produced are partly due to lack of sleep and partly to muscular fatigue.

Exhaustion and unconquerable sleepiness in man are always accompanied by extreme muscular weakness. The failure to find specific predictable changes in the visceral activities points to the absence of an effect on these activities from lack of sleep. Mental and muscular performance in various tests can be maintained at normal levels if the tests are of short duration, but sustained effort is impossible. The increased sensitivity to pain, impairment of the disposition, tendency to hallucinations, and other signs of this character are the outstanding and significant findings in all studies on lack of sleep. They suggest a fatigue of the higher levels of the cerebral cortex—the levels that are responsible for the critical analysis of incoming impulses and the elaboration of adequate responses in the light of one's previous experience.

Part 5

Spontaneous Changes in the Sleep-Wakefulness Rhythm

Chapter 23

Narcolepsy, Cataplexy, and Sleep Paralysis

One of the most suggestive spontaneous disruptions of the normal sleep-wakefulness rhythm is narcolepsy. It is characterized by repeated sudden brief attacks of sleep, occurring during the customary waking hours of the individual, usually but not always associated with attacks of muscular tonelessness known as cataplexy. Gélineau (1380), in 1880, was the first to describe narcolepsy as a distinct entity rather than a symptom of some other condition; he also gave it its name, which means "sleep seizure." He defined it as a rare neurosis manifested in an invincible need for sleep, ordinarily of short duration, occurring at longer or shorter intervals of time, often several times in the same day, forcing the subject to fall to the ground, or to lie down in order to avoid falling. Since that time many attempts have been made to differentiate between Gélineau's syndrome, or true idiopathic narcolepsy, and symptomatic narcolepsy, secondary to some other disease. Adie (17) called idiopathic narcolepsy a disease *sui generis* and suggested that the term "narcolepsy" should not be applied to other conditions involving brief attacks of arrest of consciousness which could be designated as pyknolepsy. Wenderowič (4169) distinguished three types of narcolepsy: (*a*) genuine narcolepsy, (*b*) symptomatic hypnolepsy (a postencephalitic condition), and (*c*) a symptomatic hypnoid state found in other diseases. Lafora (2322) also listed three different states: (*a*) genuine narcolepsy of Gélineau or hypnolepsy of the adolescent or adult; (*b*) pyknolepsy of early childhood; and (*c*) symptomatic lethargy or somnosia, such as sleep attacks secondary to intoxication or arteriosclerosis. Trömner (3983) distinguished four types of sleep compulsion. Lhermitte (2486) called narcolepsy paroxysmal hypersomnia, which differs from prolonged hypersomnia.

Other authors took the view that no sharp line should be drawn between true—or genuine, or essential, or Gélineau's—narcolepsy and the other symptomatic varieties. They also objected to speaking of the former as "functional" rather than "organic." Daniels (821), in a comprehensive monograph in the form of a review article, analyzing the data on 377 cases of narcolepsy, found it difficult to separate the "true" from the "symptomatic." He also raised the question whether narcolepsy should be called true if it is not accompanied by cataplexy, with the latter phenomenon considered by Wilson (4233) of greater symptomatic significance than actual sleep.

After examining a mass of contradictory statements for and against true narcolepsy, one cannot fail to conclude that though the syndrome is undoubtedly rare, it nevertheless exists, as claimed by Gélineau. The fact that true narcolepsy is of "unknown" etiology is not so significant as is the fact that attacks of sleep and of muscular tonelessness are its chief, if not its only, symptoms. True narcolepsy is less likely to be followed by recovery, and the disease may pursue a chronic course for as long as forty years, according to Doyle and Daniels (973). Indeed, the term "sleeping sickness," appropriately applied to trypanosomiasis and to epidemic encephalitis lethargica, can hardly be a description of narcolepsy: the person afflicted with narcolepsy feels and appears well, may be able to earn a living, and shows few if any signs of abnormality, aside from the attacks of sleep and muscular tonelessness.

Statistical analysis by Daniels (821), Roth and Šimon (3441, 3444), and Ganado (1349) has shown that narcolepsy usually appears during adolescence or young adulthood, with 75 to 80 per cent developing symptoms before the age of thirty. Males outnumber females 2 to 1 (821), or at least 3 to 2 (1349). No racial group is free from it, but Solomon (3750) noted an unusually high incidence of symptomatic narcolepsy among U.S. Negro recruits. Evidence of its possible hereditary or constitutional nature was offered by several authors (2258, 3441, 3444, 4296). The patients seem to conform to the athletic type but usually become obese after acquiring narcolepsy. A number of papers deal with individual cases and reviews of cases of others (440, 514, 622, 781, 786, 977, 1325, 1549, 1572, 1887, 2465, 2547, 2688, 2849, 2953, 3081, 3433, 3438, 3439, 4037, 4230, 4294).

An irresistible desire to sleep may occur several times daily. Visser's patient (4066) had ten to fifteen attacks per day. The afternoon, particularly after a heavy lunch, is a very trying time, although Lhermitte and Peyre's patient (2502) had attacks shortly after breakfast. Monotonous activity accentuates the incidence of drowsiness; diversions seem to counteract it. Generally the patient is aware of an impending attack, and some patients are able to fight off the onset of sleep more successfully than others. The degree of muscular relaxation and the depth of the ensuing sleep are not always the same, even in the same patient. Pollock (3224) held that, unlike normal sleep, narcoleptic sleep is not necessarily preceded, or accompanied, by muscular relaxation. Some narcoleptics are very easily aroused, others are not—very much as in ordinary physiological sleep. Daniels (821) was "able to confirm the experience of others that the various features of these attacks of sleep are practically identical with those observed during normal sleep. At the onset of the attack, the patient's eyes become heavy and dull, and his pupils smaller as his head inclines. He may attempt to raise his head, gazing rather stupidly at the observer meanwhile, but after a few vain efforts his eyes close and he has every appearance of being soundly asleep." The sleep may occasionally be so deep that none of the tendon reflexes can be elicited, and a positive Babinski sign may appear.

The duration of sleep varies from a few seconds to several hours, according to Johnson (1989). Wahl (4100) is the only other author who reported sleep attacks lasting a few seconds, and the upper limit for his patient was 30 minutes. Visser's patient (4066) slept from a few minutes to several hours, but several authors (1349, 1466, 1950, 3983, 4233) gave a range of 10 to 20 minutes. Some patients feel weary and mentally depressed on awakening; others feel quite refreshed. Some resent being awakened, as ordinary sleepers may under similar conditions.

Cataplexy was defined by Daniels (821) as a "state of helplessness into which a narcoleptic patient may be precipitated by emotional stress; he is not unconscious, but is a mass of toneless muscle, and he promptly recovers, none the worse for his experience." The term cataplexy literally means "being struck down," and the emotion that evokes it is most frequently accompanied by laughter. Gélineau used the terms "chute" and "astasia"; Trömner (3983) preferred "affectotonia"; Rothfeld (3452, 3453) designated as "gelolepsy" tonelessness from laughing and as "orgasmolepsy" that occurring during orgasm; other terms used by various authors are "affective adynamia," "tonus blockade," "emotional asthenia," "geloplegia," *Lachschlag,* and *Lachohnmacht.*

Wagner gave a good description of a typical attack of cataplexy (4093). The absence of warning is not characteristic of all cases. Some patients have time to sit down or lie down on the floor so that they do not fall. Although consciousness is preserved in most cases, it is lost in some; in others there is a feeling of having gone through some terrifying dream. A muscular rigidity may develop in certain parts of the body; the tendon reflexes may disappear and so may the corneal reflex; a positive Babinski sign may make its appearance; and there may be diplopia or blurring of vision.

According to Wilson (4233), a cataplectic attack seldom lasts more than 3 to 5 minutes, and others describe it as being of even shorter duration. The frequency of the attacks is related to the incidence of narcoleptic seizures. Although, according to Eley (1060), cataplexy may make its appearance several months before the development of narcolepsy, and the opposite has also been reported, they usually go together. It is often emphasized that narcolepsy occurs spontaneously but that cataplexy is provoked by some external event. Yet, as mentioned above, boredom and monotony favor narcolepsy; gaiety and excitement, cataplexy. The patient may be able to ward off an attack of narcolepsy by engaging in some form of activity; an attack of cataplexy, by learning to curb his mirth or, if he cannot suppress his sense of humor, by withdrawing from the company of friends. Conditions that help prevent narcoleptic seizures may favor cataplexy, and vice versa.

Sometimes the patient can overcome the cataplectic attack by a special muscular effort, different for different individuals; at other times a nudge or light touch by another person serves to terminate the attack. Unless the patient is active when the attack of tonelessness occurs, the attack may not be known to those present near him. As Daniels related it (821), "some narcoleptic patients describe states of powerlessness into which they pass when sitting or lying down, and in which, although entirely conscious, they are often unable for a few minutes to speak or to move a muscle. Although engaged in a terrific internal struggle to move, the patient's appearance may be that of a person sleeping."

Levin (2452) mentioned the occurrence of diplopia during cataplexy, and Ganado (1349) reported diplopia in 5 per cent of his series. The diplopia may be a manifestation of a loss of tonus in the oculomotor muscles, such as is seen in everyday life in persons who are very sleepy or under the effect of large doses of alcohol.

Although cataplexy is usually associated with narcolepsy, it occurred in only 11 per cent of the series of Solomon's Negro narcoleptics (3750), and occasionally there is cataplexy without narcolepsy (2459, 2953). There may be a confusion of cataplexy with sleep paralysis. Lhermitte and Gauthier (2498) have noted that certain cataplectic attacks occurred at the onset of sleep or at the time of awakening. Such attacks were often accompanied by hallucinations and various dream states. Brock also reported a case of this type (513) and Rosenthal (3414) described a *halluzinatorisch-kataplektische Angstsyndrom* not uncommon in schizophrenics, in which anxiety and hallucinations develop upon awakening. These attacks are called *Wachanfaelle* in German, and *crises à l'état de veille* in French. Castaigne (655) also distinguished between cataplexy associated with narcolepsy, and cataplexy of awakening and falling asleep—perhaps related to sleep paralysis. Ethelberg (1110) actually equated the terms *Wachanfaelle*, "hypnopompic sleep paralysis," *cataplexie du réveil*, and *verzoegertes psychomotorisches Erwachen*.

Rushton (3479), describing two cases of sleep paralysis, in which it was not combined with narcolepsy, defined it as "a benign, transient paralysis at the beginning or end of sleep usually associated with distressingly clear consciousness." Similar instances of isolated sleep paralysis were reported by others (2513, 2950, 3574, 3577, 3578, 4034), but Roth (3437), in a subsequent report of such cases, averred that "independent sleep paralysis has hitherto not been recorded in the literature." Roth also gathered twenty occurrences of sleep "hebriety" or drunkenness before, during, and after sleep, and found that, like sleep paralysis, it could develop independently or within the framework of the narcoleptic syndrome, idiopathic or symptomatic. Chodoff (696) and Levin (2457) also concluded that sleep paralysis could be seen independently in otherwise healthy individuals. Goode (1478) confirmed this conclusion, but noted that, in groups surveyed, males with that condition outnumbered females four to one. In a study of the relative distribution of accessory cataplexy (C), sleep paralysis (P), and hypnagogic hallucinations (H) in 390 patients with narcolepsy (N), Yoss and Daly (4296) found that 110 had N alone; 125, N + C; 10, N + P; 15, N + H; 35, N + C + P; 40, N + C + H; and 55, N + C + P + H. Thus, about two-thirds of the narcoleptics also had cataplexy, but only one-quarter suffered from sleep paralysis.

Gill (1444) considered narcolepsy not a disease, but a symptom complex. Where there is no gross pathology, there may be a history of encephalitis or other infection. Certainly many cases of symptomatic narcolepsy—confused with hypersomnia—are psychogenic in character (221, 404, 581, 749, 1491, 2305, 2421, 2844, 2850, 3083, 3703, 3731, 3732, 3768, 3891, 4024), often with a history of psychic trauma or even psychosis.

A possible kinship between narcolepsy and some forms of epilepsy has been traced by several authors (10, 382, 438, 735, 747, 1110, 1760, 2692, 2837, 2883, 3448, 3453, 3640, 3656, 3839, 3903, 3921, 3946, 4072). Others expressed doubt (359, 4315), and still others, as did Gélineau (1380) and Daniels (821), saw no connection between the two conditions (1726, 2456, 2748, 3226, 3435, 3436). Indeed, according to Daniels, "so far as the general run of cases is concerned, the attacks of sleep, from which the patient can be aroused as from normal sleep, and the cataplectic seizures, in which consciousness is not lost, are both so different from any of the usual manifestations of epilepsy that mistakes in diagnosis are easily avoided." A differentiation is particularly easy to make from a study of the patient's EEG.

Brain pathology, often of traumatic origin, has been found in certain narcoleptics (289, 953, 3444, 4023). Infections, especially encephalitis, have been shown in the history of other cases of narcolepsy (645, 2962, 3004, 3362, 3534, 3536, 4071). An association of narcolepsy with gastric complaints was also described (1466).

Of special significance is the coincidence of narcolepsy with obesity (664, 806, 2959). In one such case—really hypersomnia—a pituitary tumor was judged to be the causative agent (755). Polyuria was reported in one narcoleptic (1548) and in one case of simultaneous diabetes insipidus and narcolepsy; the former was relieved by pituitary therapy and the latter by benzedrine. Narcolepsy—again more properly hypersomnia—was linked with hypoglycemia (877, 3363), but in some narcoleptics hypoglycemia induced by insulin increased alertness and hyperglycemia caused a return of drowsiness (3731, 3733). An abnormal presence of parahydroxyphenylpyruvic acid was found in the urine of some narcoleptics (4309).

Otherwise the typical narcoleptic does not appear sick. On the contrary, he or she is often well nourished and has a florid complexion. From the data of Daniels (821) it appears that the pulse rate, basal metabolism, and body temperature are likely to be somewhat lower than normal in narcolepsy. Blood sugar and blood calcium are normal. Polycythemia has been reported by several authors as present in narcoleptics, and abnormal drowsiness has been described as a concomitant of polycythemia. Several authors (1548, 2502, 3558, 3702) have associated sleepiness with an increased red-blood-cell count, although there is not always a question of idiopathic narcolepsy.

Birchfield and associates (352, 353) detected a decrease in oxygen saturation and an increase in CO_2 in the blood of narcoleptics, compared to normal subjects, in both wakefulness and sleep.

The ESR in narcolepsy is higher than normal, according to Richter (3339). Nevertheless, an all-night sleep curve of the ESR of a narcoleptic in our laboratory was not different from that of healthy persons; nor was the EEG. In addition to earlier findings (366), waking EEGs of idiopathic narcoleptics were reported to be within normal limits (1490, 1900). However, Roth and Šimek (3443) noted an alternation of wakefulness type and sleep type EEGs in waking narcoleptic patients which they considered pathognomonic of this condition. Faure (1143), by the use of intranasal electrodes, obtained recordings of potentials from the base of the brain and observed peculiar perturbations of the EEG in narcolepsy. Others (2851, 4071) have also reported EEG abnormalities from this region in narcoleptics. Some investigators hold that EEG abnormalities are present only in symptomatic narcolepsy (1016, 1019, 1371, 1759). Similarly, EEG abnormalities have been used to differentiate between idiopathic narcolepsy and various forms of epilepsy (359, 747, 1491, 1760, 2693, 2883, 3435, 3448, 3839, 3903, 4072).

During drowsiness, narcoleptics were found by Daly and Yoss (815) to remain for abnormally long periods in the so-called floating stage and, when in that condition, to show a paradoxical alpha response: opening of eyes induced an alpha pattern, eye-closing led to its disappearance. Similar behavior in semi-sleep was noted by others during hypnosis (1469) and after sleep deprivation (129).

The night sleep of narcoleptics may be of average depth and duration, but is often deeper and longer than that of normal persons. The sleep EEG of idiopathic narcoleptics shows no abnormalities (366, 1758, 1951, 1952). Some patients complain of disturbing or short fragmentary dreams (3038, 4066), and by the use of the REM-EEG technique Vogel has found that dreaming in narcolepsy starts immediately after the onset of sleep (4075). This finding is somewhat in conflict with an older observation made by Jung (2052) that delta waves appeared in the EEG of two narcoleptics in the first minute after the onset of sleep. Penta (3150) had noted an inversion of the usual sleep-wakefulness rhythm in a narcoleptic.

In the treatment of narcolepsy, ephedrine, first introduced for this purpose by Janota (1948) and by Doyle and Daniels (973, 974), has been used with success by others (718, 1021, 1629, 4029, 4281) but benzedrine (amphetamine) was found by Prinzmetal and Bloomberg (3241) to be much more effective than ephedrine, and is now alone, or in combination with ephedrine, the drug of choice with clinicians (381, 718, 749, 1016, 1017, 1021, 1143, 1633, 3083, 3943, 4017, 4018). Among other drugs, Revoxyl, or dibenzylmethylamine (3419), and Ritalin, or methyl phenidate hydrochloride (4295, 4296), may be mentioned. Glutamic acid (1141), thyroid extract (4138), and bismuth (2079) have also been advocated for narcolepsy. Psychotherapy (1016, 2365), including psychoanalysis (2844), as well as electroshock therapy (3365), and even prolonged sleep cure (2671) were of help in symptomatic narcolepsy. The application of static sparks to the patient's head, as done by Camp in 1907 (614), or suboccipital insufflations of air, employed by Benedek and Thurzó (290) and by Nagy (2970) in the 1930's, did not seem to attract any followers.

The views concerning the nature of narcolepsy and cataplexy are varied and are undoubtedly determined partly, at least, by the available knowledge concerning the conditions that lead to symptomatic narcolepsy or other sleep-like states. These views can be divided into four groups, on the basis of the presumable localization of the postulated disorder: cortical, subcortical, definitely diencephalic, and endocrine. Levin (2444–49) published a number of papers in which he interpreted certain clinical features of narcolepsy in the light of Pavlov's teachings. Pavlov, it will be recalled, viewed sleep as a generalized cortical inhibition and cortical inhibition as localized sleep. Levin considered the military aspects of narcolepsy, giving examples of situations where the natural impulse of the combatant to run away is inhibited through cortical action. The appearance of narcoleptic symptoms in such situations Levin (2446) ascribed to cortical inhibition. In a paper on narcolepsy and the machine age, Levin (2448) pointed to the recent increase in the incidence of narcolepsy as due to an increase in cortical inhibition resulting from the exigencies of modern life.

Coodley (749) characterized psychogenic narcolepsy as a "regressive phenomenon," and Todd (3952) called it a "phylogenetic regression." Vizioli and Zappi (4073), noting that stimulation of cortical area 24 in the monkey led to a complete loss of muscle tonus, developed a "cingular hypothesis" for the origin of the narcolepsy-cataplexy syndrome.

Brailovsky (450), accepting as facts both cortical sleep and subcortical hypnogenic centers, concluded that a complicated cortical-subcortical mechanism is involved. He regarded narcolepsy, however, as subcortical in origin. Trömner (3983) localized narcolepsy, as well as the center for physiological sleep, in the thalamus. Bernardi (312) examined the brain of a woman who had suffered from narcolepsy and found no marked lesions in the hypophysis, infundibulum, tuber cinereum, and the nearby gray. He concluded that "during narcolepsy there is a partial suspension of communication between the cortex and the basal nuclei, and sleep is essentially such a suspension." Münzer (2939) discussed the pathogenesis of hypnagogic hallucinations in narcolepsy as an indication that the narcoleptic syndrome represented a primary disturbance of the mechanism governing the sleep-wakefulness rhythm. Hypnagogic hallucinations, according to Münzer, usher in a narcoleptic attack, as well as normal sleep, and in both cases they represent disintegration symptoms in the interplay between cortex and subcortex. A similar view of narcolepsy and cataplexy as "suggestive of a disjunctive psychophysical effect between the interpretive neopallic cortex and the archipallic sensory receptors in the midbrain" was expressed by Hecker and Carlisle (1676). Levin (2455) held that "the narcoleptic tendency to localized sleep . . . makes it obligatory to assume a cortical disturbance (excessive inhibitability) as the foundation of narcolepsy."

Proceeding into the subcortical region, Lhermitte and co-workers (2485, 2498, 2505) advanced the view that narcolepsy is essentially a morbid condition of the infundibular area. Khait (2151) developed the notion of "diencephalosis" for the explanation of such clinical entities as narcolepsy, pyknolepsy, paroxysmal paralysis, and migraine. Wortis and Kennedy (4281) invoked a "neurophysiological derangement probably of an organic (physicochemical) nature in the region of the floor of the third ventricle" and nearby structures. Schiff and Simon (3558) placed the causative lesion for cataplexy in the infundibular region. Others (602, 3226, 3434, 3722) variously brought in the hypophyseal-diencephalic system and the sympathetic-parasympathetic balance, and Magnussen (2622) advanced the hypothesis that "vegetative preparedness for sleep forms the introduction to—and presumably the basis of—the narcoleptic attacks." Lion (2536) found that ten out of twelve narcoleptics were "vagotonic," but Pond (3226) doubted the presence of vagotonia, and Roth (3434) decided that the sympathetic-parasympathetic tonus of narcoleptics was in the lower levels of normality.

Practically all attempts to link narcolepsy to endocrine dysfunction were related to the hypophysis. Adie (17) spoke of an endocrine-nervous system formed by the hypophysis and nearby vegetative diencephalic centers, and of narcolepsy as a disorder of this system. Serejski and Frumkin (3656) found the narcoleptic syndrome too complex to be regulated by one endocrine gland but held that the hypophysis, as the master-gland, played a dominant role. Beyermann (329) considered narcolepsy as due to hypopituitarism. According to Williams and Harding (4221), some cases of narcolepsy seem to respond to pituitary therapy.

Ionic changes in the blood plasma were also held responsible for narcolepsy. Wagner (4093) considered cataplexy as entirely different from narcolepsy and as due to a disturbance of the calcium-potassium balance affecting the hypothalamic region. Without separating narcolepsy from cataplexy, Fasanaro and Piro (1141) referred to a possible disorder of potassium, calcium, and magnesium; Hofmeister (1814), to changes in the *Kalziumspiegel;* and Fabing (1130), to a chemical disturbance without demonstrable structural change.

Karapetian (2079) noted a disturbance of carbohydrate metabolism in some narcoleptics.

As would be expected, the elucidation of the function of the BSRF brought new explanations of the narcolepsy syndrome. Stoupel (3839) postulated—and probably correctly—that the syndrome was an expression "d'une excitation paroxystique qui provoque une inhibition du système réticulé"; his view was supported by Gastaut and Roth (1371) and by Bowling and Richards (432), the latter also suggesting a neurohumoral deficiency.

The discovery of the EEG-slowing effect of carotid sinus stimulation (407, 2735) furnished powerful support to the views that the carotid sinus is involved in the etiology of narcolepsy and cataplexy. To be sure, the ancients suspected some relation of the carotid to sleep, as the name of the artery is derived from *karos*, "heavy sleep" in Greek. In present-day folk medicine there is the "strange Balinese method of inducing sleep," described by Schlager and Meier (88, 3566): specialized masseurs put a person to sleep by bilateral pressure on the carotid triangles. On the scientific side there is the 1855 report by Fleming (1208), who was able to produce sleep by pressure in the upper part of the neck. The deep sleep—perhaps syncope—never lasted more than 30 seconds. Koch (2224, 2225) associated the carotid reflex effect with the drop in blood pressure. The bearing of his findings on narcolepsy lies in the fact that, out of twenty-five men and twenty-five women tested, two-thirds of the twenty-eight who showed good responses were men; correspondingly, in Daniels' statistics of 377 cases of narcolepsy, males outnumbered females 2 to 1 (821). Weiss and associates (4153, 4154) and Buscaino (589) also dwelt on the role of the carotid sinus in fainting and loss of consciousness. Gellhorn (1385, pp. 224–25) suggested that loss of consciousness from carotid sinus stimulation may be related to "the so-called cerebral type of carotid sinus hypersensitivity." He pointed out that a loss of muscle tonus might be associated with the slowing of the EEG. The first to link the carotid reflex directly with narcolepsy were Wilson and Watson (4232), who noted a supernormal response of narcoleptics to pressure over the carotid sinus and suggested that stripping of the sinus, with cutting of its nerve fibers, might have a beneficial effect in narcolepsy. Lindsley (2528) independently linked the inhibitory effect of the carotid sinus mechanism to "unconsciousness produced in seizures, syncope and narcolepsy."

A case of a mixed salivary tumor in the right tonsil fossa near the carotid sheath was described by Bates (249) in a man with narcolepsy and cataplexy. Removal of the tumor abolished all the symptoms of this condition. A similar case was reported by Møller and Ostenfeld (2852), this time aberrant thyroid tissue pressing on the carotid sinus. Their patient suffered from clouding of consciousness and loss of muscle tonus, on occasion, several times a day. The attacks promptly stopped after the tumor was excised.

The predominance of narcolepsy among males of a tall, heavy-set, athletic type, and its tendency to run in families (2258, 3436, 3444, 4296) suggest that a particular type of neck musculature or adipose tissue may be conducive to producing pressure on the carotid sinus. It should be noted that successful elicitation of the carotid sinus reflex in normal persons is often related to the position of the head (3958) and to its turning (262). Thus, unbeknown to himself, the narcoleptic may precipitate inhibitory effects on the wakefulness system repeatedly by merely engaging in his everyday activities. As well expressed by Yoss and Daly (4296), "phenomena occurring in narcolepsy are exaggerations of similar experiences in normal persons." The exaggerations resulting in sleep are due to accidental stimulation of the vulnerable carotid sinus mechanism.

The surmise of Wilson and Watson (4232) rated only a brief footnote in the original edition of this book, and the chapter was concluded with the assertion that "when we know the exact mechanism of narcolepsy and cataplexy, we shall have the correct explanation of the operation of the mechanism of the physiological sleep-and-wakefulness cycle." It turned out to be quite the other way around. Through the discovery of the unique inhibitory effect of carotid sinus stimulation on the wakefulness system by Bonvallet and co-workers (407), rational support is given to the lucky surmise by Wilson and Watson (4232). It is now up to experimental surgeons to determine the feasibility and safety of the operation suggested to bring about the disappearance of narcolepsy and associated symptoms as clinical problems.

Chapter 24

Encephalitis Lethargica

Epidemic lethargic encephalitis, or sleeping sickness, is a disease causing a varying and complex disturbance of the sleep wakefulness rhythm acute, chronic, or acute with chronic aftereffects. Its symptoms are, in one case or another, often in the same case, hypo- and hypersomnia, sometimes verging, in extreme situations, on complete insomnia and coma, and at other times leading to a shift in the hours of sleep and wakefulness, which may amount to an inversion of the 24-hour rhythm. Gayet (1377) described the first case of *encéphalite diffuse* in 1875. According to Piéron (3192), Wernicke's report of a similar case in 1880 led to the designation of that condition as the Gayet-Wernicke syndrome. The general symptoms comprised fever, delirium, and agitation, or, instead, stupor and sometimes coma. In 1890, during the epidemic of sleeping sickness, Mauthner (2717) definitely related the symptom complex to inflammatory lesions in the periventricular gray (*Höhlengrau*). On the basis of his observations, Mauthner advanced the idea of a functional break between the cerebral cortex and the lower regions of the nervous system as an explanation of the sleep process. From that time also date the various theories concerning the existence of a sleep center in or near the periventricular gray and the adjacent portions of the aqueduct. Because there were frequently a ptosis of the upper eyelid and a paralysis of the muscles innervated by the third nerve, some authors saw a connection between the sleep center and the centers governing palpebral and ocular movements. During the epidemic of encephalitis that prevailed in Europe in World War I, it was Economo (1030) who reinvestigated this disease and related it to lesions in the floor of the third ventricle. Richter and Traut (3345) studied the case of a girl who had chronic encephalitis of the Economo type and, at the age of twenty-six, fell into unbroken sleep lasting 5 years. She awakened from time to time, learned to call for bedpan by grunting, but could not maintain wakefulness. The lesion was located in the posterior part of the hypothalamus.

Mingazzini (2835) gave a complete description of the symptomatology of the disease from his experience during the epidemic of encephalitis lethargica in Italy in the winter of 1919/20. Like Economo, he distinguished three stages: (*a*) stage of psychic symptoms, paresthesia and fever; (*b*) hyperkinetic stage of marked restlessness, lasting as long as 6 weeks; and (*c*) lethargic stage, which sets in suddenly or gradually, the restlessness and fever disappearing. The third stage may last longer than the second and then give way to an apathetic adynamic stage.

Hunt (1872) considered hypersomnia the cardinal symptom of encephalitis and found that in some cases it might set in a few days after the onset of the fever. The hypersomnia differed from stupor in that the patient could be easily aroused and, when so aroused, appeared to be in complete possession of his senses. Pollock (3224) also emphasized the prompt orientation and the unclouded consciousness of the encephalitic patient awakened from his sleep. Gelma and Hanns (1392), however, stated that encephalitis could be distinguished from normal sleep by a less complete awakening, and Good (1477) maintained that the lethargy of encephalitis might vary from a slight drowsiness to complete stupor. Richter (3339) found that the ESR was increased in encephalitic patients during the stuporous state. Cobb and Hill (726) described the "bursts" encountered in the EEGs of patients suffering from subacute encephalitis as different from the "spindles" of normal human sleep "by reason of the frequency of the rhythm, which is remarkably slow" in these patients.

Salkind (3498) considered the sleep anomalies of encephalitis as hypersomnia and hyposomnia. In the former the range was from drowsiness to lethargy, with three distinct subdivisions: (*a*) a state resembling natural sleep; (*b*) a half-delirious state, imitating the effect of scopolamine; and (*c*) a progressive somnolence ending in coma. The hyposomnia might vary from slight unrest to complete exhausting insomnia, with extra-pyramidal hyperkinesis. Between the definite hyper- and hyposomnias there were transitional states involving a disturbance of the normal sleep-wakefulness rhythm.

The ocular symptoms of encephalitis were dwelt upon by several authors. Parmenter and Cheney (3097) described the case of a young man who was drowsy during the day and wide awake at night. He suffered from diplopia and showed double choked disks. He was nearly operated upon for a suspected brain tumor, when it became apparent that he had encephalitis. A normal sleep rhythm returned at the same time that his oculomotor disturbances abated. Salkind (3498) associated the hypersomnia of encephalitis with ophthalmologic symptoms, ranging from pupillary changes to ptosis. Cestan and Sendrail (667) described a case of encephalitis in which the hypersomnia was accompanied by diplopia.

Stockert (3823, 3824) not only considered oculomotor disturbances and somnolence as the cardinal symptoms of encephalitis but showed that, in the acute stage of the disease, fixation of an object by means of the eyes caused first a convergence spasm (manifested by diplopia) and then sleep. Closing the eyes for a moment often led to loss of consciousness and sleep. It was not the absence of vision that was responsible, as the patients could keep completely awake while in the dark, provided they did not close their eyes. The Bell phenomenon—an upward and outward rolling of the eyeball on closing the lids— is the cause of the onset of sleep in these cases, according to Stockert. He was able to induce sleep in postencephalitic patients, and in persons poisoned by barbituric acid, by this method. Hyperventilation of the lungs had the same sleep- inducing properties as ocular fixation. Velhagen (4045) confirmed Stockert's ocular findings in both encephalitic and postencephalitic patients. Zeckel (4312) also succeeded in producing sleep by ocular fixation in a case of subacute en- cephalitis. Overventilation of the lungs in some patients, he found, led to a lower level of consciousness, as well as oculogyric crises, epileptic fits, and sleep attacks. Chambers (671) described a case of encephalitis in a young girl who was troubled with diplopia on awakening. Rozner (3464) related the diplopia that sometimes occurred on awakening from deep sleep (hypersomnia) to the Bell phenomenon.

According to Salkind (3498), hypersomnia occurs when the inflammatory process is localized in the central gray of the interbrain and midbrain and affects the oculomotor nuclei. Involvement of the striopallidal system does not lead to drowsiness. On the contrary, when the inflammatory process reaches this system, the hypersomnia tends to disappear and is replaced by postencephalitic parkinsonism.

Buscaino (587) saw in the parkinsonism, and in other sequels of enceph- alitis, evidence of the intoxicating effects of certain organic substances (amines?) absorbed from the intestinal mucosa. The action of these substances lowered the resistance of the mesencephalon and basal nuclei to the encephalitic infec- tion. This view was based by Buscaino on the occurrence of lesions in the mesencephalon, after animals had been poisoned by histamine and similar products.

Pette (3165, 3166) reviewed the evidence for the localization of the lesion in encephalitis and concluded that the gray matter in the floor of the third and fourth ventricles was involved. According to Pollock (3224), the pathology is limited more or less to the basal nuclei, the midbrain, and the hypothalamus. Pathological studies by Dawson (860) of the brain of an encephalitic patient led to the discovery of "inclusion bodies," suggestive of a virus disease, in the cells of the cortex, basal nuclei, and the pons. However, no such bodies could be found in the brains of two other encephalitic patients. During the St. Louis epidemic of 1934, McCordock and co-workers (2740) determined the patho- logic differences between acute encephalitis of the St. Louis type and Economo's type of encephalitis lethargica. In their specimens they found extensive in- volvement of the spinal cord and inflammatory foci spread throughout the brain rather than limited to the midbrain and basal nuclei. Curiously enough, the oculomotor nuclei rarely showed degenerative changes.

Concerning the nature of the disease, there is a variety of opinions. Schwartz (3625) ascribed the lethargy to hypopituitarism, because the anatomical closeness of the infundibulum might lead to hypophyseal involvement through the extension of the inflammatory process, but offered no anatomical evidence in support of his contention. Trömner (3979) located the lesion in the thalamus, and Pette (3166) took issue with him on that score. However, Trömner (3980) pointed out that encephalitic somnolence resembled natural sleep when there was no oculomotor involvement. The lesion was then in the thalamus. According to Trömner, when the lesion is in the periventricular gray, a condition corresponding to Wernicke's polioencephalitis develops, and the somnolence resembles coma rather than natural sleep.

Many writers, however, support Economo in localizing the lesion of encephalitis in the periventricular gray, the hypothalamus, and neighboring portions of the mesencephalon. Because of the incidence of sleeplessness as well as somnolence, Economo (1030) suggested that these symptoms might be due to involvement of different portions of the region: lesions in the anterior part produced somnolence; lesions in the posterior (caudal) part produced insomnia. In this view Economo was sustained by several investigators, among them Tsutsui (3990). These findings also led to the assumption that there were two distinct centers in the floor of the third ventricle—a sleep center and a waking center. Economo himself (1033) spoke of a "sleep-regulating center" (*Schlafsteuerungszentrum*) as being located at the junction of the diencephalon and the mesencephalon.

Rozner (3464) considered the diplopia and ptosis that accompany the somnolence of encephalitis as supranuclear phenomena. He thought that they were due to the involvement of the sleep-producing area and, therefore, were a part of the sleep mechanism.

Among the most noteworthy and, from the theoretical standpoint, intriguing sequels of encephalitis is the so-called inversion of the sleep-wakefulness rhythm: daytime drowsiness and sleeplessness at night. At first, this inversion seemed to be marked particularly in children. A number of papers on the topic appeared in 1920–21, and one as recently as 1958 (3198). Happ and Blackfan (1623) observed a change in disposition and behavior during the waking period in six children, following apparent recovery from acute encephalitis. For several months the children were awake, excitable, and restless at night, but slept so deeply in the morning that their sleep amounted to stupor. Hofstadt (1815, 1816) described similar symptoms in twenty-one children, in some of whom the symptoms set in immediately after the acute attack was over; in others, several weeks later. He did not designate the condition as an inversion of the sleep-wakefulness rhythm but more correctly as a shift or retardation (*Hinausschiebung*) of the onset of sleep. He clearly distinguished between the failure of the children to fall asleep after they were put to bed and the insomnia which accompanies the choreatic forms of encephalitis itself. During their waking hours the majority of the children behaved normally, but some, like the patients of Happ and Blackfan, showed changes of state or condition (*Wesens-veränderungen*). The total duration of sleep per 24 hours was curtailed. Therapeutically very little could be done to overcome this condition.

Fletcher (1211) had some success in restoring the normal sleep-wakefulness rhythm in a boy, suffering from postencephalitic retarded sleep onset, by the administration of tepid baths in the morning and hot baths in the evening, when large doses of bromide were previously found to be ineffective in producing sleep in the evening. Rütimeyer (3476) observed eight children, aged five to eight years, who were unable to fall asleep until the early hours of the morning for 3 to 6 months after they recovered from an acute febrile disease, encephalitis or influenza. Sedatives were of no help, but psychotherapy was. Bychowski (595), in an analysis of the postencephalitic sleep disturbances in forty patients, noted that, while some could not fall asleep in the evening, others did so but would awake 1 to 2 hours afterward and begin to move and toss around until the early hours of the morning. He, too, found this quasi-reversal of the normal rhythm to be more common in children than in adults. Leahy and Sands (2386) succeeded in restoring the normal sleep-wakefulness rhythm in six children, six to fourteen years old, by forcibly keeping them awake during the daytime hours. Saccheto (3488), like Hofstadt, noticed a decrease in the total number of hours slept, her ten patients, aged three to four years, sleeping for 4 to 6 hours in the morning, after they were fatigued by the activity they engaged in during the night. She ascribed the shift in the onset of sleep to a bacteriotoxic disturbance of the endocrine glands that regulate the metabolic rhythm. The same conclusion was reached by Roasenda (3367), who studied the "inversion" phenomenon in three adult patients.

Reports of a change in the sleep-wakefulness rhythm in adults following encephalitis were made by Janecke (1943), who restored the normal rhythm in a patient by improving his general condition through the use of quartz-lamp irradiation, and by several others (2835, 3486, 3701, 4306).

Norgate (3022) observed the sleep-wakefulness inversion in 10 cases out of 50, following encephalitis. He successfully employed fatiguing physical labor in the daytime as a means of restoring the normal onset of sleep at night. He also found that these patients were afflicted with terrifying dreams when they slept in a darkened room. These dreams did not develop when the room was brightly illuminated.

Zeiner-Henriksen (4313) gave the following "explanation" of the sleep inversion phenomenon: together with an inertia of the vital functions, especially of muscular activity, there is a hypersensitivity of the parasympathetic system, as shown by greater responsiveness to pilocarpine; at the end of the day the metabolic exchanges that follow food intake are not completed and continue into the night; the patients are therefore unable to fall asleep for several hours after the usual time of going to bed.

Stiefler (3820) described a case which he diagnosed as a circular sleep disturbance resulting from encephalitis. There was no night sleeplessness, and no daytime somnolence, but the insomnia lasted from 2 to 4 full days at a time and was followed by several days of hypersomnia, from which the patient had to be awakened. Occasionally, the insomnia and hypersomnia periods were separated by a period of normal rhythm; on rare occasions the same condition (sleeplessness or sleep) would cease and recur without an intervening period of the opposite kind. Campbell (617) also had a patient who went through 2 or 3 days of deep, continuous sleep from which he could not be aroused, but it alternated with "free" intervals, also of 2 to 3 days' duration, when the patient went about his business in the daytime and slept well at night, thus differing from Stiefler's case. Campbell's patient developed his condition five years after an attack of acute encephalitis. The onset of the coma-like sleep was preceded by a sense of difficulty in initiating movements, and, in spite of the patient's efforts to fight it off, sleep gradually overpowered him. In returning to the waking state, he went through a phase of immobile "pseudo-sleep."

Several papers dealt with the presence of hypersomnia only following encephalitis. Reichelt (3303) described the symptoms in three patients who suffered from somnolence after attacks of the grip. One of them, a woman, aged twenty-eight years, developed diplopia in addition to sleepiness. She would fall asleep while eating or talking but could be awakened by auditory stimuli. The somnolence later became continuous. A diagnosis of encephalitis lethargica was made. Although pathologic changes were found in the central gray, the neighborhood of the oculomotor nuclei, the thalamus, and the cerebral cortex, the author ascribed the condition to the lesions in the thalamus. Sittig (3721) reported a somnolence that lasted for two years and which, because of attendant symptoms, was diagnosed as encephalitis lethargica. Stiefler (3821) cited a case of deep sleep setting in from time to time and lasting weeks or even months after the acute attack of encephalitis was over. The sleep attacks did not come on suddenly, but developed over periods of several hours. Strizek (3851) mentioned two cases of parkinsonism after encephalitis in which compulsive sleep would frequently set in and the permanent somnolence continued for 2 to 4 years. Aubert (155) divided the disorders following encephalitis (*névraxite épidémique*) into two types: an inversion of the sleep-wakefulness rhythm and a hypersomnia form. The latter he subdivided into paroxysmal hypersomnia and continuous hypersomnia, or somnolence. The somnolence might be quasi-continuous, in which perceptions were confused, or vacillating between sleep and wakefulness, and might last for months or even years. He attributed the continuous somnolence to the persistence of the encephalitic virus in the centers of the infundibulotuberal system.

Koster (2248) described a peculiar recurrent hypersomnia, as a sequel to encephalitis, that continued for 5 years. At first, the sleep attacks occurred every month, then at longer intervals, up to 14 months. The sleep lasted for a week, deeper at night than in the daytime; and, after the attack was over, the patient consumed large amounts of food. Except for a facial tic, there were no other disturbances.

Gerstmann and Schilder (1409) mentioned catalepsy and akinesis as sequels to encephalitis in three patients. Sabatini (3486) and Froment and Chaix (1306), like Strizek, described the parkinsonian syndrome following encephalitis. One such patient of Sabatini was very dull during the day but could do fine work in the evening. Sabatini showed striking samples of handwriting of children that manifested similar symptoms. Their handwriting was good in the evening but poor in the morning. Froment and Chaix described a parkinson-like rigidity in the limbs of a child following encephalitis: the rigidity changed according to the position the child was made to assume (Magnus–De Kleijn reflexes).

Bonhoeffer (399) described a postencephalitic parkinsonism in which there were an isolated loss of tonus of the levator of the upper eyelid and an irresistible urge to close the eyes. When the eyes were closed, a loss of tonus of the neck muscles would cause the patient's head to droop. However, the patient did not lose consciousness, and there was no tendency to hypersomnia. Another peculiar manifestation of the delayed effects of encephalitis was found in a patient of Leonhard (2431), a woman thirty-eight years old, with parkinsonism, who suffered from *Schau,* or attacks in which she was forced to turn her head and eyes to one side and maintain that attitude for some time. She had a feeling of being paralyzed, when in this condition, and had acoustic hallucinations. She was not really asleep, was completely oriented, and the state of her consciousness was very close to, if not entirely at, the waking level. The author diagnosed the case as one of partial sleep, or sleep of the sphere of volition, akin to hypnosis.

Finally, there are reports of postencephalitic symptomatic narcolepsy and cataplexy. Adie (17) stated that postencephalitic narcolepsy might be distinguishable from true, or idiopathic, narcolepsy. Daniels (821) devoted considerable space to the discussion of this type of narcolepsy. His analysis of the reports in the literature and of the records of the Mayo Clinic showed that most of the cases comprised cataplexy in addition to narcolepsy. There may be no free interval between the recovery from encephalitis and the onset of narcoleptic attacks, or narcoleptic symptoms may make their appearance a month or two, up to several years, later. The reversal of the sleep-wakefulness rhythm that sometimes follows encephalitis often disappears when narcoleptic symptoms set in. Recovery, or considerable improvement, is more likely to occur in the postencephalitic than in essential narcolepsy. Like Adie, Daniels stated that "aside from a history of a preceding attack of acute encephalitis and the presence of signs and symptoms of the chronic stage of the disease, postencephalitic narcolepsy may be similar clinically to the ordinary variety." Daniels raised the question "whether the majority of the cases now being seen actually represent a larval form of epidemic encephalitis." He answered this question in the negative, because narcolepsy may be on the increase when there are few cases of encephalitis and because postencephalitic narcolepsy is rather rare compared to other sequels of this infection.

Individual reports on this topic were made by several authors (62, 664, 2960, 3769, 3893, 4029, 4262, 4312). Some observed narcolepsy alone; others noted clear-cut cataplectic attacks following laughter. Inversion of the sleep-wakefulness rhythm, diplopia, parkinsonism, and emotional disturbances were some of the attendant symptoms.

From a study of ten cases of encephalitis, Eaves and Croll (1022) concluded that there was no definite relationship between the sleep disturbances in that disease and alterations in the anterior lobe of the hypophysis. Lhermitte (2490) reported a case of a fourteen-year-old boy who, after recovering from encephalitis, showed precocious sexual development, obesity, and increase in stature, in addition to hypersomnia and attacks of narcolepsy and cataplexy. Lhermitte stated that, since it had been established that encephalitis does not affect either the hypophysis or the epiphysis, the sexual precocity, like the other symptoms, must be due to injury to the diencephalic-vegetative system, and particularly to the mammillary bodies.

Encephalitis lethargica thus appears to be secondary only to narcolepsy and cataplexy as a spontaneous disturbance of the sleep-wakefulness rhythm, challenging the various theories that are proposed to account for the existence and maintenance of the normal rhythm. The disease may take a hyperkinetic or lethargic form, may begin with one and end with another, may produce insomnia or somnolence, shift or invert the regular hours of sleep and wakefulness as one of its many sequels, or may lead to narcoleptic and cataplectic symptoms indistinguishable from the idiopathic types. Finally, in encephalitis, as first discovered by Mauthner (2717), there are anatomically localizable lesions in the periventricular gray matter and in neighboring parts of the diencephalon and mesencephalon. There are ocular symptoms, suggesting not only an anatomical but also a functional connection between the centers for convergence of the eyes and closure of the eyelids and those primarily injured by the infection. The pathological data pertaining to encephalitis are responsible for the development of the various theories of a sleep center or a wakefulness center, located in the region of the brain stem affected by the disease. The proximity of the hypophysis has given rise to a number of inferences concerning the role this gland plays in the function of sleep. All these matters will be further discussed in connection with the analysis of the various theories of sleep.

Chapter 25

Catalepsy and Epilepsy

Catalepsy, or "downward seizure," differs from cataplexy in that the person usually loses consciousness and often develops, along with the abolition of voluntary movement, a peculiar plastic rigidity of the limbs. In virtue of this waxy state of the muscles, or *flexibilitas cerea,* the limbs may be passively placed in any position, which they maintain for a long time. The cataleptic condition is frequently associated with hysteria and epilepsy and constitutes a definite stage in the progress of hypnosis. The condition is also found in the catatonic stupor of schizophrenics, and, in the description of the state of such patients, the terms "catalepsy" and "catatonia" are sometimes used interchangeably.

Dide (933) regarded the marked "suggestibility of posture" in catatonic patients as an elective sleep of the motor activity. Baruk and Albane (238) indicated the relation of catatonia to the sleep-wakefulness rhythm by citing the case of a woman who went into a catatonic state only upon retiring at night. Gjessing studied the pathological physiology of catatonic stupor in two groups of patients (1454). One group of nine patients showed a periodically recurring state of catatonia that lasted 2 to 3 weeks and was characterized by "critical" onset and termination. The prestuporous period was distinguished by increasing restlessness, irritability, and lack of inhibitions. At the onset of the stupor, he noted a change from a predominantly vagotonic to a sympathicotonic behavior. There were a rise in BMR, increased excretion of urinary nitrogen, hyperglycemia, and raised blood pressure and heart rate. During the stupor-free period there were changes in the opposite direction and, in addition, a leukopenia and lymphocytosis. The other group, of 10 patients, had a non-periodic recurrent catatonia, with "lytic" beginning and end. The physiological characteristics of the stuporous and stupor-free periods were the same as in the group in which the alternation of the two periods was regular. A 48-hour periodicity of catatonia in a schizophrenic was described by Stockert (3827). The stupor phase of 29 hours, with excess water excretion, alternated with a wakeful one of 19 hours, during the first part of which water was retained.

Du Bois and Forbes (996) studied the postures assumed by catatonics. Curled-up or "fetal" postures comprised only 10 per cent of the various positions. Two patients who lay curled up during the day showed the usual range of different positions during sleep. Forbes (1238) obtained photographically recorded evidence that the waxy state of catatonics disappeared with the onset of sleep. The sleep motility of such patients approached the range seen in normal sleepers. Forbes's results suggest the existence of some mechanism, perhaps related to sleep, whereby the waxy state can be quickly abolished and just as rapidly re-established. Page (3075) observed the day and night motility of four catatonic subjects, comparing it with that of normals, parkinsonians, and manics. The motility of the catatonics was by far the lowest of the four groups, in the daytime and at night. They went to sleep, on the average, quickest, and their movements were evenly distributed during the entire sleep period. Of the four catatonic subjects, only one showed *flexibilitas cerea,* and he was somewhat more active during the night than in the daytime. The three rigid catatonics were quieter at night. Sodium amytal increased the movements of the latter, compared to control nights, but it lowered the motility of the "flexible" patient. Thus, the two types of catatonia are influenced in opposite directions by sleep and by amytal.

Richter (3337) measured the palm-to-palm ESR of schizophrenics in catatonic stupor. The resistance was only 8,000–13,000 ohms, with the "normal" value around 45,000 ohms. Richter concluded that such individuals perhaps had a greater nervous activity and more contact with the environment than was generally suspected. Forbes and Piotrowski (1239) studied the ESR of ten catatonic patients and of four normal persons. There was considerably more variation, as well as more marked fluctuations, in resistance in the catatonic compared to the normal group. The authors stated that this greater resistance variability was not to be confused with GSRs to external stimulation. Ando and Ito (66) followed the EEG changes of the several stages of catatonia. Prior to the stupor there was a gradual slowing of 0.5–1.0/sec in the alpha frequencies, but the alpha rate was further decreased in the immediate prestupor stage. During the stupor there was an appearance of beta activity, as well as 6–7/sec waves. In the poststupor and recovery periods the EEG was progressively normalized.

Tomescu and Vasilescu (3954) obtained evidence of a possible endocrine factor in the production of catatonia. They described four cases in which cessation of ovarian function led to the development of a psychosis and later to catatonia. The regulation of the ovarian activity caused the catatonia, and later the psychosis, to disappear.

Of special interest are the several reports on the production of cataleptic states in animals through the action of various pharmacodynamic agents, particularly bulbocapnine, the alkaloid of *Corydalis cara.* According to Van der Horst and De Jong (1836), there is a close parallelism between clinical catatonia and bulbocapnine catatonia in cats, in which it is also possible to observe the waxy state.

De Jong himself (2012) had previously injected bulbocapnine into cats, dogs, and monkeys and produced in them a marked inhibition of movement, stupor, and a cataleptoid state. As also reported by De Jong (2013), animals without a neocortex (fishes, frogs, snakes) never develop catatonia after bulbocapnine; hyperkinetic symptoms appear instead, but only after large doses of the drug. He further found that smaller doses of bulbocapnine produced sleep in higher animals, whereas large doses might lead to epileptoid symptoms. Baruk and De Jong (239) produced sleep or catalepsy in the chicken by varying the dose of bulbocapnine from 10 to 40 mg. They concluded that catalepsy and sleep were closely related to each other, the difference between them being in degree rather than in kind. They saw the catalepsy in the chicken disappear and reappear, as it does in human catatonia. Demole (907), however, in the course of his experiments on the effect of salts on the brain stem of cats and rabbits (p. 200), encountered states resembling catatonic stupor, including the waxy state. He therefore was inclined to consider catatonia to be of organic rather than of functional origin.

Divry (950), also using bulbocapnine, obtained results that differed from those of Baruk and De Jong. In his hands the drug had the same effect on poikilothermal as it did on homoiothermal animals. From his observations he concluded that experimental catalepsy in animals was different from the clinical syndrome of catatonia because, unlike the latter, it was limited to a loss of motor initiative and a waxy plasticity. He likewise found that the electromyographic curves, as well as the chronaxie, in the two conditions were quite different.

Richter and Paterson (3343) produced a cataleptic state in monkeys by means of bulbocapnine which enabled the animals to support their weight in the air when one hand was closed over a horizontal bar. The catalepsy was proportional to the dose, with a maximum hanging time of 60 seconds reached when the dose exceeded 17 mg/kg. This hanging response was completely absent in normal adult monkeys that did not receive bulbocapnine.

Sager (3490) developed contralateral catalepsy in unilaterally decorticated cats after injecting them with bulbocapnine. The righting reflexes were also lost on the side opposite to the decortication. He interpreted his results to mean that the bulbocapnine inhibited those centers in the diencephalon and mesencephalon which, under ordinary circumstances, exerted an inhibitory effect on the myelencephalic centers. Decerebrate rigidity is due to the abolition of these inhibitory influences by surgical cutting of the brain stem; catalepsy is caused by the abolition of the same inhibitory influence through the action of bulbocapnine.

Nieuwenhuyzen (3011) could call forth bulbocapnine catalepsy in the cat after decortication, thus showing that cortical function was not necessary for the appearance of this experimental syndrome. Divry (950) had previously found that the motor inertia he produced in cats by bulbocapnine could not be obtained in decerebrated or bulbar cats. The site of action of bulbocapnine is thus rostral to the bulb, though probably subcortical. Such a conclusion was also reached by Buscaino (588), who placed the site of action of bulbocapnine in the extra-pyramidal centers of the basal nuclei. He likened the bulbocapnine effect both to the catatonia of schizophrenia and to the motor phenomena characteristic of postencephalitic parkinsonism. He further likened bulbocapnine action to that of somnifen—also an amine. Finally, he advanced the theory of the amine origin of catatonic syndromes, postulating that the chemical agents acted on the subcortical centers mentioned.

Harreveld and Kok (1637) obtained loss of motor initiative in cats under the influence of bulbocapnine, but also "negativism," which Divry did not observe under similar conditions. Their cats showed *Klimmzuhang,* i.e., they remained hanging by the front paws on the back of a chair. If a cat were blindfolded while in that condition, it would allow its head to fall back, while continuing to hang on to the chair. There was a diminution or complete abolition of labyrinthine righting reflexes exerted on the head during bulbocapnine catalepsy; but the head was maintained in the normal position, thanks to visual impulses, as demonstrated by the sinking of the head upon blindfolding. The authors concluded that there was a partial paralysis of the CNS, in the course of which certain reactions were abolished while others were not. Their results appeared to favor the interpretation of bulbocapnine catalepsy that was offered by Sager (3490). Harreveld and Kok (1636) had previously induced a cataleptoid state in the dog by passing an alternating current through its brain. When the strength of the current was gradually increased, the catalepsy changed to electronarcosis.

Katzenelbogen and Meehan (2093) noted a decrease in the calcium content of the blood in cats with bulbocapnine catalepsy but no change in the cerebrospinal fluid calcium.

Jongbloed (2014, 2015) performed a series of experiments that convinced him that experimental catatonia, however produced, and probably clinical catatonia as well, was due to anoxia of the CNS. Employing cats, rabbits, rats, and mice, he subjected them to atmospheric pressures of 150 mm Hg, and they exhibited symptoms resembling bulbocapnine catalepsy. He used other physical and chemical means of bringing about anoxia of the brain (injection of lycopodium powder into the carotid arteries, formation of methemoglobin, or cyanide) and, in all cases, developed experimental catatonia.

Baruk (236) injected attenuated *Bacillus coli* toxins into cats, mice, pigeons, and guinea pigs, producing conditions resembling narcolepsy, pathological sleep, and catalepsy. The same toxins led only to a state of torpor when injected into fishes, frogs, and lizards.

Ranson and Ingram (3269), and later, in a more extensive investigation, Ingram and co-workers (1903) were able to produce a state of catalepsy, with exaggerated muscle tonus, in cats by making bilateral electrolytic lesions in the region between the mammillary bodies and the third nerve. There were a lack of motor initiative, stolidity, and a waxy condition which caused the animals to maintain passively imparted positions for a long time. Extensive lesions in the central gray of the third ventricle and the aqueduct were without such effects. The damage had to be done to the structures in the immediate vicinity of the mammillary bodies: the posterior hypothalamic nucleus, and the supramammillary area, the local hypothalamic area, or the region just caudal to the mammillary bodies. Incidentally, under the conditions of electrolytic catalepsy, the cats showed no change in blood calcium.

A striking example of spontaneous mass catalepsy was furnished by Lush (2582) concerning a flock of "nervous" goats on a farm in Texas. These animals, when frightened, would lose consciousness and become so rigid that they could be pushed or turned over as if they were solid. The rigidity lasted only a few seconds.

Marinesco and co-workers (2680) described the case of a fourteen-year-old boy with the rare combination of acute chorea and catalepsy with *flexibilitas cerea*.

Gullota (1559) expressed an opinion that there is a close connection between sleep, catalepsy, catatonia, hypnosis, and other disturbances of the normal sleep-wakefulness rhythm. The evidence presented was contradictory in many ways. One saw that the rigidity and waxy state might disappear with the onset of sleep. The localization of the lesions appeared to be anywhere between, and including, the mammillary bodies and the corpus striatum, although there is general agreement that the cerebral cortex is not required for the development of catalepsy. The effect of bulbocapnine and anoxia indicates a depression of some centers particularly sensitive to the drug and to lack of oxygen. The rigidity is, of course, just the opposite of the muscular relaxation that characterizes cataplexy, which frequently accompanies idiopathic narcolepsy. There is a loss of consciousness in catalepsy, but not in cataplexy. The ability to maintain a certain posture for a longer than usual time shows that one is perhaps not dealing with contractile tonus which leads to fatigue, but with a special type of plastic tonus usually not shown by skeletal muscles. The waxy condition of the limbs supports the idea of a special kind of tonus. While catalepsy and catatonia are intriguing phenomena from the standpoint of the physiology of the brain stem and of skeletal muscle, the anatomical, physiological, pharmacological, and clinical data at present available fail to connect them definitely with the function of sleep.

Epilepsy represents an entirely different type of seizure, with the muscular involvement in the form of tonic or clonic convulsions rather than simply plastic rigidity and immobility, as in catalepsy, or complete relaxation and tonelessness, as in cataplexy. As regards narcolepsy, it is generally admitted that the minor form of epilepsy, or petit mal, bears only a very superficial resemblance to narcoleptic attacks, which are usually of a more gradual onset and of longer duration than petit mal. The possibility of a connection between epilepsy and narcolepsy was previously discussed (p. 237); coexistence of the two in the same patients—epileptic narcolepsy—has been reported (2506, 3664). Hypoglycemia, noted in some cases of narcolepsy (877, 3363), was also found in epileptics by Harris (1647) and by Riser and co-workers (3361). A clinical association of epilepsy with somnambulism (3018, 3185) and with enuresis (3185, 3862) was also noted. As is commonly the case with cataplexy, laughter can induce epileptic attacks in some patients (2661). Conversely, forced laughter was elicited in seven persons out of 2780 by the use of photic stimulation, with or without metrazol; out of the seven, three were epileptics (177). Krisch (2283) reported five cases of epilepsy concurrent with a "migrainous brain-stem syndrome."

Wimmer (4235) described epileptic seizures that occurred in eleven patients with chronic epidemic encephalitis. The seizures were accompanied by encephalitic ocular symptoms, such as convergence troubles. There were also significant vegetative dysfunctions: adiposity, polyuria, polydipsia, excessive sweating, and pyrexia. A more direct connection between an abnormally high body temperature and epileptic hypnolepsy was noted by Sterling (3806). His patient, a man of thirty-eight, had attacks of very profound sleep, during which his body temperature fluctuated between 37.8° and 40.2° C. The "sleep," from which he could not be awakened by most powerful stimulation, lasted from 30 to 75 minutes and was accompanied by muscular relaxation and a tachycardia (probably from the fever). Awakening was prompt, and shortly thereafter the temperature fell "lytically." The sleep attacks were preceded and followed by pain in the left parietal and frontal regions of the head. The author considered his observations as supporting the idea that the centers concerned in sleep and in fever production are located in nearby, if not the same, regions of the brain stem. It will be recalled in this connection that Ivy and Schnedorf (1926), in repeating Piéron's hypnotoxin experiments, found that deep sleep could be produced in dogs by intraventricular injection of cerebrospinal fluid only when there was a concomitant hyperpyrexia (p. 203).

The recording of the EEG furnished an enormous amount of material pertaining to the nature of epilepsy, the diagnosis of its several forms, the influence of sleep and wakefulness, of drugs, stimulations, and lesions. Gibbs and co-workers (1423) noted that the onset of grand mal seizures during sleep was "preceded by the gradual appearance of waves of somewhat higher frequency than those previously dominant." What is more, "if the patient is roused from sleep during a subclinical grand mal discharge, a clinical grand mal seizure supervenes, suggesting that during sleep the cortex is de-efferented" (1419)—the first additional evidence of cortical de-efferentation since the discovery of the positive Babinski sign in normal persons during sleep. They further reported that all types of seizure discharges were commoner during sleep than in the waking state; this finding applied particularly to psychomotor seizures. That sleep may be of help in diagnosing epilepsy was also pointed out by Passouant (3102) and Grossman and co-workers (1532). Bagchi and associates (179, 180), however, challenged this conclusion, having found that in only 10 per cent of their series did they obtain specific additional information during the patients' sleep. Pentothal-induced sleep is particularly suited for diagnosing epilepsy from the EEG (1113, 1328, 1757). Hyperventilation may in some instances be as effective as sleep for diagnostic purposes (2428, 2438).

Several authors dealt with the application of the EEG to the study of epilepsy in children—the newborn (1179, 1180, 3874), older infants (1179) and children (1667, 2122, 2123)—with good results. Sleep is not epileptogenic in infants, but may bring out epileptic EEG patterns, according to Fischgold and co-workers (1180). Kellaway (2122, 2123) found that for children, at least, sleep may be more efficaceous than hyperventilation in revealing epileptiform activity and other cerebral pathology. Davidoff (833) considered the relation of epilepsy to pathologic sleep, and Snyder (3745), epileptic equivalent in children. Jähninchen (1940) reported a very high value for the depth of sleep in epileptic children, as had been noted earlier for adult epileptics (3192).

For differentiating among the several forms of epilepsy, and also epilepsy from kindred conditions, various procedures have been suggested, mostly based on EEG (2507, 2974, 3104, 3106), but also on hypnosis (3866). For elicitation of behavioral or EEG signs of epilepsy in patients, photic stimulation during sleep was found effective (814). So was metrazol (2782, 2783), said to be superior to sleep for diagnostic purposes. In a case of psychomotor epilepsy, it had been possible to produce an attack of grand mal in a patient under light sodium amytal narcosis (224) during an intense state of rage, with the suggestion that "the violence of this subject's reaction resulted from the inactivation by sodium amytal of cortical inhibitory influences." On the other hand, noise or pain was reported to be instrumental in abolishing epileptic EEG discharges (2696). Not much difference was found between epileptics and normal persons with respect to cerebral blood flow, oxygen consumption, and blood gases (1500), the effect on blood pressure of intravenous injection of Sympathol (p-methylaminoethanol-phenol tartrate) under anesthesia (2214), and the presence of sharp EEG waves at the vertex of the head during the early stages of sleep (2155).

The incidence of epileptic attacks was increased by loss of sleep (3601, 3793), as well as by 120 hours of experimental sleep deprivation (320); in the latter case, fivefold, from once in 66 to 69 hours to once every 12 hours. The same length of sleep deprivation had no clear-cut effect on blood and urine composition of epileptics (203).

Amphetamine (882) and reserpine (2353) have been found useful in the treatment of epilepsy, and Hunter (1873) considered a variety of drugs in the handling of the several types of epilepsy.

Of particular interest to the student of sleep, wakefulness, and consciousness is the behavior of patients with psychomotor epilepsy. Gibbs and associates (1418, 1421, 1426) pointed out that during an attack the patient "is not usually unconscious." It would be more correct to say that he is usually awake, as the low level of his consciousness is betrayed by his being "confused" and amnesic—features characteristic of dream consciousness. Indeed, as the authors stated, "his general manner is that of a person acting out a bad dream" (1426). In addition, the EEG of "pure" psychomotor epileptics (no grand mal or petit mal) is usually normal during wakefulness, but shows seizure activity during spontaneous, or drug-induced, light sleep. Because this work was done before the REM-EEG technique for monitoring dreaming episodes was developed, it was not possible to determine whether the seizure activity was related to dreaming. The focus in psychomotor epilepsy, when it can be located clinically or anatomically, is in the temporal cortex, and two out of five patients have severe personality defects in interseizure periods.

Gastaut and associates (1369), from an EEG study of three hundred patients with psychomotor or temporal epilepsy, concluded that temporal psychomotor epilepsy properly so-called is extremely rare, with hippocampal psychomotor epilepsy much more frequent, and diencephalic psychomotor epilepsy intermediate between the other two in frequency. Rovetta (3456) also noted that maximum seizure activity in 16 out of 18 cases of temporal lobe epilepsy was from the hippocampus.

Quite a different picture is presented by petit mal epilepsy, in which the main, or only, abnormality is a partial or complete brief loss of consciousness, and the pathology is subcortical. Schwab (3617, 3618) showed that the RT to a light stimulus remained unchanged, or increased two to three times, during a petit mal attack, occurring spontaneously or brought on by overventilation, depending upon the degree of impairment of the patient's consciousness. Jasper and Droogleever-Fortuyn (1964) were able to reproduce the essential EEG features of petit mal (synchronization of large areas of both cerebral hemispheres into a rhythmic discharge of 3/sec, and the spike and dome complex) in cats "by rhythmic electrical stimulation by brief shocks to a small area . . . in the medial intralaminary region of the thalamus." Spiegel and co-workers (3767) then showed that metrazol brought on spike and dome discharges simultaneously in the EEG and the electrothalamogram of a petit mal patient. The thalamic discharges outlasted the cortical ones, and during general anesthesia only thalamic discharges were obtained. Sometimes the thalamic discharges appeared several seconds before the cortical ones, and at no time did discharges appear primarily in the cortex and secondarily in the diencephalon.

EEG studies revealed a number of peculiarities in petit mal patients. Cornil and co-workers (761) noted that with very brief attacks there was no change in consciousness; with longer attacks there was a loss of the higher (cognitive) form of consciousness, whereas the simpler (perceptive) one remained intact. Others have reported petit mal EEGs without loss of consciousness (2662), or the disappearance, under treatment, of both clinical symptoms and 3/sec waves, with the preservation of the dome-and-spike pattern (2884). The petit mal EEGs were found to be associated with spontaneous changes in respiratory volume (725) and could be elicited by overventilation (251), photic driving (724), or even emotional conflicts (220). An unusual case of petit mal in a child was reported by Stark (3787): "instead of a normally appearing increase in theta rhythm with eye closure and cessation of visual blocking, frank petit mal seizure bursts and clinical concomitants appeared consistently." Another peculiarity in petit mal patients, as noted by Singh (3718), is their response to a sudden noise during the spindle stage of sleep by an isolated single or double spike potential, instead of the normal initial negative sharp wave followed by a couple of broad high voltage waves.

In animal studies, Gellhorn and Ballin (1389) obtained large slow EEG waves in rats by repeated intraperitoneal injections of water and surmised that the different forms of epileptic seizures might be due to water intoxication. Blum and co-workers (383) developed unilateral Jacksonian seizures in immature monkeys, with symmetrical bilateral frontal cortex extirpation, after the administration of benzedrine. Hunter and Jasper (1874, 1875), using unanesthetized cats with previously implanted electrodes, produced a type of "arrest reaction" by thalamic stimulation. The animals "would remain immobile, with no loss of tone, and failed to respond to usually effective stimuli" (1875). The reaction resembled in many ways the petit mal seizure in man. Liberson and Akert (2512), from observations on guinea pigs, suggested that "the hippocampus may play an important role in epilepsy in general."

The connection between sleep and the incidence of epileptic attacks has already been touched upon. Earlier findings include the report on alkalosis by Stark (3786), and on blood chemistry in relation to sleep by Hopkins (1832), who noted that the acid-base and ionic changes were such as "to encourage the development of seizures during . . . sleep." Recent studies involved the utilization of the EEG. Several French authors (893, 2349, 3108) coined the term *épilepsie morphéique* to designate a type of epilepsy in which attacks occur during sleep. Delmas-Marsalet (892) described four cases in which the crises were precipitated at onset and termination of sleep, in one of the cases by sudden darkness. Dew and co-workers (929) noted an association of sleep focal abnormalities with subnormal BMRs. Brazier (466) advanced the hypothesis that "the typical epileptic spike is an abnormal discharge of apical dendrites of pyramidal cells." On the assumption that the firing of these dendrites is regulated by circuits to and from the BSRF, she suggested that "the disruption of the reticular ascending system by the sleep would unbalance this control and this might thus explain the appearance of spikes in the EEG of these patients." Rovetta (3456) referred to maximal seizure activity of 16 out of 18 cases of temporal lobe epilepsy in wakeful rest coming from the hippocampus. Kajtor and co-workers (2064) found that "foci in the hippocampus have the greatest tendency to provoke seizures during sleep," while foci on the convexity of the cortex may cause seizures mainly during sleep or during wakefulness, depending on location. Kajtor (2063) also noted that when focal seizures occurred during sleep from the motor or sensory areas, they frequently precipitated awakening, but did not do so when they arose from frontal or temporal foci. Chatrian and Chapman (681), using scalp and depth recordings, observed "a spectacular increase of the spike discharges in the amygdaloid electrodes" during sleep, together with a marked spiking on the scalp. Further, "when the patient awakened spontaneously the discharges immediately disappeared from the scalp and became infrequent in the amygdaloid region." Two cases of "retarded psychomotor awakening" were described by Rosenthal (3412) in epileptics, somewhat reminiscent of his hallucinatory-cataplectic anxiety syndrome (p. 236). There is a state of immobility on awakening, although the person is completely conscious. The author held normal awakening to be a chain phenomenon, with the impulse starting from the thalamus and reaching the cerebral cortex in a roundabout way via the striatum and the periphery. Retarded psychomotor awakening was considered by him to occur when the impulse passes directly from the thalamus to the cerebral cortex, due to a *Schaltschwäche* (circuit weakness) in the striothalamic apparatus.

Concerning the 24-hour distribution of the incidence of epileptic attacks, there is the observation of 1888 by Féré (1155) that two-thirds occurred from 8:00 P.M. to 8:00 A.M., as opposed to that of Sal y Rosas (3496) of 1957 that three-quarters of the seizures took place during the waking hours of his patients. Langdon-Down and Brain (2361) divided their patients into three groups, with seizures in each group concentrated in the daytime, at night, or diffusely through the 24 hours. A similar division was made by Patry (3116) and by Janz (1949), the latter finding that the attacks fell during sleep or shortly after awakening in the morning in 95 per cent of the cases of genuine, cryptogenic epilepsy, but in only 55 per cent of the cases of symptomatic epilepsy (including traumas). Engel and co-authors (1088) found the 24-hour eosinophil count rhythm present in epileptics, and when seizures were observed they tended to coincide with the minimum eosinophil level. Levin (2456) discussed the occurrence of fits at awakening from the Pavlovian viewpoint.

Magnussen (2620) selected 18 out of 435 patients living in a home for epileptics on the basis of a "conspicuous regularity in the occurrence of their fits at certain hours." In all 18 sleep was the most important factor among those that correlated with the regularity of the attacks. Magnussen noted that the 18 patients had a tendency to hypoglycemia. Griffiths and Fox (1518) analyzed the distribution of fits in 114 patients with a maximum incidence at 6:00–7:00 A.M., but, confirming earlier findings (2361), also smaller secondary peaks around noon and in the evening. They additionally found that "patients tend to have fits during the early part of the night when sleep is deepest, during the latter hours of the night, in the transition period from sleeping to waking, within an hour of the time of rising at the end of the sleep, or during the day when sleep is absent."

The evidence presented in the second half of this chapter fails to bring out a definite relationship between epilepsy and the sleep-wakefulness rhythm, aside from the just-mentioned tendency of the convulsions to occur, in some patients, in one or another phase of the cycle. So far as consciousness is concerned, petit mal stands for a lapse of consciousness connected with a subcortical, probably thalamic, focus; psychomotor epilepsy, for an imitation of dream consciousness during overt wakefulness. Both of these pathological phenomena must occur within the framework of the physiological mechanisms responsible for the maintenance of wakefulness and consciousness. Even the many sleep-associated manifestations of epileptic discharges may also be related to the temporary in-activity of the wakefulness-maintaining brain circuits.

Chapter 26

Hypersomnias and Comas

Hypersomnia has been defined as uncontrollable somnolence and pathologically deep and prolonged sleep, from which it is sometimes difficult to arouse the sleeper, or to keep him awake for any length of time after he has been awakened. Coma is a state of complete loss of consciousness, from which the patient cannot be aroused even by the most powerful stimulation, and is thus equivalent to spontaneously developed anesthesia. Even though theoretically the two conditions are clearly distinguishable from each other, in practice there are gradations and oscillations between them, and a condition that starts out as hypersomnia may terminate in coma (1142).

Cerebral neoplasms have been known to produce interference with the sleep-wakefulness rhythm mainly in the direction of hypersomnia. This interference is particularly marked if there is an accompanying increase in intracranial pressure, although the somnolence may appear before such an increase develops. Other lesions in different parts of the brain may also lead to hypersomnias. The anatomical findings, first of Mauthner (2717) in 1890, then of Economo (1030) in 1916, on the localization of the infection in epidemic encephalitis lethargica led to frequent searching for and finding of lesions in Mauthner's "spot" (Chap. 24) in cases of pathological sleepiness, where an anatomical diagnosis was possible. The numerous attempts to produce sleep in the laboratory by stimulation of, or injury to, Mauthner's area by pharmacological, mechanical, and electrical means have been previously recounted (Chap. 20). Clinical and anatomical findings in spontaneous hypersomnias, other than the ones discussed in the last three chapters, most frequently, though significantly not always, point to Mauthner's region as the seat of the lesion. According to Freeman (1275), continuous sleep is always symptomatic, indicating a definite anatomical lesion.

As early as in 1903 Righetti (3350) reported the case of a boy with a cerebral glioma, characterized by continuous sleep. The boy could be awakened but would soon fall asleep again. The tumor was found to have destroyed the optic chiasm and the tuber cinereum, thereby producing a distention of the third ventricle. Righetti also analyzed the case histories of 775 patients with cerebral tumors. Of these, 115 displayed pathological sleep. Hypersomnia was more or less frequent depending on the location of the tumor. For those who had tumors of the thalamus and around the third ventricle it was present in 35 per cent of the cases; tumors of the medulla, 28 per cent; tumors of the hypophysis and vicinity, 27 per cent; tumors of the corpora quadrigemina and epiphysis, 26 per cent; tumors of the cerebellum, 16 per cent; and frontal-lobe tumors, 6 per cent. In other words, although the condition of stupor, which Righetti designated as somnolence, was found in less than 15 per cent of all the cases, its incidence was twice as high in tumors involving the brain stem.

Warren and Tilney (4121) found a tumor of the pineal body that invaded the midbrain, thalamus, hypothalamus, and hypophysis in a boy who had attacks of somnolence. Francioni (1258) located destructive lesions in the mesencephalon of a child of three years and an infant of ten months, in both of whom hypersomnia was an outstanding symptom. Souques and co-workers (3754) studied the case of a woman, aged thirty-seven, who for the last three months of her life had attacks of uncontrollable sleep, with diplopia and slight fever. A diagnosis of encephalitis lethargica appeared justified by the symptoms, but necropsy revealed a cancer in the infundibular recess of the third ventricle. This patient did not develop either glycosuria or polyuria; but another woman, whose case was reported by Français and Vernier (1257), with an epithelioma involving the third ventricle and the infundibulum, showed an increasing polyuria, in addition to attacks of sleep that became longer and deeper as the condition progressed. For the last six weeks of her life she was continually asleep but could be awakened to be fed and cared for.

In 1928 Bailey (181) described four cases of third-ventricle tumors in which somnolence was one of the symptoms. One was that of a woman, aged twenty-eight, who had brief attacks of sleep, as well as polyuria, for six years prior to her death. Toward the end she was almost continuously asleep. Necropsy showed a vascular tumor of the hypothalamus. The second case was of a man, aged thirty-eight, who had only one attack of sleep, lasting a day and a half, 2 years prior to his death. A tumor was found in the third ventricle, but the latter was scarcely dilated. Another tumor, which filled the entire third ventricle but did not involve the infundibulum, led to continuous drowsiness, which was thought to be due to encephalitis. The fourth tumor, in a boy of fifteen, was a pinealoma which filled the third ventricle and involved its walls. This boy, like the first case, showed polyuria as well as somnolence. Fulton and Bailey (1320) pointed out that small tumors at the base of the brain might lead to hypersomnia, without a rise in intracranial pressure. They described a case of a slowly growing sarcoma, which was sharply limited to the region of the hypothalamus and did not lead to an increased intracranial pressure. Yet there was a five-year history of gradually increasing somnolence. Marinesco and associates (2679) reported two cases of hypothalamic tumor. In one the periaqueductal gray was also involved, but in the other it was not; pathological hypersomnia was present in the first and absent in the second. They concluded that the region around the aqueduct was more directly concerned in the sleep function than the more anterior periventricular gray.

Bürger-Prinz (562) had four patients with ventricular and intraventricular tumors who had attacks of sleep that continued uninterruptedly for days or even weeks. There was some disturbance of orientation, and at times the patients on awakening appeared to be unaware of having been asleep. Drăgănesco and Sager (976) described attacks of continuous sleep, lasting 2 to 3 days, and a growing adiposity and polyuria, in a woman who had a third-ventricle tumor. Bismuth and neosalvarsan therapy led to a temporary disappearance of the somnolence but not of the polyuria. When she was asleep, it was hard to awaken her, and, like Bürger-Prinz's patients, she showed poor orientation on awakening.

Rowe (3459) studied three cases of diencephalic tumors. Two of these were associated with somnolence, but in the third there was no change in the sleep-wakefulness rhythm. By serial sections he determined the exact location and confines of each tumor. In the two hypersomnia cases the tumor extended through the dorsal and posterior portion of the diencephalon, in one case involving the thalamus bilaterally; in the other, unilaterally and the medial thalamic nuclei chiefly. The periventricular gray, including the reuniens and the nucleus paraventricularis, was infiltrated, but the infundibular and tuberal regions and the mesencephalon were not affected. In the third case, where there was no hypersomnia, the tumor occupied almost the entire thalamus but extended into the diencephalon only unilaterally, though farther ventrally and caudally (into the mesencephalon) than did the other two tumors. Rowe concluded that the development of hypersomnia necessitated a bilateral involvement of the periventricular gray and, at least, a unilateral damage to the thalamus.

Cardona (633) studied the case of a tumor occupying the entire interpeduncular and infundibular areas, including the floor of the third ventricle, in a woman who, in addition to somnolence symptoms, had genuine non-diencephalic epilepsy. There was no complete reversibility of the sleep-wakefulness rhythm in this woman, but she was frequently somnolent during the day and wakeful at night. Zeitlin and Lichtenstein (4314) described two cases of hypersomnia due, in each situation, to pressure of cystic tumors, containing colloid material, on the floor of the third ventricle. Ford and Muncie (1240) reported three cases of pronounced somnolence, polyuria, and disturbances of temperature regulation. In each of the three patients there was a malignant tumor that invaded the ventricular walls. Monnier (2864) investigated a case of symptomatic narcolepsy, with an increase in intracranial pressure, progressive hemiplegia, trembling, and muscular rigidity. There were a tubercle in one frontal lobe and lesions in the ventriculodiencephalic region, as well as in the corpus striatum. The narcolepsy was ascribed to the diencephalic involvement.

One could cite many more examples of meso-diencephalic tumors (3817) that led to prolonged sleep states, with or without polyuria and other side effects, but the symptomatology and pathology are more or less the same as those already mentioned. In addition to Rowe (3459), several observers linked tumors in regions other than the periventricular gray with sleep pathology. Lignac (2516) had a patient with marked somnolence and paralysis of the muscles of the face and tongue. The condition had been diagnosed as encephalitis lethargica, but later a tumor in the thalamus and internal hydrocephalus were shown to be the pathology of the case. Babonneix and Widiez (170) found a glioma of the corpora quadrigemina that spread over the region of the cerebral peduncles and thalamus of a patient whose main symptom was somnolence. Hechst (1675) had four cases of pronounced somnolence, in which an anatomical diagnosis was made. In three of these the tumors involved the thalamus. The locations of these three tumors were: (*a*) the posterior third of the periventricular and the neighboring parts of the periaqueductal gray, as well as the posterior and medial parts of the thalamus; (*b*) the dorsal part of the periaqueductal gray and the medial part of the posterior third of the thalamus; and (*c*) very little of the periventricular gray and the posterior third of the left thalamus. Cox (770) described a variety of brain tumors, in the midbrain, hypothalamus, and thalamus, each having an effect on the sleep-wakefulness rhythm and on the state of consciousness during the periods of wakefulness (changes in disposition, disorientation).

Lechelle and co-authors (2393) had two cases of frontal-lobe tumors. Somnolence was the main symptom in one case and the only symptom in the other. This last patient started with brief narcoleptoid attacks, which gradually became deeper and of longer duration. McKendree and Feinier (2755) analyzed one hundred cases of cerebral neoplasms and found evidence of intracranial hypertension in most of them. Somnolence was most constantly found in such cases, particularly when there was, as a result, a marked internal hydrocephalus. Kolodny (2232) studied 38 patients with temporal-lobe tumors, and found that nine of these showed hypersomnia. He did not think that somnolence should be definitely ascribed to lesions in the periventricular gray, as in only five of the nine cases could such lesions be detected. Wodoginskaja (4249) had a similar experience. In examining five brains of patients who had sleep disturbances, she located two tumors in the region of the third ventricle, while in the remaining three, the tumors were at some distance from that region. Frazier (1268) reported 105 cases of frontal-lobe tumors; in 34, there was some form of hypersomnia, ranging from drowsiness to stupor. However, he regarded the hypersomnia as a neighborhood symptom and attributed it to the involvement of the diencephalon. Like McKendree and Feinier, he thought that the somnolence might be due to increased intracranial pressure, particularly tension within the third ventricle.

In addition to neoplasms, various destructive lesions in the periventricular gray have been found to produce hypersomnia. Luksch (2575) told of a case of *endocarditis lenta,* with aortic insufficiency and empyema. The patient slept continuously for two weeks prior to his death, could be awakened only with difficulty, and would soon fall asleep again. Necropsy revealed a suppurative destruction of the ventricular and aqueductal gray. Smaller offshoots of the focus stretched both to the medial thalamic nuclei and to the anterior corpora quadrigemina. Adler (19) described a similar case of endocarditis, with continuous sleep, very much like the one studied by Luksch. The anatomical finding was an abscess in the periventricular gray extending into the hypothalamus. Marinesco and associates (2679), in three cases of tuberculous meningitis, with hypersomnia, found changes in the periventricular gray and in the infundibulo-tuberian region. Hirsch, however (1779, 1780, 1782), reported the presence of thalamic abscesses in two patients with pathological sleep, in addition to a variety of other deficiencies. In one case, a walnut-sized abscess completely replaced the left thalamus, with the exception of the ventral portions and the pulvinar. Hirsch concluded that the thalamus, or perhaps only the medial portion of the left thalamus, was connected with sleep-and-wakefulness alternation, serving as a connection between the cortex and Mauthner's area. Ohkuma and Tuyuno (3044) found foci of softening in the ventral portions of both thalami, in a patient who died after six weeks of lethargy, accompanied by oculomotor paralysis. Stern's case (3810) of severe organic dementia and drowsiness involved a selective bilaterally symmetrical degeneration of the thalamus, and in two cases of protracted somnolence Globus (1460) found "discretely circumscribed lesions in the diencephalomesencephalic region." Schaltenbrand (3545), in a case of hypersomnia that lasted one month and then disappeared, detected a small softening focus (*Erweichungsherd*) which destroyed the mammillothalamic bundle and neighboring structures, on one side. Tretiakov (3970) studied cases of lethargic sleepiness which, because of a negative Queckenstedt sign, were interpreted to indicate an involvement of Mauthner's zone and a stoppage of the aqueduct, and he designated the condition as the symptom-complex of the aqueduct.

Perhaps the most systematic study of the effects of lesions in different parts of the brain with or without increased intracranial pressure was made by Davison and Demuth (851–57) in 50 cases that came to autopsy. In nine lesions confined to the cortex, with either hypersomnia or coma, the convolutions mainly involved were the hippocampal, cingular, frontal, prefrontal, and temporal. The frontal region was also implicated in an earlier report by Lechelle and co-workers (2393). In twenty-five cases (855) the lesions were at the corticodiencephalic level; in seventeen cases (856), the diencephalic level (hypothalamus); in a last group of eight (857), the mesencephalometencephalic level, with the hypothalamus uninjured. Davison and Demuth concluded that the hypothalamus is one of the main centers for the control of sleep and wakefulness and that "damage to the hypothalamus, especially the posterior part of the lateral hypothalamic area and of its various pathways bilaterally, causes somnolence" (856).

Several authors (399, 1142, 1303, 4022, 4025, 4322) observed hypersomnia, among other symptoms, in patients with cranial trauma. Posterior fossa compressions (1972), thrombosis at the bifurcation of the trunk of the basilar artery (1132), and apoplectic strokes (3616) were also noted as causes of hypersomnia. Buccelli (553) had seen several cases of somnolence in children, following extirpation of adenoids; Winnicott (4244), after a tonsillectomy; and Traina (3964), after a mastoidectomy. Dercum (918) and Meyer (2792) mentioned cases of hypersomnia as a sequel to grip (perhaps mild encephalitis); Castex and co-authors (658), as a result of chronic respiratory insufficiency. Sternberg (3816) had a patient with seasonal somnolence related to a pollen allergy. Troilo (3984) and Urechia (4022) had hypersomniac patients with a history of syphilis. Genoese (1394) discussed the incidence of somnolence in infants and children during the various stages of malaria. Levin (2450), from the literature and his own experience, gathered seven cases of periodic "somnolence-hunger," or attacks of somnolence, accompanied by excessive food intake, lasting several days, or even weeks. All the patients were males, and in three of them the symptoms appeared following an acute febrile condition (sore throat, grip, influenza). During the somnolence-hunger attacks the patients showed motor unrest, as well as hyperirritability, forgetfulness, incoherent speech, and hallucinations. The so-called Kleine-Levin syndrome was described and discussed by several other authors (785, 1330, 1514, 2606, 3078, 3402). Ronald (3402) and Grewel (1514) considered this syndrome to be a real entity, but Pai (3078) held that the association of hypersomnia with the morbid hunger is purely coincidental.

Valerio (4031) reported a case of hypersomnia apparently due to excessive formation of gas in the intestine. The depth of sleep at times verged upon coma. Correction of the intestinal condition abolished the sleep attacks, which at that time had continued for two years.

Metabolic conditions, especially when the liver is involved, often lead to hypersomnia. Thomson (3930) attributed a condition of hypersomnia in a boy five years old to hepatic dysfunction. Since he was weaned, the boy had recurrent attacks of sleep lasting three days, and at one time coming on every three weeks. He would fall asleep quite suddenly and, during the attack, wake up at infrequent intervals to take nourishment or empty his bladder. In between the attacks the boy behaved and slept in a normal fashion.

Elliott and Walshe (1069) obtained a positive Babinski response in toxic states, bordering on coma, due to a variety of causes, including acute and chronic impairment of liver function.

Neisser (2980), like many others, found that somnolence could be associated with a polycythemia. A patient of his, with a seven-year history of paroxysmal hypersomnia, had a red-blood-cell count of nine million but a hemoglobin of only 85 per cent. Baserga (240) reported polycythemia in a patient who had a tumor of the hypophyseal stalk. He discussed the possibility of the existence of a diencephalo-hypophyseal center regulating hemopoiesis. Lunedi and Liesch (2580) studied a family in which the father had a pyloric ulcer and polycythemia, a daughter had Fröhlich's syndrome, and two sons had duodenal ulcers. They ascribed all these ailments to diencephalic dysfunction. It will be recalled that in narcolepsy polycythemia was detected on numerous occasions and that the deprivation of sleep sometimes leads to a decrease in the red-blood-cell count.

May (2720) had a patient nineteen years old who was treated with peptone to alleviate dysmenorrhea and severe migraine. She developed attacks of somnolence after the peptone treatments were stopped. Resumption of the peptone medication abolished the hypersomnia. May attributed the sleep attacks to anaphylactic shock. Druckmann (994) observed what he called somnolence in thirty patients (out of 1,100) who were being given X-ray treatments. The somnolence abated 4 to 14 days after the irradiation, depending on the dose of X-rays. Reduction of the intensity of irradiation in subsequent treatments led to the non-appearance of the somnolence after-effect. Barré and Andlauer (229) described sudden attacks of hypersomnia, 2 to 6 hours in duration, in a patient with Thomsen's disease. Insulin therapy was followed by a temporary cessation of the hypersomnia.

There are many papers on somnolence as a symptom of endocrine dysfunction. The well-known apathy and sleepiness of persons with hypothyroidism, and the opposite for hyperthyroidism, need not be reiterated. Bonoriño (403) and Bauer (266) each had success in overcoming somnolence of hypothyroid origin by means of thyroid therapy. Dana (818), in taking up the relation of somnolence to disorders of the endocrines, found that the hypophysis was involved most frequently, and indeed most communications on the condition pertain to the hypophysis and to the gonads.

Dercum (918) ascribed a post-influenza case of somnolence to endocrine dysfunction, as the patient's extremities suggested acromegaly and his testes were atrophied. Basile (241) cited the case of a patient with almost continuous sleep. Removal of a nasopharyngeal tumor was followed by a return to normal. The author concluded that the tumor caused changes in the hypophysis which led to the ensuing morbidity. Bychowski (594) reported the presence of a large tumor of the dura mater and a hypertrophy of the hypophysis in a woman with periodic somnolence. Beckmann and Kubie (271) studied twenty-one cases of pituitary-stalk tumors. In nine of these somnolence was one of the symptoms. Children and young adults are particularly likely to show sleep disturbances in the presence of such tumors. Brouwer (527) described a case of deep hypersomnia lasting three weeks in a woman who had been somnolent for some time previously. She also gained in weight and had menstrual disturbances. The author's diagnosis of a hypophyseal tumor was confirmed by X-ray examination.

Lhermitte and co-workers (2496) relieved a case of hypersomnia, accompanied by bilateral ptosis, diplopia, polyuria, and sexual impotence, by a spinal puncture.

An unusual case of gonado-hypophyseal involvement in hypersomnia was presented by a patient of Lhermitte and Kyriaco (2501) whose history was given in detail by the latter (2312). The patient, a woman forty-six years old, had attacks of hypersomnia for three years. She also developed hemiplegia and a unilateral positive Babinski sign, which became bilateral during sleep. Her hypersomnia consisted of an attack of continuous sleep of four days' duration just prior to each menstruation. The hypersomnia was accompanied by a complete rectovesical incontinence, whereas during the normal period, which lasted 24 days, she had good control of her sphincters. The authors concluded that they were dealing with a hypersomnia of organic origin, somehow affecting also the hypophysis.

Markov (2687) studied a case of hypersomnia in a young man who was tall, obese, had infantile genitalia, and almost no secondary sex characters. There was a history of syphilis, and X-ray evidence pointed to a gumma of the hypophysis. The author believed that the hypersomnia was due either to the pressure of a gumma on the hypothalamic region or to a disturbance of hormonal correlations between the hypophysis and neighboring nervous structures. Similar cases were described by Stadler (3776). Davidoff (835), analyzing the symptomatology of one hundred cases of acromegaly, found hypersomnia in forty-two; and Léopold-Lévi (2434) noted somnolence as a symptom of the initial stage of acromegaly, but later the somnolence was replaced by insomnia, presumably when the hypophysis was destroyed. Kraus and Perkins (2267) reported a mild hypersomnia in a patient with a three-year history of unilateral muscular wasting and visceral atrophy. They found that the "hypersomnia that this patient showed has not persisted since the administration of the solution of pituitary." (The solution referred to was probably pituitrin, as it was used to control diabetes insipidus.)

McGovern (2754) noted somnolence to be associated with pituitary cachexia. The hypersomnia was of the paroxysmal type, occurring several times per day during the regular waking hours and sometimes followed by insomnia at night. The somnolence was practically abolished by treatment with anterior pituitary lobe extract, only to return when treatments were discontinued.

Engelbach and McMahon (1089) presented a case of paroxysmal hypersomnia in the daytime, and insomnia at night, in a man thirty-five years old, whose condition was diagnosed as pituitary-thyroid insufficiency. The dyssomnia was relieved by treatment with pituitary and thyroid preparations.

Other papers (891, 1162, 1525) pertain to the association of certain types of somnolence with hypophyseal dysfunction. André-Thomas and co-workers (76), however, found the hypophysis normal in the presence of a large ventricular tumor in a woman who had intermittent attacks of hypersomnia, and Fulton and Bailey (1320) also stated that a lesion at the base of the brain might cause hypersomnia without concomitant hypophyseal involvement. Parhon and Tomorug (3091), in a case of acromegaly and hypersomnia, ascribed the latter not to changes in hypophyseal secretion, but, as was shown by necropsy, to the extension of a tumor into, and destruction of, neighboring brain stem structures.

The hypophysis is also involved in hypersomnias related to the functions of the gonads. Kaplinsky and Schulmann (2077) collected a series of cases of periodic hypersomnia of 8 to 10 days' duration that began at puberty. Lhermitte and Dubois (2492, 2497) reported a bout of hypersomnia in a fourteen-year-old girl beginning in the fourth day of her third menstrual period. The sleep lasted 4 to 5 days; the girl objected to being awakened in the morning but ate voraciously when offered food, especially bread. These hypersomniac crises recurred in connection with menstruation. More striking was a single episode of 112 hours of deep sleep, involving a healthy eleven-and-a-half-year-old girl who woke up the moment she started her first menstrual period and immediately began to catch up with her homework (1985). During the ensuing three and a half years, menstruation was normal, and the hypersomnia did not recur. Several other papers deal with periodic insomnia connected with menstruation (2395, 2497, 2499, 4054), some accompanied by thirst and polyuria (879). A case of hypersomnia with amenorrhea, along with hypoglycemia and thirst (3363) is of interest, because fresh hypophysis therapy abolished the hypersomnia and thirst, but had no effect on the amenorrhea and hypoglycemia. In another woman with hypersomnia coinciding with menstruation, X-rays revealed evidence of a hypophyseal tumor (754).

Into quite a different classification fall the numerous cases of somnolence that are probably psychological in origin. Laudenheimer (2376), considering such hypersomnias as symptoms of depressive states, explained them as responses to the monotony of the environment. In some cases they were a means of avoiding, or escaping from, the difficulties of life. Biologically, Laudenheimer likened these states to a protective reaction which shields the individual from nocuous influences. Physiologically, the somnolence is lengthened and deepened normal sleep.

Willey (4216) offered an example of "sleep as an escape mechanism" in the story of a student who developed marked somnolence, especially when alone, as a result of falling in love with a girl and being too timid to tell her about it. When this personal difficulty was straightened out, the somnolence disappeared. Willey and Rice (4217) reported two additional instances of the "psychic utility of sleep." One was of a boy who would fall asleep every time he felt guilty of some infraction of the rules of conduct. The other pertained to a man who could get along on much less sleep when his wife was away than when she was at home. His "desire for sleep while his wife was with him resulted from the monotony and routine of an unadventurous marriage." The authors enlarged upon "sleep as an escape mechanism" from boredom.

Bakhtiarov (185) cited two cases of women who developed sleep attacks, resembling narcolepsy, as a means of escaping from an unpleasant situation created by domestic difficulties. One of the patients frequently fell "asleep" while sitting at the table but heard and remembered what was going on around her. She even answered questions, although often incorrectly. Removal of the unpleasantness led to a cessation of the sleep attacks, and new difficulties resulted in a return of the hypersomnia.

Jones (2009) made a detailed study of a girl twenty-two years old who had brief attacks of sleep of only a few minutes' duration and also attacks of prolonged sleep that lasted from 1 to 6 days. The somnolence during the attacks varied from mere drowsiness to deep sleep. In the latter state the corneal reflex was often absent, and it was possible to obtain a positive Babinski sign, which changed to negative on continued stimulation. On awakening she had no idea as to how long she had slept. At such times her vision was dim, and diplopia was present. The onset of the illness coincided with the development of an unhappy domestic situation, and the author concluded that the hypersomnia was due to the patient's desire to escape from reality.

One could cite other reports on psychogenic hypersomnia resulting from marital infelicity (1471, 3037, 3730), job dissatisfaction (3078), conflicts and guilt feelings (956, 3599), or retreat from unpleasantness (858). It is hard to account for a patient's falling asleep during a psychoanalytic session (354), except that he was in a state bordering on psychosis.

As with hypnosis, the question has been asked if it is possible for a hypersomniac to commit crimes when in a state of sleep-ebriety and be amnesic about the criminal act (1897, 2364, 3570). *Schlaftrunkenheitdelikte* have been tried in German military courts (1897) with varying verdicts. Schmidt (3570) gathered fifteen reports of such episodes. Compared to narcolepsy, Roth (3437) considered sleep drunkenness "an independent nosological entity." Carrot and co-workers (646) described several instances of "walking in a semi-waking state" or the "syndrome of Elpenor," named after the youngest companion of Ulysses, who fell asleep while drunk, awakened in the middle of the night, stepped out, walked over a cliff, and fell right into hell. They mentioned the accident of President Paul Deschanel of France, who fell out of a railway-car door on September 22, 1920, and referred to the medico-legal aspects of "pseudo-suicides by defenestration" from sleep drunkenness. A case of suicide in *Schlaftrunkenheit* was reported by Wagner (4099).

The EEGs of three patients with recurrent hypersomnia during menstruation were found to be abnormal by Vesely (4054) but could be changed to normal by hypnosis, suggesting a psychogenic element in what appeared to be an endocrine involvement. Roth and Tuháček (3440, 3445) recorded sleep EEG patterns during the waking state in 63 per cent of the cases classified as organic hypersomnias and in 82 per cent of the functional ones. Kennard (2135) noted a 14-and-6/sec activity in boys, six to sixteen years old, patients in a mental hospital, when they became drowsy during an EEG recording. The incidence of drowsiness under these conditions was about the same in normal controls, but the abnormal EEG activity did not appear. Roth (3442) maintained that "states of lowered vigilance are characterized by EEG rhythms . . . of transition from awakeness to sleep," distinguishing four stages of reduced vigilance; Grunewald (1544) was able to correlate RT for light and sound stimuli with similar four degrees of impaired wakefulness, and RT values were more than doubled for the whole range.

As pathological conditions conducive to hypersomnias, Kyriaco-Roques (2312) listed disseminated sclerosis, meningitis, autointoxication, and hysteria. To these conditions Daniels (821) added diabetes mellitus, obesity, deficient oxygenation, and mental deficiency. Other writers discussed hypersomnias in general (2469, 3203, 3395), some emphasizing the role of the diencephalon (288, 3063) or vegetative regulation (3432, 3442). Earlier, Rowe (3459) summarized the available evidence by listing four locations in the diencephalon that are connected with the sleep-and-wakefulness function: (*a*) the infundibular region, (*b*) the periventricular gray matter, (*c*) the medial portion of the aqueduct, and (*d*) the cephalic portion of the periaqueductal gray. The pathological findings thus appear to be in agreement with the experimental data on the importance of the thalamus, in addition to the periventricular region. Bringing the thalamus into this nexus, as was done by Hechst (1675) and others, serves to bridge the gap between the lower lying structures and the cerebral cortex. The thalamus may thus be the "missing link" between the two systems.

As indicated in the beginning of this chapter, the term coma is sometimes applied to very deep sleep from which it is difficult to awaken the patient. Zanocco and Alvisi (4308), in studying EEG and clinical changes in vigilance in six cases of pineal gland tumor, concluded that in only two did the disorder look like coma. Fau (1142) noted oscillations between semi-vigilance and deep somnolence in a case of cranial trauma. Dechaume and Jouvet (869) worked out a system of grading perceptivity, non-specific reactivity, reaction to painful stimuli, and autonomic reactivity, substituting a quantification of symptoms for the terms "unconsciousness," "hypersomnia," and "coma." Favorable or unfavorable prognosis could be made from grades on the four categories of responsiveness of the patient. Robin and associates (3374) found that the respiratory sensitivity to CO_2 was decreased in hepatic coma, though alkalosis was present. Kety (2148), summarizing the variations of oxygen consumption by the human brain, noted, as previously stated (p. 56), that sleep had little effect, that even in general anesthesia the oxygen consumption was over half the normal value, but in coma it was down to one-fourth (from 3.3 ml to 0.8 ml/100 gm of brain tissue).

French (1277) examined the brains of five patients with brain lesions result- ing in prolonged unconsciousness and concluded that the "disturbance occurred predominantly in the reticular activating system in three cases, in the subcortical radiation in one, and in its cortical terminus in one." He was able to simulate coma in man by electrolytic lesions in the central cephalic portion of the brain stem in monkeys (1284). Brockman (516) and Heid (1679) located the causa- tive lesions in coma either in the thalamus or the thalamus and hypothalamus. Jouvet and co-workers (2050) noted a decrease in the "rhombencephalic phase" of sleep in patients with injury to the pontine reticular formation, while the "telencephalic phase" continued; and, conversely, after injury to neocortex by anoxia or traumatic encephalopathy, the "telencephalic phase" of sleep was abolished, but the "rhombencephalic phase," with its associated phenomena, persisted. Thus, clinical findings confirmed those obtained experimentally in the cat (p. 213).

Dandy (819) abolished consciousness in patients by tying off the left anterior cerebral artery and concluded that the center of consciousness was located in the corpus striatum, but Meyers (2798, 2799) operated on the basal nuclei, one or the other side, without producing a permanent loss of consciousness.

The EEG in coma resulting from myxedema (3008) or that induced by insulin (401, 2686, 3292) showed the appearance of slow waves, 3–5/sec. How- ever, no definite relationship necessarily exists between the degree of coma and the type of EEG changes (2548, 2550, 2712), and even a normal EEG may be recorded in fatal coma (2578). The slow EEG waves seen in coma are per- haps associated with functional (metabolic, circulatory) or structural changes (2550, 2578) rather than absence of consciousness itself.

In general, coma represents a profound depression in the activity of the nervous system, and its concomitants furnish no information applicable to the sleep-wakefulness rhythm.

Chapter 27

Insomnia or Hyposomnia

The term "insomnia," as it is used clinically and in everyday life, refers to a hyposomnia, a lessening of the duration or depth of sleep, or both. Because of this common usage, the word "insomnia" will be employed in this and following chapters when in most cases "hyposomnia" would be a more correct designation of the condition discussed.

There are a great many classifications of insomnia, for no two writers seem to agree on the proper basis for the division or on the terminology of the different groupings. The most frequent basis for the classification is the cause of the insomnia. But there are also divisions according to the time of incidence, the degree or completeness of the insomnia, the age and health condition of the patient, and whether acute or chronic. Because of the variability in the depth and duration of sleep in different individuals, and in the same person from one season to another, there is no good objective criterion for calling a certain deviation from the normal sleep pattern "insomnia." The complaint must come from the hyposomniac himself, unless his behavior is such as to attract the attention of, or cause annoyance to, others. The subjective attitude will vary somewhat with the well-being of the hyposomniac and according to how much value he attaches to getting a certain number of hours of sleep of a "quality" satisfactory to himself. As Kingman (2161) stated, "those who sleep 8 hours and believe that they need 10 consider themselves to be suffering just as much from insomnia as others who cannot get more than 4 or 5 hours of sleep but who would be satisfied with 6 or 7."

There are more books and articles devoted entirely, or mainly, to the discussion of insomnia than to any other trouble connected with sleep (93, 160, 309, 338, 544, 737, 782, 796, 952, 1071, 1107, 1167, 1331, 1415, 1619, 1866, 1867, 1941, 1942, 2011, 2604, 2608, 2693, 2701, 2709, 2793, 2800, 2820, 2825, 2826, 2924, 2946, 3079, 3380, 3409, 3421, 3751, 4105, 4302), but they are too general to comment on. More specific writings pertain to the different types of insomnia, as a basis for a rational therapy of the condition.

Insomnias are divided into exogenous and endogenous, depending on the cause. The former have been connected with occupation and mode of living (324, 3183), faulty habits of hygiene (3848, 4215), or environmental, climatic, and meteorological conditions (55, 1023, 1446, 1447, 2709). The endogenous insomnias are usually divided into two groups, on the basis of whether or not they are caused by, or can be referred to, pathological processes in some organ or system of the body. Some authors speak of primary and secondary insomnias, while others call them essential and symptomatic. Just what primary or essential insomnia may be due to is, of course, unknown, but Hirsch (1783) thought that there might be a hereditary predisposition to insomnia, and Bettòlo (324) considered temperament an accessory factor. The subdivisions of the secondary insomnias are numerous. Mental, psychic, psychogenic, psychobiological, nervous, organic, functional, physical, physiogenic, cerebrospinal, vegetative, toxic, inflammatory, and degenerative have all been used in one or another combination by many authors (324, 744, 1023, 1446, 1447, 1485, 1554, 1700, 1880, 3132, 3848, 4215, 4280, 4283). Some apply the same term to entirely different conditions. Thus, Hutchison (1880) called an insomnia due to worry or anxiety, primary; other writers would call it secondary, albeit psychic or mental, tracing it to a definite cause. Anxiety and fear (1216, 3050, 3451, 4181), certain categories of dreams (1450), sleeping alone (2342), impending psychosis (1867), and actual psychosis (3751) have been found to produce insomnia. A case of "false insomnia" was described by Held and co-authors (1686). The patient insisted that she did not sleep, although she failed to respond to stimuli and showed a typical EEG pattern of deep sleep. There are many anecdotal accounts of this type of "pseudo-insomnia," the person incorrectly maintaining that he could not sleep, when in fact he did.

The mental state of a person with insomnia needs no special description, as everyone, at one time or another, has gone through a "torture" of sleeplessness. Actually, in the absence of overt pain, insomnia need not be terrifying, but may be so, because of what the individual has heard or read about its leading to insanity or having other dire consequences. From observations made on persons undergoing experimental sleep deprivation (Chap. 22), it can be stated with assurance that no immediate untoward developments need be feared from the loss of a night's sleep, whether it be partial or complete. Prolonged, continuous wakefulness, however, even if undergone voluntarily, may cause temporary mental deterioration (3229).

As regards the time of incidence, the insomnias are divided by Roger (3392), Worster-Drought (4280), and others into three types: initial or predormitional, where the onset of sleep is delayed; broken, choppy, intermittent, or lacunary, with one or more periods of wakefulness in the middle of the night; and terminal or postdormitional, where the sleeper wakes up too early and is not able to fall asleep again. The first type is undoubtedly the most common and is usually referred to by a person when he says that he "cannot sleep." The actual time elapsed may not be very long, but it appears to be so to the sufferer. The more he tries to fall asleep, by changing his position, adjusting his pillow and covers, the less likely he is to fall asleep quickly. He usually gets tired in the process of trying to sleep, relaxes his muscles, and in an unguarded moment eventually falls asleep. The second type may be a neurotic habit of waking up in the middle of the night (308, 920), often associated with unpleasant dreams or nightmares. The third type or terminal insomnia is more likely to occur in elderly people who need less night sleep than formerly, but who go to bed at the usual time and expect to sleep as long as younger people do. Most people, it will be recalled (p. 123), wake up spontaneously during the second half of the night but fall asleep again. When one has had "enough" sleep, one wakes up more and more frequently and finds it progressively harder to fall asleep again. When that stage is reached at 4:00 instead of 7:00 A.M., the condition is called "terminal insomnia."

A sense of fatigue usually leads to muscular relaxation and thus helps to induce sleep. But psychic fatigue, a sort of asthenia of certain neurotics, has been found to be associated with an unusual difficulty in falling asleep. Mac-Curdy (2602) gave a description of such a fatigue syndrome: the individual is restless and hyperirritable; at night he may feel exhausted and even sleepy, but the process of going to bed seems to make him tense, with disturbing thoughts interfering with the onset of sleep. Benon (296) reported on a case of asthenia and hyposomnia, of 17 years' duration, in a French peasant who showed no dementia but only a "melancholic depression." Poulin (3237) observed an insomnia of the overworked (*l'insomnie des surmenés*) among energetic or overactive people who sooner or later suffer from exhaustion and complain of not being able to sleep well. In all these cases there is no physical pain, and no special anxiety or worry, to account for the insomnia.

Organic and functional forms of ailments have been found to interfere with sleep (2651, 3073), sometimes hyposomnia alternating with hypersomnia (1133, 3004, 3817), especially where brain lesions are involved.

Poulin (3237) stated that some people could not sleep for a while after an operation, even though they were free from pain. La Cassie (2318) distinguished among types of postoperative insomnia, according to whether the insomnia directly followed the operation or was delayed by several weeks, and whether it was complete or partial.

Hepatic insufficiency was considered to be the cause of insomnia by Arullani (137), as well as by Parturier and Feldstein (3100). The latter stated that about 50 per cent of patients with liver ailments complained of insomnia. They found it hard to fall asleep, woke up at 2:00 A.M., remained awake until 4:00–6:00 A.M., then fell asleep again. Sometimes they were awakened by pain in the region of the gall bladder. Binet (346) reported awakening of patients with cholecystitis at 2:00–3:00 A.M. due to cramps from "an irritation of the abdominal sympathetic."

Insomnia may also be caused by cardiac disease (2746), especially by left ventricular heart failure (2065), sometimes unrecognized as such and inadequately treated (4184). Buscaino and Balbi (593) noted that insomnia was often associated with a high serum-magnesium value.

Service (3660) referred to five tuberculosis patients, each of whom had a different type of insomnia. The higher than normal temperature level of such patients might be partly responsible for their inability to sleep. Dutrey (1011) treated a tuberculous individual with three injections of gold salts. After each injection the patient had a period of insomnia, the last one persisting for three months. Dutrey ascribed the insomnia to the action of the gold salts on the infundibulo-hypophyseal region.

Vignes (4060) attributed the insomnia of pregnancy to nervous preoccupation and to hyperthyroidism. Wong (4271) described periods of insomnia in the same woman in two successive pregnancies. In her first pregnancy the insomnia set in during the fifth month; in her second, in the second month. The woman could not sleep more than two hours, even when she took hypnotics. Each pregnancy came to a normal termination, and with the latter the insomnia was abolished.

Kahn (2061) mentioned eyestrain as a frequent cause of neurosis with a concomitant insomnia. According to him, 50 per cent of all persons with eyestrain also have some sleep abnormality. Of 219 patients who complained of insomnia and nightmares, which seemed to be connected with eyestrain, 187 obtained relief when they were fitted with glasses. Keschner (2147) also referred to eye symptoms as accompanying insomnia. A patient of De Rivas Cherif (3364) could not fall asleep after reading but was able to sleep when he did not read. When he was fitted with corrective glasses, his insomnia disappeared.

Roger (3392) gave a systematic and exhaustive account of various other conditions that might lead to insomnia. Among the vegetative or visceral disorders, he listed digestive (dyspepsias), cardiac, hypertension, respiratory, and urinary. Autointoxicative conditions comprised uremia, diabetes, hyperthyroidism, and fatigue (from overactivity, muscular or cerebral). Intoxications included alcoholism (delirium tremens), caffeine, drugs (digitalis, belladonna), and abstention of drug addicts. Under infections, Roger listed grip, typhoid fever, tetanus, intermittent fevers, and tuberculosis. To the cerebrospinal conditions belonged pain from any peripheral source, encephalitic and other lesions in the CNS, neurosyphilis, cerebral arteriosclerosis, convulsions, and other motor disturbances.

Special attention has been given to insomnia in the very young and the very old. Although young infants sleep more than half the time, Debré and

Doumic, in their monograph (866), listed several causes of insomnia in infants under three months of age, connected with errors in handling them, rigidity of feeding schedules, and discontinuance of night feeding. In somewhat older infants insomnia may be caused by colic, infections, teething, and poor training habits (1527). In children from nine months to three years of age, motor hyperactivity and psychic excitation were causative agents (866); in older children, bad sleep routine, overtiredness, fear of the dark, and digestive disturbances (1464). In northern Norway children have difficulty in falling asleep during the winter season of darkness (928). Among suggested methods of therapy, good hygiene (63, 1554), habit training (3772), occasional judicious uses of tranquilizers (2) or hypnotics (63, 866, 3400) have been mentioned. Further, Hartmann (1655) emphasized the value of assuring clear air passages in treating insomnia in children. Some children wake up because they experience difficulty in breathing, and tonsillectomy and adenotomy have been known to improve their sleep. Brown (533) also dealt with difficulty in breathing as a cause of insomnia, but he often found it to be due, in both infants and older children, to an enlarged thymus. In six such cases he treated the thymic region with X-rays and brought relief from insomnia, presumably through easier breathing.

At the other end of the age scale, insomnia is a common complaint among the elderly, particularly retired persons with little to do, who receive no attention from others, and spend a large part of their "waking" hours in dozing (1456). Different writers pointed out the advantages of one over another hypnotic drug in the treatment of insomnia in the aged (218, 1026, 2721, 3153). By the use of the "double-blind" technique Pepino and Bare (3153) established that placebos had about as frequent a hangover effect (headache, nausea) as barbiturates, but chloral hydrate caused much less of a hangover than either placebos or barbiturates (218).

The use of hypnotics is advocated most frequently for the treatment of insomnia in young and middle-aged adults (269, 827, 1778, 1886, 2261, 2657, 2709, 2800, 3285, 3848), with hydrotherapy a close second (269, 957, 2657, 2938, 3542, 3940). Hypnosis (957, 2657, 2916, 3073) and suggestion (269, 1168), as well as psychotherapy (2820, 2964, 3073), physical (948) and hygienic (2709, 3542) measures, diet (231, 2824), vitamins (458, 593, 2083, 3744), tranquilizers (1778), and a variety of fanciful methods (1309, 1359, 1521, 3307, 3764, 3939, 4178) have also been used with success, according to their proponents.

In addition to unmixed hyposomnias, there are many reports in the literature on alternate hypo- and hypersomnias, shifted or inverted sleep rhythm, and other abnormalities. In the discussion of encephalitis it was mentioned that the disease, frequently ushered in by a period of restlessness and insomnia, was followed by a shift in the sleep-wakefulness rhythm.

Urechia and Mihalescu (4026) described the case of a girl nine years old with a three-year history of chorea, with insomnia and inversion of the sleep-wakefulness rhythm. Roger and co-authors (3393) had a young patient with spasms of the inferior oculomotor muscles. This patient had hypersomnia following a period of hyposomnia. The combination of sleep disturbances with oculogyric symptoms has been already touched upon (Chap. 23). Roger and Vaissade (3396) reported on another patient, a boy of fifteen, who had ocular paralysis and showed an inverted sleep-wakefulness rhythm.

Here, too, one could go on giving example after example from the clinical literature to show that insomnia, hyposomnia, and dyssomnia accompany a great variety of ailments. In some cases the connection is apparent; in others, obscure. Because of the frequent presence of hysterical, neurotic, or psychotic factors, as well as of external influences, the etiology of the insomnia may remain unrecognized.

Just as in experimental deprivation of sleep the subject can be kept awake only by continued exteroceptive or proprioceptive stimulation, so probably in spontaneously occurring insomnia exteroceptive, proprioceptive, and interoceptive stimulations playing on the nervous system serve to maintain the waking state, in spite of—perhaps because of—the person's efforts to fall asleep. Therein probably lies the chief contribution of secondary, or symptomatic, insomnia to the understanding of the normal operation of the sleep-wakefulness cycle.

Chapter 28

Sleep Abnormalities and Disturbances

There are a number of miscellaneous sleep abnormalities and disturbances which do not readily lend themselves to classification. Some of these also appear from time to time in apparently normal individuals, especially children, whereas others are definitely associated with pathological states, particularly neurotic and psychopathic. To this miscellaneous group of dyssomnias, or, as Roger (3392) called them, parasomnias, belong nightmares, night terrors, somniloquy, somnambulism, grinding of teeth and jactitations, enuresis, numbness and hypnalgia, and personality dissociations. The terms "oniric" and "oneirogenic" have been applied to these phenomena in order to indicate their close connection with dreaming or other cortical activity during sleep.

The commonest and most innocuous of the parasomnias are the nightmares, defined by Hadfield (1571) as "anxiety dreams of such intensity that they completely overwhelm the personality; that they give rise to exaggerated bodily sensations, of palpitation, sweating and suffocation . . . and fill us with such horror that we wake up in dread."

There is no sharp line of demarcation between the nightmare and the terrifying dream. Although it occurs in normal persons, the nightmare is often described as a companion symptom to hallucinations, somnambulism, and a variety of abnormal mental states. It is commonly agreed to be due to digestive, and occasionally to circulatory, disturbances. Distention of the stomach by food or by gases and the pressure against neighboring structures that follows such a distention are thought to be the source of afferent impulses that are sometimes interpreted by the dreamer as due to a giant pressing on his chest. The pattern of the nightmare shows considerable variations, but the terrifying factor is the distinguishing component.

Kourétas and Scouras (2255) emphasized the report of a complete absence of muscular tonus during nightmares in one of their patients, while Dereux (919) described a case of apparently symptomatic narcolepsy in which the night sleep was disturbed by nightmares, accompanied by muscular rigidity.

There is possibly no general rule for the condition of the musculature during a nightmare, and essentially different parasomnias may be put into this common classification. Hallucinations on awakening are often indistinguishable from nightmares.

In the elderly, nightmares may be associated with circulatory changes (106): "A sudden spasm of a blood vessel . . . can result in a brief pain that is interpreted by patient with a dream response." Moore (2877) suggested a simple psychotherapy for nightmares: have patient tell and retell content of dream, and associations brought out in retelling entail less and less "affect."

The night terror, or *pavor nocturnus,* unlike the nightmare, is a disturbance more peculiar to children, mostly between the ages of three and eight years, only rarely extending beyond puberty. Roger (3392) described a typical attack: "Suddenly, while fully asleep, after a short period of agitation and one or two groans, the child sits up in his bed, eyes wide-open and facial expression one of terror. Pale, covered with perspiration, he extends his trembling arms, as if to protect himself against an approaching enemy." The imaginary enemy may be the devil, a fairy-tale character, or a wild beast. The crisis rarely lasts longer than half an hour. The child may be awakened and consoled by his parents, or he may go back to sleep without completely awakening. In the morning the child does not remember the occurrences of the preceding night.

The night terror differs from the nightmare, as listed by Kanner (2073), in five respects: (*a*) the night terror is usually not followed by awakening; (*b*) the child does not recall the incident; (*c*) it is accompanied by profuse perspiration; (*d*) it lasts much longer; and (*e*) it does not occur in adults. Roger (3392) mentioned the common causes of night terrors as digestive disturbances, infectious diseases, intestinal parasites, lesions of the CNS, and, chiefly, a constitutional or hereditary predisposition (psychomotor instability, nervous temperament, alcoholic or syphilitic parents). The prognosis, however, is nearly always favorable.

Stern (3814) ascribed *pavor nocturnus* in general, and Sperling (3763), at least one type of this syndrome, to sexual trauma. Maria (2676), on the basis of the EEGs of seven patients with *pavor nocturnus,* concluded that it was an epileptic manifestation of the psychomotor type.

Talking during sleep, or somniloquy, can hardly be called an abnormality except when it is associated with other parasomnias. Walsh (4107) reported somniloquy in 8 out of 100 mental defectives, aged 6 to 40 years; and Clardy and Hill (711), in one-half of sleep difficulties among institutionalized disturbed children and delinquent boys. Cameron (613) studied sleep behavior of enlisted men during World War II, under conditions of very high temperature and humidity, hard work, poor food, and little recreation. The sleep talk he heard "was virtually normal in volume, enunciation, and general flow of content," and one has to ask if the bored men did not talk to themselves while lying awake. Indeed, it is questionable whether any groans, mumblings, or even articulate speech do not involve an interruption of sleep. By the use of the REM-EEG method, Kamiya (2069) and Rechtschaffen and collaborators (3286) determined that sleep talking was done largely during non-REM periods and in EEG stages 2, 3, and 4, and was usually accompanied by body movements. When it occurred during dreaming (3286), somniloquy "was appropriate to recalled dream in one instance when such a report was available," and there was little or no movement-artifact in the EEG record. Vocalization in non-REM conditions entailed a sudden drop in ESR, suggesting that the subject was no longer asleep.

A potentially dangerous sleep disturbance is somnambulism, or sleepwalking, with an incidence of 1 to 6 per cent, depending on whether the survey applied to the general public (838), hospital patients (3077), or was limited to children with sleep abnormalities (108, 3684). The occurrence of somnambulism in 3 per cent of narcoleptics studied by Ganado (1349) is close to its incidence in 2 out of 60 non-enuretics—as contrasted to 16 out of 60 enuretics (27 per cent)—reported by Pierce and associates (3188). That the condition may be due to some constitutional or hereditary factors was pointed out by Clerici (720) and confirmed by others (67, 838, 3187). Clerici, referring to a family of six (husband, his cousin-wife, and their four children), all afflicted with somnambulism, related one episode as follows: "One night the entire family arose about three in the morning, gathered in the servants' hall around the tea table; one of the children in moving about upset a chair. Only then did they awaken." Clerici further reported that in many cases, on the assumption that sleepwalkers are particularly sensitive to cold, pans filled with cold water were placed around their beds. It was expected that the patients would step into the water and thus awaken, but some of them soon learned to avoid the pans on getting out of bed. He also found that some persons would start their somnambulism activities at exactly the same time every night, which he interpreted as evidence of the persistence of mental activity and time sense during sleep.

All writers on the topic confirm Carpenter's statement (644) that there is an amnesia for the events transpiring during a somnambulistic episode, but there is no agreement as to the state of the sleepwalker. Clerici, as indicated, spoke of the family being "awakened." Roger (3392) gave a good description of a typical sleepwalker. The sleeper performs various acts with a certain degree of dexterity and can avoid obstacles. But his behavior is characterized by a rigidity, which gives him the appearance of an automaton. He can answer questions correctly and is quite receptive to suggestions. He obediently carries out rather bizarre orders and tends to preserve attitudes passively imposed on him, exhibiting cataleptic properties. At the end of 15 to 30 minutes of activity, he goes back to bed, sometimes fully clothed, and wakes up next morning, quite surprised to find himself dressed. He can carry out dangerous tasks, like walking along the edge of a roof, which he would be afraid to do when awake.

Seashore (3639) described the case of "a college student who formed the habit of getting up in his sleep, dressing, walking down to the river three-fourths of a mile distant, undressing, taking a deliberate and enjoyable swim, dressing, walking back to his room, undressing and retiring, only to wake up in the morning without the slightest inkling of remembrance from the escapade of the night." However, when he was awakened during his sleep-walking on one occasion, he recalled exactly what he had been doing.

Laughlin (2379) reported the case of a man who walked along the ledge of windows at the height of 12 stories and returned to bed without waking. Mayon-White (2726) noted that while, in appearance, the sleepwalker seemed to be almost awake—eyes open, pupils moderately dilated but reactive to light, movements slow and purposeful, seemingly under voluntary control—he could usually be led back to bed without being awakened. Unlike Roger (3392), Mayon-White stated that the somnambulist would not answer questions, al-though his hearing was not impaired. Pai (3077), after a study of 117 cases, concluded that "post-epileptic automatism is the only condition in which the patients may be said to be asleep. In all other cases of sleepwalking the persons are awake, although the extent and degree of awareness may vary with each patient." Thus, as in the case of somniloquy, somnambulism takes place dur-ing the night's sleep, but the individual may be asleep, half-asleep, or awake at the time.

Pierce and Lipcon (3187) noted a greater frequency of EEG abnormalities among somnambulists than in normal controls. André-Balisaux and Gonsette (67) divided one hundred sleepwalkers into three categories, based on fre-quency of occurrence and personal and family history; their EEGs varied from completely normal to markedly abnormal, depending upon the severity of the condition.

Somnambulism has been found associated with epilepsy (3018, 3659), post-encephalitic parkinsonism (3003), imminence of psychosis (1931), enuresis (3188), hypoglycemia (4319), a variety of neuroses and psychoneuroses (46, 1495, 3186, 3516, 3916), antisocial acts (949), and dissociation of personality (46, 2890). Roger (3392) held that the somnambulist was dreaming, but, in-stead of seeing or hearing the events, acted them out. Seashore (3639) also re-ferred to somnambulism as "dream action." As to the motor excitement that can break through the sleep deefferentation and lead to overt and co-ordinated locomotion, its cause is unknown. Psychologically, according to Pierce and Lipcon (3186), "sleepwalking episodes represent an attempt to solve problems through safe channels," and Teplitz (3916) looked upon the patterned motility of somnambulism "as a partial defense against sleep itself," because to the patient "sleep itself was frightening because it was associated with loss of voluntary muscular control generally, or with death or loss of identity." Earlier, De Morsier (2890) compared somnambulism with dual personality, secondary or twilight states, automatism, and other conditions involving transitory amnesia. These amnesias are due not to lesions but to temporary and reversible blocking of the pathways used in mnesic acquisitiveness. In somnambulism the blocking can be destroyed by waking the subject. This concept brings somnambulism into the realm of the psychically abnormal.

Bed-wetting, or enuresis, though it is sometimes associated with somnambulism (3188), is a much commoner sleep disturbance, occurring in 5 to 15 per cent of children (371, 1848). The incidence drops off with age (379) but sometimes persists or even develops in adults, as revealed in studies of military service personnel (1009, 2280, 3188). Normal children do not involuntarily urinate during sleep after the age of three or four years. Enuresis is more common among boys than among girls, and more siblings of enuretics wet their beds than do those of "dry" children (379, 3188, 3862). Also, enuresis is more frequent in twins than among singly-born individuals, and in girls with a male twin partner than in girls with a female partner, with no such difference seen among boys (1613). Michaels and Goodman (2802) noted not only a greater incidence of enuresis among males, but also in those with psychopathic personality, behavior problems, or mental deficiency, ranging from 16 per cent for normals to 86 per cent in extreme abnormality. Similar findings were made by others (711, 3935) among inmates of a school for mental defectives. Pierce and associates (3189) found enuretics to be small in stature, with a "Peter Pan" complex—refusing to "grow up" and to accept responsibilities. Andreev (71), by actography, determined that enuretic children moved less during sleep than did normals. Ström-Olsen (3852) reported very deep sleep in adult enuretics.

The EEGs of the majority of enuretics are likely to be abnormal (1560, 3187, 3758), bordering on the epileptogenic (1009, 3862, 3994), with the depth of sleep in EEG terms showing a wide variation during the act of bed-wetting (376, 943). By the use of the REM-EEG method, Pierce and associates (3190), on the basis of 17 enuretic episodes in 8 young boys, were able to establish that during enuresis the EEG consisted of delta waves and that at no time did dreaming precede bed-wetting. Furthermore, "the time of the first wetting coincides with the usual time for the first nightly dream" and thus appears to be "a dream substitute or equivalent."

Psychotherapy has been used successfully in the military service (2280), and long-lasting relief of symptoms in a thirteen-year-old boy with simultaneous enuresis and encopresis was achieved by psychoanalyzing his mother (2301). Good results were also reported by the use of hypnosis (666, 4200) and tranquilizers (2353, 2737), as well as by the development of a conditioned reflex through the ringing of a bell when the bedding was wetted (836, 1397, 2909, 3649, 4201).

Vulliamy (4091) established that there was no significant difference between the volumes of urine passed at night by enuretic and normal children, and thus nocturnal polyuria could not be a contributory cause. Most enuretics have a history of anxiety and fears (1398, 2909); or of rejection by, and hostility toward, parents (711, 2909); or of repressed sexuality, of which enuresis becomes a substitute form of gratification (2909). Other speculations concerning the etiology of enuresis involve a possible immaturity of the nervous system (1560) and "exterior gestation" (423).

Among other motor abnormalities during sleep is the *jactatio capitis nocturna,* or banging of the head, usually appearing in the fourth to the twelfth month (87, 102, 321, 775, 3537) and lasting till adolescence (86, 795), or even into adulthood (97, 2702). Occasionally, the body is also involved, producing a rolling or rocking movement (3, 100). The subjects are often unaware of any anomaly, as their sleep is otherwise quite normal. Children usually outgrow the habit, but, while it lasts, it may be more disturbing to others than to themselves. A somewhat different case of a girl, aged eighteen, who for fourteen years sucked and chewed her bed covers in her sleep was reported by Costa (763). The habit was abolished by hypnosis therapy.

Along with other parasomnias, Strauch (3845) listed hypnalgias, or pains occurring only during sleep, and Critchley (784) mentioned the intensification of neuralgias at the onset of sleep. Sometimes there is only numbness, experienced when one awakens during the night. This applies particularly to the hands and forearms (94, 1050) and may be a mild form of *acroparaesthesia* or *brachialgia paraesthetica nocturna.* More common in women than in men and appearing usually between the ages of forty and fifty (2278, 4030, 4242), the sensation may vary from painful tingling to burning and can be abolished by hanging the arm out of bed or rubbing the hand. There are no objective neurological or orthopedic signs (4030, 4123); the course of the condition is benign and self-limited, but when the pain is disabling, relief may be obtained by drugs (3600), injections into the stellate ganglion (2437), or cutting the transverse carpal ligament (1050, 2278) or scalenus anticus muscle (2437), depending on the location of the pain.

Aside from numbness, vascular spasms, and muscular cramps (1481), all of which increase with advancing age, the need of getting up repeatedly for micturition is a prominent cause of sleep disturbance in the elderly person (768). Otherwise, statistically, sleep disturbances and age are not correlated (1452) after adulthood is reached. At the other end of the age scale, sleep disturbances are very common between the ages of 2 and 5 (3684), or 3 and 5 (3761, 3762), during the "oedipal phase" of development. Among the disturbances discussed earlier, about two-thirds of the night terrors, nightmares, and sleepwalking occur at the ages of 4–7, 8–11, and 12–16, respectively (108, 187). Some EEG abnormalities have been found in children under 3 (367), but they were not of any diagnostic significance. Among the causes of sleep disturbances in children have been listed neurotic (2726, 4077) and emotional (559, 1187, 1501) factors, and a failure to adjust to the family routine. Vegetative lability has also been invoked (4287). As therapy, hygienic measures and sedatives (325) and love and understanding, firmness and patience (1898) have been suggested.

There is a profusion of publications dealing with neurotic disturbances of sleep (308, 920, 1153, 2581, 2615, 3050, 3347, 4237), or with sleep disturbances in general (418, 850, 2313, 2493, 2624, 2625, 2820, 3079, 3557, 3829, 3843, 4020, 4219), as well as therapy of these conditions (1104, 1802, 1807, 2926, 3629, 4078), including psychotherapy (3607, 4081, 4171), but not much that is new on the sleep of neurotics and psychotics. Among earlier authors, Epstein (1092) observed that neurotic patients fell asleep, and later went into a cataleptic state, whenever he tested them for the Aschner phenomenon (a slowing of the pulse produced by pressure on the eyeball). This sleep effect was not obtained with normal persons. Epstein considered this peculiar onset of sleep a part of a "hypnopathic syndrome." It will be recalled that Stockert (3823, 3824) was able to induce a loss of consciousness, catalepsy, and sleep in patients with acute encephalitis merely by having them fixate an object with their eyes, or close their eyes (p. 244). Birkner and Trautmann (356) reported that X-rays directed at the diencephalon affected sleep, among other functions, and suggested the use of such irradiation for therapy of sleep disorders.

Hypersomnia (1944, 1945) and hyposomnia (675) have been connected with delusions of psychotics. Courbon (764) made an extensive study of the sleep of the insane. He found hyposomnia to be the rule rather than the exception in mental patients. The hyposomnia is dysphoric in patients with anxiety neuroses, dipsomania, melancholia, psychasthenia, confusion, persecutory delusions, and hypochondria; it is euphoric in manics, who sometimes have complete insomnia; it has no effect on dementia. Hypersomnia, when present, is dysphoric in patients with brain tumors, organic dementias, epilepsy, and encephalitis. Euphoric hypersomnia is an unfavorable prognostic sign. Hypnophobia is present in psychasthenic patients, and hypnomania in those seeking an "escape."

Ladame (2319), in a statistical study of the sleep of 210 inmates of an insane asylum over a period of 18 months, found that in epileptics, idiots, and imbeciles sleep was of rather long duration. Manic-depressives' sleep was not only short but broken. Women slept more soundly, but about 30 minutes less, than men. In the interval between periods of several nights of disturbed sleep, day sleep was likely to set in. There was a "personal coefficient" of sleep made up of characteristic values of the several variables peculiar to a certain patient.

Sleep irregularities might prognosticate approaching disturbances, as, for instance, manic periods.

Muncie (2947) noted that continuity and duration of sleep in the psychopathic were influenced by mood fixations, content (toxic), support (tonic metabolic), organic (structural defect), and personality disorders. Content disorders led to difficulty in falling asleep; depression, to early awakening. Richter (3341) reported regular cyclic fluctuation in the sleep characteristics of three psychotic patients at intervals of 4 to 6 days.

The sleep motility of psychopathic patients was studied by Forbes (1238) and by Page (3075). The motility of eight non-catatonic schizophrenics was quite comparable to that of normal individuals, as noted by Forbes. Page compared the motility of five normal persons, previously described (pp. 78, 86, 149), with that of three abnormal groups: (*a*) four catatonic schizophrenics, bedridden, mute, force-fed; (*b*) five manic-depressives, showing "typical maniacal behavior—overactive, overtalkative and at times destructive"; and (*c*) five postencephalitic parkinsonians, with tremors, muscular rigidity, and a stumbling gait. "Day" motility recorded from 8:00 to 11:00 A.M. was about the same in the parkinsonians as in the normal persons; it was much smaller in the catatonics; and greater in the manic patients. The delay in going to sleep at night and sleep motility showed about the same relationship in the four groups as did daytime motility. For instance, the length of the "pre-sleep" periods in the catatonic patients was, on the average, 6 minutes; in the parkinsonians, 20 minutes; in the normal subjects, 23 minutes; and in the manic patients, 80 minutes. The parkinsonians, who showed about the same degree of motility as the normal subjects in the daytime while staying in bed, moved less than the normal persons during the night sleep. All subjects and patients but the catatonics moved more during the successive thirds of the night, thus following the normal sleep pattern; the motility of the catatonics was not only very low but also uniform throughout the night.

Our work was done on patients in the Division of Psychiatry of the University of Chicago Clinics, where two beds were equipped with our devices for recording motility in terms of time spent in movement (p. 83). In addition, the nurses and attendants kept sleep charts on each individual studied by making direct observations at half-hour intervals. Using for analysis of the sleep-motility data only those patients on whom at least ten nights' records were available, we had 408 sleep records for twenty-four patients. Classified according to the type of psychiatric disorders, there were among the patients studied ten psychoneurotics (226 nights), eight schizophrenics (95 nights), and six affective psychotics (87 nights). The motility of these patients showed considerable variation from person to person, as would be true of normal subjects. For the group as a whole it was rather low, averaging around 20 seconds of movement per hour. In each of the three classifications there was greater motility and incidence of awakening in the second half of the night compared to the first. The time taken to fall asleep was shortest for the psychoneurotics (23 minutes), longest for the schizophrenics (45 minutes), and intermediate for the affective psychotics (36 minutes). The tendency for the sleep to be interrupted by awakenings was rather small, but of the three groups was most marked for the schizophrenics. In general, the patients whom we studied differed only slightly from a similar group of normal persons with respect to the time of onset of sleep, the time spent in motility, the frequency of spontaneous interruptions of sleep, and the distribution of motility and awakenings over the two halves of the night's sleep.

According to Deglin (872), the night sleep of schizophrenics in a catatonic stupor was shallow and of short duration. Their EEG patterns were about the same around the clock. Paranoid schizophrenics slept normally and showed typical sleep EEGs. Using the REM-EEG technique, Dement (898), in a study of seventeen schizophrenics, determined that their dreaming incidence did not differ from that in normal controls. A peculiarity of dream content of schizophrenics, occurring in about half their reports, was the presence of "inanimate objects, apparently hanging in space, with no overt action whatsoever." As these "motionless" dreams were accompanied by the usual REMs, it may mean that the REMs need not always represent visual experience.

Concerning mental defectives, there are the older observations of Terman and Hocking (3918) on the duration of sleep of 193 children, aged from 6 to 19 years, who showed no age differences in the duration of sleep, except for a slight increase at the age of 14. In general, they found that low-grade mental defectives of all ages slept less than normal children of the corresponding mental-age level, whereas high-grade defectives slept as much as, or more than, normal children of the same mental age.

Mullin and Titelbaum also made sleep-motility studies of a number of feeble-minded children, subdivided into three groups as follows: 10 children, classified as idiots (mean IQ of 18), a total of 141 nights; 12 imbeciles (mean IQ of 34), 180 nights; and 14 high-grade mental defectives (mean IQ of 58), 210 nights. Here, as in the psychopaths, there was considerable individual variation in motility. Treated by groups, the sleep motility of the idiots was slightly higher during the first half of the night than it was during the second, whereas both the imbeciles and the high-grade mental defectives tended to conform to the normal pattern of greater motility during the second half of the night.

We also studied the sleep motility of a group of seven children residing at a school for the mentally and physically subnormal. Their IQs ranged from 60 upward. Their group sleep-motility curve was quite normal, but individually only five of the seven showed a definite ascending curve of motility.

It would seem that mentally ill patients need not have an abnormal sleep-motility pattern, except under special conditions of muscular hypo- or hyperactivity. Nor is the sleep motility of the mentally subnormal different from the normal—aside from the lowest-grade mental defectives, the idiots, whose motility, like that of catatonic schizophrenics, as shown by Page, follows a fairly even course throughout the night.

With respect to enuresis, the striking finding of Pierce and associates (3190) that it is not a part of a dream episode, but that the first bed-wetting coincides with the time of the first dreaming period, poses more questions than it answers. It is possible that the emptying of the bladder is a component of the basic rest-activity cycle but good sphincter control prevents its manifestation in non-enuretics.

Of the other sleep abnormalities and disturbances discussed in this chapter, the most intriguing, from the standpoint of the nature of sleep and wakefulness, is that of somnambulism. The fundamental point is whether the sleepwalker is asleep or awake. Although the descriptions of the behavior of the sleep-walker by Roger (3392) and Mayon-White (2726) differ in minor particulars, that behavior meets the criteria of wakefulness: the ability to stand and walk, to see and to hear, to avoid obstacles, to find one's way in familiar surroundings. Where it differs from daytime wakefulness of the somnambulist is in poorer critical reactivity, as in failure to recognize the danger of walking along the edge of a roof (which involves projection into the future), and complete amnesia of events, shared with psychomotor epilepsy activity and the greater part of ordinary dreaming. In other words, the wakefulness of sleepwalking is accompanied by a low level of consciousness, certainly lower than in some types of dreaming. Somnambulism occurs during the night's sleep because in that portion of the 24-hour rhythm cortical activity is at its lowest. Dream-like behavior of individuals deprived of sleep for several days manifests itself repeatedly in the early morning hours. The term sleepwalking is a misnomer if used to denote "walking while asleep," rather than walking in the course of an interruption of the night's sleep. All the characteristics of somnambulism underline the difference between wakefulness and consciousness.

Part 6

Means of Influencing Sleep and Wakefulness

Chapter 29

The Pharmacology of Sleep and Wakefulness

Among the chemical substances capable of influencing the sleep-wakefulness rhythm, there are some used in the treatment of hyposomnia, and they are the drugs upon which most of the pharmacological and therapeutic research has been done. Some of these chemical substances, however, influence the cycle in the direction of wakefulness, and they have been used in alleviating hypersomnias, particularly narcolepsy. There are still other substances (calcium and magnesium salts, urethane) which have no therapeutic application but are of value in throwing light on the mechanism of the sleep-wakefulness cycle.

Substances used as drugs to facilitate sleep are referred to as hypnotics, soporifics, or somnifacients. They may be used to hasten the onset of sleep or to increase its depth or duration. The German writers distinguish between *Hypnotica* and *Narcotica,* the latter producing an irresistible deep stupor rather than a facilitation of sleep. Another distinction is made between hypnotics and substances (volatile and non-volatile) commonly used to produce surgical anesthesia. The distinctions apply mainly to usage, as most hypnotic drugs, when taken in large enough quantities, produce narcosis or anesthesia.

Opiates are among the oldest hypnotic drugs, but their use for that purpose alone has been largely discontinued. Chloral hydrate, introduced by Liebreich in 1869, is still in use, as are a number of other aldehydes: paraldehyde, bromal, chloralose, and hypnal. The ethyl-sulphones came in as hypnotics in 1888, and the finding that their action seemed to be related to the number of ethyl radicals they contained had been applied in preparing urea derivatives, to which the majority of the various hypnotics belong. Urea itself has no hypnotic properties, but some of its salts have; among the latter are the bromine-containing carbromal (adalin, nyctal) and bromural, as well as the bromine-free sedormid. Ethyl carbamate, or urethane, is not used as a hypnotic drug, but its derivatives, hedonal and neodorm (containing Br), are. By far the largest groups of urea derivatives are the barbiturates, or barbituric acid compounds. Barbituric acid itself, diethylbarbituric acid or diethylmalonylurea (veronal, barbitone, barbital), was prepared by Emil Fischer in 1903 and became the parent substance of such well-known hypnotics as dial, luminal (phenobarbital), phanodorm, somnifen, soneryl, nembutal, amytal, evipal, allonal, and the bromide-containing homologues, pernocton and noctal. Practically every pharmaceutical firm owns, markets, and extols the virtues of one or another barbituric acid derivative.

Renner (3317) classified hypnotics as (*a*) drugs that lead to a quick onset of sleep, their action of short duration and rather mild, leaving no detectable after-effect (bromural, adalin, diogenal, aponal, alendrin, voluntal); (*b*) drugs with the same properties as those of *a,* but with an action of medium duration and intensity (paraldehyde, amylene hydrate, acetal, methylal, hypnon, urethane, and hedonal); and (*c*) drugs that act slowly, are of medium duration and intensity, but have a definite after-effect (chloral hydrate, chloralamide, and other chlorals, sulphonal, trional, tetronal, veronal, luminal, nirvanol, somnifen). Intermediate between *b* and *c* are neuronal, dormial, isopral, dial, curral, and proponal. There are many books and articles devoted largely to the therapeutics of insomnia (30, 124, 158, 174, 204, 285, 322, 324, 340, 411, 434, 579, 608, 612, 733, 744, 765, 778, 780, 787, 804, 915, 940, 963, 994, 1008, 1023, 1028, 1114, 1137, 1174, 1270, 1276, 1300, 1399, 1447, 1464, 1470, 1483–85, 1487, 1496, 1499, 1530, 1534, 1540, 1562, 1563, 1577, 1616, 1619, 1662, 1663, 1700, 1783, 1793, 1831, 1833, 1871, 1880, 2226, 2377, 2394, 2601, 2674, 2701, 2715, 2803, 2856, 3025, 3042, 3074, 3100, 3132, 3156, 3177, 3197, 3199, 3251, 3265, 3284, 3310, 3317, 3331, 3348, 3372, 3380, 3400, 3401, 3467, 3477, 3478, 3480, 3487, 3521, 3586, 3589, 3602, 3604, 3630, 3651, 3749, 3966, 4002, 4032, 4078, 4125, 4140, 4147, 4169, 4215, 4236, 4283, 4284, 4316).

The question whether a purely hypnotic effect can be produced by a drug appears to have been answered by Hondelink (1828, 1829), at least, for the experimental animal he was testing, the finch. Using a specially constructed cage, he obtained separate graphic records of the motility of the finch when the bird was on the perch or on the floor of the cage. During sleep the finch remains perched, but in the state of narcosis it lies on the floor of the cage. By determining the minimal sleep- and narcosis-producing doses of a certain drug, Hondelink was able to establish the degree of spread between the two. The greater the ratio of the narcotic dose to the hypnotic one, the more satisfactory was the drug as a hypnotic. By this test, urethane was the least satisfactory drug, and somnifen and barbital-sodium not much better. Chloralose was good, but best of all was somnacetin—a mixture of barbital-sodium, phenacetin, and codeine. Renner (3317) stated that "most hypnotics do not produce sleep in the daytime when given in doses that are effective at night." The importance of being sleepy, or physiologically ready for sleep, in the enhancement of the effect of a certain hypnotic was also demonstrated by Hondelink, when he exposed the finches to continuous weak light. Like most birds, finches are decidedly monocyclic, but under continuous illumination they become polycyclic, with continual activity interrupted by short periods of sleep. Under these special conditions much smaller doses of the hypnotics produced sleep, but the narcotic doses remained practically unchanged—another proof of the essential difference between facilitating the onset of sleep and eliciting a stuporous condition.

Dost (964, 965), using Hondelink's method, studied the action of hypnotics and "vegetative poisons." Apomorphine, pictrotoxin, ergotamine, physostigmine, and betatetra-hydronaphthylamine were found to produce sleep in birds when injected intramuscularly. Ephetonine and atropine, when given in large doses, also produced sleep. Regelsberger (3294, 3297), by the method of continuously and automatically recording the CO_2 content of alveolar air (p. 110), observed the effects produced by various influences and suggested that this method was also applicable to the objective estimation of the action of hypnotic drugs. For instance, he found that scopolamine changed the depth-of-sleep curve, as regards both the general level and the occurrence of the peak or peaks, in a patient with a pallidal syndrome. Other methods of evaluating the action of hypnotics have been used by several investigators (690, 2442, 3587, 3667, 3668).

A classification of hypnotic drugs according to the site of their alleged action was made by Molitor and Pick (2860), who showed that different hypnotics act on different parts of the nervous system. In general, bromides, alcohol, and aldehydes influenced the cortex, while the urea derivatives affected the subcortical centers. Decortication abolished the action of some hypnotics while enhancing the action of others. Experiments were made to test the classification of Molitor and Pick (2119, 2120, 2172, 3163, 3340, 3802, 4289), with many investigators in favor of it (526, 935, 1034, 1276, 3151, 3177, 3322, 3403, 3493) and others against (992, 1450, 2235, 2236, 3042, 3563, 4206). The matter is now of historical interest only.

Various hypnotic agents were tested for their effect on the onset of sleep and motility during sleep. Gerber and Rembold (1401) employed a motility-recording device and found bromural to increase the ability to fall asleep in nervous and neurasthenic patients. After large doses, the sleep induced was of long duration and very quiet. Page (3075), in the study referred to in the preceding chapter (p. 287), also observed the effect of therapeutic doses of amytal on sleep motility in four groups of patients. The motility of catatonics was actually increased by amytal (10 per cent), but the drug caused a decrease in motility in normal individuals (14 per cent), in parkinsonians (16 per cent), and in manics (35 per cent), the quieting effect in the latter manifesting itself especially in the first third of the night.

Some of the psychiatric patients whose motility we studied (p. 287) were given hypnotic drugs (luminal, amytal, and bromides) as a part of their treatment. On seventeen patients we obtained 318 control-night records, and 273 postmedication records, of motility during sleep. In all patients the time of on-set of sleep was reduced by the hypnotics (17 per cent for schizophrenics, 33 per cent for others); the motility was smaller, and the awakenings fewer, for each of the two halves of the night. Data we (2200) published on the effects of two barbiturates, amytal (100 mg) and evipal (260 mg), on a number of sleep variables in twenty-one normal individuals showed that both drugs de-creased motility, but not significantly. On the other hand, evipal increased the ease of going to sleep, while amytal, but not evipal, significantly lengthened the duration of sleep (by over 30 minutes), the only two of the different ex-perimental conditions to have such effects. Maliniak (2640), with herself as subject, found that therapeutic doses of opium decreased motility during sleep (from 4.8 to 3.9 movements/hour) without a change in the general shape of the motility curve.

Early EEG studies were made by Bremer (473), who established that the EEG pattern of the cat, produced by the action of barbiturates, did not differ from the pattern characteristic of normal deep sleep, whereas the EEG changes resulting from ether anesthesia did not resemble those of sleep. During the two types of narcosis there was also a disparity in the response pattern to sound (476, 477) and to saphenous nerve stimulation (1684). Derbyshire and asso-ciates (917) studied the effects of three drugs on the EEG of the cat: ether, avertin (tribromethanol), and pentobarbital sodium. Under light and mod-erate avertin and pentobarbital anesthesia, the EEG differed little from those found in the unanesthetized animal, but under deep anesthesia the EEG changes became infrequent. Under ether anesthesia, there was a marked change in the basal EEG pattern, with the appearance of small, rapid waves which did not change in frequency but were further decreased in amplitude as the ether anes-thesia became deeper. The authors concluded that avertin and pentobarbital "suppress activity in the cortex without blocking the sensory paths leading to it, whereas ether blocks these paths before cortical activity is wholly suspended." Adrian (24) also saw a resemblance between the cortical potential changes occurring in sleep and those produced by the barbiturate, dial, in the monkey. Gibbs and co-workers (1428) have found that, in general, in man sedatives and hypnotics produce EEG changes that are comparable to sleep-EEG changes. The same authors (1429), having observed a certain EEG pattern in epileptics only during sleep, were able to duplicate it during the waking state by the injection of phenobarbital.

Many papers were published on different EEG patterns and the site of their appearance in connection with the depth of sleep or anesthesia produced by one or another drug (273, 464, 468, 668, 714, 736, 816, 991, 1322, 1431, 1705, 1967, 3109, 3556, 3595, 3681, 3688, 3887, 3888, 4229) or on the use of hypnotic agents for obtaining EEGs for diagnostic purposes (1326, 1424, 1799, 2461, 3992). Fischgold and co-workers (1185, 3620) noted a dissociation between behavior and EEG pattern in some patients who were given about 300 mg of nembutal. With objective and EEG signs of sleep there was a preserved ability to communicate with the experimenter or a denial of having slept.

Soskin and Taubenhaus (3753) reported that sodium succinate was a safe and effective antidote against toxic doses of nembutal. The experiment has been repeated on man and animals, using a variety of barbiturates, and the analeptic properties of sodium succinate confirmed (230, 609, 3205), refuted (762, 2369, 3538), or left in doubt (327, 865, 1169, 3991, 4334). Potentiating effects or prolongation of "sleeping time" has been reported for barbiturates (but not for ether, chloral hydrate, or chloralose) in dogs and guinea pigs by intravenous injections of glucose (2355); in mice, by certain cholinesterases (3408); and in rats, by septal lesions, but not by similar lesions in the cerebral cortex or caudate nucleus (1694). Cerebral blood flow (1910, 4136) and oxygen consumption (1775, 4136), eye positions (471) and movements (573, 3258), development of conditioned reflexes (3710, 3805), and a variety of other conditions affecting, or affected by different stages of, anesthesia (649, 746, 802, 1290, 1954, 2297, 2677, 2764, 2915, 3324, 3783, 4187, 4203) in man and animals have been studied by many investigators.

From the time that barbiturates had been classified by Molitor and Pick (2860) with subcortically acting hypnotics, their site and mode of action have been under experimental scrutiny. Keeser and Keeser (2119) combined barbiturates (barbital, luminal, and dial) with ferric chloride chemically. Rabbits were injected with non-lethal doses of these compounds at intervals of 1 to 3 hours. Then the anesthetized rabbits were killed by bleeding 8 to 9 hours after the first injection. After having been hardened, the brains were treated with potassium ferrocyanide and, by the blue color developed, the hypnotics injected were located in the thalamus and corpus striatum but not in the cerebral cortex, mesencephalon, cerebellum, pons, or medulla. Koppanyi and co-workers (2236) took issue with the Keesers. By their quantitative method these investigators found that barbiturates were distributed equally through all parts of the CNS. Forbes and Morison (1235) studied the "secondary discharge" appearing in both hemispheres, in regions remote from the primary sensory projection area, as a response to the stimulation of one sciatic nerve. Under deep barbital anesthesia, "the secondary discharge fades out completely on repetition of the afferent stimuli at frequencies above about 4/sec," and this fading out was ascribed to a raised threshold or rapid fatigue of a pacemaking mechanism in the thalamus or some other subcortical centers. French and co-workers (1282, 1287) noted a blocking of impulses propagated through the BSRF of monkeys by pentothal sodium, whereas "laterally conducted impulses reached the sensory cortex with unimpaired, or even augmented, intensity." The authors suggested, as a neural basis for the anesthetic state, that "the central-brain-stem system has a multisynaptic interneuronal organization, making it more susceptible to anesthetic blockade than the paucisynaptic lateral pathways." This view found support in observations made on the cat and man by other investigators (116, 488, 567, 1384, 2557, 4070), and seems to be applicable to ether anesthesia as well (116, 1287). On the other hand, the cortical desynchronization occurring in the early stages of ether anesthesia, according to Rossi and Zirondoli (3429), "may be due to an excitatory influence upon the BSRF," and in large doses barbiturates were thought by King and co-workers (2159) to "exert a depressant influence directly upon thalamic relay nuclei." Brazier (465) has advanced a hypothesis that "the initial action of barbiturates is on neurones in the cortex," and Himwich (1773) stated that barbiturates "in general act most strongly on the later-developed parts of the brain—the cortex of the cerebral hemispheres—and least so on the more primitive medulla oblongata." Species of animal, dosage, and, perhaps, type of barbiturate preparation are to be considered when one evaluates somewhat conflicting findings of different investigators.

A state presumably comparable to that produced by chemical anesthetic agents, electronarcosis was induced in the rabbit in 1902 by Leduc (2398, 2399). With the positive electrode on the back of the animal's neck and the negative one on the vertex of its head, a direct current was passed at the rate of 100/sec, with a pulse duration of 1 msec. The strength of the current was gradually increased, and when it reached 1–2 ma, there was a loss of body righting and of motility, with a suppression of all reflexes. This condition could be maintained for several hours, and abdominal operations were performed without any evidence of pain or discomfort on the part of the animal. When the current was turned off, the animal at once recovered from the narcosis. A similar condition was produced in the dog (1634) with 30–80 ma, increased to 100–200 ma, whereas a current of 10–20 ma led to the development of a catatonia, resembling the effect of bulbocapnine. Gualtierotti and co-workers (1545, 1546, 2698, 2699) and others (574, 575, 913, 3405) induced electronarcosis in a variety of animals, but specified the use of pulsed or rhythmical stimulation rather than of a continuous current. Because electronarcosis was, in certain situations, accompanied by convulsions in animals (913) and man (1545), it has been likened to electroshock. Simon and co-workers (3704), in treating patients, observed a greater hyperglycemia from electronarcosis than from electroshock. Tietz and associates (3941, 3942) found electronarcosis to be "a safe and practical method of treating schizophrenia," and the results were "definitely superior to those obtained by electroshock." Monro (2871), who administered 2,443 electronarcosis treatments to 152 patients, including 105 schizophrenics, pointed out the difficulties and dangers involved, and Bowman and Simon (433), because of the extreme rise in blood pressure accompanying it, regarded electronarcosis as more dangerous than electroshock. Rees (3289, 3290), after a comparative study, concluded that both electronarcosis and electroshock were far less effective than insulin therapy in schizophrenia.

Electrosleep differs from electronarcosis in that it continues for some time after the current has been cut off, resembling, in this respect, sleep induced in animals by weak currents (p. 204). Gilyarovski and associates (1451) specified that the sleep-inducing device must supply "pulsating current of constant polarity, rectangular in form, pulse duration of 0.2–0.3 msec, and frequency 1–20/sec." Others indicated a voltage of 0.5–2.5 (4089) and milliamperage of 0.2–1.5. Electrosleep is made easier when subclinical doses of hypnotics are administered at the same time (1152, 3661, 3662, 3913). When a conditioned stimulus is also used repeatedly, it permits a reduction in both the electric and pharmacological factors. Kleinsorge and co-authors (2175) obtained only drowsiness in animals and indicated that electrosleep in human subjects might be due to suggestion, rather than to the current applied. As this type of current induces sleep in animals, irrespective of the part of the brain stem the current is passed through (p. 204), there is no reason why it should not have the same effect when surface electrodes are used. The procedure is the reverse of obtaining EEG or EKG records from the surface of the body instead of directly from the brain or heart.

Among the drugs that are used to prevent sleep or to antagonize the action of hypnotics are caffeine, ephedrine, and benzedrine. Almost any drug capable of stimulating the CNS can be used as an antihypnotic. Picrotoxin has been employed successfully as an antidote in barbiturate poisoning, but it is too toxic to be used to promote wakefulness. Caffeine also has analeptic properties, although one hardly thinks of it as a powerful drug because it is taken regularly in common beverages—coffee, tea, and a variety of soft drinks.

The effects of caffeine on body temperature and on motility were described in Chapters 8 and 10 (pp. 61, 87). In human subjects caffeine, in amounts contained in one or two cups of coffee, decreases RT slightly (689, 1835, 3937), improves performance in tests requiring muscular strength and speed of movement, but has an adverse affect on steadiness (3937). Caffeine also delays fatigue (1541) and tends to shift the EEG to a higher frequency (1431). In experiments on the intact and CI rabbit, Krupp and co-workers (2290) found that caffeine produced an EEG arousal pattern not by stimulating the ARAS, but by inhibiting the intralaminary mediothalamic recruiting system. Whatever its mode of promoting wakefulness, caffeine, because of its availability and safety, is an excellent antihypnotic agent.

Ephedrine, chemically related to epinephrine and having, like it, a stimulating effect on the sympathetic system, has been, in crude form, a constituent of the Chinese pharmacopeia for many centuries. Within the last forty-five years it has also been used in the Occident as a substitute for epinephrine for a variety of conditions, among them asthma and hay fever. Many hay-fever patients noticed that ephedrine induced wakefulness, but it was not until 1931 that Janota (1948) and Doyle and Daniels (973, 974) applied it to the treatment of narcolepsy. Hypersomnias have also been reported to respond to ephedrine therapy (731, 743, 4248, 4281). Wortis and Kennedy (4281) obtained more complete relief of cataplexy than of narcolepsy itself by means of ephedrine. Vadàsz (4029) suppressed sleep attacks by ephedrine in a case of postencephalitic narcolepsy, but the concomitant cataplexy responded better to a hyoscyamine derivative. These differences in results with ephedrine therapy are in line with the finding (p. 236) that, although narcolepsy and cataplexy usually appear together, they need not always do so and therefore may involve somewhat different processes in the CNS. Simonson and Enzer (3711) found that pervitin, or desoxyephedrine, increased the critical flicker frequency—an objective sign of relief of fatigue.

Benzedrine (benzyl methyl carbinamine), or as it has been designated by the non-proprietary name of amphetamine, when given by mouth, was found by Prinzmetal and Bloomberg (3241) to be three times as effective as ephedrine in preventing narcoleptic sleep attacks. When sniffed into the nose, benzedrine tends to cause a vasoconstriction, drying up the nasal mucous membrane and affording relief from head colds. Persons using a benzedrine inhaler have reported an inability to fall asleep at their usual bedtime. Among other symptoms that followed benzedrine medication, Ulrich and co-authors (4017, 4018) noted a palpitation of the heart, a slight rise in arterial blood pressure, occasional nausea and vomiting, and a loss of appetite. The latter led to the extensive use of benzedrine in the treatment of obesity. Benzedrine has no therapeutic value for the relief of catatonic stupor (1676) and appears to be more stimulating to normal persons than to depressed patients (834). Tihen (3943) stated that benzedrine was an effective means of combating narcoleptic attacks in patients who had been unsuccessfully treated with thyroid and pituitary extracts, ephedrine, and a ketogenic diet.

Experimentally, benzedrine bettered performance and delayed the onset of fatigue (635, 3712). Unlike caffeine, benzedrine also improved steadiness (3937). Like caffeine, benzedrine tended to shift the EEG to a higher frequency (1431), and during sleep following benzedrine administration the delta waves were diminished in length and amplitude, particularly in narcoleptics (365, 366). After electroshock convulsions, the phase of extreme EEG slowing was eliminated in monkeys, in 11 out of 19 trials, when they received 1–3 mg/kg of benzedrine 10–15 minutes prior to the shock, and the animals appeared more alert (2427). In the conscious cat, benzedrine produced not only an "alerting" LVFA, but enhanced the EEG response to photic stimulation (443) and led to excited behavior (441).

Our interest in benzedrine was aroused by the possibility of using it to maintain prolonged wakefulness. It will be recalled (p. 220) that, after remaining awake for more than one night, it was progressively harder to keep awake on successive nights and that walking, or engaging in some other muscular activity, was the means of preventing the onset of sleep. Prior to the employment of benzedrine the longest I ever remained awake was for 5 days (115 hours). By taking 10–30 mg of benzedrine sulphate every night, I kept awake, on one occasion, for 8 days; and, instead of being half-asleep all the time, as one usually gets to be after 65 hours of continuous wakefulness, I was fairly alert at the end of this period of sleeplessness. Other subjects in our laboratory had similar experiences. Sixty-odd hours of sleeplessness, such as they were required to undergo on numerous occasions, were rendered more supportable with, than without, benzedrine. The procedure, usually, was to take 10 mg of benzedrine sulphate every 4–8 hours, or else only when one felt unusually sleepy. Of ten subjects, eight men and two women, who had undergone periods of wakefulness with and without benzedrine, only one complained of frequent micturition following benzedrine; another subject was eliminated, because benzedrine made him nauseated. Practically all our subjects had definite palpitation of the heart and developed a dryness of the mouth which made it impossible to give placebos to those who had once before taken benzedrine. At the time of going to bed, after 65 hours of sleep deprivation, the subjects who had taken benzedrine were usually not very sleepy, and their motility during the subsequent sleep was not only greater than after prolonged wakefulness without benzedrine but in several subjects was higher than during an ordinary night's sleep. Kornetsky and associates (2240) tested the effect of benzedrine on the performance of nineteen subjects, after 44 and 68 hours of sleep deprivation. Out of a battery of psychological tests, only the least-impaired performances were brought up to the control levels by 10–15 mg of benzedrine. In a field study of military personnel (805) benzedrine caused a greater inability to fall asleep in the open after a 23-mile march, but "in spite of poor quality or absence of sleep the benzedrine group rose in the morning feeling less fatigued than controls."

Somewhere between the hypnotic and antihypnotic drugs in affecting CNS processes are the tranquilizers which, as the term indicates, have a calming effect, without either producing sleep or enhancing alertness. Unlike barbiturates, tranquilizers do not depress the neocortex, but they differ widely in their influence on the limbic system and on the different subcortical structures. The most powerful of these psychopharmacological agents are the phenothiazines, such as chlorpromazine (largactil), which depresses the BSRF and blocks sensory-produced arousal (446, 448, 887, 1761, 2150, 2324), as well as the sympathetic mechanisms of the hypothalamus (1773, 3358). Chlorpromazine may interfere with the spontaneous activity of the thalamo-cortical complex (830) and increase the activity of the amygdaloid complex which has an "inhibitory influence over wide areas of the brain" (3239). A therapeutic dose of 25 mg of chlorpromazine affected the performance of subjects in the Minnesota Multiphase Personality

Inventory (MMPI), also producing sedation and mental clouding (1668); in much larger doses (200 mg) it impaired attention in a continuous performance test, comparable to the effect produced by 66–70 hours of sleep deprivation (2838). Although it did not cause distinctive EEG changes (1463, 2872), chlorpromazine slowed down the alpha pattern by as much as 1.5/sec (2838, 3894). In cats with permanently implanted electrodes, spike discharges from the lateral geniculate nucleus during the LVFA phase of sleep were abolished for 4–5 hours after the administration of 4 mg/kg of chlorpromazine.

Reserpine, a Rauwolfia alkaloid, like chlorpromazine, does not produce any distinctive EEG changes (2872). It is said to stimulate subcortically the BSRF (3354, 3358), or at least not to depress it (2868), and therefore to have no hypnotic effect; it is said to alter neither the threshold for BSRF stimulation nor the behavioral arousal threshold (448, 2153); and to have a "mode of action of a fundamentally new type," as "only certain selected and specific functional systems within both the autonomic and somatic systems are susceptible to its action" (278, 279). Likewise, it has been stated that the action of reserpine is due to a release or depletion of serotonin (and norepinephrine) stores from the brain (1773, 3215, 3686) or to a change in brain serotonin from a bound to a free state (1730), but an opinion has been expressed that depletion of serotonin does not play a part in this action (1123). Behaviorally, reserpine has been reported to decrease the speed of establishment of conditioned responses in monkeys (4150); to suppress the pugnaciousness of Siamese fighting fish, without impairing their sensitivity and motor activity (4104); to produce an acute hypersecretion of ACTH in rats (4162); and to decrease selectively the rate of self-stimulation of rats with electrodes implanted in several regions of the brain (3051). The last-mentioned effect is somewhat different after chlorpromazine, and the suggestion was made that the self-stimulation procedure could be applied to the screening of tranquilizers. In the hypothalamus, reserpine, like chlorpromazine, suppresses the sympathetic mechanisms, but it additionally stimulates the parasympathetic ones (1774).

Reserpine is less powerful than chlorpromazine, and the weakest of the tranquilizers is the substituted propanediol, meprobamate, which affects neither the BSRF nor the neocortex, but has a slight depressing effect on the thalamus and on the limbic system that is related to the emotional aspects of behavior (1774, 2208). Meprobamate was shown to inhibit the adrenocortical response to psychic stress in rats under acute experimental conditions, but the effect disappeared on repeated trials (2614). In man, therapeutic doses of 200 mg of meprobamate had little effect on performance (1668), but 800 mg impaired learning, and 1600 mg also impaired motor co-ordination and RT (2239). Doses of 400–800 mg exerted a hypnotic action, compared to a placebo; 800 mg, but not 400 mg, reduced motility during sleep. Meprobamate (2737), like reserpine (2353), has been used with some success in the treatment of enuresis.

Lysergic acid–diethylamide, or LSD 25, a semisynthetic derivative of ergot, in extremely small doses produces visual hallucinations and other psychic disturbances in man. In the rabbit it causes a suspension of spontaneous rhythmical activity of the brain (881), and in the cat and rabbit it acts somewhat like amphetamine (441, 1134, 2150), producing behavioral excitement and fast "alerting" cortical activity. However, LSD 25 does not change the EEG response to photic stimulation, probably differing from amphetamine in its mode of action. In rabbits and mice, the site of the excitatory action of LSD 25 is subcortical, probably diencephalic (2989). In man, LSD 25 impairs attention and abstract thinking but increases the alpha pattern by 0.5–4/sec (1368). It has also been found to counteract the effects of barbiturates and chlorpromazine (867). The peyote alkaloid mescaline, which also causes visual hallucinations, decreases the amplitude of the alpha EEG in man (702). The psychological effects of ACTH and cortisone on patients have been described as "heightened alertness and keenness of perception" and "a sense of increased energy for physical or intellectual activities" (1256). The EEG effects of ACTH, in thirteen out of fifteen patients, were a reduction in alpha activity—in one case a change from 12–13/sec to 7–8/sec (1798), whereas cortisone caused "a slight but definite increase in the alpha frequency" (1297).

The study of the behavioral and EEG effects of a variety of sympathomimetic and parasympathomimetic drugs on animals and man has given rise to the conceptions of adrenergic and cholinergic mechanisms in the operations of the systems concerned in furthering wakefulness and sleep. The action of epinephrine on the EEG resembles that of benzedrine (886, 887, 1431), but direct (3308) and indirect (2354) evidence has been presented that epinephrine potentiates the hypnotic effects of barbiturates in mice and guinea pigs, respectively. Mantegazzini and co-workers (2656) have concluded that the results they obtained in the curarized EI cat "do not seem to support the hypothesis that adrenaline and nor-adrenaline, intravenously injected, would act as chemical mediators on the synapses of the ascending activating system." Guillemin (1552) made the same conclusion on the role of these two substances in the hypothalamic-pituitary activation by neurotropic stress. Longo and Silvestrini (2556) in an intact non-curarized rabbit obtained EEG activation from acetylcholine, eserine, and benzedrine but not from adrenalin. Frommel and co-workers (1308, 1311–14) failed to detect any barbiturate-potentiating effect in sympathomimetic drugs but noted that pilocarpine, acetylcholine, anti-cholinesterase, and other vagotonic drugs did potentiate barbiturate action. Rinaldi and Himwich (3355–57) produced a stable sleep EEG in the rabbit by atropine, resistant to "all types of stimulation, including the direct electrical one of the midbrain reticular formation." They concluded that "the function of the mesodiencephalic activating system is cholinergic in nature," and this conclusion has found support among others (2555, 3120, 3494). The sleep EEG effects of atropine are not matched by behavioral ones, as pointed out by several investigators (442, 444, 445, 1321, 4207) ; to complicate matters, in man atropine causes drowsiness and other behavioral effects consistent with the EEG changes (3066, 3895). Atropine has been shown to neutralize the alerting action of methedrine, closely related to benzedrine and an adrenergic agent (868). In the decerebrated cat, after an injection of epinephrine, single neurones in the BSRF showed "an increase in their discharge rate, a decrease, or were unaffected by the drug" (449). In the same preparation acetylcholine also produced facilitation, inhibition, or a mixed response in a single neurone. Thus, there may be cholinergic and adrenergic mechanisms in the BSRF, synergistic or antagonistic, depending on conditions (449, 1134).

Bradley (441), Verdeaux and Marty (4046), and Himwich (1774) prepared tables showing the comparative behavioral and EEG effects of a number of psychopharmacological agents, as well as the sites of their action in the CNS. Considering the multiplicity of species of animals, and the variety of preparations (intact, anesthetized or not, curarized or not, EI, decerebrated, CI) tested, and that injected epinephrine does not duplicate its neurohumoral role in the organism, the lack of consistency in the findings reported is not surprising. The operation of a single adrenergic or cholinergic mechanism, or a combination of the two, as related to the possible functioning of a single wakefulness or sleep center, or sleep-wakefulness regulating system, is discussed in the last part of this book.

Chapter 30

The Hygiene of Sleep and Wakefulness

How much sleep does one need? What can one do to improve the quality of sleep? How can one get the greatest benefit from a certain amount of sleep? Is it harmful to one's health to cut down on the time allotted to sleep? Can one sleep too much? Is "tossing and turning" during sleep beneficial or harmful? Is it desirable to eat or drink shortly before going to bed? These and dozens of similar questions concerning beds, bedding, bedroom conditions, reading in bed, use of an alarm clock, going to bed early or late, are constantly being asked, and very few of them can be answered adequately at the present time. There are many and diverse opinions on the topic but not many established facts.

The disparity between the number of hours of sleep infants "should" have (89, 1004) and the number of hours they actually sleep was already dwelt upon (p. 114). Still some authors (3002, 4247) maintain that infants do not get enough sleep. Although there are circumstances that interfere with the sleep of infants (621, 975, 1793, 2665, 3064, 3867, 3928, 3929, 3988), under equal environmental conditions, individual infants have a tremendous range in the hours of sleep, as shown in Table 13.1 (p. 116) Sarylowa (3525) stressed habit-training, or a conditioning process, as an aid to proper sleep in infants and children, but in the 1890's Manacéine (2643) condemned "all methods of putting infants to sleep artificially by . . . lullabies and the rocking of infants in cradles." What has been said about body weight or the time of eruption of the first tooth also applies to tables of sleep hours for infants based upon means, modes, or medians obtained on groups.

The same considerations hold for the hours of sleep of older children. Although Kotsovsky (2252) found a relation between sleep and the rate of growth in puppies, Anderson (60) admitted that there was "no evidence to show a direct relation between hours of rest in bed and the general nutrition of children." Burn (577) noted that "a large number of children do not readily show signs of fatigue, even when the amount of sleep is markedly inadequate." Reynolds and Mallay (3327) observed that, in spite of large daily fluctuations in the amount of sleep taken by individual children, over long periods each child seemed to find its own norm for the duration of sleep. Bowers (430) considered that sleep has the same value whenever taken and that it does not make any difference at what hour a child goes to bed. Manacéine (2643) stated that "the wish of grown-up persons to arrange their evenings as freely and quietly as possible has led to the widespread custom of sending children to bed at a very early hour." Reese (3291) found that daylight-saving time had no effect on the duration of sleep in young children who lived in an institution where the mode of existence was strictly routinized. For the "underrested" child Ramsay (3264) suggested, in addition to correction of dietary and hygienic faults, a rest cure in bed, involving a 2-hour rest in the afternoon and a 15-hour (7:00 P.M.–10:00 A.M.) stay in bed at night, followed by breakfast in bed. It is doubtful if any but a sick child would submit to such a routine. The cure may be worse than the disease of "underresting." Despert (924) suggested that parental attitude toward children's sleep should not be rigid, as many sleeping problems are initiated by undue stress on the need for obtaining an arbitrary number of hours of sleep.

The problem (for such it is sometimes) of the daytime nap for older children has been discussed (p. 117). As there is no general rule about the total duration of sleep per 24 hours for the individual child, there can be none for the afternoon nap. Aron (136) recommended 1 to 2 hours for pre-adolescent children. It will be recalled, however, that children take or give up their naps on an all-or-none basis rather than by a gradual shortening, as they might be expected to do. Sherman (3678) observed no connection between the duration of the afternoon nap and the activity, as well as the behavior, of preschool children. Staples and Anderson (3785) could not detect any relation between the length of the afternoon nap and the time it took preschool children to fall asleep in the evening, although for some children, particularly older ones, such a relationship may exist. A safe rule with respect to afternoon naps may be that they should be encouraged, unless (and until) they can be seen to delay the onset of sleep in the evening. Anything that causes a child to remain awake after going to bed is undesirable, as it may lead the child to play while in bed, and thus destroy the conditioning process of associating bedtime with sleep time. Usually, dispensing with the afternoon nap meets with the enthusiastic approval of the child, who may be easily induced, by way of compensation, to go to bed a little earlier, should he show signs of sleepiness before his customary bedtime.

According to Boynton and Goodenough (437), children who usually assume definite positions on going to bed fall asleep more readily. As pointed out (p. 11), the position of the child may influence the jaws and the teeth system, but there is no agreement on the seriousness of these influences, nor on the means of avoiding them (2653, 3626, 3771).

Heavy evening meals have a disturbing effect on the sleep of children, as judged by increased motility (1433, 1434, 2344). Karger (2081) found mental work and exciting games in the evening, and Renshaw and co-workers (3320) certain types of moving pictures, disturbing to the subsequent sleep. Giddings (1435) noted no change in the sleep motility of children after an hour of study or of outdoor exercises, but emotional states (fear, worry, disappointment, or pleasant anticipation) increased the number of movements during sleep (1435, 1437). In general, emphasis is placed on the proper distribution of work, play, and rest, and the development of habits that are conducive to regularity in eating and in bedtime hours as means of "improving" children's sleep (286, 323, 372, 577, 612, 674, 924, 1210, 1253, 1324, 1457, 1528, 1529, 1687, 1691, 1692, 1800, 1801, 2188, 2738, 2961, 3371, 3653, 3741, 3773, 3774, 4078, 4137, 4189, 4277).

What constitutes the proper duration of sleep has no more been decided for adults than for children (3236). Several authors (2070, 2161, 2226) came to the conclusion that not only do different individuals require varying amounts of sleep, but that certain persons may get enough sleep and think that they do not. Camp (615) maintained that many people sleep too long and that oversleeping is just as reprehensible as overeating. Although it is said that it is not the duration of sleep but its quality that counts, there is no agreement on what constitutes good quality of sleep.

The daytime nap for adults was condemned because it destroys the depth of the night sleep (2226) or because one's mood is worse on awakening (1718). It was held to be desirable, and refreshing out of proportion to its duration, as a "pick-me-up" (3175, 3796).

The timing of sleep was crucial, according to Stöckmann (3830–34), who presented evidence that a shortening of sleeping time could best be accomplished by changing the hours of going to bed to about 7:00 P.M. One could then get up at 11:00 P.M. or midnight and feel more refreshed and be more efficient than one was previously on 8 to 10 hours of sleep during the conventional hours. Stöckmann (3832) attempted to rationalize his "discovery" by pointing out that the earth is governed by the rising and setting of the sun, through which life is alternately stimulated and depressed. Sunset is the best time for going to bed, as it insures a quick recovery sleep. These views were criticized by Laudenheimer (2378), mainly because Stöckmann was not a physician but only a teacher and, as such, had no business to meddle with the sleep problem.

In actual practice the time of going to bed is often related to an individual's occupation, and, if the latter is not restrictive, to one's personal 24-hour rhythm. Wuth (4283) distinguished two types of sleepers: one type is tired in the evening, quickly falls asleep, soon reaches the greatest depth of sleep, and wakes up refreshed and well rested; the other type is alert in the evening, does not fall asleep easily, achieves the greatest depth of sleep toward the morning, and wakes up feeling tired. Schultz (3604) also acknowledged the existence of two types, but he based his division on different grounds. One type he designated as a monocyclic sleeper, who sleeps well through the entire night and needs no daytime nap. He called the other type of sleeper dicyclic—such people have two periods of deep sleep; they are ready to get up after 4 to 5 hours of sleep; but, if they do not, they have a second period of deep sleep; if they cannot get a second period of sleep during the night, they need an afternoon or twilight (6:00 P.M.–8:00 P.M.) nap. This dicyclic type is close to the young child, with its daytime nap, and Schultz designated such persons' sleep pattern as "sleep infantilism."

Léopold-Lévi (2435), as mentioned (p. 161), divided mankind into four types, related to propensities for going to bed early or late, and for rising early or late. The "to-bed-late, rise-early" type needs little sleep and has overactive endocrine and sympathetic nervous systems. The "to-bed-early, rise-late" type suffers from an endocrine-sympathetic asthenia, is obese, always tired, and can sleep 10 to 14 hours. The "to-bed-early, rise-early" or "morning" type conforms to the "law of nature," follows the sun, like "animals and peasants." The "to-bed-late, rise-late" or "evening" type needs no excessive sleep, but is unhappy because he does not conform to the social habits of the majority of the population. He seeks night work. If he is an intellectual, he does his best work in the evening or at night. Sheldon (3676) worked out only three extreme body-build and temperament combinations (p. 120), lacking the "to-bed-early, rise-early" type of Léopold-Lévi. Of course, both classifications apply to extreme types and by Sheldon's scheme nearly everyone has viscerotonic, somatotonic, and cerebrotonic components in varying proportions in his temperamental makeup. Bingel (347) noted that schizophrenics are often of the morning type, whereas cyclothymics and manic-depressives are likely to be of the evening type. Volkind (4083) found that the time of onset, the duration, and the depth of sleep of dogs were also related to the types of nervous system they possessed. Geyer (1414) reported that identical twins, in addition to the presence or absence of a positive Babinski sign (p. 17), showed several other sleep characteristics in common and even awakened in the same manner. As everyone is born with certain hereditary bodily and temperamental characteristics, there may be a limit to the degree of modification that can be accomplished by training and experience.

Much has been written on the setting that is conducive to good sleep. After a day of sustained activity, the motility of the sleeper may be greater than normal (2004). Evening activity may also have a deleterious effect on sleep (2963), because the individual cannot properly prepare himself for sleep. Our subjects (2200), likewise, did not sleep well when their usual evening routine was upset. Cultivation of regularity and avoidance of excitement are undoubtedly beneficial for those who are temperamentally inclined to a "vegetative" existence and enjoy their evenings at home, reading a book or listening to music.

The matter of evening meals was stressed by some writers, who ascribed restlessness during sleep and bad dreams not so much to eating as to unwise eating or overeating (3332); or stated that more restful sleep can be obtained if nothing is eaten just before going to bed (3782); or found that a light snack at bedtime decreased the motility of their subjects (by 6 per cent), compared to control nights when nothing was taken (2344). It is probably true that one person will sleep better if he eats or drinks something before going to bed, whereas another will do better if he takes nothing at that time.

The alleged benefits of the proper bedspring and mattress have been emphasized, mainly by the makers of such equipment. Instead of offering the consumer a well-made article which can be expected to last for a number of years, the advertiser attempts to make the buyer good-sleep-conscious by extolling the "sleep-improving" properties of one or another type of bedding equipment. Bowers (431) traced the evolution of the bed from a pile of leaves, skins of beasts, framework interlaced with thongs, through the ornate beds of Cleopatra and of the Roman emperors, the couch, the bedstead, the twelfth-century high-post canopy-top beds, down to the iron beds of the eighteenth century and the modern folding cot.

The substitution of the vertical coil spring and mattress for the horizontal coil (hammock-type) spring and plain felt mattress has been considered a tremendous improvement, as it prevents the weight of the body from producing a sagging in the middle of the bed. Diagrams have been prepared to show how curvature of the spine is prevented by the individual vertical coils giving way only in certain places and conforming the contour of the bed surface to that of the body. Aside from the fact that the spine has a couple of natural curves, there is no evidence that a change in curvature is produced in the cat, which sleeps curled up; in the Japanese, who sleep on the ground, which usually does not conform to the curves of the body; or in sailors, who often sleep in bona fide hammocks, with a considerable sag in the middle. The sagging of the mattress and bedspring may discourage frequent changes in position in some people, but that is an individual matter. Likewise, some persons prefer a softer mattress than do others. It is all a matter of individual likes and dislikes and, except through suggestion, the type of mattress used has little, if any, influence on the "quality" of sleep. Indeed, Suckling and associates (3863), who compared the effects of hard, medium, and soft mattresses on sleep and found that hard surfaces tended to increase motility and decrease the depth of sleep, as well as the subjective estimates of the quality of sleep, concluded that "the differences in these variables were not large and were not always statistically significant."

Even the placing of the bed in a certain way, usually with its head in the direction of north, had been advocated and practiced by Charles Dickens, according to Sarton (3524). Stopes (3838) not only insisted on this orientation, but could "feel" or "magnatate" the north and claimed to be able to detect a deviation of only 4° off the true north-south meridian.

The matter of bedcovers is also one for the individual to decide. With the rooms at the same temperature some people will sleep without covers, while others feel that they must have something, if only a sheet, over their bodies. In cold weather, also, there are great differences in the number of blankets one would consider just enough to make one comfortable. In this connection, Hellmuth and De Veer (1695), it may be recalled (p. 87), recorded the skin (thigh) and bed temperatures, as well as the movements of the sleeper, in 90 experiments on several women, and found the level of the skin temperature to have little influence on motility, provided the difference between the bed and skin temperatures was not too small. This difference usually amounted to 4°–5° C., but, if it got to be 1°, or smaller, the motility was increased. On the other hand, too great a difference between these two temperatures prevented the onset of sleep. A low bed temperature also discourages changes in position, as in the wintertime, because the sleeper finds that any movement beyond the confines of the area warmed by his body brings him into an "arctic" zone; he therefore immediately retreats into the previously occupied warmed part of the bed. The sleep paralysis, described by Stockmann (3828) as occurring on awakening, and evidently due to lying too long in one position, is much more frequent in the winter than in the summer. A way to make conditions favorable for motility is either to keep the room warm or else to use an electric blanket to keep the bed warm. Prewarming the bed on a cold night also makes it more pleasant to get into and thus contributes to the removal of a possible source of annoyance that may interfere with the onset of sleep. On the other hand, some of our subjects reported that, on getting into an ice-cold bed, they were constrained to lie still, and thus fell asleep quickly. Evidently, it is again a matter of individual preference, and it makes little difference what one does about the temperature of the bedding.

The position in which one is to sleep and the use of pillows have come in for their share in the discussion of the hygiene of sleep. Earlier writers weighed all the arguments for and against lying on one's back or abdomen, in left- and right-side position, but as early as in 1834 Macnish (2610) knew that the sleeper changes his position during the night. In 1897 Manacéine (2643) observed that "to maintain the regular nutrition of all the tissues and organs of the body it is important to change the position of the body as often as possible during sleep, and to take advantage of each awakening during the night to sleep in turn on the right side, the left side, and the back." But it was Szymanski (3897) who gave an impetus to the study of the motility of sleepers, and through the work of Johnson and associates (2003) there is not only a better knowledge of the frequency with which one changes positions during sleep but also photographic evidence of the multiplicity of positions a particular sleeper may assume during a single night's sleep. Later observations only confirmed the universality of sleep motility, and subsequent evaluations of beds and bedding have been largely based on whether this or that construction encourages or discourages changes in position during sleep. Our results differed from those of Johnson and co-workers on the question of the distribution of the movements through the night. All our normal subjects showed a gradually increasing frequency of movement—certainly a greater motility during the second half of the night than during the first. Remaining too long in one position, as happens after a large dose of alcohol (p. 61), is likely to produce a feeling of discomfort and stiffness in the musculature, or may lead to temporary paralysis. Too much motility, on the other hand, denotes disturbed sleep. The difficult question to answer is how much one should move and what the normal range is for motility figures. In this connection, from our data on seasonal variation in motility it can be seen that our subjects moved 50 per cent more in the autumn than they did in the spring (2200), and yet, until they were told about it, they themselves did not know it. It is therefore fair to conclude that the permissible (and the naturally occurring) variation in motility is rather large and the night-to-night variability in the motility of a partcular subject is even greater than the mean seasonal variation for the group as a whole.

Ventilation of the sleeping quarters is advocated by some and condemned by others; likewise, the sharing of a bed by two sleepers, or even the presence of more than one sleeper in the same bedroom; and the taking of exercise before going to bed. The undesirability of setting a certain hour for awakening as a disturbing influence on sleep was mentioned by Omwake and Loranz (3056). Boigey (395) condemned early-morning exercises as a menace to health, or even life, particularly in elderly persons. He saw danger in quickly getting out of bed on awakening, as practiced by "energetic" people.

Among the conditions required to insure a good night's sleep, darkness and quiet have been stressed by Vorwahl (4085), but Johnson (1998) considered light and noises inconsequential, and Craig (771) found that his subjects fell asleep sooner under the influence of disturbing sounds than in perfect quiet. Production of monotonous sounds, as a soporific agent, is, of course, an ancient procedure.

In addition to all the other measures, or in their default, various suggestions that can best be characterized by the term "rituals" have been offered for improving the quality of sleep. They involve doing certain things which, the prospective sleeper must believe, will make him fall asleep and sleep well. Drinking or eating or taking a warm bath—anything that could be called a conditioning process—may solve the problem. If not, progressive relaxation (1936, 4276) or passive relaxation by means of Rosett's apparatus (3416) is said to be of help. Iselin (1920) has proposed that a subject lie on his back, hold his head free in a lateral position (to diminish the arterial blood supply to the head) and direct his eyes inward and upward, inhaling and exhaling deeply— then he will fall asleep. Evans (1114) recommended taking two deep breaths before an open window, or some rhythmical physical exercise, and Kennedy (2138) suggested a combination of muscular relaxation and rolling the eyes into the upward position they are supposed to assume in sleep as the best procedure for inducing sleep. "Psychological" rituals have also been proposed. Binns (348) referred to a story told by Rabelais concerning "some monks, who, oppressed with wakefulness, resolutely addressed themselves to prayer, and before they had concluded half a dozen aves, or pater-nosters, we forget which, they all fell asleep." Evans (1114) also suggested prayer as an alternate ritual for breathing exercises, declaring: "This ritual at its best involves body, mind and soul in its performance. It is for this reason that prayer has satisfied human nature for centuries of time." Farrow (1140) offered a psychoanalytical method of going to sleep: all one has to do is to paint large imaginary figure 3's extremely slowly on a large imaginary black wall by means of an imaginary brush and a tin of white paint. Anyone who painted three of these 3's in this very slow manner would find it quite impossible to remain awake. Tichenor (3938) recommended turning one's thoughts to trivial things such as naming objects of different categories following the alphabet (example: ape, bear, cat, dog, elephant, fox, goat). The autosuggestion of Coué could probably also be placed in the ritual classification.

Additional information and advice on the hygiene of sleep have been offered by many authors (45, 47, 127, 152, 348, 578, 627, 693, 728, 789, 1042, 1214, 1267, 1516, 1604, 1649, 1938, 2332, 2337, 2338, 2341, 2343, 2564, 2607, 2610, 2643, 2947, 2984, 2985, 3026, 3119, 3182, 3200, 3489, 3521, 3561, 3651, 3694, 3742, 3795, 3841, 3936, 3963, 4078, 4218, 4297).

In our subjects (2200) we studied six characteristics which, we thought, might collectively determine the quality of sleep: (*a*) the ease of going to sleep; (*b*) motility during sleep; (*c*) sleeping continuously; (*d*) incidence and character of dreaming; (*e*) the duration of sleep; and (*f*) the subjective feeling of being well rested on awakening. The most striking feature of the results obtained on 36 subjects, with a mean number of 179 nights per subject, was that, with respect to every sleep characteristic, there was a considerable variation from subject to subject, and in the same individual from night to night.

Having obtained a control pattern of our subjects' sleep, we then studied its modification by various external and internal conditions, such as: (*a*) environmental conditions not under the control of the individual; (*b*) daytime and evening activities, entirely or partly under his control; (*c*) feelings, moods, attitudes, state of health, perhaps partly dependent upon the individual's actions but not under his control; and (*d*) imposed or prescribed conditions, when the individual was instructed to eat, drink, or swallow certain materials. From an analysis of the results we concluded that "none of the foregoing influences on the several sleep characteristics affected all our subjects in the same way, or a particular subject to the same extent on different nights. They represent shifts in the general tendencies which determine the quality of sleep characteristics of the group studied." Concerning the significance of the changes produced in the sleep of the group as a whole, some were definitely without significance, and others could be considered significant.

Another sleep variable is the "quantity" of sleep, as the product of its depth and duration (1081, 3346), based on the assumed correctness of the depth-of-sleep curve drawn by Kohlschütter (2228). On this premise, the amount of sleep obtained during the first 2 hours exceeded that furnished by the remaining 6 hours. Therefore, ran the argument, by sleeping for 2 hours, then staying awake for 4 and sleeping for 2 hours once more, one could obtain as much sleep in 4 hours as one usually gets from continuous sleep of 8 hours' duration. Many people have tried this scheme at one time or another and have given it up as unworkable. Husband (1876, 1877) studied his own performance during a month on a normal sleeping routine of 8 continuous hours, and then during a second month, when he slept from 11:00 P.M. to 2:00 A.M. and from 5:00 A.M. to 8:00 A.M., a total of 6 hours. He felt well, and his health was unimpaired. Physiological measures, such as blood counts and BMR, showed no deviation from the normal. His performance suffered some slight deterioration in tests pertaining to hand steadiness (tremor), body steadiness (ataxia), and speed of tapping. In spite of the absence of untoward symptoms, Husband did not adopt divided sleep as a permanent routine.

We had two subjects, O and T, follow the divided sleep routine for about a month. They slept for two 2.5-hour periods, separated by a 4-hour interval of wakefulness. They compared their motility during the two portions of divided sleep with that prevailing during a normal night's sleep of 7 to 8 hours' duration, as well as with the incidence of movements during a sleep period of only 5 hours per night, or the sum of the two periods of divided sleep. Both subjects had a somewhat greater motility during the second 2.5-hour period of sleep than during the first, suggesting a lack of equivalence between the two. But for both sleep periods the motility figures were within the normal range and did not differ much from the corresponding figures for the 7- to 8-hour or the curtailed 5-hour sleep. Subjectively, both individuals reported a very low capacity for work during the 4-hour interval separating the two "sleeps." They happened to be of the type who feels tired on getting up in the morning, and getting up twice did not improve matters. The routine definitely did not appeal to them as a time-saving proposition.

A hygiene of wakefulness is even more requisite than a hygiene of sleep. Much as one should like to insure the euphoria said to follow a "good" night's sleep (427, 428), it is capacity for performance during the hours of wakefulness that one seeks to achieve by the proper kind of sleep. Rowe (3458) found no relation between the length of his sleep and the amount of daily work he performed. Viaud (4056, 4057), noting that performance immediately upon getting up in the morning was often poorer than it was just before retiring the night before, chose afternoon hours for testing five subjects, whose sleep hours varied widely. For a sleep duration of 1 to 6 hours, afternoon performance improved almost linearly with the length of sleep. Beyond a duration of 6 hours

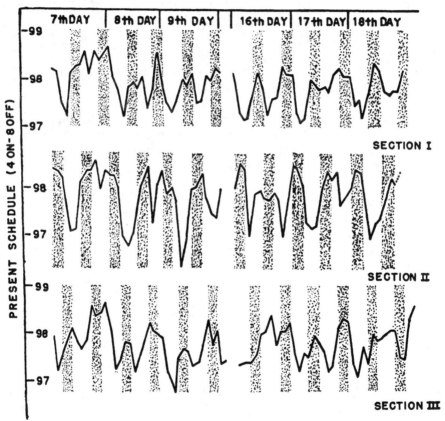

FIG. 30.1—Samples of group mean 24-hour body-temperature curves of three sections (10, 11, and 8 men, respectively) of a submarine crew during a 19-day simulated wartime patrol, reported by Utterback and Ludwig (4028). Watch-standing time of 8 hours out of 24 consisted of two 4-hour watches (shaded bands), separated by two 8-hour "off" duty periods (white spaces between bands)—a 12-hour routine of activity and rest. The 24-hour body-temperature curves of each of the three sections were irregularly bimodal.

of sleep, improvement was less marked, and it was completely absent when sleep was lengthened from 8 to 10 hours.

Efficiency of performance during the 15 to 17 hours of daily wakefulness follows the 24-hour rhythm, with an initial ascent, a terminal descent, and a crest or plateau in the middle (p. 151). Driving late at night (1165, 2752, 3944), or a rapid transfer by air into a distant time zone (3253, 3855, 3856), as well

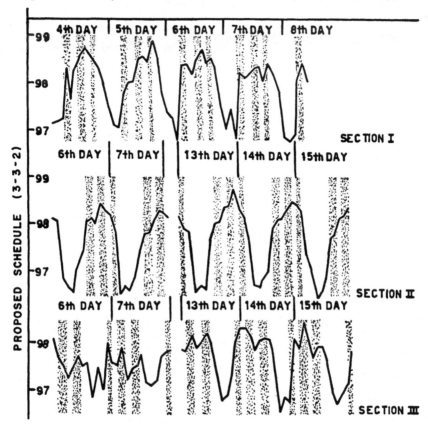

Fig. 30.2—Samples of group mean 24-hour body-temperature curves of three sections (8, 10, and 10 men, respectively) of a submarine crew during a 21-day simulated war-time patrol, reported by Utterback and Ludwig (4028). Watch-standing time of 8 hours out of 24 was divided into three 2 to 3 hour fractions (shaded bands), close together, thus allowing for a 12-hour period of freedom from duty daily. Distinct 24-hour body-temperature curves were in evidence in the fourth and sixth 24 hours in Sections I and II, but were also established later in Section III whose watch-standing hours were at night, necessitating an inversion of the customary 24-hour shore routine of living. The adjustment of the members of the crew to three different "time zones" is shown in the 8-hour shifts in maxima and minima of the body-temperature curves of the three sections, the maxima corresponding to the hours of duty, and the minima to the duty-free intervals.

as working during the night without adjusting the 24-hour rhythm (2563, 2903, 3778) may result in a greater number of errors (361, 362, 541) and accidents (2773, 2775, 4285). The round-the-clock operations of certain industries, public utilities, transportation and communication companies, police and fire departments, hospitals and military services necessitate the employment of multiple shifts with a dislocation from the customary acquired 24-hour rhythm of wakefulness and sleep. Night workers often get less sleep than day workers (2773, 3778) and complain of fatigue (501, 2903, 3183) and a variety of ailments, particularly digestive ones. Reports of a greater incidence of gastric ulcers among night and shift workers (1449, 2381, 3890), however, have been denied (3922, 3923). The timing of the shifts is unfortunate. When a second shift is required, in addition to the usual day shift, hours of 8:00 A.M. to 4:00 P.M. and 4:00 P.M. to midnight are logical, as both shifts then allow for sleep at night. However, that leaves only the hours from midnight to 8:00 A.M. for a third shift, which necessitates daytime sleep and working during the part of the 24-hour rhythm when temperature is lowest and sleepiness greatest (p. 157). A more physiological timing would provide for shift hours of 4:00 A.M. to noon, noon to 8:00 P.M., and 8:00 P.M. to 4:00 A.M. (2184), doing away with the "graveyard" shift entirely.

Work-rest alternation of 4 hours on and 4 hours off (3801) and 4 hours on and 2 hours off (13) has been tried experimentally, but the most common division, as practiced on U.S. submarines, is the "4 on, 8 off" schedule of watch-standing which is essentially an operation on an artificial 12-hour cycle. It may be recalled that it is practically impossible to establish such a rhythm in man (p. 175). A study of members of a submarine crew, with three watch-standing sections (2187) revealed that meals, recreation, and sleep were all skewed to correspond, as much as possible, to the regular "shore" routine of living. The body-temperature curves of members of the three sections were shown by Utterback and Ludwig (4028) to be unequally bimodal, but somewhat closer to the ordinary 24-hour body-temperature curve in the section whose hours of duty were 8:00 A.M. to noon and 4:00 P.M. to 8:00 P.M. (Fig. 30.1). A "close" watch schedule, with the 8 hours of duty divided into three parts and a free period of at least 12 hours for each section, led to the establishment of three distinct 24-hour rhythms, as shown by the body-temperature curves of members of the three sections operating on this schedule (Fig. 30.2). The "close" watch system was acceptable to the crews of several submarines, but has not been adopted by the U.S. Navy, even for the Polaris-type submarines which travel submerged for many weeks. It should be added that "unphysiological" as the "4 on, 8 off" system of watch-standing may be, it is much superior to the daily rotation of the "dogged" watches as practiced on large U.S. Navy surface vessels (p. 157). Daily rotation was a necessity when members of the crew slept in hammocks, strung in the large mess area, and daytime sleep was impossible. Now that separate sleeping quarters allow for a fixed system of watches, there is every reason for instituting a "close" watch-standing schedule which would give each man 12 hours free of duty daily.

Another solution to the multiple-shift problem, when fixed or permanent hours of work are not practicable, is to rotate the shifts as infrequently as possible (99, 362, 380, 1449, 2184, 2562, 2903, 4048).

The maintenance of a stable sleep-wakefulness rhythm, as indicated by a superimposable 24-hour body-temperature curve, serves a double purpose: (a) it makes for alertness and efficiency during working hours, and (b) it insures an easy onset of sleep and a "good" night's sleep, when they coincide with the drop in body temperature at certain hours of the evening and a low temperature during the night. The rhythm can be disrupted by irregularity and fortified by regularity in one's schedule of work, meals, recreation, and sleep. Children in particular can be more easily induced to follow a repetitive routine of living (4078).

It must be conceded that some persons are temperamentally more suited to a regular mode of living than are others. Morning persons have an advantage over evening ones, as the "early-to-bed, early-to-rise" system, upon which the working hours of society are largely based, fits in with their natural inclination. Certain individuals are capable of incurring a "sleep debt" by going to bed much later than usual for several nights in succession, but getting up at the customary hour. Such persons develop a feeling of lassitude and manifest a decreased alertness during their regular period of wakefulness. Those who are capable of accumulating a sleep deficit of several hours liquidate the debt by allowing themselves to sleep longer during the weekend. The ability to remain asleep much beyond one's customary getting-up time indicates a failure to establish and maintain a sleep-wakefulness rhythm.

The 24-hour routine of sleep and wakefulness, linked to living on the surface of the earth, may not be the optimal routine under conditions of isolation where day-night alternations are absent. In studies of non-24-hour schedules (p. 177), it was shown that the longer the sleep-wakefulness cycle the greater the body-temperature range. This finding suggests that, by operating on a longer than 24-hour routine, one may expect to reach a higher degree of alertness and level of performance, on the one hand, and a more complete muscular relaxation, perhaps better sleep, on the other.

Whatever one's temperament and disposition may be, it should be remembered that the 24-hour rhythm is an individually acquired, learned process, depending upon the presence and functional participation of the cerebral cortex. Physiology can contribute to hygiene by rationalizing the development of regular habits with respect to sleep and wakefulness.

Part 7

States Resembling Sleep

Chapter 31

Hibernation

Hibernation, as distinguished from prolonged winter sleep of some species, like the bear, or the nightly torpor of others, like the bat, is a biological adjustment of the highest order. It enables some homoiothermal animals to survive a season of cold and paucity of food by setting their thermostatic controls at very low levels and decreasing activity almost to the vanishing point. Attempts have been made to draw analogies between seasonal lethargy and nightly sleep, with respect to both cause and mechanism.

The entrance into hibernation, like drowsiness before the onset of sleep, is preceded by a number of changes, particularly in the vegetative nervous system and endocrine glands (2097, 2101, 2596). Gelineo (1381) noted that in the gopher heat production dropped markedly several days before the beginning of hibernation. According to Lyman (2590), golden hamsters, when brought into a cold environment, increase their food intake and lay on fat before they enter hibernation, whereas ground squirrels hibernate within 24 hours after exposure to cold. Even for ground squirrels, Johnson (1991) found that starvation or limited rations accelerated and prolonged hibernation. Petzsch (3172) also considered hunger an impetus to hibernation, but Pengelley and Fisher (3149) noted that the golden-mantled ground squirrel hibernated from October to May, even if kept in a warm room with 12 hours of artificial daylight and given an unlimited supply of food and water. Thus, environmental temperature and availability of food may be decisive external factors for some species and not for others (2591).

The ability to revert to a poikilothermal condition is the *sine qua non* of hibernation. A non-hibernator, including man, will consume more fuel in maintaining its body temperature at the normal level when the outside temperature becomes lower; and in extreme cold, when the body begins to lose heat at a greater rate than it produces it, the body temperature may fall sufficiently to produce a state of lethargy, usually terminating in death. The hibernating animal, however, as observed by Herter (1719), behaves in a different manner.

The hedgehog, whose normal body temperature varies from 33.5° to 35.5° C., becomes partly poikilothermal when the environmental temperature falls below 17° C., and, as long as the latter is above 14.5° C., will remain "half-asleep," with the body temperature fluctuating between 30° and 15° C. When the environmental temperature is below 14.5° C., the animal definitely hibernates, keeping its body temperature about 1° above the environmental temperature, down to 6° C. If the temperature falls below 5.5° C., the hibernating hedgehog either maintains its own temperature at the 6° level or awakens. It is this latter thermogenetic property that caused Uiberall (4003) to reject the interpretation of hibernation as a simple failure of body-temperature regulation. The great resistance to cooling-off below 5°–6° C. enables the hibernating animal to survive. It may be said to remain poikilothermal when it economizes fuel by doing so but not when its life is endangered.

The blood of hibernating animals has been analyzed for a variety of constituents. Prompted, no doubt, by the theory of Dubois (998) that hibernation is brought about by an accumulation of CO_2 in the blood, Endres (1076) looked for and found an increase in the CO_2-combining power of the blood, as well as an increased amount of physically dissolved CO_2 in the blood of hibernating hamsters. This greater CO_2-combining power of the blood Endres ascribed entirely to the low body temperature. But the increase in free CO_2 is even greater, and the disturbance in the ratio of free to combined CO_2 is responsible for the greater acidity of the blood, compared to normal. The degree of oxygen saturation remains unchanged, confirming much earlier findings of Dubois (997).

The blood sugar of hibernating animals has been studied by several workers, with varying results. Endres and co-workers (1082) reported a blood-sugar concentration of 71–96 mg per cent for the hibernating marmot, or not much lower than normal. Dische and collaborators (942) could likewise detect no pronounced hypoglycemia in the hibernating squirrel and dormouse; but Britton (508) stated that the blood sugar of the marmot was lowered by 31 per cent in hibernation, and Feinschmidt and Ferdmann (1149) found a decrease of 27 per cent in the hibernating ground squirrel and a lesser fall in the marmot. Similar decreases in blood sugar were reported by others (336, 351, 2599, 2736, 3860). Although Lyman (2599) did not consider hypoglycemia as essential for the maintenance of hibernation, Kayser (2104) emphasized the hyperactivity of the pancreas. Further, Dworkin and Finney (1013) caused a woodchuck to hibernate by the administration of insulin and terminated the hibernation by the injection of glucose. Similar results were obtained by Dische and co-workers (942). Suomalainen and Saure (3873) noted an increase in the beta cells of the pancreas during hibernation and were also able to induce artificial hibernation in the hedgehog with insulin.

Among other constituents of the blood plasma, hibernation entails no change in chloride concentration (2170), an increase in both magnesium and potassium (2736), a slight rise in calcium (3870), with a marked elevation of both the K:Ca and the Mg:Ca ratios (1149, 3870). There is a decrease in bromide (3868), creatinine, and hemoglobin (3860).

For the formed elements of the blood, the earlier findings of a leucopenia by Fleischmann (1206) were confirmed by several others (351, 2736, 3275, 3860), though there were some differences with respect to the relative changes in the differential white blood cell count. The erythrocyte count is decreased during hibernation (3860).

In deep hibernation, the heart rate may decrease from 300 to 2 per minute in the ground squirrel (3397), and from 500 to 4 per minute in the golden hamster (678). According to Buchanan (554), there is a dissociation of auricles and ventricles in the heart of the hibernating dormouse, and Landau and Dawe (2356) noted a cardiac arrhythmia in the hibernating ground squirrel; but Tait (3901) found the action of the isolated heart of the woodchuck to be fully co-ordinated when cold slowed it down to 2 beats per minute. The slowing of the heart, as would be expected, lengthens the various EKG waves and intervals between them. Thus, when a hibernating woodchuck was cooled from 37° C. to 7° C., the duration of the P wave was increased by 350 per cent, that of the QRS complex by 425 per cent, and the P-R and Q-T intervals were lengthened 6 times (656, 2593, 3520). Dawe and Morrison (859), studying hibernating woodchucks, also observed a lengthening of the several components of the EKG, though the order of magnitude change was not the same. It should be noted that even at the very low rates prevailing during hibernation, cardiac acceleration can be obtained in the ground squirrel by raising the CO_2 content of the air above 2.5 per cent; in the hamster, above 5 per cent.

The blood pressure of the hibernating hamster is very low (678), but direct observation revealed no intravenous agglutination of red blood cells in the hibernating groundhog at 5° C. (2736).

Like the heart rate, the respiratory rate is greatly slowed during hibernation, going down to 1–3 per minute in the hibernating ground squirrel (2356), and to 23–45 per hour in the marmot (961). Kayser (2096) considered the periodic respiration seen during hibernation as a sign of the relative inexcitability of the medullary centers at low temperature. Like Endres and co-workers (1082), Kayser (2098) found no hyperventilatory response to CO_2 accumulation during hibernation, and Biörck and co-workers (350) noted that hibernating hedgehogs tolerated anoxia for 1 to 2 hours, as contrasted to 3 to 5 minutes for non-hibernating ones. Lyman and Hastings (2597) found "little evidence for the profound loss of sensitivity in respiratory center" during hibernation. Lyman (2589) could increase the respiratory rate of hibernating hamsters and ground squirrels by CO_2 concentrations above 2.5 per cent, thus differing from

Endres and co-workers (1082) with respect to their observations on the hibernating marmot.

Friedman and Armour (1299) found that the gastric mucosa of the hibernating groundhog continued to secrete, but the juice was of low acidity and contained almost no pepsin. Histamine increased the acid content but not the pepsin, while stimulation of the vagus increased both. The oxygen consumption drops greatly during hibernation (2103, 2588), and the law of surfaces no longer applies in this condition (2111). The RQ was reported by Dontcheff and Kayser (961, 2096) to vary from 0.65 to 0.72, but Schenk (3553) gave much lower values—0.41 to 0.65. Urinary nitrogen partition resembles that of starvation (643). There is also some adjustment in liver function (1639, 4321).

Hibernation affords an opportunity to study the effect of great variations in body temperature on the excitability of the nervous system. Cipiccia (704) studied cold-numbed amphibia; Merzbacher (2784) and Eisentraut (1056), stuporous bats. The latter, however, are in a sense poikilothermal (568), and their activity is related to external temperature at all times. In truly hibernating mammals, Barelli (219) found a greatly diminished response of the temperature-regulating mechanism to the injection of a fever-producing drug during hibernation. By the use of implanted thermocouples, Strumwasser (3857) was able to show that the squirrel did not enter hibernation in one simple decline of brain temperature. At a room temperature of 5.5°–8.0° C., and light on for 13 hours daily, there were distinct 24-hour brain temperature curves, with progressively, but irregularly, lower minima. When a critical brain temperature of 8.8° C. was reached in 6 days, hibernation definitely set in. Endres (1082) reported a tenfold increase in the threshold stimulus required to elicit movement during hibernation, as compared to ordinary sleep.

Cortical electrical activity was studied by Kayser and co-workers (2117, 3397), by Lyman and Chatfield (2595), and most intensively by Strumwasser (3858, 3859), all of whom used implanted electrodes. Spontaneous EEGs were present in some hibernators at brain temperatures of 5°–7° C., and desynchronization of the EEG by sensory stimulation was possible, even at a "90 per cent reduction of amplitude of general brain activity present at those temperatures" (3859). In very deep hibernation, there is variously reported to be an "EEG silence" (2117) or cortical and subcortical neuronal activity comparable to "that of an alert squirrel brain at merely reduced amplitude" (3859).

Histological studies indicated some chromatolysis of nerve cell bodies, particularly in the ventral horn of the spinal cord (228), and changes were reported in the chemical composition of brain tissue, with a number of differences (1149), including a decrease in ascorbic acid content (1230), during hibernation. According to Borak and Uiberall (412), dormice did not hibernate after they were irradiated by certain doses of X-rays, while unirradiated controls did. The hibernation-preventing effect of X-rays was less marked, both qualitatively and quantitatively, at lower environmental temperatures, and it was completely absent at temperatures near 0° C.

In addition to the pancreas, other glands of the endocrine system have engaged the attention of several investigators. Cushing and Goetsch (803) noted a great resemblance between the physiological phenomena accompanying hibernation and those associated with a retardation of tissue metabolism and inactivity of the gonads, seen in clinical states of hypopituitarism, as well as in experimentally induced hypophyseal deficiency. In hibernating animals Cushing and Goetsch detected histological changes in several endocrine glands but particularly in the hypophysis. This gland decreases in size, and the cells of the anterior lobe lose their characteristic staining reactions to basic and acid dyes. Toward the end of hibernation, the hypophysis swells, and the cells enlarge and recover their differential affinity for dyes. These authors were therefore inclined to seek the cause of hibernation not in external factors, such as cold and lack of food, but in a seasonal variation in endocrine function, with the hypophysis, as the master-gland, foremost in the group. Rasmussen, however, stated that hibernation produces no change in the size of the hypophysis or in its histological structure if comparison is made with the condition of the gland before, instead of after, hibernation (3274).

Britton published several papers on the relation of the adrenal gland to hibernation (506–9). He thought he could see a possible explanation of hibernation in a natural autumnal diminution of sympathico-adrenal activity affecting relatively unstable hibernating organisms. Conversely, recovery of hibernating animals from their winter stupor, as well as of homoiothermal animals from the effects of low body temperatures induced by artificial cooling, was presumably due to an increased activity of the sympathico-adrenal mechanism. Adrenalectomy, which was as rapidly fatal to hibernating species as to other mammals during the summer season, had no effect during the hibernating season, even when the animals did not actually hibernate. They would usually succumb to the effects of the operation in the spring, at the time at which they would normally awaken from their winter stupor. Kayser and Petrovic, and others (2108, 2109, 2115, 4059), however, reported that adrenalectomy impeded hibernation, shortening the number of days spent in stupor. Cortisone, and more effectively desoxycorticosterone, when injected into adrenalectomized hamsters, partially restored the number of hibernation days. It is generally agreed (1207, 2112, 3869, 4305) that the adrenalin content of the adrenal gland is lowest during hibernation.

In the numerous experimental attempts to induce or prevent hibernation, administration of gland extracts occupied a prominent place. Adler (20) noted that injection of thyroid extracts into hibernating marmots caused awakening in 2 hours, with a rise in body temperature from 6.5° to 29°, and later to 34.5° C. However, the animals would be found asleep the following morning. Epinephrine had the same effect as thyroid extract, but thymus preparations were less effective (animals aroused in 5 hours, but asleep 2 hours later). Zondek (4327) ascribed the effects observed by Adler to the temperature of the solution injected. When the liquid was more than 8° C. warmer than the rectal temperature of the hibernating animal, the latter would wake up, but not otherwise. Likewise, Johnson and Hanawalt (1993) reported that neither feeding of desiccated thyroid or thymus nor injection of huge doses of thyroxin or pituitrin produced any difference in the tendency of ground squirrels to hibernate when compared with controls. On the other hand, Schenk (3553) seemed to confirm Adler's findings not only for extracts of thyroid, adrenal medulla, and thymus, but also for those of anterior lobe of hypophysis. He also found thyroid extract best, as it had the greatest effect on metabolism.

On the supposition that hibernation may be related to the presence of a brown fatty body in hibernating animals, Wendt (4170) prepared an extract of that body taken from a hibernating hedgehog and injected it into rats. The animals became apathetic in 2 to 3 hours and showed a drop of 20–30 per cent in BMR. Control injections of olive oil had no such effects. Similar results were obtained by Hook (1830). The role of the brown fatty body as a possible "hibernation gland" (391, 2171) was disputed by Kayser (2109), who looked upon it as a fat reserve which melts away during the winter, though more slowly than other adipose tissue reserves.

Among other extracts tested was one made of lymphatic tissue ("P-substance"), which is very toxic, producing a loss of appetite and a marked fall in body temperature and in BMR. Because the effects of this extract resembled in many respects the condition of hibernation, Nitschke and Maier (3015) tried it on dormice and, with appropriate doses, produced typical hibernation. These authors pointed out that there is an increase in lymphoid tissue in the wintertime and suggested that this condition as well as hibernation may be due to a lack of vitamin D. Nitschke (3014) tested the suggestion by giving three captured hedgehogs daily doses of irradiated vigantol. Although these animals were kept in a dark room at 5°–10° C. for 3 winter months, they did not hibernate, but a fourth animal captured at the same time promptly fell into hibernating stupor, as did one of the treated animals when the vigantol feeding was stopped.

In the arousal from hibernation, the increase in the heart rate precedes that of the body temperature (859, 2594). The electrical activity is restored to normal at different temperature levels in the several parts of the brain, as recorded by indwelling electrodes (679, 3276), reaching the waking level in the cortex at 20° C. in some species (3397) and only at 30° C. in others (59, 680). Chatfield and Lyman hold that "the process of arousal is initiated when the limbic system is activated" (679). Arousal from hibernation was found by Suomalainen and Herlevi (3871) to induce the "alarm reaction," and Lyman and co-workers (678, 2598), as well as Raths (3275), emphasized the role of the sympathico-adrenal system in this process.

The nature of hibernation becomes clearer when one compares the behavior of various systems in hibernators and non-hibernators. Under curare and artificial respiration, the hearts of anesthetized cats, guinea pigs, and rats stopped beating at 11°–17° C.; those of hamsters and ground squirrels, at 1°–5° C. (2105, 2106). The temperature-heart rate curves are linear at higher temperatures (20°–36° C.) and curvilinear at lower temperatures (6°–20° C.) in hibernators (1762, 2593), but are almost entirely linear through the somewhat smaller temperature range in non-hibernators. But even the excised heart, or auricle alone, of hibernators stops beating at 1.5°–6° C. (1784, 3901); that of non-hibernators, at 16°–18° C. Tait, who stated that the woodchuck heart ceases to beat only when it freezes (3901), called attention to the less solid fats in the tissues of hibernators. The latter point was also noted by Fawcett and Lyman (1146). Further, peripheral nerves of the cat, dog, rat, and rabbit stop conducting at 8°–9° C.; those of the hamster continue to function below 4° C. (677, 1236).

The lethal temperature is, of course, much lower for hibernators than for non-hibernators, but in either type of mammal it is lower in the young than in the adult. Adolph (21) gave the age-related span of lethal temperatures for the cat as 7° to 18° C., and for the hamster, 1° to 4° C. This preservation and accentuation of embryonic ability to survive low temperatures may be the chief distinction between hibernators and non-hibernators. Other peculiarities, such as resistance to anoxia, more liquid fats, brown-fat endocrine properties, special enzyme systems connected with cardiac and nerve tissue activity, and a lesser homoiothermality, may be instrumental in permitting the hibernator to function at temperatures that are lethal to non-hibernators.

Hypothermia, as distinguished from true hibernation (2106, 2113), can be induced in non-hibernators, including man, and is entirely safe, if not too profound or too prolonged. In the rat, the EEG seems to be entirely normal at body temperatures between 32° and 39° C., but at about 30° C. marked changes appear (662, 1837). Similar data for the cat were reported by Koella and Ballin (2227), who obtained a straight line by plotting EEG frequencies against the reciprocal value of the absolute body temperature from 37° C. to 30°–28° C. As in the rat, a typical break occurs in the slope of the curve at 28°–30° C. Scott (3633) reduced the body temperature of anesthetized patients to 28° C. and also noted a voltage drop and irregularity of EEG pattern below 30° C.

Fedor and co-workers (1148, 1189, 1198) kept anesthetized dogs for 6 to 31 hours at body temperatures of about 24° C. and found that the percentage of survivals was related inversely to the duration of the hypothermia. In the animals that recovered there were no morphological changes in the heart, lungs, kidneys, and pancreas. Niazi and Lewis (2997, 2998) chilled dogs and monkeys to a temperature below 10° C., with survival, even though cardiac standstill was produced in the process. They also lowered the temperature of a terminal cancer patient—with the latter's consent—to 9° C. (48° F.), her heart stopping at 10.5° C. Revived after one hour, the patient made an immediate recovery from the chilling. In this connection, it should be noted that Andjus (64) could revive completely frozen rats, provided he induced in them an anoxia and carboxemia, by confining them to a small space during the chilling. The recovered rats lived only a few days, but when they were cooled to only 7°–9° C., survival was prolonged.

In therapeutic hypothermia, the anesthetized patient's body temperature is usually kept at the 27°–30° C. level (298, 2316, 2317, 4043). Though some pattern changes—sinus tachycardia, extrasystoles—may occur at the induction of the hypothermia, a normal cardiac pattern prevails during the maintenance of these low body temperatures, with the heart rate reduced, Q-T interval lengthened, and a lowering of the arterial and venous pressures (4063).

Therapeutic hypothermia is quite harmless, as is the winter sleep of the bear, whose body temperature is held at the 27° C. (81° F.) level for many weeks. The bear, however, is quite lethargic during his pseudo-hibernation, whereas Strumwasser (3858) noted that a true hibernator, like the squirrel, is "perfectly capable of getting up and moving to a new nest site while entering hibernation even at a brain temperature of 27°–28° C."

Camp (614) and Claparède (707) saw a connection between hibernation and sleep—both regarded as instincts. Rosenthal (3413) likened hibernation to the relatively dominant sleep phase of infants, and Hughes (1861) maintained that hibernating ancestors have left their mark on seasonal variations one can find in man today. In the reviews of Lyman and Chatfield (678, 2592, 2596) and Kayser (2100, 2107, 2110) various theories of hibernation are considered. Whether it is a reversion to the infantile ability to withstand anoxia and hypothermia, or a possession of enzymes which enable the heart and nervous system to operate at temperatures lethal to non-hibernators, the stupor of hibernation is what permits a limited group of mammals to survive long periods of cold and starvation. There is no evidence of a common cause in the onset of sleep and the entrance into the state of hibernation.

Chapter 32

Hypnosis

Braidism, hypnotism, mesmerism, and magnetism are names given to a process whereby a sleeplike trance, or hypnosis, can be induced in an individual by appropriate means, such as ocular fixation, "passes," or verbal suggestions. Charcot and his "Salpêtrière school" distinguished three phases in hypnosis: (*a*) a lethargic phase, which, paradoxically, was like real sleep, but with neuromuscular hyperexcitability; (*b*) a cataleptic phase, characterized by muscular rigidity and maintenance of imposed body positions; and (*c*) a somnambulistic phase, into which the subject might pass from either of the first two, manifested by extreme suggestibility to commands of the operator. Bernheim and the "Nancy school" did not accept this rigid subdivision but, instead, described a number of stages, from drowsiness through light and later deep sleep, but also ending with somnambulism and extreme suggestibility. Forel, according to Schultz (3603), discerned the following three hypnotic stages: (*a*) drowsiness, suggested sleepiness, heaviness of limbs and eyes; (*b*) hypotaxy or *charme,* an acceptance of suggestion, catalepsy, automatism, often analgesia and hallucinations, but no amnesia; and (*c*) somnambulism, with all the phenomena of hypotaxy, but with amnesia, and often posthypnotic suggested acts and posthypnotic hallucinations. The battles over the symptomatology and terminology of hypnosis are of little interest today, except that Bernheim (316) always maintained that he produced natural physiological sleep in the hypnotized subject. The main reason for considering this sleeplike state is to discover if there is any clue to the nature of physiological sleep in the mass of observational and experimental data pertaining to hypnosis.

The visceral and somatic concomitants of hypnosis in man have been studied by many investigators (772). Some (1472, 4102, 4337) found that the heart was slower during hypnosis, while others (1978, 1981, 2425, 4199) reported no change in heart rate as compared to the waking state. Bier's results indicate that some subjects will show a rise in the pulse rate, and others a fall, under hypnosis (332). There is also disagreement with respect to blood pressure: Walden (4102) and Zynkin (4336) found a fall; Lenk (2425), a rise; and Goldwyn (1472) and Bier

(332), no constant change. No changes have been noted in peripheral circulation (967), nor in the cerebral one (3031), although complicated fluctuations in plethysmographic tracings were described (3902, 4001, 4102). Qualitative and quantitative changes in leucocytes have been reported (2991).

Klemperer and Weissmann (2207) could detect no differences in the oxygen and CO_2 content of the blood during hypnosis, but Doust (969), as he did for sleep, reported a decrease in oxygen saturation from about 95 per cent to about 90 per cent.

Jenness and Wible (1978, 1981, 4199) compared hypnosis not only with wakefulness but also with normal sleep. In sleep they saw occasionally periodic respiration resembling the Cheyne-Stokes type, but never in the waking state or in hypnosis. They suggested that the apparent disagreement between their findings and those of other investigators, who reported a slowing of the heart and respiration in hypnosis, might be due to the fact that these other workers really studied sleep, instead of hypnosis, since they took no precautions to prevent their subjects from passing from hypnosis into sleep.

The BMR may remain unchanged (4194), or fall slightly, if hypnosis is associated with mental and physical inactivity (1472). There is a decrease in sweat (2667) as well as non-digestive gastric secretion (2007).

The ESR level is markedly increased during hypnosis, according to some authors (540, 1109); is unchanged, according to others (215, 2464).

Mayorov (2728, 2729) studied the chronaxies of antagonistic muscles in man during hypnosis and found them to resemble his Phase II of sleep. Nevsky and Zrjacick (2992), measuring muscular power with a dynamometer in the waking state and in hypnosis, reported a progressive depression, up to the point of adynamia, with increasing depth of hypnosis.

Numerous reports deal with the EEG during hypnosis. In addition to earlier fragmentary findings (365, 2559) suggesting that the EEG is that of wakefulness, there are reports confirming this view (692, 930, 1018, 1241, 1683, 3211), others that link the EEG to the phase of hypnosis (2579, 2670–73), and still others that find sleep or wakefulness EEGs (222, 223, 1469, 2260, 2669). Finally, there are those investigators who recorded sleep EEGs during hypnosis (2994, 3688) to the point of distinct delta wave patterns (1259, 1262). Darrow and associates (825, 826) noted that the parallelism between the EEG activities in the frontal and motor areas increased in hypnosis, as compared to normal wakefulness. Ravitz (3283) measured standing potential differences between forehead and palms, and concluded that "when they decrease in voltage, D.C. hypnotic records cannot be distinguished from D.C. sleep records."

Aside from the concomitants of hypnosis, the latter's influence on evoked responses and suggested performance affords a comparison with similar activities during normal wakefulness. A most remarkable series of physiological changes was produced in a twenty-six-year-old girl during hypnosis by Benedek (287).

By appropriate suggestion of emotional states, he produced an increase in heart-rate from 82 to 146, in blood pressure from 104 mm to 136 mm, hyperidrosis of the face and forehead, salivation, and a rise of 3° C. in skin temperature (by suggesting that her hand was placed in hot water). He could change neither her blood sugar nor her blood calcium by these methods. Bennett and Scott (294) produced bradycardia and EKG abnormalities in subjects by suggesting anxiety; Lauber and Pannhorst (2375) elicited changes in heart rate and cardiac output by arousing a feeling of joyfulness; and Raginsky (3259) was able to induce symptoms of syncope and temporary cardiac arrest in a patient. Stokvis (3836) studied the effect of suggested muscular work, joy, pain, anger, and fear on blood pressure during hypnosis, by an automatic recording method: all sent the blood pressure up, but suggested muscular exercise was less effective than suggested emotional states; and, of the latter, pain and anger caused greater rises than joy and fear. Vasoconstrictor effects from suggested cold were observed by Talbert and co-workers (3902), using an arm plethysmograph. Bigelow and associates (337) noted greater changes in the peripheral pulse and finger volume during hypnosis, as did Uhlenbruck (4001). Schliffer (3685) tested the effect on blood pressure of injecting adrenalin during hypnosis. The effect was insignificant when compared to that obtained in the waking state (4–5 mm *versus* 24–58 mm). Suggestion of pain by Hadfield (1569) resulted in blisters appearing on the hypnotized subject's skin. Ullman (4006) produced a similar effect by suggesting a burn on the dorsum of a patient's hand.

Hypnosis reduced the plasma hydrocorticosterone level, but there was a significant difference between the sexes in response to the induction of anxiety (3160). An increase in oxygen consumption was observed in one subject by inducing anxiety (4195) but not by creating moods of elation or depression. Gastric hunger contractions were inhibited by feeding a fictitious meal to hypnotized subjects (2476). Peiper (3134) and Levine (2463) were able to elicit a marked GSR to the suggestion of a painful stimulus, but here, too, as in the case of plasma hydrocorticosterone level, there was reported to be a sex difference (3637).

According to Bass (243) and Brown (540), the knee jerk and other tendon reflexes, which usually disappear during sleep, remain undiminished in hypnosis, no matter how deep the stage. There is no change in auditory acuity (3579).

Williams (4223) obtained an increase in the work done by five subjects in hypnosis by appropriate positive suggestions, but Nevsky and Zrjacick (2992) were unable to increase muscular power by such means, although they were able to decrease it by suggestion. Mead and Roush (2759) could increase the strength of the arm but not of the hand. The suggestion of a shining light to a hypnotized person kept in a dark room abolished the EEG alpha pattern (365, 2559), but the reverse change could not be produced by suggesting darkness in the presence of light. Goldie and Green (1469) elicited a paradoxical EEG effect in a drowsy hypnotized subject—the alpha pattern appearing on opening his eyes. It will be recalled that similar paradoxical alphas may be seen in sleep-deprived subjects when they become drowsy (129), as well as in drowsy narcoleptics (815).

Platonov and Matzkevich (3213), having observed that hypnosis abolished the effects of acute alcoholic intoxication, gave two normal subjects several mental performance tests, first, while they were intoxicated, and later, after they had been hypnotized. The scores were much lower than normal after alcohol but returned to normal levels as a result of hypnosis. If the subjects were given intoxicating doses of alcohol while hypnotized, but were told they were drinking water, they showed no signs of intoxication in the posthypnotic state and performed at their normal levels.

Sears (3638) employed suggested anesthesia in one leg and reported weaker cardiac responses and GSRs to painful stimulation of the "anesthetic" leg. Doupe and associates (967) rendered one side of the body analgesic by hypnotic suggestion. Pinpricks then elicited a weaker vasoconstrictor response in an analgesic limb than in the "normal" one.

Erickson (1098) hypnotically induced color-blindness; Deely (870), however, showed that similar effects could be produced by suggestion without hypnosis. Pattie convinced himself of the genuineness of hypnotically induced deafness (3118), but questioned the nature of the anesthesia of the skin produced by the same method (3117).

Mental work, as well as learning and relearning lists of numbers, was not improved during the hypnotic trance over that prevailing in the waking state, according to Mitchell (2845) and Das (829).

The ability to evoke conditioned responses already established, and to develop new ones, has been tested by a number of investigators. Fisher (1200), working on the knee jerk, obtained negative results; but Nevsky and Levin (2993) could get conditioned secretory reflexes. Levin (2462), Pen and Jagarov (3142), and Traugott and Poworinsky (3965) found a relationship between the depth of the hypnosis and the persistence of the conditioned reflex. Levin observed also a marked dissociation between motor and secretory conditioned responses, the former persisting longer than the latter, as well as a difficulty in developing conditioned inhibitions. Pen and Jagarov obtained a depth of trance in which the reactions to verbal stimuli disappeared, but conditioned responses to direct stimuli were preserved.

Scott (3632) developed motor conditioned responses during hypnosis, as did Levin (2462) and Pen and Jagarov (3142); the latter pointed out that the hypnosis must be rather light in order to develop new conditioned reflexes, as well as to elicit old ones.

Some investigators (3142, 3632, 3965) evoked conditioned reflexes, established in the trance, during the succeeding waking state, although the subject showed complete posthypnotic amnesia. Scott emphasized this finding as proving that the amnesia was not really complete in hypnosis.

Subjects can also be put into a hypnotic trance by the conditioned-reflex method, as shown by Narbutovich (2972). In a certain room thirty-two patients were repeatedly hypnotized by verbal suggestion, during which they could hear the beat of a metronome. Then, in the absence of the hypnotizer, the sound of the metronome, or the setting of the room alone, was sufficient to induce hypnosis in the patients. Dehypnotization could also be conditioned. In some cases one metronome frequency could be made to produce hypnotic sleep, and another frequency, dehypnotization.

Wilson (4234) produced a suggestible state akin to hypnosis, without loss of consciousness but with complete analgesia, by the administration of proper mixtures of N_2O and air or oxygen. The exact proportions varied for different people, but in the author's own case this condition could be invoked through breathing a mixture of 60 per cent N_2O, 32 per cent air, and 8 per cent oxygen. When he inhaled a mixture of 80 per cent N_2O and 20 per cent oxygen, the suggestible state vanished, and with it the analgesia. Oxygen limitation seemed to be the prerequisite for inducing complete analgesia. Sumbajew (3864) employed a combination of different drugs with hypnosis, and he designated the resulting state as hypnarcosis or narcohypnosis, depending upon which of the two means was used first. Certain hypnotics, such as alcohol, chloral hydrate, morphine, and barbital, had a much stronger effect when used with hypnosis, while bromides did not. Through hypnosis he could destroy the sleep-inducing action of barbital or chloral hydrate and (as could Platonov and Matzkevich) antagonize the effect of alcohol.

Hypnotic age regression is a reversion to an early age, while under hypnosis, on the appropriate suggestion of the hypnotist (2121, 3986, 4291). Kupper (2310) was able to produce—as well as to stop—a convulsive seizure in a man of twenty-four, who started to have tonic and clonic convulsions at eighteen, by regressing him to the age of ten, when he had had an unhappy experience. Gidro-Frank and Bowersbuch (1439) obtained infantile plantar responses in two subjects whom they regressed to the age of a few months, and so did True and Stephenson (3987), although the latter did not note any EEG changes corresponding to the regressed age. Schwarz and associates (3628) reported no profound change in EEG during hypnotic age regression. Others (2742, 2785, 3034) likewise reported no effects of age regression on subjects' alpha frequency, though childish handwriting was achieved (3034). As a result, the question has been raised whether hypnotic age regression is not an artifact—a disorientation of the subject (2211), or a mere role-playing (3060, 4300).

Posthypnotic phenomena, including the induction of sleep and production of dreams, have engaged the attention of many investigators (1102). A subject of Thomson and associates (3931) was able to induce in himself, at will, trancelike states, similar to light sleep, with an appropriate EEG pattern. Dreaming during hypnotically caused sleep (2008, 2739, 3532, 3576, 3719, 3889, 3951) has been compared to natural dreaming and found to be similar (3532, 3719), or not quite so (2733). Klein (2173) reported that posthypnotic dreams lasted only about half a minute, and Welch (4159) found both time and space of induced hypnotic dreams to be greatly condensed. Using the REM-EEG technique, Stoyva (3840) confirmed earlier findings that persons could be made to dream on specific topics, with the unexpected addition that "when instructed to do so, certain subjects will dream on the suggested topic in every dream of the night." Stoyva's posthypnotic sleepers had shorter REM periods, though not to the extent of the very short dreaming episodes of the subjects of Klein and Welch. Schiff and co-workers (3559) not only observed REMs during posthypnotic dreaming but were able to associate the eye movements with the dream occurrences. Scantle-bury and collaborators (3532) noted that posthypnotic dreams, like ordinary ones, had an inhibitory effect on hunger contractions of the stomach.

Grassheim and Wittkower (1502), using twenty subjects in hypnotic trance, produced posthypnotic satiety, increased secretion of digestive juices, and a char-acteristic leukocytosis by suggesting the consumption of a meal during hypnosis but could not evoke a specific dynamic action by such fictitious feeding. Instead, they observed a fall in BMR amounting to 14 per cent. Marcus and Sahlgren (2664), after establishing that there was no change in blood sugar and that the individual responded normally to a sugar-tolerance test during the hypnotic trance, tried the effect of giving a sugar solution but suggesting to the subject that he was getting water. This suggestion did not affect the usual rise in blood sugar. However, they obtained a lesser than usual hyperglycemia upon the in-jection of adrenalin by suggesting that it was water; they also obtained a lesser hypoglycemia by injecting insulin and telling the subjects that they were inject-ing water (a drop of 10 mg per cent, instead of 29).

A posthypnotic effect on mental and physical efficiency was observed by Matz-kevich (2713) in a group of thirty-four adult subjects, normal and abnormal. The performance in a number of tests before and after hypnosis (or before and after a rest of similar duration, as a control) was determined. There was a marked improvement of efficiency after hypnosis, provided the experimenter was able to develop a state of euphoria in the subject by means of instructions given during the hypnosis.

Whether susceptible individuals can be induced to commit antisocial and criminal acts posthypnotically was discussed by several authors (214, 1097, 4155, 4164), and the conclusion was that such behavior was very unlikely. In this con-nection, it should be noted that the personality of the subject plays a part in determining the degree of hypnotic suggestibility that can be developed in him, even with his complete co-operation. Cannon (623) stated that extroverts could not be put into as deep a trance as introverts. According to Nachmansohn (2967), anyone can be brought into the light stages of hypnosis, but deepest somnam-bulistic trance can be induced only in individuals with certain constitutional characteristics. Biermann (334) indicated that differences in hypno-suggestibility are due to peculiarities of the subject's cortical dynamics and the mutual relation between cortex and subcortex, and that testing the reaction to hypnotism can be used to determine whether a person is normal or neurotic. Ananyev and Dubrovski (58), by means of the conditioned-reflex technique, worked out differences among their subjects, whom they divided into three groups and, apparently borrowing their terms from the Salpêtrière school, designated as (*a*) lethargics, who show inhibition predominantly; (*b*) somnambulists, rather excited; and (*c*) cataleptics, occupying an intermediate position.

Personality traits which govern hypnotic susceptibility were investigated by Davis and Husband (845) and by White (4190, 4191). The latter divided subjects into active ones, with tendencies toward deferential behavior, and passive ones. Motivation was emphasized by White (4193), as "no one can be hypnotized against his will." The attitude of the subject to the operator—amiability (1295), co-operation (1100, 1128), expectation (945), previously mentioned role-taking (3522), knowledge of what to do (3062)—may determine hypnotizability.

Hypnotism in the general practice of medicine and surgery has been discussed in several books (1101, 4264) and articles (691, 2704, 2806, 3196, 3819, 4129). The percentage of persons who can be hypnotized is estimated to vary from 85–90 (2704, 3819) all the way to 100 (4299), but a deep trance can be produced in a much smaller fraction of the population (2704, 4129, 4299). Anesthesia deep enough to permit surgery can be achieved in some 10–20 per cent. Consent of the patient is essential, though Oswald (3069) reported that a patient was rehypnotized despite her lack of co-operation. Hypnosis is useful in diagnostic procedures (1241, 3161, 3837, 3866), but its main employment is in the treatment of nervous and mental disorders (495, 4263). Thus, it has been possible to abolish or diminish the tremor of Parkinson's disease (560); restore vision in hysterical blindness (4006); stop an eighteen-year-old girl from chewing her bed-covers during sleep (763); cure enuresis (666, 4200); relieve neurotic (1190, 3573) and hysterical conditions (2520, 2521); and overcome sleep disturbances (763), most particularly insomnia (496, 957, 1084, 2916). Posthypnotic dreams have been analyzed both for diagnostic (2075) and therapeutic (493, 1138) purposes.

So much for hypnosis in man. But, since Athanasius Kircher performed his *experimentum mirabile* in the seventeenth century, many immobilization experiments have been made on animals which were said to be thus hypnotized. This animal hypnotism, induced or spontaneously developed, has also been known under the names of catalepsy and cataplexy, death-feigning and sham death, still reaction and immobilization reflex, rigidity and akinesis. It has been seen in many invertebrates and vertebrates. In the former the condition is hard to distinguish from sleep. According to Hoffmann (1813), natural sleep of certain insects is characterized by a waxy condition and complete anesthesia. Steiniger (3800) also differentiated between hypnosis in vertebrates and catalepsy in invertebrates. Babák (167) considered immobilization effects in fishes as hypnosis, and so did Reisinger (3309) in birds. Pavlov and Petrova (3129, 3130) claimed to have observed the finest shades of hypnosis in dogs, as a result of repeated application of one and the same conditioned stimulus. They went into great detail concerning the dissociation phenomena, responses to weak but not to strong stimuli, etc. On the other hand, Sumbajew (3864) held that hypnosis in dogs differed from that in human beings, because dogs reacted differently from people to NaBr.

Producing the hypnotic state in hens and rabbits, Rijlant (3352) could decrease or abolish the action potentials of the skeletal musculature by varying the depth of hypnosis. Bonnet and Saboul (402) studied the reflex responses of the frog after immobilization by fitting a rubber ring behind its jaws. They obtained evidence of a depression in the central parts of the reflex arc in this condition. Hoagland (1786), in investigating the mechanism of tonic immobility in a species of lizards, came to the conclusion that epinephrine was excreted in excess in this animal following immobilization.

Among more recent studies of animal hypnosis, using EEG recordings, Gerebtzoff (1403) found that, in the rabbit, cataleptic immobility by fascination (approaching bright object to animal's eyes) was accompanied by slow waves; and hypnosis by turning the animal over on its back, by fast waves. Similar results were obtained by him on EI cats. Other investigators pointed out the similarity between the hypnotic EEG and that of drowsiness (3627) or sleep (3697). Liberson (2510) could prolong the immobility of guinea pigs by repeated daily hypnotization. Svorad (3881–83), working on rabbits, found that the EEG pattern of hypnosis was identical with that of sleep, and that the EEG changes from stimuli abolishing the hypnosis were the same as those accompanying the arousal from sleep. He considered animal hypnosis to be "a paroxysmally initiated central inhibition, which originates in the subcortical regions of the brain and from there spreads to the cerebral hemispheres."

The literature on hypnotism is extensive. In addition to monographs by Lecron and Bordeaux (2397), Weitzenhoffer (4156), Gill and Brenman (1445), and the collected papers, edited by LeCron (2396) and Kuhn and Russo (2299), there are numerous general reviews and discussions (40, 284, 699, 760, 1489, 1665, 2296, 3212, 3643, 3825, 4301). Concerning the nature of hypnosis, one should mention the old view of Brown-Séquard (543), seconded by Pavlov (3123) and others (335, 828, 2241, 2244, 3875), that hypnosis is simply a matter of cortical inhibition. Arnold (133, 134) held that in the decision to co-operate with the hypnotist, there occurred in the subject "an inhibition of every other action impulse" (134). Others saw in hypnosis a return to a more primitive level of mental activity (2760, 3575); a similarity with schizophrenia (2160, 3125); or a "controlled dissociated state" (4179). At the other extreme is the view of Bernheim (316) that all the phenomena of hypnosis can be produced in wakeful susceptible individuals. In a series of papers Barber (208–13) adheres to the thesis that hypnosis is not a state of consciousness, but merely "a descriptive abstraction referring to an interpersonal relationship" (208) requiring "only appropriately predisposed persons" (212). Barber thinks that the analgesic effect of hypnotic suggestion is that of a placebo. Glass and Barber (1456) have tested the hypothesis and concluded that "a placebo administered by a physician as a 'hypnosis-producing' drug is as effective as a formal 20-minute procedure in enhancing 'suggestibility.' " That simple suggestion may be as effective as instructions under hypnosis was also reported by others (870, 1570, 2958).

What is the relation of hypnosis to normal sleep? There are two definite trends toward and away from the notion that sleep and hypnosis are identical, with some authors occupying an intermediate position. In his review, Schultz (3603) was inclined to look for a common mechanism for these two states. The views of Pavlov (3121) on this topic are well known. He considered hypnosis as an inhibition limited to usually active points in special areas of the cerebral cortex, and sleep as generalized inhibition involving the whole cortex. Thus, sleep and hypnosis and central inhibition are all identical, varying only in extent. Biermann (333) defined human hypnosis as "a partial conditioned-reflex sleep" but stated that, whereas sleep involves a diffusion of inhibition throughout the cortex, hypnosis requires the maintenance of a waking point which serves to insure a rapport between the subject and the hypnotist. Thooris (3933) accepted Pavlov's views *in toto,* and so did Mishchenko (2842).

On the other hand, in examining the view of hypnosis as partial sleep, Nachmansohn (2967) decided that they were not identical, since hypnosis, unlike sleep, does not involve an assimilatory metabolic phase and has no regulatory function in the body. Pilcz (3196) pointed out that awakening from hypnosis requires suggestion, as opposed to the spontaneous awakening from normal sleep. Coriat (758), in studying muscular tonus and relaxation as related to sleep, found that hypnotized persons behaved like waking subjects. Bass (243), comparing the two states, concluded that "sleep is not hypnosis and that hypnosis is neither a suggested sleep nor a modified sleep nor anything between sleep and the normal waking state." That hypnosis is not sleep is also the opinion of Heimann (1682), Walter (4110), and Barber (212). Koster (2249), however, considered hypnosis a special sleeping condition; Bellak (281), that it was similar to the process of falling asleep; and Brenman (494), that it was like sleep psychologically but perhaps not physiologically. Fujisawa and Obonai (1319) distinguished two stages of hypnotic sleep, different in EEG terms, and also with respect to EKG, GSR, and patellar reflex. Stage II is like natural sleep. Barber (205–7) compared the behavior of subjects when lightly asleep and when hypnotized and found that those "who were most suggestible when awake were also the most suggestible during the sleep experiment" (207). With respect to the hypnotic state itself, Barber (212) failed to find a physiological index which could differentiate it from the waking state.

Whether animal hypnosis is analogous to human hypnosis is not clear. Nor is it helpful to throw together such heterogeneous phenomena as the state induced in dogs by conditioned stimuli, sham death evoked by sudden fright, and normal sleep in animals produced by gentle restraint. Hoffmann (1813) pointed out that, whereas sleep is produced by a decrease in external stimuli, just the opposite is true of so-called reflex immobilization. In the opinion of Coriat (759), although many animals become motionless in response to a frightening stimulus, these reactions do not have "the biological importance of sleep." However, Byrne (598) attempted to prove that the still reaction and physiological sleep are closely related to each other. The still reaction is evokable in all animals. In birds and mammals it is associated with an acute consciousness of the situation and is perhaps a voluntary act. Death-feigning is a lower form of the still reaction and corresponds to a primitive form of sleep, as distinguished from a more advanced form in higher animals and in man. According to Byrne, "the purposivity of the still reaction and that of sleep are identical, viz., the maintenance or refitting of the organism for the adequate performance of the dynamic functions," and "sleep may be considered as a specialization of the still reaction."

What is known of human and animal hypnosis indicates that it is a state of hyperexcitability which by appropriate means can be lowered so much as to change it into a depression resembling sleep or narcosis. It sometimes passes into real sleep, thus creating confusion concerning the relation of these states to each other.

Part 8

Theories of Sleep

Chapter 33

Neural Theories of Sleep

Many theories have been proposed from time to time to account for the alternation of sleep and wakefulness. A theory may be a working hypothesis, predicting the results of future investigations and susceptible of experimental verification; or it may be "a scheme of things," based upon existing information and the imagination of the author. In either case, the theory must be in agreement with known facts and formulated in understandable terms in order to be acceptable.

Piéron (3192) discussed the theories of sleep proposed up to 1912, and with respect to these older theories I shall limit myself to brief statements of their salient points and to critical objections offered to them, for both of which I shall draw freely on the material presented by Piéron.

Theories of sleep that attempt to account for the existence of the sleep-wakefulness cycle itself, for the necessity of sleep, were designated by Piéron as complete theories; and those explaining not why one sleeps but how one falls asleep, partial theories. Authors of partial theories are often content to elucidate the mechanism of the change from wakefulness to sleep, but disregard the reverse process of awakening. Complete theories, explaining why one sleeps, more frequently also explain why the sleeper awakens, or, in general, the alternation of the two phases. Complete theories usually also account for the "how," or the onset of sleep, sometimes borrowing the mechanism of some partial theory. Structural elements characterize the different theories as complex and simple, multiple factor and single factor, polygenic and monogenic. Depending upon the mechanism invoked, the theories may also be designated as neural, humoral, or a combination of the two; and "biological," or an instinct involving the activity of the organism as a whole.

Since newly discovered facts render previously accepted alleged facts obsolete, the theories based on the latter are mentioned here only for their historical interest or for their amusing aspects. The oldest theories pertain to a shifting of the blood, their authors postulating either a congestion or an anemia of one part of the body or another, usually the brain. These theories date back to the period when the brain was not suspected of being an organ of analysis and integration of incoming and outgoing impulses, respectively. Piéron credited the Croton physician, Alcmeon, a contemporary of Pythagoras, who lived in the sixth century b.c., with the first theory of sleep on record. Sleep, according to Alcmeon, is due to a retreat of the blood into the veins, and awakening to venous disgorgement; this statement was as often interpreted as signifying that sleep is due to anemia as that it is caused by venous congestion.

Aristotle (125) considered sleep a necessity, related to the activity of the heart from which "both motion and sense-perception originate." He envisaged sleep as arising from

> the evaporation attendant upon the process of nutrition. The matter evaporated must be driven onwards to a certain point, then turn back, and change its current to and fro, like a tide-race in a narrow strait. Now, in every animal the hot naturally tends to move upward. . . . This explains why fits of drowsiness are especially apt to come on after meals; for the matter, both the liquid and the corporeal, which is borne upwards in a mass, is then of considerable quantity. . . . It also follows certain forms of fatigue; for fatigue operates as a solvent, and the dissolved matter acts, if not cold, like food prior to digestion. . . . Extreme youth also has this effect; infants, for example, sleep a great deal, because of the food being borne upwards—a mark whereof appears in the disproportionately large size of the upper parts compared to the lower during infancy. . . .

It can be seen that Aristotle did not merely offer an explanation of sleep but tried to show how it fitted even then well-known facts, such as the tendency to sleep after a heavy meal or when one is fatigued, and the preponderance of sleep in the existence of the infant. One can only hope that current explanations will appear a little less fantastic to readers who may come upon them 2,300 years from now.

With a better understanding of the circulation and of the functions of the brain, vascular theories, ascribing sleep to either congestion (Willis, Morgagni) or anemia (Blumenbach) of the brain, came into their own. Piéron mentioned Donders, Kussmaul and Tenner, Durham, Hammond, and others, but Mosso was undoubtedly the most prominent advocate of the cerebral anemia theory of sleep, followed by Hill and by Howell (1846), who attributed the anemia of the brain to splanchnic and cutaneous vasodilatation, respectively. Brodmann (519), and later Shepard (3677), demonstrated the development of a plethora, instead of an anemia, of the brain during sleep, and Mangold and associates (2649) found that sleep led to a statistically significant increase in cerebral blood flow.

The oldest group of partial theories might be called humoral, although not in the modern endocrine sense of the term. With the development of knowledge concerning the existence of vasomotor nerves, these theories appear to be oriented toward the neural, rather than humoral, classification. Another group of partial theories, more strictly neural, gained considerable popularity in the nineties of the last century. They pertained to histological changes in the neurones of the cerebral cortex as the cause of the onset of sleep. Duval (1012) suggested that the dendrites of cortical cells could be retracted by a sort of ameboid movement, thus breaking the contacts between neighboring neurones. Powerful afferent impulses allegedly led to an elongation of the dendrites and to re-establishment of the broken contacts, resulting in awakening. Lépine (2436) claimed priority for the dendrite retraction idea, as he had written on that topic six months before Duval. There were several variants of the dendritic theory, among them the idea of Legendre (2401) that vacuolization of dendrites led to the retraction of the nerve cell, and the modification, made by Cajal, who suggested that the neuroglia cells might be endowed with ameboid motion and by the movements of their pseudopodia separate adjacent neurones. Aside from the inability of several authors to substantiate the existence of ameboid movement in either neurones or neuroglia cells, nothing was heard about these dendritic theories till 1956, when Purpura (3250), from observations on unanesthetized paralyzed cats, concluded that there was an indication that "high frequency stimulation of the ascending bulbar reticular system alters synaptic activity of cortical dendrites." By Purpura's scheme, "persisting dendritic inhibition resulting from reticulo-cortical synaptic excitation is believed to underlie the alternation in electrocortical activity associated with behavioral arousal."

A different group of neural theories, the inhibitory, which appeared earlier than the dendritic, is still current. The first proposal of an inhibitory theory of sleep was made by Brown-Séquard (543) in 1889 (although there were vague proposals earlier). The onset of sleep, accompanied as it is by closure of the eyelids and changed position of the eyes, appeared to Brown-Séquard to be an inhibitory reflex. Because decerebrated pigeons sleep, he postulated the center of this reflex to be in the base of the brain, without indicating the source of the afferent impulses responsible for the liberation of the sleep reflex. Like the dendritic theories, the inhibitory theories had nothing factual in their favor, but they apparently appealed to, and were adopted by, a number of subsequent workers, sometimes as a link in a complete theory, to account for the mere onset of sleep. The greater popularity of the inhibitory theories was probably due to their being considered more "physiological" than were the histological theories. Further, each author could have his own idea of how the inhibition performed its task.

Shepard (3677), who was instrumental in demolishing the anemia theory of sleep, proposed an inhibitory theory of his own. On the basis of introspective analysis, he concluded that "as we go to sleep we become absorbed in a mass or complex of fatigue sensations. These tend strongly to inhibit other processes, especially motor activity and consciousness of strain sensations from the muscles."

The chief exponent of the inhibitory nature of the onset of sleep was Pavlov

(3122–28), who concluded from the study of conditioned reflexes that cortical inhibition was localized sleep and that sleep was due to widespread cortical inhibition. This sleep by cortical inhibition was usually brief, a few seconds to a few minutes. Its termination, like its onset, was often very sudden. That abrupt change suggests more a condition of animal hypnosis than of physiological sleep. Here is a description of the behavior of a dog, subjected to the action of a "delayed" conditioned stimulus—a stimulus acting continuously for the duration of the "delay" between its beginning and the application of the unconditioned stimulus—as such conditioned stimuli were said by Pavlov to be particularly effective in producing sleep during the "delay" (3124, p. 261):

> It sometimes happens that the reverse, namely a pure replacement of inhibition by sleep, is obtained with the long delay of 3 minutes, or even with delays so short as 30 seconds. The animal, which has previously kept fully alert in its stand during the experiment, now falls asleep, each time exactly at the beginning of the action of the conditioned stimulus. The eyes close, the head droops, the whole body relaxes and hangs on the loops of the stand, and the animal emits an occasional snore. After a lapse of a definite period of time—in the short delay 25 seconds or in the case of the long delay 1½–2 minutes—the animal quickly and spontaneously awakens and exhibits a sharp alimentary motor and salivary reaction. It is clear that in this case an inhibition which is generally concentrated becomes replaced by diffused inhibition, i.e. sleep.

What maintains the alleged inhibition for a definite and rather short period of time? If inhibition is a result of exhaustion, why does it set in all of a sudden, at the exact moment of the beginning of the conditioned stimulation? Is the short interval of sleep sufficient to produce a recovery of the cells from the sudden functional exhaustion? One could go on asking such questions, but, instead, a phenomenon should be mentioned that was seen not only by Pavlov and his co-workers but by many others who had occasion to note the behavior of dogs placed in a stand for observation. Such animals usually fall asleep, particularly if they are subjected to the action of a monotonous sound or, as in Pavlov's laboratory, are kept in a soundproof chamber. The production of sleep under such circumstances has already been touched upon and has nothing to do with conditioned inhibition or any other conditioned phenomenon. I should perhaps mention again that we (2180) observed dogs fall asleep while they were "conditionally" secreting saliva, and sleep in these cases entailed a cessation of the conditioned salivation rather than developed as a result of such a cessation.

Pavlov's views of the nature of sleep onset won many adherents (37, 72, 597, 661, 1031, 1275, 1888, 1925, 2057, 2058, 2079, 2087, 2391, 2448, 2454, 2455, 2460, 2685, 2975, 3070, 3230, 3282, 3398, 3432, 3463, 3933, 4004), who usually left the burden of proof to the master, limiting themselves to the acceptance of his theory. Pavlov started with the intention of dealing in physiological facts, shunning the psychologist's analysis and formulation of results, but ended by spinning a complex web of terms created *ad hoc*, such as external and internal inhibition, inhibitory after-effect, positive and negative induction, irradiation and concentration of excitation and inhibition.

A distinct "personality cult" is revealed in the attitude to Pavlov of some of his disciples. Statements like "many scientists attempted to explain the essence of sleep, but only the prominent Russian scientist I. P. Pavlov succeeded" (4004) or "until Pavlov there was no physiology of sleep, as there was, in general, no 'real' physiology of the cerebral cortex" (3230) are not uncommon. The extreme of chauvinism was shown by the editors of the volume of articles on sleep compiled by Bogorad (392) who declared in their introduction:

> The forthcoming compilation will contain only works which throw light on the sleep problem from the position of the teachings of I. P. Pavlov concerning higher nervous activity. Works treating sleep from another point of view, propounding different theories of sleep, stemming mainly from foreign [beyond-the-border] scientists, are not included in this compilation. The editors find that, making this type of selection, the compiler has acted correctly. Among the more widely disseminated theories of sleep proposed by foreign bourgeois scientists, it is necessary to point to (1) the theory of a subcortical sleep center . . . (2) toxemic theory of sleep . . . (3) endocrine theory. . . . These as well as many other theories of sleep, proposed by foreign scientists, can in no way stand up to the many-sided teachings concerning sleep developed by I. P. Pavlov. Inclusion of the works of these authors, as well as of others who treat sleep not from the Pavlovian positions, would deprive this compilation of its harmoniousness and structural sequence, would correspond to the harmful tendency of combining eclectically the teachings of Pavlov concerning sleep with any one of the enumerated theories. This attitude does not mean, however, that the critical attitude toward the theories of sleep, proposed by foreign scientists, should entail a disregard of those facts which might serve as a basis for any one of these theories. On the contrary, it is very important to juxtapose to the incorrect interpretation of the particular facts, on which these theories are based, the proper correct explanation leaning on the teaching of I. P. Pavlov concerning sleep. This method of criticism one must recognize as most correct and that is just what I. P. Pavlov did. . . .

> The division dealing with the physiological mechanisms of dreams includes . . . a small number of papers. A series of investigations by Soviet clinicians (M. I. Astvatsaturov, A. M. Grinstein, and others) representing a certain value, as regards the factual findings, were not included in this compilation, however, because the authors of these papers in their totality throw light on the problem of dreams not from the positions of Pavlovian teachings.

In December, 1935, shortly before he died, Pavlov gave his definitive views on the various aspects of the sleep problem in a lecture (3128) which he prefaced by stating that "for such an important scientific problem as sleep . . . my view is not without a certain significance as I and my collaborators have been thinking of the phenomenon of sleep for 35 years." Recognizing that the idea of a subcortical sleep center rivaled his own notion that sleep originates in the "cerebral hemispheres," Pavlov declared that such an idea was too crude, "the existence of a special center of sleep being 'out of the question.' In my opinion, the crude idea that there is a special group of cells which produces sleep, while another group produces wakefulness, is physiologically contradictory. When we see sleep in every cell, why speak about some special group of cells which produces sleep? Once a cell is there, it creates an inhibitory state, and the latter, by irradiation, creates a state of inactivity in neighboring cells, and when the inhibition spreads farther, it causes sleep." To a member of the audience who wondered why such an important function as sleep should not have a center, Pavlov repeated: "It is very simple. Inhibition and sleep exist in every cell. Why then should there be a special group of cells?" Asked to explain the regular succession of sleep and wakefulness, Pavlov replied: "It is clear that our daytime work represents the sum total of excitations which entail a certain amount of exhaustion, and the latter, carried to a certain point, calls forth automatically, by an internal humoral means, the condition of inhibition, accompanied by sleep." How did he account for the sleep of dogs following decortication? "It is clear that since sleep is a widespread inhibition, and this inhibition spreads through the nervous system to the lower end of the spinal cord, then as long as there is a central system and a nerve fiber, there must also be inhibition. If there are no big hemispheres (cerebral cortex) why can there not be inhibition in the lower parts of the CNS, now concentrated, now irradiated?" Pavlov explained dreaming by invoking "a new fact," positive induction: "When one point becomes inhibited, another point enters into the reverse —an excitatory state. If one admits this, i.e., assumes positive induction, it makes the fact of dreaming particularly clear." Thus, from cortical inhibition Pavlov changed in the direction of an inhibition involving the entire nervous system, and from generalized inhibition he passed to inhibition here and excitation there. The final departure from his original stand came when Pavlov admitted the possible existence of two kinds of sleep: "One sleep is passive, resulting from a falling off of the mass of stimuli usually arriving in the large hemispheres, and another, active sleep, as I envisage it, is an inhibitory process, because an inhibitory process must, of course, be regarded as an active process, and not as a state of inactivity." Like Humpty Dumpty in *Through the Looking-Glass*, Pavlov, in effect, said, "When *I* use a word, it means just what I choose it to mean."

Piéron (3193) doubted whether the investigations and theoretical views of Pavlov were essential contributions to the clarification of the process of inhibition which is presumably involved in the onset of sleep. So did Nachmansohn (2965), and Liddell and co-workers (2515), who, from results obtained in conditioned responses of sheep, "failed to support Pavlov's conception of sleep as summation and irradiation of internal inhibition." Roger and Gastaut (3385) refused to accept Pavlov's idea of intracortical connections, or cortico-cortical bonds across the cerebral cortex. Severe criticism of Pavlov's notion of the spread of inhibition was also expressed by Hilgard and Marquis (1768). A complete refutation of Pavlov's theory came from factual data on the spontaneous and evoked discharges of individual subcortical and cortical neurones. Huttenlocher (1884) found that a majority of 77 single units in the BSRF and superior colliculi of the cat showed more spontaneous activity during both LVFA and HVSA sleep than in wakefulness. Evarts and associates (1120) confirmed this finding not only for the BSRF, but also for the visual cortex, and Evarts (1119) concluded that LVFA sleep, "which is the deepest stage of sleep in the cat, is not associated with generalized inhibition of cortical activity, but . . . on the contrary . . . with high rates of discharge of the visual cortex neurons." Fleming and co-workers (1209), studying cortical responses to lateral geniculate stimulation in the cat, noted that the excitability of the visual cortex was increased during sleep, and Evarts (1117), observing photically evoked responses in man, determined that "the shortest latency deflections did not change significantly with the onset of sleep."

Into an entirely different category fall the partial theories which account for the onset of sleep by the supposition that there is an interruption in the afferent pathways to the cerebral cortex, or a cortical deafferentation. Purkinje, writing in Wagner's *Handwörterbuch der Physiologie*, in 1846, proposed a theory, which, in a sense, is also a vasomotor theory, Piéron (3192) referring to it as a "congestive" one. It postulated that the onset of sleep was due to a hyperemia of the basal nuclei, resulting in a compression of the corona radiata, which contains the thalamocortical tracts. As the thalamus is the last cell station of the afferent pathway to the cortex, the interruption of communication between the thalamus and the cortex should deprive the latter of sensory impulses and produce sleep. In 1849, Osborne offered "some considerations to prove that the choroid plexus is the organ of sleep," which was presumably accomplished through a swelling of the plexus and distention of the ventricles, thus mechanically blocking the corticopetal impulses. In 1890, Mauthner (2717), on the basis of his clinical observations, as well as pathological findings in cases of encephalitis lethargica, proposed the theory that

> sleep is to be considered as a fatigue phenomenon of the periventricular gray. Through temporary cessation of function of the central gray there occurs a break in the conducting pathways to and from the cerebral cortex. Therefore sensory stimulations do not reach consciousness, even though the sensory

organs, on the one hand, and the cerebral cortex [dreaming], on the other, have not lost their activity. In the same way, the motor centers may be stimulated during dreams, but, because of a break in conduction in the central gray, no movements are produced, even though the peripheral nerves are capable of conducting.

In 1916, Dana (818), discussing several cases of morbid somnolence, came to the conclusion that in sleep there might be a blocking of the sensory inflow and of many association paths; also that drowsiness might be due to "pressure on great sensory stations, like the optic thalami." Lignac (2516) made a similar inference from the study of a case of a thalamic tumor and internal hydrocephalus. Jelliffe (1975), discussing third-ventricle tumors, and Pick (3177), analyzing the action of hypnotics, postulated the necessity of an afferent functional block at the level of the thalamus for the onset of sleep. But it is mainly because of the striking results of Bremer (474–77) that in a sense functional deafferentation of the cortex during sleep may be considered established. It will be recalled (p. 205) that Bremer could obtain the same EEG patterns in the cat's cerebral cortex, after "isolating" it by cutting through the brain stem just behind the origin of the third nerves, as those which prevailed during sleep. That finding suggested to him that in normal sleep, by some mechanism, the cortex becomes deafferented. Adrian (24) came to the same conclusion from a study of the EEG of monkeys subjected to dial anesthesia.

On the efferent side, indirect evidence of a functional, easily reversible, block between the cortex and the subcortical regions is afforded by the presence of the big-toe extension phenomenon, or positive Babinski sign, in deep sleep. As pointed out (p. 16), the phenomenon itself was observed in sleep much earlier than its pathological significance was elucidated by Babinski. It was shown (2176) that during sleep the positive Babinski sign could easily be converted into a negative one by scratching the sole of the foot at frequent enough intervals, and Tournay (3960) described its spontaneous reversal during the alternate phases of Cheyne-Stokes breathing. More striking was the finding of Gibbs and Gibbs (1419) that epileptics showed seizure discharges in their sleep without overt convulsions, but "if the patient is roused from sleep during a subclinical grand mal discharge, a clinical grand mal seizure supervenes, suggesting that during sleep the cortex is de-efferented."

A possible mechanism for the functional break—both motor and sensory—between the brain and periphery was suggested by Chauchard (682–86) on the basis of chronaximetric studies (pp. 14, 73). The constitutional chronaxies of cortical neurones, it will be recalled, are very long; of the peripheral neurones, very short. A center of subordination in the red nucleus produces an isochronism, with both chronaxies even shorter than the constitutional one of peripheral neurones. During drowsiness there is a gradual increase of both chronaxies, with the isochronism preserved, but at the onset of sleep heterochronism sets in, the cortical chronaxies continuing to rise in proportion to the depth of sleep; the chronaxies of the peripheral neurones, however, drop abruptly, reaching and remaining at their low constitutional values. According to Chauchard (685), "in putting into play the center of subordination, stimuli from the external environment, or from the body itself, maintain wakefulness, whereas deafferentation stops the subordination and creates chronaxic conditions of sleep."

Another theory that would fit into the humoral group as easily as into the neural one is the biological theory, first advanced by Claparède in 1905, according to which sleep is an "instinct." This theory has nearly as many adherents as Pavlov's cortical inhibition theory. It is a complete theory, by Piéron's classification, since it purports to explain why one sleeps, and is definitely "a scheme of things," based on imagination rather than on a working hypothesis susceptible of experimental testing. Claparède (705–10) considered sleep not a passive but an active function, protective in character, in that it prevents possible intoxication or exhaustion from continued wakefulness. "We sleep not because we are intoxicated or exhausted, but in order to prevent our becoming intoxicated or exhausted." Sleep is achieved by the active interest and will of the animal, obeying the "law of momentary interest," which can be formulated thus: "At each moment the instinct which is of greatest importance predominates over the other instincts." Sleep, according to Claparède, results from a loss of interest in the environment (*réaction de désintérêt*), and one wakes up because one becomes tired of sleeping. In the meantime, there has been a restoration of the organism through rest. One has thus done something positive to avoid eventual breakdown from autointoxication or exhaustion. As a mechanism for the onset of sleep, Claparède postulated a general inhibition of reactivity, which is the best that can happen to the organism at the time, when there is nothing of interest going on. And then, just as one stops eating when one has had enough to eat, one wakes up because one has had enough sleep. Of course, stating that one eats in order not to starve to death, or breathes in order not to die of asphyxia, tells nothing concerning the mechanism of hunger or of respiration.

Sleep was also looked upon as an instinct, or an essential biological reaction, by several other authors (48, 578, 614, 1083, 1783, 3498, 3978, 4152, 4318). Ley (2483) declared that there is a dynamogenic element, a particular activity, in sleep, rather than a simple diminution or cessation of psychic activity. Legendre (2402) held that sleep is an absolute necessity—"a function of a vital principle alternating with being awake." Bechterev (268) regarded sleep "as a kind of defensive or protective reflex inhibitory in character—a reflex which has been biologically evolved for the purpose of protecting the brain from further poisoning by the products of metabolism, and which may be evoked as an association reflex, under conditions of fatigue." Murray (2954), from observations of the behavior of, and the conflicts developed in, sleep-deprived subjects, concluded that "sleep may be construed as a physiological drive with a number of learned components." It may be said of all the different biological theories that they emphasize the usefulness of sleep and account for it in general terms of protective instincts or reactions without an adequate explanation of the mechanism underlying the alternation of sleep and wakefulness.

Chapter 34

Humoral Theories of Sleep

The common feature that characterizes humoral theories of sleep is the production and accumulation of certain substances, usually end-products of metabolism, either in the tissues, in general, or in certain organs, such as the brain. When a definite concentration of such substances has been reached, the activity of the brain is depressed either directly, or through indirect influences, like vasoconstriction or asphyxia. The gradual removal of these substances during sleep leads to a return to the waking state.

Piéron (3192) listed a number of such theories. Preyer thought that the accumulation of lactic acid led to its taking up the available oxygen supply of the blood, thus causing a cerebral asphyxia and making it impossible to maintain the waking state. Brissemoret and Joanin (502) ascribed the onset of sleep to the accumulation of cholesterol, as the latter, in certain concentrations, produced narcosis in guinea pigs. Marchand (2659) found no somniferous effects from cholesterol. Dubois (1000) developed the theory (or rather theories) of CO_2 autonarcosis, according to which CO_2 accumulates in sufficient quantities to slow up the oxidative processes of the nervous system, producing sleep; CO_2 goes on accumulating during sleep, and, having reached a higher concentration, causes awakening. His three successive theories have been summarized by Piéron as follows: (*a*) there is only one sleep center, which is excited by a certain concentration of CO_2, producing sleep, and paralyzed by a higher concentration, causing awakening; (*b*) there are two centers, one of sleep, the other of awakening, and a certain concentration of CO_2 stimulates the former, while a higher concentration stimulates the latter; (*c*) there is a center of wakefulness which is paralyzed by a certain concentration of CO_2 and stimulated by a higher one. How the high level of CO_2 at the time of awakening is brought down again so that it can begin to accumulate toward the concentration needed to produce sleep once more was not explained. Legendre and Piéron (2407) could detect no change in the CO_2 content of the blood of dogs deprived of sleep for several days, destroying the basis of the CO_2 theory of sleep. As a variant of this theory, Straub (3844) suggested that the accumulation of CO_2

is responsible for a number of phenomena accompanying sleep. Wuth (4282) accepted Straub's view concerning the role of CO_2 in sleep and attributed the so-called acidosis of sleep to a lowering of the irritability of the respiratory center. Amsler (56) wrote of acidosis of sleep and alkalosis of the waking state.

Errera (1105) postulated the accumulation of toxic products, "leucomaines," as responsible for sleep through their depressing effects on the nervous tissues. Bouchard (425) ascribed sleep to "urotoxins," having observed that daytime urines had narcotic properties, and that night urines, on the contrary, were convulsive. Litwer (2539, 2540) showed the baselessness of Bouchard's contention. Trew and Fischer (3973) found that urinary glycine content was higher at night than in the daytime and related this finding to a possible faulty detoxication connected with the 24-hour rhythm.

Legendre and Piéron (2402–13), having obtained what they called "hypnotoxin" (p. 203) from animals kept awake for a long time, did not attribute the onset of sleep to the direct action of hypnotoxin but to an inhibition of the CNS, the hypnotoxin thus acting as an accessory influence. Piéron (3193) expressly repudiated the view often attributed to him that normal sleep was due to the action of a toxin but stated that hypnotoxin releases an inhibitory process which is responsible for the onset of sleep.

Cabitto (600) postulated the existence of fatigue toxins, although he admitted the contribution of a nervous factor in the production of sleep. Economo (1035) also emphasized the role of alleged fatigue substances in the sleep function. Kroll (2287, 2288) not only extracted a "sleep substance" from the brains of rabbits put to sleep by a variety of means, but also found a different kind of substance in the brains of waking animals. Thus, according to Kroll, the brain produces two kinds of substances during the two states of sleep and wakefulness.

Bancroft and Rutzler (198, 199) advanced a theory that "sleep must be due in part to a reversible agglomeration of some proteins in the centers of consciousness." They did not know "what the agglomerating substance or group of substances is." They called it X, while another substance that accumulated during sleep they called Y. "A peptizing agent, such as sodium rhodanate, will decrease this irritability (of the sensory nerves) and make sleep possible though not causing it. A larger dose of the peptizing agents may act also on the centers of consciousness and thereby prevent sleep." Psychosis, according to Bancroft and Rutzler, "is due unquestionably to an overdispersed state," and if persons suffering from a psychosis nevertheless sleep normally, "one portion of the brain must be over-agglomerated at times, even though another portion is overdispersed." Henderson's comment (1699) on Bancroft's theory of sleep and insanity was that "the claims made on such a slender foundation and with such inadequate knowledge of physiology, pharmacology and other fundamental sciences, might be ignored were not the author so eminent a chemist."

Cloetta (721), as indicated (p. 35), attributed sleep to a shift of calcium ions from the blood into the tissues, among others, the infundibular portion of the hypothalamus, and his theory has been accepted, with some modifications, by other investigators (195, 2932, 3322, 3815). The decrease in blood calcium is supposed to be due to a passage of calcium into the tissues, but in hypoparathyroidism the low blood calcium is interpreted to reflect a low tissue calcium. Which is the correct interpretation? Obviously the second one, as by parathormone one can raise the blood-calcium concentration and at the same time increase the tissue-fluid calcium (referring, of course, to the soft tissues of the body). Furthermore, it was conclusively shown by Cooperman (p. 36) that the ionizable calcium is not decreased but may actually be somewhat increased during sleep, and the ionizable calcium is the only portion that can pass in and out of the blood stream. There is thus no factual or theoretical basis for Cloetta's calcium theory of sleep.

Stern (3811, 3812), it may be recalled (p. 217), ascribed the onset of sleep to changes in the permeability of the blood–cerebrospinal-fluid barrier and in the composition of the cerebrospinal fluid. Mueller (2918, 2919) advanced the idea that the secretion of cerebrospinal fluid into the third ventricle induced sleep by an increase in intraventricular pressure and that the reabsorption of the fluid led to awakening. Gans (1353, 1354), discussing a "third circulation," offered a working hypothesis that sleep influences the flow of the cerebrospinal fluid so that it passes from the ventricles to the subarachnoid spaces, entirely or partly, by a transcerebral route, bringing nourishment (glucose) to, and removing waste products (neurotoxins) from, the brain cells. Friede (1291) assumed that sleep is produced by the release of a stimulating substance into the cerebrospinal fluid.

Kalter and Katzenstein (2066) suggested that sleep may be due to the action of products of intermediary metabolism, such as alcohol and ureides. Dienst and Winter (935), like Amsler (56), supposed that "through metabolic activity of the organism there occur shifts in the acid-base equilibrium which result in a tonus change of the autonomic system which, in turn, activates the sleep center" to cause the onset of sleep. Mueller (2928) discussed the possibility that cerebral cortical cells are charged with "bioelectric energies" during sleep, and McCormick (2741) thought that sleep led to a replenishment of the B1 reserves of brain cells.

The general criticism of toxin or metabolic waste-product theories is that they do not explain why a certain concentration of the alleged sleep-producing substances at one time results in sleep; at another, in wakefulness. The same individual, in an equal state of intoxication, may sleep or remain awake, according to external or internal circumstances. Newborn infants, who are relatively inactive, sleep the greater part of the time. The adherents of such theories point out that even bona fide hypnotics produce sleep only when conditions are favorable, and that neonates have such a low resistance to the action of hypnogenic substances that they cannot remain awake for any length of time. By the same reasoning, the behavior of parabiotic "monsters," infants with two heads and a common body and, of course, a common circulation, can be used as an argument against toxic theories. Such an infant was observed by Geoffrey Saint-Hilaire in 1836; while one of the "twins" was nursing, the other was often fast asleep. Similar reports were made about the behavior of Siamese twins, exhibited by Barnum and Bailey in the beginning of this century, and of two pairs of non-disjointed twins by Alekseyeva (37). One twin usually slept longer than the other, and, if fed in succession, the satiated twin slept while her partner was being nursed. Demikhov (906) grafted the head and forepart of a puppy onto the neck of an adult dog, connecting the arch of the puppy's aorta to one carotid artery, and its superior vena cava to one jugular vein, of the dog. Several such transplanted heads survived for 1 to 7 days (one for 29 days), retaining their functions. As described by Demikhov, the transplanted head usually "reacted briskly to the surroundings, had an intelligent expression and eagerly lapped up milk or water." Further, "the transplanted head fell asleep irrespective of whether the recipient dog was awake or asleep." The reported behavior of the joined twins and the "two-headed" dogs seems at first glance to contradict the view that circulating waste products can produce sleep. If, on the other hand, one considers that the condition of the nervous system undoubtedly determines its irritability and thus its resistance to the action of chemical agents, it is quite conceivable that, with a certain concentration of hypnogenic substances in the circulation, one brain may be depressed to the point of sleep, while the other is not. The twin that had been fed and had no hunger pangs could easily succumb to the action of the particular concentration of toxins, while the hungry one would remain wide awake under these conditions. For the same reason, the cross-circulation experiments that Neri and co-workers (2986, 2987) performed on dogs (p. 203), the results of which they interpreted to mean that "sleep is produced by a purely nervous, probably inhibitory, mechanism," need not at all be interpreted as militating against the toxin theories.

A strong argument against the toxin theories is that, on staying awake for several days, one does not get continuously sleepier but follows a periodic curve of greater sleepiness at night and lesser sleepiness in the daytime. As has been pointed out (p. 220), one is less sleepy on the afternoon of the third day of sleep deprivation than in the middle of the second night. Another reason for rejecting the toxin theories is the poor performance of an individual on getting up in the morning, when he presumably has attained a low level of concentration of these hypothetical substances, followed by an improved performance in the afternoon. Support for the toxin theories, on the other hand, may be found in the action of some drugs, stimulating when in low concentrations and depressing in higher ones. Thus, it may be argued, the individual on getting up in the morning has none of the waste products and performs at a certain rate. Later in the day, as these waste products accumulate, they act as stimulants, gradually bettering the performance (and perhaps also raising the body temperature). At an optimum concentration of metabolic products one's performance is best. Later in the afternoon and in the evening the further increase of these substances gradually produces a greater and greater depression, until the maintenance of the waking state is well-nigh impossible. The scheme, up to this point far from unacceptable, fails when one considers that in the middle of the night, as the waste products are being eliminated or destroyed, a person should have about the same concentration of waste products as in the middle of the afternoon, and yet the temperature is low and the ability to remain awake and to perform is least. For this reason, even though an accumulation of certain end products of metabolism should become an established fact instead of a mere assumption, such an accumulation could not account for the alternation of sleep and wakefulness.

Another group of humoral theories of sleep is that of endocrine functional periodicity. The thyroid and hypophysis were the glands most frequently linked with sleep. The earliest theory of this type attributed sleep to thyroid activity, but later, when hypothyroidism was found to produce apathy and somnolence, the hypofunction of the gland was considered responsible for the onset of sleep. The chief protagonist of the hypophyseal theory—really a combined toxin-and-secretory theory—was Salmon (3499–3511). The theory postulates that the anterior lobe of the hypophysis produces an antitoxic hormone that prevents the toxins formed during wakefulness from affecting the diencephalic wakefulness centers, whereas the posterior lobe produces a vasoconstrictor hormone which inhibits the activity of these centers and leads to sleep. Thus both the anterior and the posterior lobes contribute to the welfare of the infundibulo-tuberal centers, the former protecting them during wakefulness; the latter, through the production of sleep. The role of the posterior lobe was held by Salmon (3500) to be amply supported by laboratory and clinical findings. Salmon considered sleep to be a "vegetative function" destined for the reparation of the CNS, fatigued and intoxicated by wakefulness. When Zondek and Bier (4330–32) reported the presence of a bromine-containing hormone in the anterior lobe of the pituitary gland, Salmon adopted that hormone for his antitoxic factor, which supposedly protected the wakefulness centers. Alvarez (49) did not accept Salmon's original hypothesis of a specific hypophyseal hypnotic hormone, and Kovàcs (2257) brought forward a number of arguments against the hypothesis that sleep is produced by a local vasoconstriction in the diencephalon, through the action of a posterior pituitary secretion. Kovàcs, on the contrary, proposed the view that "sleep is connected with general metabolic activity and that it is the expression and the result of the anabolic phase of metabolism." Gélyi (1393) interpreted sleep as due to the exhaustion of a wakefulness-producing hormone which is restored during sleep: a toxin theory "in reverse."

With reference to the posterior lobe of the hypophysis, Schutz (3615), from experiments on rats and human subjects, concluded that the antidiuretic principle is instrumental in producing sleep, as caffeine and other diuretic drugs promote wakefulness. Garcia (1358), however, held that extracts of the posterior lobe of the hypophysis promoted wakefulness, whereas extracts of the anterior lobe induced sleep.

Salmon later amended his theory (3512, 3513) by suggesting that the physiology of sleep is dominated by three factors: (*a*) the infundibular nuclei, (*b*) the hypophysis, and (*c*) the cerebral cortex. The infundibular nuclei, as regulators of wakefulness, stimulate metabolic processes and psycho-affective reactions, which result in the production of toxic products. The hypophysis is very sensitive to these toxic products, and their accumulation leads to hypophyseal hyperactivity which serves to depress the infundibular nuclei. Cortical activity stimulates the infundibular nuclei via the fronto-diencephalic pathways and contributes to wakefulness. Thus, there is an antagonism between the hypophyseal hormones and cortical activity in their influence on the infundibular nuclei.

In Salmon's scheme there is no mention of a possible secretory activity of the infundibular nuclei, but evidence has accumulated to indicate that something like a "diencephalic gland" does exist (2904, 3279, 3547). Harris (1643) suggested that "the hypothalamus may influence the secretion of the adenohypophysis by means of a neurovascular link," liberating, upon excitation, some chemical transmitter which is carried by the hypophyseal portal vessels to the pars distalis of the gland. In addition, the anterior lobe activity may be influenced by the purely humoral transmission of substances in the systemic circulation (1249). There is thus a double, perhaps multiple, control of the liberation of ACTH (1047, 1640–43, 1901, 2812, 3462), as well as of other hypophyseal hormones. That hypophyseal activity may be affected directly or indirectly by the natural alternation of light and darkness has been suggested by several authors (110, 1045, 2026, 2213, 3222), but the striking findings of Rahn and Rosendale (3260), previously mentioned (p. 172), prove that a 24-hour skin coloration rhythm depends upon the hypophysis for its continuance. The work of Halberg and associates (1583, 1592, 1597) brought the adrenal cortex into the chain of command through their study of the 24-hour eosinophil curve, which is abolished in hypopituitarism, in Addison's disease, as well as after bilateral adrenalectomy. Whether the 24-hour rhythm is charted by the eosinophil count, plasma corticosteroid level, or urinary excretion of ketosteroids, the role of the hypophysis is unmistakable. As expressed by Halberg and associates (1592):

In comparing the time course of the daily changes in the blood level of hormone with those in motor activity of the body as a whole, we may infer that the adrenal cortex not only reacts to the activities of daily life, as has been amply demonstrated, but what is equally important, the periodicity of the gland underlies our preparation for daily activity as well. Thus, . . . a new sequence of metabolic events is being initiated in the cell once a day, under at least partial corticoid control. Normally, such metabolic arousal occurs *before* the reticular activating system starts us on our daily activities; in other words the adrenal cortical and metabolic "arousals" ordinarily precede in time cerebral cortical arousal.

The last sentence applies also to the body-temperature curve, which, as an index of the 24-hour rhythm, is far easier to follow than are the three manifestations of hypophyseal-adrenocortical activity. Although the latter is connected with the 24-hour rhythm, it must be remembered that neither the removal of the hypophysis or adrenal glands nor their extreme hypofunction abolishes the alternation of sleep and wakefulness.

Vegetative theories based on the antagonism between the sympathetic and parasympathetic divisions of the visceral nervous system contain elements of both neural and humoral mechanisms, as they involve discharges of groups of cells and the production and liberation of adrenergic and cholinergic substances.

Denisova and Figurin (914) ascribed the peculiar periodicity in the breathing of infants to an insufficient co-ordination of the activity of the sympathetic and parasympathetic systems. Kikuchi (2152), accepting the view that "sleep leads to an excitation of the parasympathetic system," maintained that sleep "does not always diminish the irritability of the sympathetic system, but rather alternately increases and decreases it." Zondek and Bansi (4329) believed that the inhibition of the action of certain hormones is necessary for narcosis and perhaps also for normal sleep. Vagotonic conditions, they held, are associated with an inhibition of the absorption of these hormones, while sympathicotonic conditions have the opposite effect. Molfino (2859) claimed that in endocrine disturbances there is often a vagotonia or sympathicotonia. Ewen (1124) observed signs of parasympathetic overreaction in ten schizophrenics and postulated that the mechanism responsible for sleep may also be operating to produce schizophrenia. Dikshit (937, 938), having produced sleeplike states through the action of acetylcholine on the hypothalamus, was also inclined to consider sleep a parasympathetic function. The chief advocate of the vegetative theory of sleep is Hess (1731–52), whose name is as frequently associated with it as Pavlov's is with the cortical inhibition theory or Claparède's with the biologic or instinct theory. Hess holds (1731) that during sleep the "animal" apparatus loses its freedom of function not because of exhaustion but because the rest phase of the "vegetative" apparatus places inhibitory influences in the path of the "animal" conduction pathways. Sleep, according to Hess, is an excellent example of parasympathetic function, a manifestation of which is the constriction of the pupils, which insures (and also compels) a functional rest of the eyes. The waking stimulus comes from the sympathetic system, bringing about a disinhibition of the animal elements of the organism's functions. As already stated (p. 204), Hess obtained real physiological sleep in the cat by the stimulation of a definite area of the diencephalon with currents of certain pulse durations, intensities, and frequencies. The area "is situated lateral to the massa intermedia and is limited caudally by the habenulo-interpeduncular tract and rostrally by the mammillo-thalamic bundle," and in it "there exists a functional center whose activity leads to a general depression and it appears justified to assume that this center is in action at the onset of sleep" (1751). Hess called this system "trophotropic," in contrast to the "ergotropic" or arousal system that is brought into play by the "stimulation in the 'dynamogenic field,' which is situated in the posterior and mesial part of the hypothalamus, and extends to the central gray matter of the mesencephalon and anterior rhombencephalon." Many investigators (173, 193, 195, 937, 938, 1044, 1124, 1453, 1462, 1504, 1803, 2868, 3512, 3650, 4181, 4186) supported the general thesis of Hess, implicitly or explicitly, using such terms as double mechanism, see-saw principle, reciprocal activity, mutual antagonism, or inhibition-facilitation, with reference to sympathetic-parasympathetic systems, ergotropic and trophotropic influences, dynamogenic and hypnogenic areas in the mesodiencephalic region. Ax and Luby (161), from changes in twelve physiological variables in five subjects during prolonged sleep deprivation, interpreted their results as evidence of "profound sympathetic fatigue." Less consistent are the conclusions with respect to cholinergic and adrenergic mechanisms controlling sleep and wakefulness, respectively (449, 4036).

It is obvious, whether one accepts the emergency theory of adrenal function or not, that in states of excitation and marked animalistic activities there is usually a simultaneous stimulation of the sympathetic innervation. This simultaneity does not mean that sympathetic stimulation is the cause of the excitement any more than the predominance of parasympathetic activity, during rest and relative absence of animalistic activity, denotes that rest is due to parasympathetic dominance. It is putting the cart before the horse to say that animalistic activity is due to sympathetic dominance and vegetative activity to parasympathetic dominance. There may be a concomitant relative hyperactivity of the sympathetic nervous system in wakefulness, and of the parasympathetic system during sleep, without the dependence of the sleep-wakefulness cycle itself upon sympathetic or parasympathetic influences.

It appears that the vegetative theories, like the toxin and endocrine theories, do not offer a satisfactory explanation of the alternation of sleep and wakefulness, although some of the facts they are based upon are well established and have to be accounted for in any acceptable theory that might be proposed.

Chapter 35

The Sleep-Center Problem

Mauthner (2717) located a sleep-regulating center in the periventricular gray and postulated for it the ability to influence the passage of impulses to and from the cerebrum through its action on the thalamus (p. 243). Little more was done or said about this center until Economo (1030), on the basis of his studies on encephalitis, revived the idea of a center in Mauthner's area capable of regulating sleep. Rather than a single nucleus, this center was envisaged by Economo to involve a large area in the mesodiencephalic transitional region which spreads out anteriorly in the hypothalamus up to the region of the basal nuclei. Inhibitory influences pass from this central region to the cerebrum, on the one hand, and to the midbrain, on the other. Wakefulness is produced by disinhibition from the same source. In some papers Economo (1031, 1034) referred to two centers or areas: an anterior portion, close to the basal nuclei, where disturbances lead to pathological wakefulness; and a posterior part, where disease processes produce oculomotor disturbances and pathologic sleep (as in encephalitis). Economo (1031) further distinguished between "brain" sleep—disturbances of consciousness, and "body" sleep—the "physical" accompaniment. The former, according to Economo, is due to inhibitory influences on the thalamus and cortex and may well involve the type of inhibition postulated by Pavlov, while the latter is brought about through the inhibition of the neighboring vegetative centers. Economo therefore suggested the existence of two apparently antagonistic sleep centers and of two different kinds of sleep. It should be added that Economo considered brain sleep and body sleep to be two distinct entities rather than two aspects of the same phenomenon. Thus he spoke of a dissociation between the two—the existence of brain sleep without a concomitant body sleep, and vice versa.

Economo had many adherents for the theory of dual cortical-subcortical control of sleep (1930, 2440, 3220, 3221, 3990), as well as for his notions of brain sleep and body sleep (1046, 1275, 1414, 2266, 2391, 2440, 2685, 3282). The concept of a subcortical sleep center was accepted by several investigators (927, 2487, 2498, 3391, 3616, 3654), and Adler (19), referring to the fact that decorticated animals sleep, suggested an independence of the center, in the sense of freedom from cortical control. Koslowsky (2246) saw the importance of the subcortical sleep center in its influence on the parasympathetic system. Pette (3167, 3168), on the assumption that centers for metabolism, water balance, and temperature regulation are located in the diencephalon, stated that one must postulate the existence of centers in the same region for regulating both sleep and wakefulness. He assumed a connection between these centers and the endocrine system. Skliar (3723) stressed the inhibitory influence of the periventricular gray on the cerebral cortex, but Rétif (3324) thought that there is a reciprocal inhibition between the mesencephalic center and the cerebral cortex. Marinesco and co-workers (2684) held that parasympathicotonia is a condition of sleep and not a result of it; that the endocrine glands act as sensitizers of the vegetative centers; and that sleep is a combination of conditioned (quiet, darkness, position) and unconditioned (humoral-vegetative) reflexes.

Despite the vogue of the mesodiencephalic localization of the sleep center, Trömner (3979–83) advanced reasons for the localization of the sleep center in the thalamus. The afferent impulses to the cortex can be most completely blocked from the cortex in the thalamus, and yet without a cortex the thalamic sleep center can still periodically depress the activity of lower-lying parts of the CNS. Even lesions in the Mauthner-Economo area may, according to Trömner, exert a pressure on the thalamus and thus produce sleep. He also postulated the possible existence of "partial" sleep centers acting together as one sleep-regulating complex. Friedemann (1292) and Tizzano (3949) accepted Trömner's thalamic localization of the sleep center, but Hirsch (1780) confined it to the medial portion of the left thalamus, admitting the existence of a hypothalamic center as well. Real pathological sleep, according to Hirsch, occurs when both centers are injured. Spiegel (3765), like Trömner, took issue with the adherents of periventricular gray localization theories and placed the sleep-regulating center in the thalamus. Spiegel located a primitive center of consciousness in the thalamus, which in turn transmits impulses to the higher centers of consciousness located in the cerebral cortex. Conversely, the cortex can influence the thalamus, either in an excitatory or in an inhibitory manner. Spiegel explained pathologic sleep as the "putting-out-of-function" of the thalamic center.

There were investigators who thought that neither the localization of the sleep center in the hypothalamus and neighboring portions of the mesencephalon nor its placement in the thalamus corresponds to the available physiological and pathological data on sleep. Luksch (2575) held that both of the foregoing areas, though each is concerned with sleep, are under the control of the cerebral cortex. Brailovsky (450), accepting the existence of brain sleep, nevertheless considered sleep to be governed by a complex cortico-subcortical mechanism, starting with cortical inhibition. Hechst (1675) postulated the existence of three equally active centers, none of which is in the cortex: a disturbance in any one of the three centers (periaqueductal, periventricular, or thalamic) would lead to somnolence. Salmon, as indicated in the preceding chapter, located his three factors in the cortex, infundibulotuberal nuclei, and the hypophysis. All these views were evidence of a dissatisfaction with unitary centers, no matter where they were placed by the respective authors. There were also those (2484, 2819, 3084, 3892) who would not commit themselves to a particular localization, although they admitted that a "sleep center" regulated the sleep-wakefulness rhythm. Others (17, 48, 598, 2695, 2792, 3498, 3756, 4134), on the contrary, rejected the very concept of a circumscribed sleep center.

Keeser and Keeser (2120), on the basis of their barbiturate studies, regarded the diencephalon as least important for sleep and the cerebral cortex as most important. Fraser-Harris (1267) held it as "psychologically incorrect" to assume that any part of the CNS lower than the brain proper went to sleep. His views might be interpreted to mean that body sleep, in the sense in which the word was used by Economo, is simply the manifestation of brain sleep, since the body in its somatic activity depends upon brain function.

Considering sleep as a specialized function, Johnson (1994) started with the assumption that there must be a special apparatus responsible for the change from wakefulness to sleep. This apparatus consists of "sleep" neurones, having the same properties and obeying the same laws as do other neurones. The special neurones are in the cerebral cortex, because sleep shows the features of learning by experience and habit formation, and these features are characteristic of cortical activities. Catabolic products activate the "sleep" neurones which inhibit the other cortical neurones—a meaningful difference from Pavlov's concept of a generalized cortical inhibition. In fact, Johnson thought that "the relations between the sleep system and the whole of the CNS, concerned only in elaborating the reactions of the waking state, are mutually antagonistic."

The connection between sleep and oculomotor phenomena, first pointed out by Mauthner, himself an ophthalmologist, has been emphasized by several authors as indicating a localization of the sleep center in the vicinity of the oculomotor nuclei. The drooping of the eyelids and diplopia are accepted as signs of drowsiness. Frank (1263) suggested that the pars lateralis of the nucleus subfascicularis belongs to the sleep-regulating center and that in it is localized the most characteristic sleep component, the eyelid paresis. Stockert (3826) also saw a connection between sleep and the movements and positions of the eyes. He called attention to the fact that the oculomotor apparatus is constantly active during the waking state, even when the other muscles of the body are at rest, and the continuation of wakefulness is bound to lead to a strain of the oculomotor muscles, which can be relieved only by sleep.

Through the years of continuous searching for a center whose spontaneous or induced activity led to sleep, there have been many expressions of views that sleep is a passive state, requiring no special mechanisms for its onset. In 1860, Longet (2554) cited opinions for and against the concept of sleep as an elementary state of the organism. In 1901, Dubois (999), who ascribed multiple functions to the CO_2 concentration in the blood, preferred the name of waking center for the region of the CNS affected. Bérillon (307), in 1909, stated that the phenomena connected with the onset and cessation of sleep suggested the operation of a waking center. Later Kahn (2061) referred to sleep as the normal state of life; Haenel (1576) advanced the view that the primary state of psychic life is the absence of consciousness, and that the cortical neurones are made to function only through the stimulating effects of afferent impulses.

If there is a center, it is a waking one, concerned with the maintenance of cortical activity. Support for the concept of the passivity of sleep and the probable operation of a wakefulness center may be found in the writings of other clinical and laboratory investigators (25, 1094, 1955, 2248, 3266, 3270, 3910), and in going through the enormous accumulation of articles and books dealing with the theoretical aspects of sleep (45, 85, 131, 153, 154, 156, 157, 578, 598, 608, 616, 660, 664, 706, 708, 709, 796, 1023, 1025, 1036, 1038, 1039, 1062–64, 1083, 1164, 1243, 1251, 1275, 1348, 1446, 1447, 1510, 1783, 1806, 1946, 1971, 1974, 1995, 2055, 2253, 2505, 2533, 2565, 2608, 2632, 2805, 2894, 2917, 2996, 3013, 3028, 3134, 3157, 3169, 3232, 3246, 3293, 3351, 3380, 3470, 3541, 3554, 3605, 3616, 3635, 3736, 3775, 3832, 3847, 3878, 3896, 3949, 4110, 4241, 4284), one can find any number of arguments for or against a particular view. On the factual side, there are the findings of Hess, Nauta, and Jorda and Manceau suggesting the existence of both a sleep center and a wakefulness one. Hess (1751) admitted that one can awaken a cat, put to sleep by electrical stimulation, by applying a higher voltage to the same spot, or "to any part of the brain." He also stated that "there is little evidence, so far, of sleeplessness consequent to destructions in the areas of the 'sleep center,'" and that "this might be due to the anatomical scattering of this functional unit whose elements cannot be put out of action in sufficient number by lesions compatible with life." It will be recalled that Nauta's rats, with the sleep center destroyed, did not live for more than a day, and that of the guinea pigs of Jorda and Manceau with similar lesions, only one lived for 26 days. The proof of the presence of an anatomically separate sleep center at present rests on that one guinea pig's induced 26-day sleeplessness.

Several authors (958, 3271, 3582) offered experimental evidence in support of Hess with respect to a sleep center, and others (480–83, 2867, 2902, 3427) accepted his views on the dynamogenic and hypnogenic mechanisms. The suggestion that another sleep center, or, at least, a synchronizing influence, might be located in the lower brain stem (252, 253, 2616, 2619, 2899)—the two sleep centers straddling both the mesencephalic wakefulness center and the pontine centers responsible for the "paradoxical phase" of sleep (p. 212)—adds to the multiplicity of structures and mechanisms possibly involved in the alternation of sleep and wakefulness.

Whether one accepts the subcortical localization of a sleep center, a wakefulness center, or centers for both, the cerebral cortex is not required for the functioning of such a center or centers. The contribution of the cerebral cortex to the 24-hour sleep-wakefulness rhythm is discussed in the next and last chapter.

Chapter 36

The Evolutionary Theory of Sleep and Wakefulness

Which came first—the hen or the egg? In the alternation of sleep and wakefulness, which of the two states interrupts the other? Is the onset of sleep an active process or a mere cessation of wakefulness? By an evolutionary theory presented in the first edition of this book, sleep is a passive condition, and the phylogenetic and ontogenetic development of the CNS is reflected mainly in the characteristics of induced wakefulness: the subcortically controlled wakefulness of necessity gradually evolves into a cortically regulated wakefulness of choice, along with the establishment of the 24-hour sleep-wakefulness rhythm. A certainty was expressed at that time that, as new facts were brought to light, modifications would have to be made in the theory. Discoveries made since 1938 suggest that there are evolutionary changes in sleep as well as in wakefulness, and this chapter deals with revisions of the theory dictated by these discoveries.

The onset and continuation of sleep, as well as awakening and the maintenance of wakefulness, can conceivably be explained by postulating the stimulation and inhibition, or activity and rest, of a sleep center, wakefulness center, or two reciprocally innervated centers, as discussed in the preceding chapter. Similarly, in astronomy the older Ptolemaic or geocentric theory accounted for the alternation of day and night and the apparent movements of the fixed stars just as satisfactorily as the newer Copernican or heliocentric theory. The movements of the planets, however, appeared to follow no systematic course by the geocentric theory, whereas the heliocentric one easily explained the planetary "retrogressions" as perspective effects resulting from the combination of the movements of the earth and other planets around the sun. Therefore, the heliocentric theory was accepted and the geocentric theory rejected. Examining findings with respect to destructive lesions in the brain stem, the conclusion must be made that the principal, if not the only, mechanism involved is a BSRF center or system whose activity induces and maintains wakefulness and whose inactivity leads to sleep. The possible existence of accessory or secondary hypnogenic systems, rostral, caudal, or within the BSRF, does not affect this conclusion fundamentally. In the medulla, for instance, one can stimulate certain spots to produce vasoconstrictor effects and others to cause vasodilation; but cutting the cervical spinal cord leads to a profound drop in blood pressure, showing that the principal tonic influence is a vasoconstrictor one. In any case, there is general agreement that the primitive sleep-wakefulness system or systems are subcortical in their location. Cortical processes are influenced by, and, in turn, influence, the mesodiencephalic centers, although they are not needed for the centers' elementary functioning in producing an alternation of sleep and wakefulness.

An innate alternation of primitive sleep and wakefulness can be seen in anencephalous children and in decorticated dogs. In these creatures there is no consciousness, as defined in the introductory chapter of this book—nothing to learn individually. A similar sleep-wakefulness cycle prevails in the normal human neonate. The temporal aspects of the cycle are: (a) sleep duration of 2 to 4 hours, bearing little relation to the succession of night and day; and (b) dominance of the sleep phase, with a sleep-to-wakefulness ratio of two-to-one. The criteria for the repetitive passage from primitive wakefulness to primitive sleep are: (a) a decrease or cessation of muscular activity and (b) a raised threshold of reflex excitability. The periodic awakening is adjusted to the organism's nutritional needs and is essentially a gastric cycle. Either hunger contractions or some humoral agents furnish the internal stimulus, in the absence of external disturbances. The length of the cycle represents a coalescence of several basic short-term rest-activity periodicities of 50–60 minutes' duration, as first described by Denisova and Figurin (914) and later observed in our laboratory (150). On a self-demand infant feeding routine, the interfeeding interval is usually an integer of these basic activity cycles. If the infant is not aroused through external or internal stimuli during the shallow phase of the periodicity, he is not likely to awaken till the shallow phase recurs.

The relatively short primitive wakefulness is maintained through the activity of the wakefulness center or system of the BSRF which, independently of its ability to arouse the cortex, has extensive feedback connections via the DRAS with caudal regions of the nervous system and peripheral receptors and effectors. After feeding is completed, and other general body needs or animalistic functions fulfilled, the activity of the wakefulness system abates, and sleep sets in. Primitive sleep, though undoubtedly dreamless, is not of uniform depth, for it is subject to the influences of the basic rest-activity periodicity; it is more easily terminated at certain intervals, but semi-awakening or full awakening can and does occur at any time, if the external or internal stimuli are of proper magnitude and duration.

The basic periodicity does not disappear with the development of the advanced types of sleep and wakefulness. As with other cycles, the wave length increases with age from 50–60 minutes in the young infant to 60–70 minutes in children of nursery-school age (1364), and 80–90 minutes in the adult. This periodicity has been detected by several investigators; it may be discerned in findings of others who themselves did not notice it; and it appears in the REM-EEG cycles which are associated with dreaming in advanced sleep. In the cat the basic periodicity manifests itself in cortical activation and associated phenomena that make up the "paradoxical phase" of sleep (p. 212), with a wave length of 20–30 minutes in the kitten, and 30–45 minutes in the adult cat. There is a suggestion of a 3–5 minute EEG periodicity during sleep in the rat (4141), which has 12–16 major activity cycles in 24 hours. The mechanism of this basic periodicity in the cat appears to be neurohumoral (p. 213). In embryos of Amblystoma punctatum Coghill and Watkins (727) noted a periodicity in the sensitivity to touch which appeared to be of endogenous origin and not attributable to fatigue. The authors surmised that such an intrinsic periodicity might be "the primary factor in the activities and sleep of animals generally."

The basic rest-activity periodicity which appears in advanced sleep as a series of dreaming episodes may also manifest itself in the advanced wakefulness phase of the 24-hour rhythm in recurrent fluctuations in alertness. Postprandial letdowns and bouts of weariness at the end of the working day, often coinciding with the crest of the 24-hour rhythm, would be difficult to explain but for the relief afforded by a 15–30-minute catnap, which may be long enough to tide one over the lowest part of the 80–90-minute periodicity.

The functional element which changes the innate primitive sleep and wakefulness alternation into the acquired advanced 24-hour sleep-wakefulness rhythm is consciousness or critical reactivity. If sleep and wakefulness may be crudely likened to the dichotomy of solid ice and liquid water (p. 4), which can be distinguished from each other by mere inspection, levels of consciousness are analogous to the degrees on a thermometer scale. There is only one dimension of consciousness running through sleep and wakefulness. As the freezing point of water is lowered by substances dissolved in it, so may the level of consciousness at which advanced wakefulness passes into sleep be affected by the condition of the individual. In other words, under certain circumstances, the degree of critical reactivity may be lower in wakefulness than it ordinarily is in certain stages of sleep.

The level of consciousness associated with wakefulness shows many gradations, and the transition from the primitive non-conscious wakefulness of the neonate to the fully-conscious midday wakefulness of the adult does not occur all at once. The beginning of the evolution of advanced wakefulness in the human infant can be seen in Table 15.1 (p. 134). For the group of infants we studied, the day-night sleep-wakefulness disparity, amounting to 2 hours in the third week of life, gradually increased to 5 hours by the fourteenth week. This evidence of acculturation to the family and community routines of living was not, however, associated with any increase in wakefulness capacity, as the total number of hours of wakefulness (and sleep) per 24 hours remained unchanged during that period:

the 1.5 hours of increased wakefulness from 8:00 A.M. to 8:00 P.M. were matched by increased sleep at night. During the second trimester, as Gifford (1442) put it, there is a "beginning of object relations," with the appearance of an occipital EEG pattern, and the added one hour of daytime wakefulness is not compensated for by an hour of night sleep. This added daytime hour represents a net gain in relative wakefulness capacity. It will be recalled that with the doubling of hours of wakefulness in the course of human ontogenetic development, the relative wakefulness capacity is quadrupled, as the ratio of the wakefulness fraction to that of sleep is reversed from 1:2 to 2:1. The absolute wakefulness capacity expressed as the number of hours of continuous wakefulness eventually reaches 15–17, for it is linked to the 24-hour day-night alternation.

By establishing artificial sleep-wakefulness over-24-hour rhythms of increasing length it should be possible to determine the absolute wakefulness capacity of man. The 28-hour rhythm that has been successfully developed (p. 177) is certainly not the upper limit for such artificial rhythms. It should be pointed out that sleep deprivation experiments do not furnish information concerning the absolute wakefulness capacity as a part of a new sleep-wakefulness rhythm. The ability to endure long stretches of enforced wakefulness without permanent damage to the nervous system shows the great margin of safety allowed by the usual 15–17 hours of wakefulness associated with the 24-hour rhythm. It may be added that the only effect of keeping rats awake for 20 hours daily for many weeks (2514) was an extreme irritability of the animals—a prominent feature in the behavior of persons during sleep deprivation.

Individual variation in the length of the wakefulness fraction may be dependent upon one's relative and absolute wakefulness capacity but is also affected by environmental happenings. The environment, however, may be of neutral or negative, as well as of positive, interest. Boredom and monotony of surroundings tend to favor sleep, but unusual excitement or worry may prolong wakefulness, in spite of a desire for sleep. Such protracted, unwanted wakefulness is definitely not of one's choice, and, therefore, "advanced wakefulness" is a better, more comprehensive term than "wakefulness of choice," which I formerly used to denote the addition of a certain level of consciousness to the primitive innate "wakefulness of necessity."

The effect of environmental conditions on the length of the wakefulness phase has also been observed in animals. It may be recalled that, according to Rioch (3359), normal cats kept in the dark were quiescent for 18–20 hours out of 24, and that a herd of monkeys watched by Slonim and Shcherbakova (3727) appeared to sleep 8.5 hours per night in the summer and 14.5 hours in the winter, seasonal differences comprising air temperatures as well as duration of daylight. No comparative data are available on the wakefulness capacity of infra-human species living in their natural habitat, but it is a fair surmise that unfavorable circumstances, such as paucity of food, would tend to prolong the wakefulness phase of the cycle. It is doubtful if curiosity alone would suffice to keep any animal awake for two-thirds of the time, as is the case with man.

The ontogenetic evolution of advanced wakefulness manifests itself not only in a total increase in duration but also in a consolidation of the wakefulness phases into three, two, finally one continuous stretch, as the morning and later the afternoon naps are given up (Fig. 36.1). For this evolution the presence of a maturing and functioning cerebral cortex is indispensable. In addition to the feedback circuits through the DRAS, involved in the maintenance of a primitive wakefulness, there are developed (*a*) circuits via the ARAS and DTPS to the cerebral cortex and back to the mesodiencephalic wakefulness system, and (*b*)

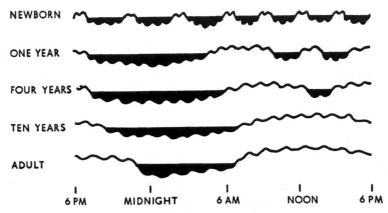

Fɪɢ. 36.1—A schematic representation of the ontogenetic transition from the primitive polycyclic alternation of sleep and wakefulness in the newborn infant to the monocyclic sleep-wakefulness rhythm in the adult. The 50–60-minute basic rest-activity periodicity in the infant, shown in the secondary undulations, is gradually lengthened to 80–90 minutes in the adult. Black areas represent sleep.

circuits from the cerebral cortex to the skeletal musculature and back to the cortex directly and via the BSRF. Thus, the cortex participates in furthering its own activity of continuously analyzing the stream of impulses arising from the sense organs, particularly the distance receptors, and integrating appropriate responses, in the light of previous experience.

The characteristic desynchronized LVFA EEG of wakefulness and synchronized HVSA EEG of sleep are not infallible signs of these two states, unless they reflect influences from the mesodiencephalic wakefulness system. Dissociation between behavioral wakefulness or sleep and the corresponding EEGs has been discussed (p. 30), and in any such conflict the behavioral signs are decisive. The failure to recognize the association of LVFA of the "paradoxical phase" with a deepening of sleep was due to the assumption that cortical activation from any source stands for arousal. As shown by Jouvet (2033), the LVFA of the cortical

EEG during the "paradoxical phase" is not suppressed by the interruption of the BSRF at the level of the midbrain tegmentum.

Unreliable though it is as an unsupported criterion of wakefulness, LVFA in the form of the alpha-pattern frequency, when obtainable, is an excellent index of the evolution of consciousness and variations in its levels (p. 31). The maximal alpha frequency reached during ontogenetic development of cortical function varies from person to person and is of less significance than the changes associated with fluctuating levels of consciousness. Decreases in the alpha frequency per second from 12 to 11 in one individual and from 10 to 9 in another are equally indicative of a lowering of the level of consciousness. Dreaming is associated with an emergent stage 1 EEG which is essentially a somewhat irregular alpha pattern, a fraction of a cycle slower than the waking alpha. The lower level of consciousness during dreaming is revealed by the poor analysis and integration, as well as the short memory span, characteristic of events in the hallucinatory episode of a dream. From the standpoint of ontogenetic development, dreaming is nothing else than the recurrence of LVFA of the "paradoxical phase" of the basic 80–90-minute rest-activity periodicity with the element of crude consciousness added. The dream contents, often emotionally tinged, are probably responsible for the features distinguishing dreaming from mere LVFA as seen in the cat. These features are: (*a*) a regularity of REMs; (*b*) cardiac acceleration; (*c*) increased tonus of certain muscles (cessation of snoring); and (*d*) lesser depth of sleep. The incorporation of some or all of these features can be used as an indication of the first appearance of dream activity during the sleep of the infant and child. As with wakefulness-consciousness, there is probably no precise age at which sleep-consciousness or dreaming begins. Advanced sleep, with dreaming, is as inevitable a consequence of cortical development as is advanced wakefulness, with thinking; teleological explanations are as superfluous for one as for the other.

Of pathological conditions, idiopathic narcolepsy seems to be a unique inhibition of the wakefulness system from carotid sinus stimulation. The frequent association of cataplexy with narcolepsy indicates that a center for the maintenance of muscle tonus may be a part of, or closely related to, the wakefulness system. Encephalitis lethargica is not only a prime example of the effect of injury to the wakefulness system, but also points up the inability of cortical activity alone to maintain a state of wakefulness. It may be possible to arouse the sleeping patient, but not to keep him awake, suggesting that the mesodiencephalic system is one of wakefulness, rather than of waking. Psychomotor epilepsy and somnambulism underline the possible association of a level of dream consciousness with overt wakefulness in the human adult. Absolute insomnia, unlike continuous sleep, does not exist as a disease entity, in spite of anecdotal reports to the contrary. Insomnia, in the sense of hyposomnia, is nearly always traceable to some disturbing factor acting on the wakefulness system or on the cortex.

Aside from their consciousness component, advanced sleep and wakefulness differ from primitive sleep and wakefulness in duration and in adjustment to the 24-hour astronomical and social order of living. As indicated, the consolidation of several short sleep periods into a long night sleep is probably one of the first manifestations of cortical activity. Favored by darkness and quiet, and influenced by the parents' failure to respond to nighttime feeding demands, the newborn infant learns to sleep for 10 hours at night at the age of five to six weeks. It may take the child five to six years to consolidate the several short stretches of primitive wakefulness into an unbroken 12–14-hour period of advanced wakefulness. The effort required is to a large extent muscular. The skeletal muscles are both effector and receptor organs. When they receive efferent impulses and execute tonic and phasic contractions, muscles, in return, send afferent proprioceptive impulses to the CNS, specifically to the mesodiencephalic wakefulness system and the cerebral cortex. Cortical activity is thus sustained by, and sustains, the wakefulness system and the skeletal musculature. In the operation of the multiple feedback circuits, wakefulness capacity is limited by muscular endurance. As was shown by the course of events in sleep-deprivation experiments (p. 220), the subjects could maintain wakefulness as long as they were able and willing to maintain muscular activity. Even a well-rested person may have difficulty in remaining awake, if, in addition to the removal of, or decrease in, stimulation through other sense organs, he allows his skeletal musculature to relax. Conversely, tense muscles may be responsible for "insomnia."

The attainment of an absolute advanced wakefulness capacity of 15–17 hours by the human adult is associated with the concurrent maintenance of the 24-hour sleep-wakefulness rhythm. The body-temperature curve enables one to follow the development, continuation, modification, or deterioration of the 24-hour rhythm. It must be remembered that body temperature, like other physiological constants, has a range within which it can fluctuate without eliciting any corrective adjustment. Inside of this "thermostatic band" of 2°–3° F. lie the values that make up the 24-hour body-temperature curve. Although a number of factors—known and unknown—may affect the body temperature, variations in muscle tonus are promptly reflected in changes in body temperature. The numerous findings with respect to variations in alertness and efficiency of performance, both under the regular routine of living and during sleep deprivation, support the view that the 24-hour body-temperature curve charts a regular repetitive oscillation in muscle tonus. Similar 24-hour curves for the eosinophil count, plasma cortico-steroids, and urinary ketosteroids suggest that hypophyseal-adrenocortical activities may also participate in influencing the muscle tonus or the CNS in the operation of the 24-hour sleep-wakefulness rhythm. That other, at present unknown, elements may be instrumental in developing and maintaining the wavelike rhythmical changes is shown by the lack of synchronicity in the fluctuations of the several concomitants of sleep. It is therefore impossible to ascribe the operation of the rhythm to any one conditioning nervous or endocrine mechanism. It must be emphasized, however, that the presence of a functioning cerebral cortex is indispensable for both the establishment and maintenance of the rhythm.

In sum, according to the evolutionary theory, in man the innate two-to-one polycyclic alternation of dreamless sleep and primitive wakefulness is a subcortical, probably mesodiencephalic, function, and the individually acquired one-to-two 24-hour rhythm of sleep with dreaming and advanced wakefulness is a cortical function.

EXPLANATORY NOTE

Items in the Bibliography of the first edition are integrated in the present Bibliography and Author Index, with the exception of some seventy titles which were deleted for a variety of reasons. Newly included are close to one hundred pre-1912 classical papers previously omitted because they appeared in the bibliography of Piéron's *Le Problème Physiologique du Sommeil* (3192), which is no longer easily obtained.

The system of assigned numbers precluded the addition of new bibliographical entries after May, 1962, except where definitive papers replaced preliminary communications or complete information became available for articles "in press." While the number of bibliographical items is more than three times that of the first edition, no claim of complete coverage of the literature is made.

Titles of individually published bibliographical references have principal words capitalized.

Unless written in English, French, German, Italian, or Spanish, the language of the publication is given in parentheses followed by the English translation of the title.

When several papers constitute chapters of one book, form parts of a collection of articles, or make up a report of a conference, the publication details are replaced by a number in parentheses (4, 392, 875, 1357, 2299, 3021, 3747, 4036, 4270) referring to the parent volume, listed in the Bibliography under its editors or compilers.

Abbreviations of periodical titles follow no one system, but combine good features of several. Prepositions (of, *de, für, di*) and conjunctions (and, *et, und, e, y*) are generally omitted. In citing similar journal names, or unfamiliar periodicals, the city of publication is given in parentheses.

The Author Index is incorporated into the Bibliography, making the combination a publication index: it identifies the page or pages (shown as underlined numbers after the items) on which the particular publications are referred to in the text. Following the bibliographical item(s) of each sole or senior author are the bibliographical numbers of other publications of which he is a joint author.

Bibliography and Author Index

1. Aagren, G., O. Wilander, and E. Jorpes. Cyclic changes in the glycogen content of the liver and muscles of rats and mice: their bearing upon the sensitivity of the animals to insulin and their influence on the urinary output of nitrogen. Biochem. J., 25:777-85, 1931. <u>165</u>

2. Aas, K. (Norw.) Sleep disorders in little children; observations in general practice. Tskr. Norske Laegerforen., 79:389-93, 1959. <u>278</u>

3. A. B. C. Rocking movements in sleep. Brit. Med. J., I:246, 1945. <u>285</u>

4. Abramson, H. A., Ed. Problems of Consciousness. New York: Josiah Macy Found. I, 1950, pp. 200; II, 1951, pp. 178; III, 1952, pp. 156; IV, 1953, pp. 177; V, 1954, pp. 180. <u>30</u>

5. Abuladze, K. S. (Russ.) Sleep during negative induction. In: The Sleep Problem, 1954 (392), pp. 147-53.

6. Achard, C., R. Demanche, et L. Faugeron. L'élimination rénale pendant le jour et la nuit. C. R. Soc. Biol., 61:466-67, 1906.

7. Achelis, J. D., und H. Nothdurft. Ueber Ernaehrung und motorische Aktivitaet. Pfluegers Arch., 241: 651-73, 1939. <u>149</u>

8. Ackner, B., and G. Pampiglione. Combined EEG, plethysmographic, respiratory and skin resistance studies during sleep. EEG Clin. Neurophysiol., 7:153, 1955. <u>47</u>

Ackner, B., co-author: 3087.

9. Adam, J. M., and H. M. Ferres. Observations on oral and rectal temperatures in the humid tropics and in a temperate climate. J. Physiol. (London), 125:21P, 1954. <u>191</u>

10. Adam-Falkiewiszowa, S. De la localisation nosologique des attaques de sommeil et de tonus musculaire. Rev. Neurol., 63: 579, 1935. <u>237</u>

11. Adams, C. L., E. L. Gibbs, and F. A. Gibbs. Asynchronism of electrical activity of frontal lobes during sleep: A late sequel of frontal lobotomy. A.M.A. Arch. Neurol. Psychiat., 77: 237-42, 1957.

12. Adams, J. K. Laboratory studies of behavior without awareness. Psychol. Bull., 54:383-405, 1957. <u>31</u>

13. Adams, O. S., J. T. Ray and W. D. Chiles. Prolonged human performance as a function of the work-rest cycle. Aerospace Med., 32:218, 1961. <u>184</u>, <u>316</u>

14. Adey, W. R., and D. F. Lindsley. On the role of subthalamic areas in the maintenance of brain-stem reticular excitability. Exp. Neurol., 1:407-26, 1959.

15. _____, N. C. R. Merrillees, and S. Sunderland. The entorhinal area; behavioural, evoked poten-

tial, and histological studies of its interrelationships with brainstem regions. Brain, 79:414-39, 1956. 211

16. ____, J. P. Segundo, and R. B. Livingston. Corticofugal influences on intrinsic brain stem conduction in cat and monkey. J. Neurophysiol., 20:1-16, 1957. 211

17. Adie, W. J. Idiopathic narcolepsy: a disease sui generis, with remarks on the mechanism of sleep. Brain, 49:257-306, 1926. 233, 240, 249, 361

18. Adler, A. On the interpretation of dreams. Internat. J. Indiv. Psychol., 2:3-16, 1936. 103

19. Adler, E. Zur Lokalisation des "Schlafzentrums." Med. Klin., 20:1321-22, 1924. 266, 359

20. Adler, L. Der Winterschlaf. Handb. norm. path. Physiol., 17: 105-33, 1926. 325

21. Adolph, E. F. Responses to hypothermia in several species of infant mammals. Am. J. Physiol., 166:75-91, 1951. 327

22. ____, and M. J. Gerbasi. Blood concentration under the influences of amytal and urethane. Am. J. Physiol., 106:35-45, 1933. 37

23. ____, and J. Richmond. Rewarming from natural hibernation and from artificial cooling. J. Appl. Physiol., 8:48-58, 1955.

24. Adrian, E. D. Berger rhythm in the monkey's brain. J. Physiol. (London), 87:83-84, Proc., 1936. 296, 348

25. ____. The physiology of sleep. Lancet, 232(II):1296, 1937. 362

26. ____. The physiology of sleep. Irish J. Med. Sci., No. 138:237-48, 1937.

27. ____, and B. H. C. Matthews. Berger rhythm: potential changes from the occipital lobes in man. Brain, 57:355-85, 1934. 25

28. ____, and K. Yamagiwa. The origin of the Berger rhythm. Brain, 58:323-51, 1935. 25

29. Agostini, C. Sui disturbi psichici e sulle alterazioni del systema nervoso centrale per insonnia assoluta. Riv. Sper. Freniat., 24: 113-25, 1898. 215, 228

30. Ainley, A. B., and C. Kaligman. Clinical observations on the somnifacient efficacy of heptabarbital (Medomin) in mentally disturbed

patients. J. Nerv. Ment. Dis., 123:125-29, 1956. 294

31. Ajmone Marsan, C. Recruiting response in cortical and subcortical structures. Arch. Ital. Biol., 96:1-16, 1958. 210 Ajmone-Marsan, C., co-author: 1091, 1961, 1962, 3262.

32. Akert, K., und B. Andersson. Experimenteller Beitrag zur Physiologie des Nucleus caudatus. Acta Physiol. Scand., 22: 281-98, 1951. 204

33. ____, W. P. Koella, and R. Hess, Jr. Sleep produced by electrical stimulation of the thalamus. Am. J. Physiol., 168:260-67, 1952. 204 Akert, K., co-author: 1727-29, 2512.

34. Akimoto, H., N. Yamagouchi, K. Okabe, T. Nakagawe, I. Nakamura, K. Abe, H. Torii, and K. Masahashi. On the sleep induced through electrical stimulation on dog thalamus. Folia Psychiat. Neurol. Jap., 10:117-46, 1956. 204

35. Alajouanine, T. Les altérations des états de conscience causées par des désordres neurologiques. First Internat. Congress Neurol. Sci., Seconde Journée Commune. Brussels: Acta Med. Belg., 1957, pp. 19-41. Alajouanine, co-author: 2393.

36. Aleksandrova, L. I. (Russ.) The Role of Normal Sleep in the Prevention of Neuroses. Moskva: Centr. Sci. Investig. Inst. Sanit. Enlight. Min. Health Protection SSSR, 1955. Pp. 8.

37. Alekseyeva, T. T. (Russ.) Correlation of nervous and humoral factors in the development of sleep in non-disjointed twins. Zh. Vysshei Nerv. Deiat., 8(6): 835-44, 1958. 344, 354

38. Alella, A., e E. Meda. Comportamento della saturazione dell'emoglobina in un soggetto normale con respiro di Cheyne-Stokes durante il sonno. Boll. Soc. Ital. Biol. Sper., 22:836-37, 1946. 49

39. ____, e ____. Respiro di Cheyne-Stokes nel sonno fisiologico e suoi rapporti colla saturazione dell'emoglobina. Minerva Med., 2:396-402, 1947. 49

40. Alexander, L. Hypnosis. North

Carolina Med. J., 3:562, 1942. 336

41. Alfano, V. Sopra un caso di narcolessia apparentemente essenziale. Ann. Med. Nav. Colon., 42(II):140-50, 1936.

42. Alford, L. B. Localization of consciousness and emotion. Am. J. Psychiat., 89:789-99, 1933.

43. _____. The localization of the mental functions: a new conception. South. Med. J., 43:262-65, 1950.

44. Allcroft, W. M. Diurnal variations in the blood sugar level of the lactating cow. Biochem. J., 27: 1820-23, 1933. 166

45. Allen, E. C. H. Sleep: normal and abnormal. Dublin J. Med. Sci., 140:73-96, 1919. 47, 312, 362

46. Allen, I. M. Somnambulism and dissociation of personality. Brit. J. Med. Psychol., 11:319-31, 1932. 283

47. Allers, R. Ueber neurotische Schlafstoerungen. Dsche med. Wschr., 54:817-19, 1928. 312

48. Altschuler, I. M. Sleep and epidemic encephalitis. J. Neurol. Psychopath., 9:222-27, 1929. 349, 361

49. Alvarez, B. G. Reflexiones sobre la hipótesis de Salmon sobre el sueño. Siglo Méd., 64:886-87, 1917. 355

50. Alvarez, C. Physiologic studies on the motor activities of the stomach and bowel in man. Am. J. Physiol., 88:650-62, 1929. 55

51. Alvarez, W. C. Psychogenic fever. J. Am. Med. Ass., 175:530, 1961. 145

52. Alvarez de Toledo, L. S. de. Sobre los mecanismos del dormir y del despertar. Rev. Psicoanal., 8:152-72, 1951. 106

53. Amassian, K. E., and R. V. Devito. Unit activity in reticular formation and nearby structures. J. Neurophysiol., 17:575-603, 1954. 209

54. Ambrosetto, C. Aspetti moderni di problemi antichi: basi neurologiche dello stato di coscienza. Rass. Clin.-Sci., 33:10-18, 1957; also Resenha Clin.-Cient. (São Paulo), 26:119-25, 1957. 31

55. Amelung, W., F. Becker, J. Bender, und C. A. Pfeiffer. Stoerungen des vegetativen Nervensystems und Wettergeschehen (neue Arbeitsmethoden meteoropatholo-gischer Forschung). Arch. phys. Therap. (Leipzig), 2:181-91, 1950. 275

56. Amsler, C. Zur Pharmakologie und Pathogenese der Entzuendung. III. Ueber die Entzuendungshemmende Wirkung des Schlafes und ueber diesen selbst. Arch. exp. Path. Pharmakol., 171: 170-73, 1933. 34, 352, 353

57. Anand, B. K. Somnolence caused by destructive lesions in the hypothalamus in cat. Indian J. Med. Res. (Calcutta), 43:195-99, 1955. 206

58. Ananyev, B., and A. Dubrovski. (Russ.) Essay toward a reflexological study of hypnosis. Nov. Refl. Fiziol. Nerv. Sistemy, 3: 447-58, 1929. 335

59. Andersen, P., K. Johansen, and J. Krog. Electroencephalogram during arousal from hibernation in the birchmouse. Am. J. Physiol., 199:535-38, 1960. 326

60. Anderson, A. An inquiry into the hours of rest (sleep) of 1,600 school children. Med. Officer, 55:147-48, 1936. 117, 118, 305

61. Anderson, D. V. The Effect of Relaxation on the Recall of Nonsense Syllables, Words, and Poetry. Unpublished Doctor's Thesis, UCLA, 1952. Pp. 93. 72

62. Anderson, F. N. Report of a case of narcolepsy with cataplectic attacks. J. Nerv. Ment. Dis., 74:173-74, 1931. 250

63. Anderson, O. W. The management of "infantile insomnia." J. Pediat., 38:394-401, 1951. 278

64. Andjus, R. Sur la possibilité de ranimer le rat adulte refroidi jusqu'à proximité du point de congélation. C. R. Acad. Sci. (Paris), 232:1591-93, 1951. 328

65. Andlauer, P., et B. Metz. Variations nycthémérales de la fréquence des accidents du travail. Acta Med. Scand., Suppl. 307: 86-94, 1955.

Andlauer, P., co-author: 2786.

66. Ando, M., and K. Ito. Clinical and electroencephalographical studies on catatonia. Folia Psychiat. Neurol. Jap., 13:133-42, 1959. 252

67. André-Balisaux, G., et R. Gonsette. L'électroencéphalographie dans le somnambulisme et sa valeur pour l'établissement

d'un diagnostic étiologique. Acta Neurol. Psychiat. Belg., 56:270-81, 1956. 282, 283

68. Andreev, B. V. (Russ.) Investigation of the dynamics of sleep in man by means of recording eyelid movements. Fiziol. Zh., 36:429-35, 1950. 90

69. _____. (Russ.) Actograph applicable in the clinic for the objective study of sleep. Klin. Med. (Moskva), 29(6):81-82, 1951. 86

70. _____. (Russ.) Investigation of the dynamics of normal sleep in man by means of actography. Zh. Vysshei Nerv. Deiat., 1:500-505, 1951; also in The Sleep Problem, 1954 (392), pp. 249-55. 86

71. _____. (Russ.) Investigation of the dynamics of sleep in children by means of actography. Trudy Inst. Fiziol. Pavlova, 1:339-44, 1952. 89, 284

72. _____. Sleep Therapy in the Neuroses. New York: Consult. Bureau, 1960. Pp. 114. 206, 207, 344

73. _____, and B. I. Ivanov. (Russ.) Technique of recording eyelid movements by means of a new cathode device. Fiziol. Zh. SSSR, 36:243-48, 1950. 90

74. _____, and E. A. Karapetian. (Russ.) Characteristics of night sleep in narcolepsy from actographic data. Trudy Inst. Fiziol. Pavlova, 1:376-80, 1952.

75. Andress, J. M. An investigation of the sleep of normal school students. J. Educ. Psychol., 2:153-56, 1911. 99, 118

76. André-Thomas, J. Jumantié, et Chausseblanche. Léthargie intermittente traduisant l'existence d'une tumeur du IIIe ventricule. Rev. Neurol., II:67-73, 1923. 269

77. Andrieu, R. Du sommeil quotidien au sommeil éternel. I. Le sommeil. II. La narcose et ses mécanismes. Rev. Pat. Gén. Physiol. Clin., 60:201-13; 869-93, 1960.

78. Angel, J.-M. La Thérapeutique par le Sommeil. Pathologie, Technique, Indications. Paris: Masson, 1953. Pp. 152. 206
Angel, J., co-author: 4177.

79. Angyal, A. Der Schlummerzustand. Z. Psychol., 103:65-99, 1927. 79

80. _____. Sullo stato del dormiveglia. Arch. Ital. Psicol., 8:89-94, 1930; also Atti VII Convegno Psicol. Sper. Psicotecn. (Torino),

1929, pp. 88-90. 79

81. Anokhin, P. On the specific action of the reticular formation on the cerebral cortex. EEG Clin. Neurophysiol., Suppl. 13:257-70, 1960. 209

82. Anon. A study in experimental insomnia. George Washington Univ. Res. Bull., 1(1), 1925. 224

83. _____. Physiology of sleep. J. Am. Med. Ass., 109:609, 1937.

84. _____. Posture and sleep. Lancet, I:178, 1942.

85. _____. Sleep, dreams and terrors. Lancet, I:436, 1943. 362

86. _____. Grinding of the teeth. J. Am. Med. Ass., 141:1196, 1949. 285

87. _____. Habit disorder in infant. J. Am. Med. Ass., 143:694, 1950. 285

88. _____. Sleeping and waking. South Afr. Med. J., 25:669-71, 1951. 241

89. _____. Infant Care. Washington, D.C.: U.S. Department of Health, Education and Welfare, Children's Bureau Publ. No. 8, 1955. Pp. 106. 114, 305

90. _____. Physiology of sleep. Brit. Med. J., I:475-76, 1952.

91. _____. Joint-strain in sleep. Lancet, I:756, 1952.

92. _____. Sleep. Med. J. Australia, II:249-50, 1952.

93. _____. Insomnia. Med. Illust. (London), 9:260-61, 1955. 274

94. _____. Numbness of hands at night. J. Am. Med. Ass., 159:1077, 1955. 285

95. _____. Sleep and Children. The application of our knowledge about sleep to the needs of children and youth. Washington, D.C.: Nat. Educ. Ass. & Am. Med. Ass., Joint Committee, 1956. Pp. 16.

96. _____. Ueber den Sitz des Bewusstseins. Dsche med. Wschr., 81:1281-82, 1956. 31

97. _____. Head rolling. J. Am. Med. Ass., 160:818, 1956. 285

98. _____. Failure of eyelids to close during sleep. J. Am. Med. Ass., 165:764, 1957. 11

99. _____. Les rythmes du travail. Hyg. Ment. (Paris), 46:36-67, 1957. 317

100. _____. Rocking during sleep. J. Am. Med. Ass., 163:796, 1957. 285

101. _____. Learning during sleep. J. Am. Med. Ass., 166:987-88,

1958. 125
102. ____. Head-banging. J. Am.
Med. Ass., 167:926, 1958. 285
103. ____. Sleeping positions of children. J. Am. Med. Ass., 168:
1592, 1958. 9, 11
104. ____. Sleep. Lancet, I:82-83,
1959.
105. ____. Jerks on falling asleep.
Brit. Med. J., No. 5140:44, 1959.
75
106. ____. Nightmares. J. Am. Med.
Ass., 173:1871, 1960. 281
107. ____. Prone or supine? Brit.
Med. J., I:1304, 1961. 9
108. Anthony, J. An experimental approach to the psychopathology of childhood, sleep disturbances.
Brit. J. Med. Psychol., 32:19-37,
1959. 282, 286
109. Antrobus, J. S. Patterns of Dreaming and Dream Recall. Columbia Univ.: Doctoral Diss.,
1962, 98, 100
110. Appel, W., und K. J. Hansen. Lichteinwirkung, Tagesrhythmik der eosinophilen Leukozyten und Hypophysennebennierenrindensystems. Dsch. Arch. klin. Med.,
199:530-37, 1952. 170, 356
111. Apter, I. M., Z. N. Bolotova, and I. G. Sineiko. (Russ.) On the effect of combined employment of electroshock and prolonged interrupted sleep on the higher nervous activity of dogs. Zh. Vysshei Nerv. Deiat., 5:70-75, 1955. 206
112. Araki, C., K. Sakata, and M. Matsunaga. Recruiting response-like EEG changes induced with extrathalamic stimulation of cat. Acta School Med. Kioto, 34:100-122,
1956. 30, 210
113. Arborelius, M. Die klinische Bedeutung der menschlichen Rhythmik. Dsche med. Wschr., 64:993-95, 1938. 131
114. Ardis, J. A., and P. McKellar. Hypnagogic imagery and mescaline. J. Ment. Sci. (London), 102:
22-29, 1956. 80
115. Arduini, A. Lente oscillazioni di potenziale della corteccia cerebrale per stimolazione dei sistemi a proiezione diffusa. In: Problemi di fisiologia e clinica dei sistemi a proiezione diffusa dell'Encefalo (Atti del Convegno di Parma). Parma: Maccari,
1957. Pp. 83-101. 210
116. ____, and M. G. Arduini. Effect of drugs and metabolic alterations

on brain stem arousal mechanism. J. Pharmacol. Exp. Therap.
110:76-85, 1954; prelim. commun., Fed. Proc., 12:6, 1953.
298
117. ____, and T. Hirao. On the mechanism of the EEG sleep patterns elicited by acute visual deafferentation. Arch. Ital. Biol.,
97:140-55, 1959. 212
118. ____, e ____. Sonno elettroencefalografico prodotto da illuminazione continua nel preparato mediopontino. Boll. Soc. Ital. Biol. Sper., 35:1743-44,
1959. 212
119. ____, et G. C. Lairy-Bounes. Action de la stimulation electrique de la formation réticulaire du bulbe et des stimulations sensorielles sur les ondes strychniques corticales chez le chat "encéphale isolé." EEG Clin. Neurophysiol., 4:503-12, 1952.
209
120. ____, and G. Moruzzi. Olfactory arousal reactions in the "cerveau isolé" cat. EEG Clin. Neurophysiol., 5:243-50, 1953.
30
121. ____, e ____. Analisi elettrofisiologica dei rapporti talamo-corticali in rapporto all'azione del sistema reticolare ascendente. In: Psychotropic Drugs,
1957 (1357), pp. 185-92. 210
122. ____, and C. Terzuolo. Cortical and subcortical components in the recruiting responses. EEG Clin. Neurophysiol., 3:189-96,
1951. 210
Arduini, A., co-author: 521, 522,
1511, 4196.
123. Arfel-Capdevielle, G., et H. Fischgold. Initiations électroencéphalographiques. Variations sur l'E.E.G. du sommeil. Presse Méd., 61:1211-12, 1953.
Arfel-Capdevielle, G., co-author:
1186.
124. Arian, E., e V. Bergamini. Osservazioni elettroencefalografiche sul sonno terapeutico da alcool etilico. Neurasse, 7:83-86, 1958. 294
125. Aristotle. Parva Naturalia. Translated by J. I. Beare. Oxford: Clarendon Press, 1908. Pp.
436a-646b. 3, 99, 106, 342
126. Arkhangelski, G. V. (Russ.) Sleep and dreams. Feldsher Akush. (Moskva), No. 9:15-20,

No. 10:18-21, 1951. 99

127. _____. (Russ.) Sleep and Its Meaning in the Life of Man. Moskva: Medgiz, 1955. Pp. 30. 312

128. Armington, J. C., W. R. Biersdorf, and L. D. Mailloux. An apparatus for scoring electroencephalograms. Am. J. Psychol., 71: 594-99, 1958.

129. _____, and L. L. Mitnick. Electroencephalogram and sleep deprivation. J. Appl. Physiol., 14: 247-50, 1959. 226, 238, 332
Armington, J. C., co-author: 2139, 2846, 4225.

130. Armour, P. Clinical disturbances of sleep. Bull. Acad. Med. Toronto, 9:248-55, 1936.

131. Armstrong-Jones, R. The value of sleep. Practitioner, 122:1-11, 1929. 362

132. Arndt, M. Ueber taeglichen (24-stuendigen) Wechsel psychischer Krankheitszustaende. Allg. Z. Psychiat., 92:128-50, 1930.

133. Arnold, M. B. On the mechanism of suggestion and hypnosis. J. Abnorm. Soc. Psychol., 41:107-28, 1946. 336

134. _____. Brain function in hypnosis. Internat. J. Clin. Exp. Hypn., 7:109-19, 1959. 336

135. Aron, C., et C. Kayser. Sommeil hivernal et pancréas endocrine. C. R. Soc. Biol., 150:410-13, 1956.

136. Aron, H. Ueber den Schlaf im Kindesalter. Mschr. Kinderheilk., 26:209-16, 1923. 306

137. Arullani, F. Insufficenza epatica ed insonnia. Gazz. Osp., 39:215-16, 1918. 276

138. Aschoff, J. Ueber die Interferenz temperaturregulatorischer und kreislaufregulatorischer Vorgaenge in den Extremitaeten des Menschen. Pfluegers Arch., 248: 197-207, 1944. 62

139. _____. Einige allgemeine Gesetzmaeszigkeiten physikalischer Temperaturregulation. I. Mitteilung. Pfluegers Arch., 249:125-36, 1947.

140. _____. Die 24-Stunden-Periodik der Maus unter konstanten Umgebungsbedingungen. Naturwissenschaften, 38:506-7, 1951.

141. _____. Zeitgeber der tierischen Tagesperiodik. Naturwissenschaften, 41:49-56, 1954. 131

142. _____. Exogene und endogene Komponente der 24-Stunden-Periodik bei Tier und Mensch. Naturwissenschaften, 42:569-75, 1955. 132

143. _____. Der Tagesgang der Koerpertemperatur beim Menschen. Klin. Wschr., 33:545-51, 1955. 131

144. _____. Tierische Periodik unter dem Einfluss von Zeitgebern. Z. Tierpsychol., 15:1-30, 1958. 132

145. _____, und J. Meyer-Lohmann. Die 24-Stunden Periodik von Nagern im natuerlichen und kuenstlichen Belichtungswechsel. Z. Tierpsychol., 11:476-84, 1954.

146. _____, und _____. Die Aktivitaetsperiodik von Nagern im kuenstlichen 24-Stunden-Tag mit 6-20 Stunden Lichtzeit. Z. vergl. Physiol., 37:107-17, 1955. 175

147. Aserinsky, E. Effects of illumination and sleep upon amplitude of electro-oculogram. A.M.A. Arch. Ophthalm., 53:542-46, 1955.

148. _____, and N. Kleitman. Regularly occurring periods of eye motility, and concomitant phenomena, during sleep. Science, 118:273-74, 1953; prelim. commun., Fed. Proc., 12:6, 1953. 93

149. _____, and _____. Two types of ocular motility occurring in sleep. J. Appl. Physiol., 8:1-10, 1955. 90, 93, 96, 112

150. _____, and _____. A motility cycle in sleeping infants as manifested by ocular and gross bodily activity. J. Appl. Physiol., 8:11-18, 1955. 88, 91, 93, 112, 133, 364

151. Asher, E. J., and R. S. Ort. Eye movement as a complex indicator. J. Gen. Psychol., 45:209-17, 1951.

152. Ask-Upmark, E. (Swed.) Sleep and Sleep Disturbances. Stockholm: C. E. Fritzes, 1948. Pp. 25. 312

153. Atkinson, F. P. An inquiry as to the cause of sleep. Edinb. Med. J., 16:109-13, 1870. 362

154. Atkinson, J. B. The anatomy and physiology of the sleep mechanism. MD, 2:9-15, 1947. 362

155. Aubert, M. La forme somnolente prolongée de la névraxite épi-

démique. Thèse, Montpelier, 1928. Pp. 73. 248

156. Aubert, V., and H. White. Sleep and Society: An Exploration. Center for Advanced Study Behav. Sci., Stanford, Calif., Prelim. draft, 1957. Pp. 67. 362

157. _____, and _____. Sleep: a sociological interpretation. Acta Sociol., 4(2):46-54, 4(3):1-16, 1959. 362

158. Augustin, H. Die Behandlung der Schlaflosigkeit in der taeglichen Praxis. Schweiz. med. Wschr., 62:817, 1932. 294

159. Austin, G., and H. Jasper. Diencephalic mechanisms for facilitation and inhibition. Fed. Proc., 9: 6, 1950. 209

160. Austregesilo, A. (Portug.) On insomnia. Cultura Méd., 2:317-20, 1940. 274

161. Ax, A., and E. D. Luby. Autonomic responses to sleep deprivation. A.M.A. Arch. Gen. Psychiat., 4: 55-59, 1961. 173, 225, 226, 229, 358

162. Azima, H. Prolonged sleep treatment in mental disorders (some new psychopharmacological considerations). J. Ment. Sci., 101: 593-603, 1955. 206, 207

163. _____. Sleep treatment in mental disorders. Results of four years of trial. Dis. Nerv. Syst., 19:523-30, 1958. 207

164. _____, and F. J. Cramer. Effects of partial perceptual isolation in mentally disturbed individuals. Dis. Nerv. Syst., 17:117-22, 1956. 199

165. _____, _____, et H. Faure. Le système réticulé activateur central: son rôle en psychopathologie. Evolut. Psychiat., No. 1:121-43, 1955.

166. Azzali, G. Il comportamento dell'apparato neurosecretorio ipotalamo-ipofisario nell'ibernazione e nell'ipotermia artificiale. Acta Neuroveget. (Wien), 11:72-89, 1955.

167. Babák, E. Bemerkungen ueber die Hypnose, den Immobilisations oder Sich-Totstellen-Reflex, den Schock und den Schlaf der Fische. Pfluegers Arch., 166:203-11, 1916-17. 336

168. Babinski, J. Sur le réflexe cutané plantaire dans certaines affections organiques du système nerveux central. C. R. Soc. Biol., 3:207-8,

1896. 16

169. _____. Du phénomène des orteils et de sa valeur sémiologique. Sem. Méd., 18:321-22, 1898. 16

170. Babonneix, L., et A. Widiez. Gliome des tubercules quadrijumeaux, avec, comme principal symptôme, la somnolence. Rev. Neurol., I:832-35, 1927. 265

171. Bach, L. M. N., H. B. Kelly, Jr., and R. Staub. Effect of lesions in reticular activating system. Am. J. Physiol., 183:594, 1955. 30, 206

172. Baege, M. H. Die Lebensverrichtungen im Schlaf. Psychol. Rundschau, 3:13-15, 1931.

173. Baender, A. Die Beziehungen des 24-Stunden-Rhythmus vegetativer Funktionen zum histologischen Funktionsbild endokriner Druesen. Z. exp. Med., 115: 229-50, 1950. 358

174. Baer, H. Psychophysische Erregungszustaende und ihre Behandlung durch neue Schlafmittelkombinationen. Schweiz. med. Wschr., 76:582-83, 1946. 294

175. _____. Die Schlafkur. Ein Beitrag zu ihrer Methodik und Technik. Schweiz. Arch. Neurol., 64:17-54, 1949. 206

176. Baerensprung, F. [W. F.] von. Untersuchungen ueber die Temperaturverhaeltnisse des Foetus und des erwachsenen Menschen im gesunden und kranken Zustaende. Arch. Anat. Physiol. wissen. Med., 126-75, 1851. 138

177. Bärtschi-Rochaix, W., und H. Sutermeister. Zur Pathophysiologie des Lachens, zugleich ein Beitrag ueber licht-aktivierte Lachanfaelle. Confinia Neurol., 15:10-32, 1955. 256

178. Bagby, E. Dreams during periods of emotional stress. J. Abnorm. Soc. Psychol., 25:289-92, 1930. 103

179. Bagchi, B. K., and N. N. Das. The distribution of EEG sleep cycle with its areal transients in normals and abnormals. EEG Clin. Neurophysiol., 2:232, 1950. 257

180. _____, and E. V. Jones. Variable temporal lobe foci in waking and sleep. EEG Clin. Neurophysiol., 3:384, 1951. 257

181. Bailey, P. Some unusual tumors of the third ventricle. Arch. Neurol. Psychiat., 20:1398-1402,

1928. 263
182. ____. Neurosurgical data on states of consciousness. First Internat. Congr. Neurol. Sci., Seconde Journée Commune. Brussels: Acta Med. Belg., 1957, pp. 135-40. Bailey, P., co-author: 1320.

183. Baker, C. H. Attention to visual displays during a vigilance task. II. Maintaining the level of vigilance. Brit. J. Psychol., 50:30-36, 1959.

184. ____. Towards a theory of vigilance. Canad. J. Psychol., 13:35-42, 1959.

185. Bakhtiarov, V. A. (Russ.) On narcolepsy. Soviet. Nevropat. Psikhiat. Psikhogig., 1:405-8, 1932. 271

186. Bakuradze, A., and S. Narikashvili. (Russ.) Spontaneous electrical activity of the brain during sleep. Trans. Beritashvili Physiol. Inst. SSSR, 6:377-401, 1945.

187. Bakwin, H. Sleep disturbances in childhood. Practitioner, 160:282-86, 1948. 286

188. Balard, P. Des variations du pouls et de la tension artérielle chez le nouveau-né, étudiées comparativement à l'état de veille et pendant le sommeil par l'oscillométrie. C. R. Soc. Biol., 72:998-99, 1912. 41, 43

189. Balch, C. C. Sleep in ruminants. Nature, 175:940-41, 1955. 10

190. Baldauf, L., und A. Pincussen. Untersuchungen ueber den Jod- und Bromgehalt des Blutes. Klin. Wschr., 9:1505, 1930.

191. Baldwin, D. S., J. H. Sirota, and H. Villarreal. Diurnal variations of renal function in congestive heart failure. Proc. Soc. Exp. Biol. Med., 74:578-81, 1950. 64
Baldwin, D. S., co-author: 3720.

192. Ballet, G. Le sommeil provoqué par occlusion des oreilles et des yeux chez les individus affectés d'anesthésie hystérique généralisée. Progr. Méd., 2ᵉ Série, 15:497-501, 1892. 199

193. Balter, V. Signification biologique du sommeil normal. Paris: Libr. M. Lac., 1930, Thèse. Pp. 56. 358

194. Balthazard, V. Variations horaires de l'excrétion urinaire chez l'homme normal. C. R. Soc. Biol., 53:163-64, 1901. 166

195. Ban, T., H. Masai, A. Sakai, and T. Kurotsu. Experimental studies on sleep by the electrical stimulation of the hypothalamus of rabbits. Med. J. Osaka Univ., 2:145-61, 1951. 204, 353, 358

196. Bancaud, J., V. Bloch, et J. Paillard. Contribution E.E.G. à l'étude des potentiels évoqués chez l'homme au niveau du vertex. Rev. Neurol., 89:399-418, 1953.

197. Banche, M. La secrezione gastrica notturna durante il sonno. Minerva Med., 1:428-34, 1950. 54

198. Bancroft, W. D. The agglomeration theory of sleep. Science, 76:522, 1932. 352

199. ____, and J. E. Rutzler, Jr. The agglomeration theory of sleep. Proc. Nat. Acad. Sci., 19:73-78, 1933. 352

200. Bañuelos, M. Patología y Clínica del Sueño y Estados Afines. Barcelona: Ed. Cient. Méd., 1940. Pp. 191.

201. Barad, M., K. Z. Altshuler, and A. I. Goldfarb. A survey of dreams in aged persons. A.M.A. Arch. Gen. Psychiat., 4:419-24, 1961. 102

202. Barahal, H. Dream structure and intellect. Psychiat. Q., 10:660-66, 1936. 103

203. Baraldi, M. Le modificazioni umorali indotte nell'organismo di epilettici sottoposti ad insonnia sperimentale. Riv. Sper. Freniat., 64:165-72, 1940. 227, 257

204. Barbé, A. Les hypnotiques en psychiatrie. Médicine, 13:105-6, 1932. 294

205. Barber, T. X. "Sleep" and "hypnosis": a reappraisal. J. Clin. Exp. Hypn. 4:141-59, 1956. 337

206. ____. Comparison of suggestibility during "light sleep" and hypnosis. Science, 124:405, 1956. 337

207. ____. Experiments in hypnosis. Sci. Am., 196(4):54-61, 1957. 337

208. ____. The concept of "hypnosis." J. Psychol., 45:115-31, 1958. 337

209. ____. Towards a theory of pain: relief of chronic pain by pre-frontal leucotomy, opiates, placebos, and hypnosis. Psychol. Bull., 56:430-60, 1959. 337

210. _____. Dream deprivation. Science, 132:1417-18, 1960. 337

211. _____. "Hypnosis," analgesia, and the placebo effect. J. Am. Med. Ass., 172:680-83, 1960. 337

212. _____. Physiological effects of "hypnosis." Psychol. Bull., 58: 390-419, 1961. 337, 338

213. _____. Death by suggestion. A critical note. Psychosom. Med., 23:153-55, 1961. 337

214. _____. Antisocial and criminal acts induced by "hypnosis." A.M.A. Arch. Gen. Psychiat., 5: 301-12, 1961. 334

215. _____, and J. Coules. Electrical skin conductance and galvanic response during "hypnosis." Internat. J. Clin. Exp. Hypn., 7:79-92, 1959. 330

Barber, T. X., co-author: 1456.

216. Barbizet, J. Yawning. J. Neurol. Neurosurg. Psychiat., 21:203-9, 1958. 71, 72

217. Barcroft, J., and C. S. Robinson. A study of some factors influencing intestinal movements. J. Physiol. (London), 67:211-20, 1929. 55

218. Bare, W. W., and A. T. Pepino. A new tablet form of chloral hydrate (WM-1127) in the treatment of insomnia in the aged. Am. Geriat. Soc. J., 9:686-93, 1961. 278

Bare, W. W., co-author: 3153.

219. Barelli, L. Ricerche sperimentali sulla febbre negli animali ibernanti. Boll. Soc. Ital. Biol. Sper., 7:1507-10, 1932; also Arch. Internat. Pharmacodyn., 45:172-88, 1933. 324

220. Barker, W. Studies in epilepsy: the petit mal attack as a response within the central nervous system to distress in organism-environment integration. Psychosom. Med., 10:73-94, 1948. 259

221. _____. Studies in epilepsy: Personality pattern, situational stress, and the symptoms of narcolepsy. Psychosom. Med., 10: 193-202, 1948. 237

222. _____, and S. Burgwin. Brain wave patterns accompanying changes in sleep and wakefulness during hypnosis. Psychosom. Med., 10:317-26, 1948. 330

223. _____, and _____. Brain wave patterns during hypnosis, hypnotic sleep and normal sleep. Arch. Neurol. Psychiat., 62:412-20, 1949. 330

224. _____, and S. Wolf. Studies in epilepsy. Experimental induction of grand mal seizure during hypnoidal state induced by sodium amytal. Am. J. Med. Sci., 214: 600-604, 1947. 257

225. Barmack, J. E. The effect of benzedrine sulphate (benzyl-methyl-carbamine) upon the report of boredom and other factors. J. Psychol., 5:125-33, 1938.

226. Barnes, T. C., and H. Brieger. Electroencephalographic studies of mental fatigue. J. Psychol., 22:181-92, 1946.

227. _____, and _____. Bioelectrical studies on fatigue: II. Students' electroencephalograms taken at 8 am and 5 pm. Fed. Proc., 5: 5-6, 1946.

228. Baroncini, L. et A. Beretta. Recherches histologiques sur les modifications des organes chez les mammifères hibernants. Arch. Ital. Biol., 35:295-96, 1901. 324

229. Barré, J. A., et M. Andlauer. Crises d'hypersomnie dans la maladie de Thomsen: action remarquable de l'insuline. Rev. Neurol. I:474-75, 1930. 268

230. Barrett, R. H. The analeptic effect of sodium succinate on barbiturate depression in man. Current Res. Anesth., 26:74-81, 105-13, 1947. 297

231. Barrington, G. G. How To Cure Insomnia. London: Lutterworth's, 1926 (?). Pp. 31. 278

232. Barry, J., and W. A. Bousfield. A quantitative determination of euphoria and its relation to sleep. J. Abnorm. Soc. Psychol., 29: 385-89, 1935. 119, 120

233. Bartlett, M. R. Curve of response to auditory stimuli preceding sleep. Psychol. Bull., 33:790-91, 1936. 76

234. _____. Minimal auditory stimuli during the onset of sleep. Am. J. Psychol., 54:109-12, 1941. 76

235. Bartley, S. H., and E. Chute. Fatigue and Impairment in Man. New York: McGraw-Hill, 1947. Pp. 429.

Bartley, S. H., co-author: 1684.

236. Baruk, H. Catatonie, sommeil pathologique et onirisme par intoxication colibacillaire. Paris Méd., 2:278-79, 1933. 254

237. _____. Le sommeil et l'onirisme. Progr. Méd., 79:584-88, 1951. 103

238. _____, et A. Albane. Catatonie intermittente suivant le rythme du sommeil. Ann. Méd.-Psychol., 89:439-46, 1931. 251

239. _____, et H. de Jong. Etudes sur la catatonie expérimentale. II. L'épreuve de la bulbocapnine chez la poule; catalepsie et sommeil. Proc. Roy. Acad. Amsterdam, 32:947-50, 1929. 253
Baruk, H., co-author: 716, 717, 3754.

240. Baserga, A. Poliglobulie da lesioni diencefalo-ipofisarie. Policlinico (Sez. Med.), 41:17-24, 1934. 268

241. Basile, G. Altro contributo sulla natura ipofisaria. Policlinico (Sez. Med.), 24:458-62, 1917. 268

242. Bass, E., und K. Herr. Untersuchungen ueber die Erregbarkeit des Atemzentrums im Schlaf—gemessen an der Alveolarspannung der Kohlensaeure. Z. Biol., 75: 279-88, 1922. 51, 110

243. Bass, M. J. Differentiation of the hypnotic trance from normal sleep. J. Exp. Psychol., 14:382-99, 1931. 331, 337

244. Bast, T. H. Morphological changes in fatigue. Wisconsin Med. J., 24:271-72, 1925. 217

245. _____, and W. B. Bloemendal. Studies in experimental exhaustion due to lack of sleep. IV. Effects on the nerve cells in the medulla. Am. J. Physiol., 82:140-46, 1927. 217

246. _____, and A. S. Loevenhart. Studies in exhaustion due to lack of sleep. I. Introduction and methods. Am. J. Physiol., 82:121-26, 1927. 217

247. _____, F. Schacht, and H. Vanderkamp. Studies in exhaustion due to lack of sleep. III. Effect on the nerve cells of the spinal cord. Am. J. Physiol., 82:131-39, 1927. 217

248. _____, J. S. Supernaw, B. Lieberman, and J. Munro. Studies in exhaustion due to lack of sleep. V. Effect on the thyroid and adrenal glands with special reference to mitochondria. Am. J. Physiol., 85:135-40, 1928. 217

249. Bates, C. E. H. Mixed salivary tumor in the right tonsil fossa with narcolepsy and cataplexy. Ann. Otol. Rhinol. Laryngol., 54: 812-17, 1945. 241

250. Bates, J. Posture during sleep. Lancet, I:186, 1942. 9

251. Bates, J. A. A technique for identifying changes in consciousness. EEG Clin. Neurophysiol., 5:445-46, 1953. 259

252. Batini, C., F. Magni, M. Palestini, G. F. Rossi, and A. Zanchetti. Neural mechanisms underlying the enduring EEG and behavioral activation in the midpontine pretrigeminal cat. Arch. Ital. Biol., 97:13-25, 1959. 212, 362

253. _____, _____, _____, e _____. Ricerche sull'origine della persistente sindrome di veglia del preparato mediopontino. Dati a favore dell'esistenza di una influenza sincronizzante di strutture bulbo-pontine sull'attività elettrica cerebrale. Riv. Neurol., 29:126-29, 1959. 212, 362

254. _____, G. Moruzzi, M. Palestini, G. F. Rossi, and A. Zanchetti. Persistent patterns of wakefulness in the pretrigeminal midpontine preparation. Science, 128:30-32, 1958. 212

255. _____, _____, _____, _____, and _____. Effects of complete pontile transection on the sleep-wakefulness rhythm: The midpontine pretrigeminal preparation. Arch. Ital. Biol., 97:1-12, 1959. 212

256. _____, M. Palestini, G. F. Rossi, and A. Zanchetti. EEG activation patterns in the midpontine pretrigeminal cat following sensory deafferentation. Arch. Ital. Biol., 97:26-32, 1959. 212

257. Batsel, H. L. Electroencephalographic synchronization and desynchronization in the chronic "cerveau isolé" of the dog. EEG Clin. Neurophysiol., 12:421-30, 1960. 211

258. Baudouin, A. Avant-Propos [to: Le Sommeil et ses Troubles]. Rev. Prat. (Paris), 4:1525-26, 1954.

259. _____, et H. Fischgold. L'électroencéphalogramme humain et son utilisation clinique. Biol. Méd. (Paris), 29:617-64, 1939. 29

260. _____, _____, R. Causse, et J. Lerique. Une vieille notion trop oubliée: La différence de potentiel rétino-cornéenne. Son intérêt théorique et pratique. Bull.

Acad. Méd., 121:688-93, 1939.
93

261. Bauer. Ueber Ermuedung und Schlaf als Arrangement des Neurotikers. Arch. Psychiat., 86: 318-21, 1929.

262. Bauer, R. B., N. Wechsler, and J. S. Meyer. Carotid compression and rotation of head in occlusive vertebral artery disease. Ann. Int. Med., 55:283-91, 1961. 242

263. Baumann, R. Physiologie des Schlafes und Klinik der Schlaftherapie. Berlin: VEB, Verlag Volk und Ges., 1953. Pp. viii + 227. 206

264. _____. Schlaf und Dauerschlafbehandlung. Berlin: VEB, Verlag Volk und Ges., 1955. Pp. 19. 206

265. Baumecker, W. Die Schlafzeit des Kleinkindes. Dsch. Gesundhwes., 13:496-99, 1958. 117

266. Bauer, J. Zur Schliddruesentherapie abnormer Schlafsucht. In: Libman Anniv. Vols., 1:181-85, New York: Internat. Press, 1932. 268

267. Bazett, H. C., S. Thurlow, C. Crowell, and W. Steward. Studies on the effects of baths on man. II. The diuresis caused by warm baths, together with some observations on urinary tides. Am. J. Physiol., 70:430-51, 1924. 64, 65

268. Bechterev, V. M. General Principles of Human Reflexology. New York: Internat. Publ., 1932. Pp. 467. 349

269. Becker, W. H. Zur Bekaempfung der nervoesen arteriosklerotischen Schlaflosigkeit. Wien. med. Wschr., 90:979-80, 1940. 278

270. Beckmann, A. Schlaftherapie. Zbl. Gyn., 76:1460-64, 1954. 206

271. Beckmann, J. W., and L. S. Kubie. Clinical study of 21 cases of tumor of the hypophyseal stalk. Brain, 52:127-70, 1929. 268

272. Beecher, H. K. Anesthesia's second power: probing the mind. Science, 105:164-66, 1947.

273. _____, and F. K. McDonough. Cortical action potentials during anesthesia. J. Neurophysiol., 2: 289-307, 1939. 296
Beecher, H. K., co-author: 467.

274. Béhague, P. Le sommeil durant les grands raids d'aviation. Rev. Neurol., I:880, 1927.

275. Beigel, H. Mental processes during the production of dreams. J. Psychol., 43:171-87, 1959. 104

276. Beilin, P. E. (Russ.) An attempt to organize medical treatment by conditioned reflex sleep in the Makarov hospital. In: The Sleep Problem, 1954 (392), pp. 543-52; also Klin. Med., (9):50-58, 1952. 206

277. _____. Curing Body and Mind with Sleep. Toronto: Northern Book House, 1958. Pp. 221.

278. Bein, H. J. Effects of reserpine on the functional strata of the nervous system. In: Psychotropic Drugs, 1957 (1357), pp. 325-31. 302

279. _____, F. Gross, J. Tripod, und R. Meier. Experimentelle Untersuchungen ueber "Serpasil" (Reserpin), ein neues wirksames Rauwolfiaalkaloid mit neuartiger zentraler Wirkung. Schweiz. med. Wschr., 83:1007-12, 1953. 302

280. Belaval, J. Y. Sur les sources sensorielles des visions du demi-sommeil. J. Psychol. (Paris), 30:812-26, 1933.

281. Bellak, L. An ego-psychological theory of hypnosis. Internat. J. Psycho-anal., 36:375-78, 1955. 337

282. Belluc, S., J. Chaussin, H. Laugier, et T. Ranson. Les variations nycthémérales dans l'élimination des principales substances de l'urine. C. R. Acad. Sci. (Paris), 207:90-92, 1938. 166, 167

283. Bellville, J. W., W. S. Howland, J. C. Seed, and R. W. Houde. The effect of sleep on the respiratory response to carbon dioxide. Anesthesiology, 20:628-34, 1959. 51

284. Beltran, J. R. La sugestión hipnótica. Rev. As. Méd. Argentina, 56:514-16, 1942. 336

285. Benda, C. E. Der Schlaf und das vegetative Nervensystem. Med. Welt, 9:1267-71, 1935. 294

286. Bénech, J. Algunos trastornos del sueño en los niños de las escuelas. Méd. Niños, 31:19-20, 1930. 307

287. Benedek, L. (Hungar.) Influence of hypnosis on the vegetative nervous system. Gyógyászat, 14:1-2, 1933. 330

288. _____, und A. Juba. Beitraege zur Pathologie des Dienzephalon. Psychiat.-Neurol. Wschr., 44: 409-12, 1942; also Z. ges. Neurol. Psychiat., 175:765-78, 1943. 272

289. _____, und _____. Beitraege zur Pathologie des Diencephalon. II. Narkoleptisches Syndrom mit histologischem Befund. Z. ges. Neurol. Psychiat., 176:586-95, 1943. 237

290. _____, e J. Thurzó. La narcolessia genuina e la sua terapia; utilizzazione del'insufflazione di aria per via suboccipitale quale efficace metodo di cura. Riforma Med., 47:443-47, 1931. 239

291. Benedict, F. G. The measurement and significance of basal metabolism. Mayo Found. Lect., 45-47, 1924-25. 55

292. _____, und J. F. Snell. Koerpertemperaturschwankungen mit besonderer Ruecksicht auf den Einfluss welchen die Umkehrung der taeglichen Lebensgewohnheit beim Menschen ausuebt. Pfluegers Arch., 90:33-72, 1902. 173
Benedict, F. G., co-author: 2705, 4194.

293. Benjamin, B., and F. A. Nash. Sleep and tuberculosis. Tubercle (London), 34:50-53, 1953. 121

294. Bennett, L. L., and N. E. Scott. The production of electrocardiographic abnormalities by suggestion under hypnosis: a case report. Am. Practitioner, 4:189-90, 1949. 331

295. Benoit, O., et V. Bloch. Seuil d'excitabilité réticulaire et sommeil profond chez le chat. J. Physiol. (Paris), 52:17-18, 1960. 212

296. Benon, R. Asthénie et insomnie. Rev. Gén. Clin. Thérap., 47:182-84, 1932. 276

297. Bentley, M. The study of dreams. Am. J. Psychol., 26:196-210, 1915. 100, 101

298. Bérard, E., et G. C. Lairy. Quelques remarques sur l'électroencéphalogramme au cours de l'hibernation artificielle. EEG Clin. Neurophysiol., 7:545-52, 1955. 328

299. Berg, H. Exogener oder endogener 24-Stunden-Rhythmus. Grenzgebiete Med., 2:386-88, 1949. 131

300. Berger, E., et R. Loewy. L'état des yeux pendant le sommeil et la théorie du sommeil. J. Anat.

Physiol. (Paris), 34:364-418, 1898. 106

301. Berger, H. Ueber das Elektroenkephalogramm des Menschen. J. Psychol. Neurol., 40: 160-79, 1930. 25

302. Berger, R. J. Tonus of extrinsic laryngeal muscles during sleep and dreaming. Science, 134:840, 1961. 50, 98

303. _____, P. Olley, and I. Oswald. EEG and eye-movements and dreams of the blind. EEG Clin. Neurophysiol., 13:827, 1961. 98, 102

304. Berggren, S., und E. Moberg. Experimentelle Untersuchungen zum Problem des Schlafes. Acta Psychiat. Neurol., 4:1-46, 1929. 200

305. Bergson, H. The World of Dreams. New York: Philosoph. Library, 1958. Pp. 58. 106

306. Bergström, J. A. An experimental study of some of the conditions of mental activity. Am. J. Psychol., 6:247-74, 1894. 150

307. Bérillon, [E.] Le centre du réveil. Interprétation anatomophysiologique de l'hypnotisme. Lancette Franç. Gaz. Hôp., 82: 483-85, 1909. 362

308. Berliner, B. Neurotic disturbances of sleep. Internat. J. Psycho-anal., 23:64, 1942. 276, 286

309. Berman, S. Insomnia. South African Med. J., 9:37-40, 1935. 274

310. Bernal, P. Traitement de l'hypertension artérielle par le sommeil. In: La Cure de Sommeil, 1954 (3021), pp. 149-56. 207

311. _____, et P. Lévy. Cure de sommeil et infarctus du myocarde. In: La Cure de Sommeil, 1954 (3021), pp. 176-84. 207

312. Bernardi, R. Gli accessi di sonno incoercibilli. Cervello, 12: 337-54, 1933. 239

313. Bernhard, C. G., E. Bohm, L. Kirstein, and T. Wiesel. The difference in action on normal and convulsive cortical activity between a local anaesthetic (lidocaine) and barbiturates. Arch. Internat. Pharmacodyn., 108: 408-19, 1956.

314. _____, and C. R. Skoglund. On the alpha frequency of human brain potentials as a function of age. Skand. Arch. Physiol.,

82:178-84, 1939. 28

315. Bernhaut, M., E. Gellhorn, and A. T. Rasmussen. Experimental contributions to problem of consciousness. J. Neurophysiol., 16: 21-35, 1953.
Bernhaut, M., co-author: 1390.

316. Bernheim. Définition et valeur thérapeutique de l'hypnotisme. Rev. Psychiat. Psychol. Exp., 15: 402-15, 1911. 329, 336

317. Berrien, F. K. Recall of dreams during the sleep period. J. Abnorm. Soc. Psychol., 25:110-14, 1930. 100

318. _____. A statistical study of dreams in relation to emotional stability. J. Abnorm. Soc. Psychol., 28:194-97, 1933. 101

319. _____. A study of objective dream activity in abnormal children. J. Abnorm. Soc. Psychol., 30:84-91, 1935.

320. Bertolani del Rio, M. Si possono provocare negli epilettici accessi convulsivi impedendo per un certo tempo il sonno? Riv. Sper. Freniat., 64:159-64, 1940. 227, 257

321. Bertoye, P. Sur un trouble rare du sommeil chez l'enfant: la jactatio capitis nocturna. Bull. Soc. Pédiat. Paris, 25:61-66. 1927. 285

322. Besold, F. Der Schlaf unter dem Gesichtspunkt der intravenoesen Narkose. Wien. med. Wschr., 92: 697-700, 1942. 294

323. Bettelheim, B. Does your child fight sleep? Parents Mag., 26:54-55, 83-100, 1951. 307

324. Bettòlo, A. L'insonnia e sua importanza clinica: le sue cause predisponenti e determinanti, i suoi caratteri nelle diverse malattie, la sua importanza prognostica ed il suo trattamento generale e speciale. Studium, 21:54-65, 1931. 275, 294

325. Beucher, M. Traitement des troubles du sommeil chez l'enfant. Rev. Neuro-Psychiat. Infant. Hyg. Ment. Enfance (Paris), 5:677-84, 1957. 286

326. Bexton, W. H., W. Heron, and T. H. Scott. Effects of decreased variation in the sensory environment. Canad. J. Psychol., 8:70-76, 1954. 198
Bexton, W. H., co-author: 3634.

327. Beyer, K. H., and A. R. Latven. An evaluation of the influence of succinate and malonate on barbiturate hypnosis. J. Pharmacol. Exp. Therap., 81:203-8, 1944. 297

328. Beyer, P., et C. Kayser. Etablissement du rythme nychtéméral de la sécrétion urinaire chez le nourrisson. C. R. Soc. Biol., 143:1231-33, 1949. 166

329. Beyermann. Ueber pathologische Schlafzustaende, insbesondere narkoleptische Anfaelle, in ihrem Zusammenhange mit Funktionsstoerungen der Hypophyse. Z. ges. Neurol. Psychiat., 128:726-50, 1930. 240

330. Bickel, A. Der Babinski'sche Zehenreflex unter physiologischen und pathologischen Bedingungen. Dsche Z. Nervenheilk., 22:163-65, 1902. 17

331. Bickford, R. G. New dimensions in electroencephalography. Neurology, 7:469-75, 1957.
Bickford, R. G., co-author: 1522, 3382, 3627, 3628.

332. Bier, W. Beitrag zur Beeinflussung des Kreislaufes durch psychische Vorgaenge. Z. klin. Med., 113:762-81, 1930. 329, 330

333. Biermann, B. Der Hypnotismus im Lichte der Lehre von den bedingten Reflexen. J. Psychol. Neurol., 38:265-81, 1929. 337

334. _____. (Russ.) Hypno-susceptibility in neuroses and its physiological basis. Arkh. Biol. Nauk, 36(I):3-12, 1934. 335

335. _____. (Russ.) Experimental Sleep. Leningrad: Gosizdat, 1925. Pp. 65; also in: The Sleep Problem, 1954 (392), pp. 98-99. 197, 336

336. Bierry, H., et M. Kollmann. Activité endocrine du pancréas et îlots de Langerhans. Cas de l'hibernation. C. R. Soc. Biol., 99: 456-59, 1928. 322

337. Bigelow, N., G. H. Cameron, and S. A. Koroljow. Two cases of deep hypnotic sleep investigated by the strain gauge plethysmograph. J. Clin. Exp. Hypn., 4:160-64, 1956. 331

338. Bijlsma, U. G., E. I. van Itallie, P. Ruitinga, P. van der Wielen, and E. D. Wiersma. The Treatment of Insomnia. 'sGravenhage: Rijks. Inst. Pharm. Therap. Onderzoek, 1931. Pp. 88. 274

339. Bilancioni, G. Su due casi di ipersonnia in soggetti otitici

d'antica data. Quad. Psichiat., 9: 161-71, 1922.

340. Billings, E. G. A new method of administering hypnotics for the purpose of controlling sleep disorders characterized by early morning awakening. Dis. Nerv. Syst., 3:38-47, 1942. 294

341. Bills, A. G. The influence of muscular tension on the efficiency of mental work. Am. J. Psychol., 38: 227-51, 1927.

342. ____. Blocking: a new principle of mental fatigue. Am. J. Psychol., 43:230-45, 1931. 155, 225

343. ____. Some additional principles of mental fatigue. Psychol. Bull., 31:671, 1934. 155

344. ____. Fatigue in mental work. Physiol. Rev. 17:436-53, 1937. 155

345. Binet, L. Données récentes sur la physiologie du sommeil. J. Méd. Franç., 15:433-38, 1926.

346. Binet, M. E. L'insomnie chez les entéro-hépatiques. Acta Gastroentér. Belg., 12:66-68, 1949. 276

347. Bingel, A. Ueber die Tagesperiodik Geisterkranker dargestellt am Elektrodermatogramm. Z. ges. Neurol. Psychiat., 170:404-40, 1940. 308

348. Binns, E. The Anatomy of Sleep; or The Art of Procuring Sound and Refreshing Slumber at Will. London: John Churchill, 1842. Pp. x + 394. 312

349. Binz, C. Ueber den Traum. Bonn: Adolph Marcus, 1878. Pp. 55. 100, 106

350. Biörck, G., B. Johansson, and H. Schmid. Reactions of hedgehogs, hibernating and non-hibernating, to the inhalation of oxygen, carbon dioxide, and nitrogen. Acta Physiol. Scand., 37:71-83, 1956. 323

351. ____, ____, and S. Veige. Some laboratory data on hedgehogs, hibernating and non-hibernating. Acta Physiol. Scand., 37:281-94, 1956. 322, 323

352. Birchfield, R. I., H. O. Sieker, and A. Heyman. Alterations in blood gases during natural sleep and narcolepsy. A correlation with the electroencephalographic stages of sleep. Neurology, 8:107-12, 1958. 51, 238

353. ____, ____, and ____. Alterations in respiratory function during natural sleep. J. Lab. Clin.

Med., 54:216-22, 1959. 51, 238

354. Bird, B. Pathological sleep. Internat. J. Psycho-anal., 35:20-29, 1954. 271

355. Birdsall, S. E. Sodium soneryl as a basal hypnotic. Brit. Med. J., I:871-72, 1933.

356. Birkner, R., und J. Trautmann. Ueber die Abhaengigkeit psychischer, Schlaf- und genitaler Funktionen von den vegetativen Steuerungszentren im Hypothalamus und die Beeinflussbarkeit dieser Funktionen durch Roentgenbestrahlungen des Zwischenhirngebietes mit kleinen Dosen. Strahlentherapie, 91:321-50, 1953. 286

357. Birns, M. Les Troubles du Sommeil dans l'Encéphalopathie Traumatique. Genève (Ambilly-Annemasse): Imprim. Franco-Suisse, 1955. Pp. 51.

358. Bizette, A. Remarques sur les phases du présommeil. J. Psychol. (Paris), 28:647-51, 1931. 79

359. Bjerk, E. M., and J. J. Hornischer. Narcolepsy: a case report and a rebuttal. EEG Clin. Neurophysiol., 10:550-52, 1958. 237, 238

360. Bjerner, B. Alpha depression and lowered pulse rate during delayed actions in a serial reaction test. A study in sleep deprivation. Acta Physiol. Scand., 19, Suppl. 65, 1949. Pp. 93. 158, 226

361. ____, Aa. Holm, and Aa. Swensson. Diurnal variation in mental performance; a study of three-shift workers. Brit. J. Indust. Med., 12:103-10, 1955. 316

362. ____, und Aa. Swensson. Schichtarbeit und Rhythmus. Acta Med. Scand. Suppl. 278:102-7, 1953. 316, 317

363. Blacker, C. P. A patient's dreams as an index of his inner life. Guy's Hosp. Rep., 78:219-44, 1928. 103

364. Blake, H. Brain potentials and depth of sleep. Am. J. Physiol., 119:273-74, 1937.

365. ____, and R. W. Gerard. Brain potentials during sleep. Am. J. Physiol., 119:692-703, 1937. 26, 223, 300, 330, 331

366. ____, ____, and N. Kleitman. Factors influencing brain poten-

tials during sleep. J. Neurophysiol., 2:48-60, 1939. 26, 75,
95, 223, 238, 300

367. Blanc, C., P. Kramarz, N. Monod,
and C. Dreyfus-Brisac. Abnormalities of sleep potentials in
children of less than three years
of age. EEG Clin. Neurophysiol.,
9:567, 1957. 286
Blanc, C., co-author: 980-83, 985

368. Blanchard, P. A study of subject
matter and motivation of children's dreams. J. Abnorm. Soc.
Psychol., 21:24-37, 1926. 102

369. Blank, H. R. Dreams of the blind.
Psychoanal. Q., 27:158-74, 1958.
102

370. Blankenhorn, M. A., and H. E.
Campbell. The effect of sleep on
blood pressure. Am. J. Physiol.,
74: 115-20, 1925. 40, 44, 45,
109
Blankenhorn, M. A., co-author:
618

371. Blau, A. Nocturnal enuresis. J.
Am. Med. Ass., 154:1116, 1954.
284

372. Bleckmann, K. H. Der Schlaf des
Kindes. Med. Welt, 20:1019-24,
1951. 307

373. _____. Der Schlaf als biologisches
und anthropologisches Problem.
Med. Mschr., 6:247-51, 1952.

374. _____. Der Schlaf des Kindes.
Goettingen: Verlag f. med. Psychol., 1955. Pp. 213.

375. Bleckwenn, W. J. Production of
sleep and rest in psychotic states.
Arch. Neurol. Psychiat., 21:365-
72, 1930; also J. Am. Med. Ass.,
95:1168-71, 1930. 206

376. Blinn, K. A., and K. S. Ditman.
The sleep EEG in enuresis. EEG
Clin. Neurophysiol., 5:474, 1953.
284
Blinn, K. A., co-author: 943.

377. Bliss, E. L., L. D. Clark, and C.
D. West. Studies of sleep deprivation—relationship to schizophrenia. A.M.A. Arch. Neurol. Psychiat., 81:348-59, 1959. 225, 226,
228
Bliss, E. L., co-author: 2810.

378. Bloch, V., et M. Bonvallet. Le
contrôle inhibiteur bulbaire des
réponses électrodermales. C. R.
Soc. Biol., 154:42-45, 1960. 209
Bloch, V., co-author: 196, 295,
406.

379. Blomfield, J. M., and J. W. B.
Douglas. Bedwetting prevalence
among children aged 4-7. Lancet,

270:850-52, 1956. 284

380. Bloom, W. Shift work and the
sleep-wakefulness cycle. Personnel, 38:24-31, 1961. 317

381. Bloomberg, W. End results of
use of large doses of Amphetamine sulfate over prolonged periods. New Engl. J. Med., 222:
946-48, 1940. 239
Bloomberg, W., co-author: 3241.

382. Blotner, H., and M. Bacon. Nar-
colepsy, cataplexy and epilepsy.
Report of a case. J. Maine Med.
Ass., 38:264-67, 1947. 237

383. Blum, R. A., J. S. Blum, and K.
L. Chow. The production of unilateral epileptiform convulsions
from otherwise quiescent foci
by the administration of benzedrine. Science, 108:560-61, 1948.
259

384. Blume, J. Ueber die Beeinflussung des Grundrhythmus der
Koerpertemperatur durch rhythmische Aenderungen der Wach-
und Schlafzeiten. Z. ges. exp.
Med., 128:452-57, 1957.
Blume, J., co-author: 2779, 2780.

385. Blume, P. (Swed.) On the blood
pressure of sleepers. Ugeskr.
Laeger, 84:1126-32, 1922. 43

386. Boas, E. P. The heart rate during sleep in Graves' disease and
in neurogenic sinus tachycardia.
Am. Heart J., 8:24-28, 1932-33.
41

387. _____, and E. F. Goldschmidt.
The Heart Rate. Springfield, Ill.:
Thomas, 1932. Pp. 166. 40, 42,
43, 74, 109, 123, 163

388. _____, and M. Weiss. The heart
rate during sleep. J. Am. Med.
Ass., 92:2162-68, 1929. 41

389. Bochnik, H. J. Mehrgleisig-si-
multane Untersuchungen sponta-
ner Tagesschwankungen sensi-
bler, motorischer und vegetativer Funktionen. Ein Weg zur
Aufklaerung funktioneller Ord-
nungen. Nervenarzt, 29:307-13,
1958. 169

390. Bodenheimer, A. R. Ueber die
Schlafinversion der Greise.
Therap. Umschau (Bern), 11:57-
58, 1954. 174

391. Boerner-Patzelt, D. Das braune
Fett der sogenannten Winter-
schlafdruese des Igels. Z. mikr.-
anat. Forsch., 63:5-34, 1957. 326

392. Bogorad, S. I., Compiler. (Russ.)
The Sleep Problem—A Compilation. Moskva: Medgiz, 1954. Pp.

xiv + 620. 345

393. Bogoslovsky, A. I. Diurnal changes in the electrical sensitivity of
the eye. Bull. Biol. Méd. Exp.
URSS, 3:127-29, 1937. 159

394. _____. Changes in the electrical
sensitivity of the eye during visual activity. Bull. Biol. Méd. Exp.
URSS, 3:130-32, 1937. 159

395. Boigey, M. Hygiène du réveil et
exercice. Bull. Acad. Méd. Paris,
117:67-70, 1937. 311

396. Bolli, L. Le rêve et les aveugles.
I. Le rêve et les aveugles-nés. J.
Psychol., 29:20-73, 1932. 100, 102

397. Bolton, E. B. A concrete case for
Woodworth's hypothesis on the
cause of dreams. J. Psychol., 16:
273-84, 1943. 103

398. Bond, N. B. The psychology of
waking. J. Abnorm. Soc. Psychol.,
24:226-30, 1929.

399. Bonhoeffer, K. Ueber Dissozia-
tion der Schlafkomponenten bei
Postencephalitikern. Wien. klin.
Wschr., 41:979-81, 1928. 249, 267

400. Bonjour, J. Pourquoi nous dor-
mons. Rev. Méd. Suisse Rom., 53:
876-81, 1933.

401. Bonnet, H., and G. Malpertuy.
Electrographic, biochemical and
clinical correlations during the
course of therapeutic insulin "comas" in 18 mental patients. EEG
Clin. Neurophysiol., 7:151-52,
1955. 273

402. Bonnet, V., et R. Saboul. Contribution à l'étude de l'hypnose animale. Modifications nerveuses et
phénomène de subordination dans
l'hypnose chez la grenouille. J.
Physiol. Path. Gén., 33:887-906,
1935. 336

403. Bonoriño Udaondo, C. Hipersomnia e insuficiencia tiroidea. Rev.
Asoc. Méd. Argent., 33:413-23,
1920. 268

404. Bonstedt, T. Emotional aspects of
the narcolepsies; with report of a
case of sleep paralysis. Dis.
Nerv. Syst., 15:291-97, 1954. 237

405. Bonvallet, M., D. Albe-Fessard,
et A. Fessard. Quelques expériences de contrôle à propos de variations de chronaxies nerveuses
périphériques. Arch. Internat.
Physiol., 54:119-24, 1946. 14

406. _____, and V. Bloch. Bulbar control of cortical arousal. Science,
133:1133-34, 1961. 209

407. _____, P. Dell, et G. Hiebel. Tonus sympathique et activité électrique corticale. EEG Clin. Neurophysiol., 6:119-44, 1954. 213,
241, 242

408. _____, A. Hugelin, et P. Dell.
Sensibilité comparée du système
réticulaire activateur et du centre respiratoire aux gaz du sang
et à l'adrénaline. J. Physiol.
(Paris), 47:651-54, 1955.

409. _____, _____, et _____. Milieu
intérieur et activité automatique
des cellules réticulaires mésen-
céphaliques. J. Physiol. (Paris),
48:403-6, 1956. 209

410. _____, E. Morel, et P. Benda.
Sur quelques épreuves suscepti-
bles de déclencher une éosino-
pénie d'origine émotionelle, chez
le chien. C. R. Soc. Biol., 145:
1051-55, 1951. 170
Bonvallet, M., co-author: 378,
886-89, 1761, 1856-58.

411. Bonzanigo, C. Klinisch-experi-
mentelle Untersuchungen der
Ephetonin-Wirkung im Kindesalter. Arch. Kinderheilk., 94:15-
45, 1931. 294

412. Borak, J., und H. Uiberall. Ueber
den Einfluss der Roentgenstrah-
len auf winterschlafende Tiere.
Wien. klin. Wschr., 49:109-11,
1936. 324

413. Bordeleau, J.-M. Une nouvelle
technique pour provoquer des
psychoses expérimentales: la
privation de sommeil. Un. Méd.
Canad., 88:976-78, 1959.

414. Boring, E. G., and L. D. Boring.
Temporal judgment after sleep.
In: Studies in Psychol., Titche-
ner Commem. Vol., 1917, pp.
255-79. 126

415. Born, W. A history of dream interpretation. Ciba Symposia, 10:
926-39, 1948. 99

416. _____. The dream and art. Ciba
Symposia, 10:940-51, 1948. 99

417. Bornstein, A. Einfluss von
Schlafmitteln auf den Grundum-
satz beim Basedow. Dsche med.
Wschr., II:1861-62, 1930.

418. Boss, M. Die funktionellen
Schlafstoerungen in der Schizophrenie (Ein Beitrag zum Problem der vegetativen Regulationsstoerungen animaler Funktionen). Schweiz. med. Wschr.,
22:390-91, 1941. 286

419. _____. Der Traum und seine
Auslegung. Bern: Hans Huber,
1953. Pp. 239. Also: The Analysis of Dreams. New York: Philo-

soph. Library, 1958. Pp. 223. 106

420. Bossard, R. Psychologie du Rêve. Paris: Payot, 1953. Pp. 228. Also: Psychologie des Traumbewusstseins. Zuerich: Rascher Verlag, 1951. Pp. vii + 419. 99

421. Bostock, J. An Elementary System of Physiology. London: Henry G. Bohn, 1836. Pp. 887.

422. Bostock, J. Sleep. Med. J. Australia, II:614-15, 1940.

423. _____. Exterior gestation, primitive sleep, enuresis, and asthma: a study in aetiology. Med. J. Australia, II:149-53, 185-88, 1958. 285

424. Bouchard, C. Sur les variations de la toxicité urinaire pendant la veille, et pendant le sommeil. C. R. Acad. Sci., 102:727, 1886. 64, 200

425. _____. Sur la théorie toxique du sommeil et de la veille. C. R. Acad. Sci., 152:564-65, 1911. 64, 352

426. Bourguignon, G., et J. B. S. Haldane. Evolution de la chronaxie pendant le sommeil. C. R. Soc. Biol., 107:1365-66, 1931. 14

427. Bousfield, W. A. Further evidence of the relation of the euphoric attitude to sleep and exercise. Psychol. Rec., 2:334-44, 1938. 314

428. _____. Relation of euphoric attitude to quality of sleep. J. Psychol., 9:393-401, 1940. 119, 120, 314

Bousfield, W. A., co-author: 232.

429. Bowen, J. H., S. Ross, and T. G. Andrews. A note on the interaction of conditioned inhibition in pursuit tracking. J. Gen. Psychol., 55:153-62, 1956. 226

430. Bowers, E. F. How can we get enough sleep? New York Med. J. Med. Rec., 108:796, 1918. 306

431. _____. Sleeping for Health. London: George Routledge & Sons, 1920. Pp. 128. 309

432. Bowling, G., and N. G. Richards. Diagnosis and treatment of the narcolepsy syndrome; analysis of seventy-five case records. Cleveland Clin. Q., 28:38-45, 1961. 241

433. Bowman, K. M., and A. Simon. Studies in electronarcosis therapy. I. Clinical evaluation. Am. J. Psychiat., 105:15-27, 1948. 298

Bowman, K. M., co-author: 196.

434. Boyd, L. J., W. Gittinger, and J. Schwimmer. Sleep induction with combined administration of sali-cylamide and acetophenetidin. New York State J. Med., 57:924-28, 1957. 294

435. Boyer, P. Du Sommeil dans les Maladies. Thèse, Nîmes, 1879. Pp. 66.

436. Boynton, M. A. The postural habits of nursery school children during sleep. Proc. IX Internat. Congr. Psychol., 1929, pp. 93-94. 9, 186

437. _____, and F. L. Goodenough. The posture of nursery school children during sleep. Am. J. Psychol., 42:270-78, 1930. 8, 9, 90, 306

438. Bozzi, R. Contributo clinico allo studio della patogenesi della narcocatalessia. Note Psichiat. (Pesaro), 70:163-94, 1941. 237

439. Brabant, J. A propos du ronflement. Arch. Stomatol. (Liège), 4:205-8, 1949; 10:53-54, 1955. 50

440. Brading, E. T. Narcolepsy. South. Med. J., 38:838-41, 1945. 234

441. Bradley, P. B. The effect of some drugs on the electrical activity of the brain of the conscious cat. EEG Clin. Neurophysiol., Suppl. 3:21, 1953. 300, 303, 304

442. _____. Recent observations on the action of some drugs in relation to the reticular formation of the brain. EEG Clin. Neurophysiol., 9:372-73, 1957. 304

443. _____, and J. Elkes. The effect of amphetamine and D-lysergic acid diethylamide (LSD 25) on the electrical activity of the brain of the conscious cat. J. Physiol. (London), 120:13P-14P, 1953. 300

444. _____, and _____. Effect of atropine, hyoscyamine, physostigmine, and neostigmine on the electrical activity of the brain of the cat. J. Physiol. (London), 120:14P-15P, 1953. 30, 304

445. _____, and _____. The effects of some drugs on the electrical activity of the brain. Brain. 80:77-117, 1957. 30, 304

446. _____, and A. J. Hance. The effect of chlorpromazine on the electrical activity of the brain of the conscious cat. J. Physiol. (London), 129:50P-51P, 1955. 301

447. _____, and B. J. Key. The effect

of drugs on arousal responses produced by stimulation of the reticular formation of the brain. EEG Clin. Neurophysiol., 10:97-110, 1958; prelim. commun., XX Internat. Physiol. Congr. Abstracts, Brussels, 1956, pp. 124-25.

448. _____, and _____. A comparative study of the effects of drugs on the arousal system of the brain. Brit. J. Pharmacol. Chemotherapy, 14:340-49, 1959. 301, 302

449. _____, and A. Mollica. The effect of adrenaline and acetylcholine on single unit activity in the reticular formation of the decerebrate cat. Arch. Ital. Biol., 96:168-86, 1958; prelim. commun., Boll. Soc. Ital. Biol. Sper., 33:1627-29, 1957. 209, 304, 358
Bradley, P. B., co-author: 2150.

450. Brailovsky, V. Ueber die pathologische Schlaefrigkeit und das Schlafzentrum. Z. ges. Neurol. Psychiat., 100:272-88, 1926. 239, 360

451. Brain, W. R. Sleep: normal and pathological. Brit. Med. J., II:51-53, 1939.

452. _____. The cerebral basis of consciousness. Brain, 73:465-79, 1950. 31

453. _____. The cerebral basis of consciousness (abridged). Proc. Roy. Soc. Med., 44:37-42, 1951. 31

454. _____. The physiological basis of consciousness: a critical review. Brain, 81:426-55, 1958. 31
Brain, W. R., co-author: 2361.

455. Braines, S. N. (Russ.) Experience with artificial sleep in the biological experiment. Zh. Vysshei Nerv. Deiat., 2:381-87, 1952. 207

456. Bram, I. How much sleep do you need? Med. Rec. (N.Y.), 150:219-22, 1939. 120

457. Bramesfeld, E., und H. Jung. Unfallverursachende Daemmerzustaende bei Fahrzeugfuehrern. Indust. Psychotech., 9:193-210, 1932.

458. Brandenburg, K. Ueber die Behandlung der Schlaflosigkeit. Med. Klin., 36:19-20, 1940. 278

459. Brandrup, E. (Norw.) Problems of consciousness from a neurological view. Nord. Med. (Stockholm), 60:1593-96, 1958.

460. Brandt, S., and H. Brandt. The electroencephalographic patterns in young healthy children from 0 to five years of age. Their practical use in daily clinical electroencephalography. Acta Psychiat. Neurol. Scand., 30:77-89, 1955. 27, 28, 76

461. Brauchi, J. T., and L. J. West. Sleep deprivation. J. Am. Med. Ass., 171:11-14, 1959. 228

462. Brauchle, A. Die naturgemaesse Behandlung der Schlaflosigkeit. Dsche med. Wschr., 66(II):1289-92, 1940.

463. Brazier, M. A. B. The electrical fields at the surface of the head during sleep. EEG Clin. Neurophysiol., 1:195-204, 1949. 26, 75

464. _____. Physiological problems arising from the study of natural and sedate sleep, and of anesthesia in man. EEG Clin. Neurophysiol., 5:465, 1953. 296

465. _____. The action of anesthetics on the nervous system with special reference to the brain stem reticular system. In: Brain Mechanisms and Consciousness, 1954 (875), pp. 163-99. 298

466. _____. Neuronal structure, brain potentials and epileptic discharge. Epilepsia, 3rd Ser., 4:9-18, 1955. 259

467. _____, and H. K. Beecher. Alpha content of the electroencephalogram in relation to movements made in sleep, and effect of a sedative on this type of motility. J. Appl. Physiol., 4:819-25, 1952. 26, 28

468. _____, and J. E. Finesinger. Action of barbiturates on the cerebral cortex. Arch. Neurol. Psychiat., 53:51-58, 1945. 296
Brazier, M. A. B., co-author: 1169, 3114, 3991.

469. Bredland, E. Effect of sleep deprivation on certain human activities. Ph.D. Thesis, New York Univ., 1955. Pp. 170.; also Dissert. Abstr., 15:1781-82, 1955. 226

470. Brehmer, G., und K.-T. Ruckdeschal. Zur Technik der Winterschlafbehandlung. Dsche med. Wschr., 78:1724-25, 1953. 206

471. Breinin, G. M. The position of rest during anesthesia and sleep. Electromyographic observations. A.M.A. Arch. Ophthal., 57:323-26, 1957. 297

472. _____. Quantitative electronic techniques in ocular motility.

Trans. New York Acad. Sci., Ser. 2, 21:605-8, 1959. 93

473. Bremer, F. Cerveau "isolé" et physiologie du sommeil. C. R. Soc. Biol., 118:1235-41, 1935. 26, 205, 296

474. _____. Nouvelles recherches sur le mécanisme du sommeil. C. R. Soc. Biol., 122:460-64, 1936. 26, 205, 348

475. _____. Action de différentes narcotiques sur les activités électriques spontanées et réflexes du cortex cérébral. C. R. Soc. Biol., 121:861-66, 1936. 26, 205, 348

476. _____. Etude oscillographique des activités sensorielles du cortex cérébral. C. R. Soc. Biol., 124:842-46, 1937. 26, 205, 296, 348

477. _____. Différence d'action de la narcose éthérique et du sommeil barbiturique sur les réactions sensorielles acoustiques du cortex cérébral. Signification de cette différence en ce qui concerne le mécanisme du sommeil. C. R. Soc. Biol., 124:848-52, 1937. 26, 205, 296, 348

478. _____. L'activité cérébrale au cours du sommeil et de la narcose: contribution à l'étude du mécanisme du sommeil. Bull. Acad. Roy. Méd. Belg., 4:68-86, 1937. 12, 26

479. _____. Effets de la déafferentation complète d'une région de l'écorce cérébrale sur son activité électrique spontanée. C. R. Soc. Biol., 127:355-59, 1938. 12, 211

480. _____. L'activité électrique de l'écorce cérébrale et le problème physiologique du sommeil. Boll. Soc. Ital. Biol. Sper., 13:271-90, 1938. 362

481. _____. Le problème physiologique du sommeil. Medicina, 1:589-612, 1951. 362

482. _____. Considérations sur les interrelations de l'écorce cérébrale et des structures sous-corticales. Gaz. Méd. Portug., 7:127-30, 1954. 362

483. _____. The neurophysiological problem of sleep. In: Brain Mechanisms and Consciousness, 1954 (875), pp. 137-62. 362

484. _____. Quelques aspects physiologiques du problème des relations réciproques de l'écorce cérébrale et des structures sous-corticales. Acta Neurol. Psychiat. Belg., 55:

947-65, 1955.

485. _____. De quelques problèmes posés par la physiopathologie des altérations de la conscience. First Internat. Congr. Neurol. Sci., Seconde Journée Commune. Brussels, 1957. Acta Med. Belg., pp. 49-66. 31

486. _____. Analyse des processus corticaux de l'éveil. EEG Clin. Neurophysiol., Suppl. 13:125-36, 1960. 211

487. _____, et N. Stoupel. De la modification des réponses sensorielles corticales dans l'éveil réticulaire. Acta Neurol. Belg., 58:401-3, 1958; also Arch. Internat. Physiol., 67:240-75, 1959. 211

488. _____, et _____. Etude pharmacologique de la facilitation des réponses corticales dans l'éveil réticulaire. Arch. Internat. Pharmacodyn., 122:234-48, 1959. 298

489. _____, et C. Terzuolo. Rôle de l'écorce cérébrale dans le processus du réveil. Arch. Internat. Physiol., 60:228-31, 1952. 211

490. _____, et _____. Interaction de l'écorce cérébrale et de la formation réticulée du tronc cérébral dans le mécanisme de l'éveil et du maintien de l'activité vigile. J. Physiol. (Paris), 45:56-57, 1953. 211

491. _____, et _____. Nouvelles recherches sur le processus physiologique du réveil. Arch. Internat. Physiol., 61:86-90, 1953. 211

492. _____, et _____. Contribution à l'étude des mécanismes physiologiques du maintien de l'activité vigile du cerveau. Interaction de la formation réticulée et de l'écorce cérébrale dans le processus du réveil. Arch. Internat. Physiol., 62:157-78, 1954. 211

493. Brenman, M. Dreams and hypnosis. Psychoanal. Q., 18:455-65, 1949. 335

494. _____. The phenomena of hypnosis. In: Problems of Consciousness I, 1950 (4), pp. 123-63. 337

495. _____, and M. M. Gill. Hypnotherapy. A Survey of the Literature. New York: Internat. Univ. Press, 1947. Pp. 276. 335

496. _____, and R. P. Knight. Hypnotherapy for mental illness in the aged; case report of hysterical

psychosis in a 71-year-old woman. Bull. Menninger Clin., 7:188-98, 1943. 335

497. _____, and S. Reichard. Use of the Rorschach test in the prediction of hypnotizability. Bull. Menninger Clin., 7:183-87, 1943. Brenman, M., co-author: 825, 826, 1445, 1862.

498. Breuninger, M. Ueber den Schichtschlaf. Z. ges. Neurol. Psychiat., 171:591-606, 1941.

499. _____. Schlaf und seelische Harmonie. Gedanken zur praktischen Schlafpsychologie. Stuttgart: Dsch. Verlags-Anstalt, 1942. Pp. 279.

500. Bridger, W. H. Sensory habituation and discrimination in the human neonate. Am. J. Psychiat., 117:991-96, 1961. 210

501. Brindley, G. S. Intrinsic 24-hour rhythms in human physiology, and their relevance to the planning of working programmes. Flying Personnel Res. Comm., FPRC 871, April 1954. Pp. 5 + charts. 316

502. Brissemoret, A., et A. Joanin. Sur les propriétés pharmacodynamiques de la cholestérine. C. R. Soc. Biol., 72:824-25, 1912. 351

503. Brisset, C. Réflexions sur la cure de sommeil et les thérapeutiques voisines. Evolut. Psychiat., No. 2:241-45, 1957. 206

504. _____, et V. Gachkel. Cure de sommeil et psychothérapie. In: La Cure de Sommeil, 1954 (3021), pp. 13-22. 206, 207

505. _____, R. Gault, et V. Gachkel. Position actuelle des problèmes du sommeil. Evolut. Psychiat., No. 1:51-62, 1956.

506. Britton, S. W. Studies on the conditions of activity in endocrine glands. XXII. Adrenin secretion on exposure to cold, together with a possible explanation of hibernation. Am. J. Physiol., 84:119-31, 1928. 325

507. _____. Adrenal insufficiency and related considerations. Physiol. Rev., 10:617-75, 1930. 325

508. _____. Seasonal variations in the survival after adrenalectomy. Am. J. Physiol., 94:686-91, 1930. 322, 325

509. _____. Observations of adrenalectomy in marsupial, hibernating and higher mammalian types. Am. J. Physiol., 99:9-14, 1931. 325

510. Broadbent, W. H. On Cheyne-Stokes' respiration in cerebral haemorrhage. Lancet, I:307-9, 1877. 49

511. Broadhurst, H. C., and J. B. Leathes. The excretion of phosphoric acid in the urine. J. Physiol. (London), 54:28-29, 1920. 167

512. Brock, R. B. The effect of motion pictures on body temperature. Science, 102:259, 1945. 145

513. Brock, S. Idiopathic narcolepsy, cataplexia and catalepsy associated with an unusual hallucination: a case report. J. Nerv. Ment. Dis., 68:583-90, 1928. 236

514. _____, and B. Wiesel. The narcoleptic-cataplectic syndrome—An excessive and dissociated reaction of the sleep mechanism—and its accompanying mental states. J. Nerv. Ment. Dis., 94:700-12, 1941. 234

515. Brockhurst, R. J., and K. S. Lion. Analysis of ocular movements by means of an electrical method. A.M.A. Arch. Ophthal., 46:311-14, 1951. 93

516. Brockman, N. W. Site of minimal lesion to produce coma. Bull. Los Angeles Neurol. Soc., 11:90-91, 1946. 273

517. Brodal, A. The Reticular Formation of the Brain Stem. Anatomical Aspects and Functional Correlations. London: Oliver & Boyd, 1957. Pp. vii + 87. 209

518. _____, and G. F. Rossi. Ascending fibers in brain stem reticular formation of cat. A.M.A. Arch. Neurol. Psychiat., 74:68-87, 1955. 209
Brodal, A., co-author: 3424.

519. Brodmann, K. Plethysmographische Studien am Menschen. I. Untersuchungen ueber das Volumen des Gehirns und Vorderarms im Schlafe. J. Psychol. Neurol., 1:10-71, 1902. 46, 342

520. Brody, M. The biological purpose of the dream. Psychiat. Q., 22:64-65, 1948. 106

521. Brookhart, J. M., A. Arduini, M. Mancia, e G. Moruzzi. Potenziali lenti corticali evocati da stimolazione talamica. Boll. Soc. Ital. Biol. Sper., 33:1629-30, 1957. 210

522. _____, _____, _____, e _____. Risveglio elettroencefalografico da

stimolazione talamica. Boll. Soc. Ital. Biol. Sper., 33:1631-32, 1957. 210

523. _____, and A. Zanchetti. The relation between electrocortical waves and responsiveness of the cortico-spinal system. EEG Clin. Neurophysiol., 8:427-44, 1956.

524. Brooks, C. McC., B. F. Hoffman, E. E. Suckling, F. Kleyntjens, E. H. Koenig, K. S. Coleman, and H. J. Treumann. Sleep and variations in certain functional activities accompanying cyclic changes in depth of sleep. J. Appl. Physiol., 9:97-104, 1956. 112
Brooks C. McC. co-author: 3863.

525. Brooks, H., and J. H. Carrol. A clinical study of the effects of sleep and rest on blood pressure. Arch. Int. Med., 10:97-102, 1912. 43, 44, 163

526. Broun, D., J. Lévy, et P. Meyer-Oulif. Influence de la scopolamine sur l'action des hypnotiques corticaux et basilaires. C. R. Soc. Biol., 107:1522-25, 1931. 295

527. Brouwer, B. (Dutch) Clinical demonstration of organic nervous diseases. A. Hypophyseal sleeping sickness. Ned. Tschr. Geneesk., 74:683-85, 1930. 268

528. Brouwer, E. (Dutch) Harmonic analysis of temperature curves. Ned. Tschr. Geneesk., 72:5319-42, 1928. 138

529. Browman, L. G. Light in its relation to activity and estrous rhythms in the albino rat. J. Exp. Zool., 75:375-88, 1937. 172, 173

530. _____. The effect of bilateral optic enucleation on the voluntary muscular activity of the albino rat. J. Exp. Zool., 91:331-44, 1942. 172

531. _____. The effect of controlled temperatures upon the spontaneous activity of the albino rat. J. Exp. Zool., 94:477-89, 1943. 173

532. _____. Artificial sixteen-hour day activity rhythms in the white rat. Am. J. Physiol., 168:694-97, 1952. 175

533. Brown, A. Discussion of disorders of sleep in childhood. Brit. Med. J., II:525, 1930. 278

534. Brown, A. E. Dreams in which the dreamer knows he is asleep. J. Abnorm. Soc. Psychol., 31:59-66, 1936. 101

535. Brown, F. A., Jr. Biological clocks and the Fiddler crab. Sci. Am., 190(4):34-37, 1954. 132

536. _____. Living clocks. Science, 130:1535-44, 1959. 131

537. _____, and E. D. Terracini. Exogenous timing of rat spontaneous activity periods. Proc. Soc. Exp. Biol. Med., 101:457-60, 1959. 132

538. Brown, H. E., and T. F. Dougherty. The diurnal variation of blood leucocytes in normal and adrenalectomized mice. Endocrinology, 58:365-75, 1956. 162, 169

539. Brown, R. Sound sleep and sound scepticism. Austral. J. Philos., 35:47-53, 1957. 106

540. Brown, W. Sleep, hypnosis and mediumistic trance. Charact. Person., 3:112-26, 1935. 15, 330, 331

541. Browne, R. C. The day and night performance of teleprinter switchboard operators. Occup. Psychol., 23:121-26, 1949; also in: Rep. 5th Conf. Soc. Biol. Rhythm, 1961 (3747), pp. 61-64. 316

542. Brownlee, A. Studies in the behaviour of domestic cattle in Britain. Bull. Animal Behav., No. 8:11-20, 1950. 10

543. Brown-Séquard, C. E. Le sommeil normal, comme le sommeil hypnotique, est le résultat d'une inhibition de l'activité intellectuelle. Arch. Physiol. Norm. Path., 1:333-35, 1889. 336, 343

544. Bruce, H. A. Sleep and Sleeplessness. Boston: Little Brown & Co., 1915. Pp. 219. 274

545. Bruce, L. C. Some observations upon the general blood pressure in sleeplessness and sleep. Scot. Med. Surg. J., 7:109-17, 1900. 74

546. Bruin, M. de. Respiration and basal metabolism in childhood during sleep. Acta Paediat., 18: 279-86, 1936. 50, 56

547. Brumann, F. Experimenteller Beitrag zur Physiologie des Winterschlafes. Z. vergl. Physiol., 10:419-30, 1929.

548. Brunelli, B. Contributo alla fisiopatologia dei centri vegetativi del diencefalo con speciale riguardo al centro per la regolazione del sonno e della veglia. Riv. Biol., 14:375-461, 1932. 201

549. Brunschweiler, H. Sur le sommeil. Rev. Neurol., I:879-80, 1927.

550. Brunton, C. E. The acid output of the kidney and the so-called alkaline tide. Physiol. Rev., 13:372-99, 1933. 64

551. Brush, C. E., and R. Fayerweather. Observations on the changes in blood-pressure during normal sleep. Am. J. Physiol., 5:199-210, 1901. 44, 109

552. Brush, E. N. Observations on the temporal judgment during sleep. Am. J. Psychol., 42:408-11, 1930. 126

553. Buccelli, A. Il sonno consequente all'adenotomia. Riv. Oto-Neuro-Oftal., 5:434-36, 1928. 267

554. Buchanan, F. Dissociation of auricles and ventricles in hibernating dormice. J. Physiol. (London), 42:XIX-XX, 1911. 323

555. _____. Elektrocardiograms. (Démonstration de graphiques). Arch. Internat. Physiol., 14:41, 1914.

556. Buchwald, N. A., G. Heuser, C. Hull, and E. J. Wyers. Blocking of "caudate-spindles" by stimulation of lateral geniculate body. Fed. Proc., 20:327, 1961.

557. Buckell, M., and F. A. Elliott. Diurnal fluctuation of plasma-fibrinolytic activity in normal males. Lancet, I:660-62, 1959. 162

558. Buehler, C. The First Year of Life. New York: John Day Co., 1930. Pp. x + 281. 114

559. _____, and M. Greenberg. Emotional sleep disturbances in childhood. Nervous Child, 8:47-49, 1949. 286

560. Buell, F. A., and J. P. Biehl. The influence of hypnosis on the tremor of Parkinson's disease. Dis. Nerv. Syst., 10:20-23, 1949. 335

561. Buendia, N., M. Goode, and G. Sierra. Behavioral and EEG study of pitch discrimination in naturally sleeping cats. Fed. Proc., 21:347B, 1962. 29

562. Bürger-Prinz, H. Ueber das Zwischenhirnsyndrom and das Problem des Schlafes. Mschr. Psychiat. Neurol., 85:304-21, 1933. 264

563. Bull, N., and L. Gidro-Frank. Emotions induced and studied in hypnotic subjects. II. The findings. J. Nerv. Ment. Dis., 112:97-120, 1950.

564. Bunch, M. E., A. Cole, and J. Frerichs. The influence of 24 hours of wakefulness upon the learning and retention of a maze problem in white rats. J. Comp. Psychol., 23:1-12, 1937. 218

565. _____, J. B. Frerichs, and J. R. Licklider. An experimental study of maze learning after varying periods of wakefulness. J. Comp. Psychol., 26:499-514, 1938. 218

Bunch, M. E., co-author: 2514.

566. Buondonno, E., e C. Fiore. Ricerche sulle variazioni biologiche nel sonno: fluttuazioni nictemerali della glicemia. Osp. Psichiat. (Napoli), 23:65-82, 1955. 34

567. _____, e F. Pariante. Narcosi barbiturica. Variazioni seriche del calcio e del potassio in soggetti nevrotici. Risultati clinico-terapeutici. Acta Neurol. (Napoli), 8:1036-55, 1953. 298

Buondonno, E., co-author: 4310, 4311.

568. Burbank, R. C., and J. Z. Young. Temperature changes and winter sleep of bats. J. Physiol. (London), 82:459-67, 1934. 324

569. Burch, N. R., and T. H. Greiner. Drugs and human fatigue: GSR parameters. J. Psychol., 45:3-10, 1958. 226

570. _____, and _____. A bioelectric scale of human alertness: concurrent recordings of the EEG and GSR. Psychiat. Res. Rep., 12:183-93, 1960. 73

571. Burckard, E., L. Dontcheff, et C. Kayser. Le rythme nycthéméral chez le pigeon. Ann. Physiol., 9:303-68, 1933. 56

572. _____, et C. Kayser. L'inversion du rythme nycthéméral de la température chez l'homme. C. R. Soc. Biol., 141:1265-68, 1947. 174

573. Burford, G. E. Involuntary eyeball motion during anesthesia and sleep; relationship to cortical rhythmic potentials. Curr. Res. Anesth. Analg., 20:191-99, 1941. 297

574. Burge, W. E., and E. L. Burge. Electrical theory of sleep, consciousness, and unconsciousness. Am. J. Physiol., 133:P231-32, 1941. 298

575. _____, and E. G. Koons. Electric anesthesia in relation to brain potential. Curr. Res. Anesth. Analg., 27:290-92, 1948. 298

576. _____, and M. J. Vaught. Effects of exercise, rest, and sleep on scalp potential. Am. J. Physiol.,

133:P232-33, 1941. 32

577. Burn, J. L. An inquiry into the hours of sleep of 2,000 school children. Med. Officer, 53:207-9, 1935. 305, 307

578. Burnham, W. H. The hygiene of sleep. Pedagog. Semin., 27:1-35, 1920. 312, 349, 362

579. Burns, C. Sleep: physiology, pathology and groups of therapeutic agents. New Zeal. Med. J., 58: 584-95, 1959. 294

580. Burns, N. M. Apparent sleep produced by cortical stimulation. Canad. J. Psychol., 11:171-81, 1957. 204

581. Burr, C. B. Narcolepsy. J. Abnorm. Psychol., 13:185-89, 1918, 307

582. Burr, H. S., and D. S. Barton. Steady-state electrical properties of the human organism during sleep. Yale J. Biol. Med., 10:271-74, 1938. 113

583. Burrow, T. The physiological basis of neurosis and dreams. J. Soc. Psychol., 1:48-65, 1930. 106

584. _____, and W. Galt. Electroencephalographic recordings of varying aspects of attention in relation to behavior. J. Gen. Psychol., 32: 269-88, 1945. 31

585. Burton, A. C. The clinical importance of the physiology of temperature regulations. Canad. Med. Ass. J., 75:715-20, 1956. 174

586. Busalow, A. A. Die schonende Schlaftherapie in der Vor- and Nachoperationsperiode nach I. P. Pawlow. Z. aerztl. Fortbild., 46: 652-61, 1952. 206

587. Buscaino, V. M. Contributo allo studio della patogenesi della encefalite epidemica e delle sindromi croniche postencefalitiche. Riv. Pat. Nerv., 31:116-60, 1926. 245

588. _____. Catatonia sperimentale negli animali e nell'uomo. Boll. Soc. Ital. Biol. Sper., 5:1053, 1930; also Riv. Pat. Nerv., 36:593-603, 1930. 254

589. _____. Perchè l'epilettico perde la coscienza al momento dell'accesso? Acta Neurol. (Napoli), 1: 455-56, 1946. 241

590. _____. Das Bewusstsein und seine neurologische Grundlage. Aerztl. Forsch., 7:II/1-2, 1953. 31

591. _____. Traumi cranio-encefalici e perdita di coscienza. Acta Neurol. (Napoli), 9:628-29, 1954.

592. _____. Fondements neurologiques des phénomènes de conscience. First Internat. Congr. Neurol. Sci., Seconde Journée Commune. Brussels. Acta Med. Belg., 1957. pp. 219-33. 30

593. _____, e R. Balbi. Ricerche sulla genesi del sonno—magnesiemia e vitamina B_6. Acta Neurol. (Napoli), 7:1-7, 1952; also Boll. Soc. Ital. Biol. Sper., 28:113-14, 1952. 277, 278

594. Bychowski, G. Ueber einen Fall von periodischer Schlafsucht mit anatomischen Befund. Dsche Z. Nervenheilk., 78:113-22, 1923. 268

595. Bychowski, Z. Ueber den Verlauf und die Prognose der Encephalitis lethargica. Neurol. Zbl., 40: 46-59, 1921. 247

596. Bykov, K. M. The Cerebral Cortex and the Internal Organs. Moskva: For. Lang. Publ. House, 1959. Pp. 458. [Also, New York: Chem. Publ., 1957.]

597. Bykov, V. A. (Russ.) Physiological mechanism of sleep. Fiziol. Zh. SSSR, 42:597-603, 1956. 344

598. Byrne, J. G. Studies on the Physiology of the Eye: Still Reaction, Sleep, Dreams, Hibernation, Repression, Hypnosis, Narcosis, Coma, and Allied Conditions. London: H. K. Lewis & Co., 1933. Pp. 428. 12, 16, 113, 211, 338, 361, 362

599. Caballero, R. El sueño y los sueños: comparición de las ideas de Aristoteles con las teorías de la fisiología moderna. Sem. Méd., 2:1441-49, 1932.

600. Cabitto, L. Sulle cause che provocano il sonno. Note Riv. Psichiat., 11:95-114, 1923. 352

601. Cadilhac, J., T. Passouant-Fontaine, et P. Passouant. Modifications de l'activité de l'hippocampe suivant les divers stades du sommeil spontané chez le rat. Rev. Neurol., 105:171-76, 1961; also EEG Clin. Neurophysiol., 14:138, 1962. 211
Cadilhac, J., co-author: 668, 747, 876, 2314, 3103-6, 3108, 3112, 3353, 3619.

602. Cahana, M. G., e T. Cahana. Gli stati narcolettici e le ghiandole endocrine. Riforma Med., 56: 1600-1606, 1940. 240

603. Cahn, R. Les troubles du sommeil chez l'enfant. Strasbourg Méd., 8:751-55, 1957.

604. Cairns, H. Disturbances of consciousness with lesions of the brain-stem and diencephalon. Brain, 75:109-46, 1952.

605. ____, R. C. Oldfield, J. B. Pennybacker, and D. Whitteridge. Akinetic mutism with epidermoid cyst of the 3rd ventricle (with report on associated disturbance of brain potentials). Brain, 64:273-90, 1941. 206

606. Calef, V. Color in dreams. J. Am. Psychoanal. Ass., 2:453-61, 1954. 102

607. Calhoun, J. B. Diel activity rhythms of the rodents, Microtus ochrogaster, and Sigmodon hispidus hispidus. Ecology, 26:251-73, 1945. 172, 173

608. Callender, E. M. Insomnia. Lancet, 213(II):1280-83, 1927. 294, 362

609. Cambridge, G. W., and B. D. Wyke. Some electrographic changes induced in the narcotized cat by injection of succinate. EEG Clin. Neurophysiol., 5:472, 1953. 297

610. Camden, C., Jr. Shakespeare on sleep and dreams. Rice Inst. (Houston, Texas) Pamphlet, 23: 106-33, 1936. 4

611. Cameron, D. E. Studies in senile nocturnal delirium. Psychiat. Q., 15:47-53, 1941.

612. Cameron, H. C. Sleep and its disorders in childhood. Brit. Med. J., II:717-19, 1930; also Canad. Med. Ass. J., 24:239-44, 1931. 294, 307

613. Cameron, W. B. Some observations and a hypothesis concerning sleep talking. Psychiatry, 15:95-96, 1952. 281

614. Camp, C. D. Morbid sleepiness (with a report of a case of narcolepsy and a review of some recent theories of sleep). J. Abnorm. Psychol., 2:9-21, 1907. 239, 328, 349

615. ____. Disturbance of sleep. J. Michigan Med. Soc., 22:133-38, 1923. 119, 307

616. ____. The question of the existence of a separate sleep center in the brain. J. Nerv. Ment. Dis., 92: 5-7, 1940. 362

617. Campbell, D. Periodische Schlafzustaende nach Enzephalitis epidemica. Mschr. Psychiat. Neurol., 65:58-60, 1927. 248

618. Campbell, H. E., and M. A. Blankenhorn. The effect of sleep on normal and high blood pressure. Am. Heart J., 1:151-59, 1925. 40, 45, 109

Campbell, H. E., co-author: 370.

619. Campbell, J. A., and T. A. Webster. Day and night urine during complete rest, laboratory routine, light muscular work, and oxygen administration. Biochem. J., 15:660-64, 1921. 64, 65, 66, 167

620. ____, and ____. Urinary tides and excretory rhythms. Biochem. J., 16:507-13, 1922. 66, 167

621. Campbell, J. R. Duration of night feeding in infancy. Lancet, I:877, 1958. 305

622. Cancela d'Abreu, A. F. (Portug.) Narcolepsy. Apropos of four cases of pathological sleep. Lisboa Méd., 20:205-26, 1943. 234

623. Cannon, A. Notes upon hypnotic states. Lancet, 223(II):1103-5, 1932. 334

624. ____. Sleeping Through Space. Woodthorpe, Nottingham: Walcot Publ. Co., 1938. Pp. 131. [Also, New York: E. P. Dutton & Co., 1939.]

625. Canziani, G. Sull'inversione temporale dei sogni da stimoli sensoriali. Boll. Soc. Ital. Biol. Sper., 26:324-26, 1950.

626. Capecchi, T. Variazioni della pressione arteriosa, della frequenza del polso, e della temperatura nei fanciulli. I. Azione del sonno e del pasto. Fisiol. Med., 7:687-709, 1936. 41, 43, 44, 109

627. Capo, N. Comment Bien Dormir sans Drogues. Paris: Revue "Bionaturisme," 1956. Pp. 26. 312

628. Cappon, D., and R. Banks. Preliminary study of endurance and perceptual change in sleep deprivation. Percept. Motor Skills, 10: 99-104, 1960. 228

629. ____, and ____. Studies in perceptual distortion: opportunistic observations on sleep deprivation during a talkathon. A.M.A. Arch. Gen. Psychiat., 2:346-49, 1960. 228

630. Capra, P. Il sonno. (Cenni di fisiologia e fisiopatologia). Policlinico (Sez. Prat.), 66:168-74, 1959.

631. Caprio, F. S. Bisexual conflicts and insomnia. J. Clin. Psychopath 10:376-79, 1949.

632. Cardin, A. Il tono muscolare non

è di natura riflessa. Boll. Soc.
Ital. Biol. Sper., 27:1178-81, 1951.

633. Cardona, F. Epilessia e disturbi
psichici nei tumori di Erdheim
interessanti il diencefalo. Riv.
Pat. Nerv., 49:85-111, 1937. 264

634. Carey, R. J. Sleep. Boston Med.
Q., 6(2):54-56, 1955.

635. Carl, G. P., and W. D. Turner.
The effects of benzedrine sulfate
(amphetamine sulfate) on performance in a comprehensive psychometric examination. J. Psychol., 8:165-216, 1939. 300

636. Carleton, A. A rhythmical periodicity in the mitotic division of
animal cells. J. Anat., 68:251-63,
1934. 172

637. Carlill, H. Hysterical sleeping attacks. Lancet, 197(II):1128-31,
1919.

638. Carlson, A. J. The Control of
Hunger in Health and Disease.
Chicago: University of Chicago
Press, 1916. Pp. 319. 53
Carlson, A. J., co-author: 1939.

639. Carlson, V. R. Effects of sleep-
deprivation and chlorpromazine
on size-constancy judgments. Am.
J. Psychol., 74:552-60, 1961. 227

640. Carmichael, L., and J. L. Kennedy. Some recent approaches to the
experimental study of human fatigue. Science, 110:445, 1949. 226

641. _____, _____, and L. C. Mead.
Some recent approaches to the experimental study of human fatigue.
Proc. Nat. Acad. Sci., 35:691-96,
1949. 226

642. Carnicero, C. Das Blutbild im
Schlaf. Med. Klin., 40:103-4,
1944. 39

643. Carpenter, T. M. The partition of
urinary nitrogen of fasting and hibernating woodchucks (arctomys
monax). J. Biol. Chem., 122:343-
47, 1938. 324

644. Carpenter, W. B. Principles of
Mental Physiology. New York: D.
Appleton & Co., 1874. Pp. xxi +
737. 100, 282

645. Carrara, E. Sindrome narcolet-
tica preparalitica. Riv. Pat. Nerv.
Ment., 56:298-308, 1940. 237

646. Carrot, J. Velluz, et Rigal. "Syndrome d'Elpénor." Presse Méd.,
55(II):573, 1947. 271

647. Caspers, H. Periodizitaetser-
scheinungen bei Tieren und ihre
kausale Deutung. Studium Gen., 2:
78-81, 1949. 131

648. _____. Die Aktivierung corticaler
Krampfstromherde im natuerli-
chen und elektrisch induzierten
Schlaf beim Tier. Z. ges. exp.
Med., 124:176-88, 1954.

649. _____. Ueber die Ausloesung
corticaler Krampfpotenziale und
ihre Beziehungen zu vegetativen
Tonusschwankungen im Schlaf.
Z. ges. exp. Med., 125:596-613,
1955. 297

650. _____. Changes of cortical D.C.
potentials in the sleep-wakefulness cycle. In: A CIBA Found.
Symposium on the Nature of
Sleep, 1961 (4270), pp. 237-53.
32

651. _____, H. Grueter, und E. Lerche.
Ueber den Weckeffekt knackfreier
Tonimpulse bei der nicht narko-
tisierten Ratte. Pfluegers Arch.,
267:93-105, 1958.

652. _____, _____, und _____. Adap-
tationserscheinungen der akus-
tisch ausgeloesten Weckreaktion
bei Reizung mit definierten
Tonimpulsen. Pfluegers Arch.,
267:128-41, 1958.

653. _____, und H. Schulze. Die Veraenderungen der corticalen
Gleichspannung waehrend der
natuerlichen Schlaf-Wach-Perio-
den beim freibeweglichen Tier.
Pfluegers Arch., 270:103-20,
1959. 32

654. _____, und K. Winkel. Die Beeinflussung der Grosshirnrinden-
rhythmik durch Reizungen im
Zwischen- und Mittelhirn bei der
Ratte. Pfluegers Arch., 259:334-
56, 1954.
Caspers, H., co-author: 3595,
4141.

655. Castaigne, P. Narcolepsie et
cataplexie—Syndrome de Gélineau. Rev. Prat. (Paris), 4:1551-
62, 1954. 236

656. Castellano, M., F. Penati, e R.
Videsott. Osservazioni cardiore-
spiratorie ed elettrocardiogra-
fiche nella marmotta in ibernazione e durante la fase di risveglio. Cuore Circol., 41:129-50,
1957. 323

657. Caster, J. E., and C. S. Baker,
Jr. Comparative suggestibility
in the trance and waking states—
a further study. J. Gen. Psychol.,
7:287-301, 1932.

658. Castex, M. R., E. L. Capdehou-
rat, y G. Orosco. La somnolencia en la insuficiencia respira-
toria crónica. (Plétoricos abdo-

minales y cardíacos cianóticos).
Prensa Méd. Argentina, 27:387-400, 1940. 267

659. Castle, M. E., A. S. Foot, and R. J. Halley. Some observations on the behaviour of dairy cattle with particular reference to grazing. J. Dairy Res., 17:215-30, 1950. 10

660. Cate, J. ten. Zur Frage der Entstehung des Schlafes beim Menschen. Z. ges. Neurol. Psychiat., 122:175-86, 1929. 362

661. _____. (Dutch) The sleep problem. Mansch Maatschap., 5:304-20, 1929. 344

662. _____, G. P. M. Horsten, and L. J. Koopman. The influence of the body temperature on the EEG of the rat. EEG Clin. Neurophysiol., 1:231-35, 1949. 327

663. Cathala, H.-P., et A. Guillard. La réactivité au cours du sommeil physiologique de l'homme. Pathol. Biol. (Paris), 9:1357-75, 1961. 26, 48, 49, 86, 98
Cathala, H. P., co-author: 1551.

664. Cave, H. A. Narcolepsy. Arch. Neurol. Psychiat., 26:50-101, 1931. 237, 250, 362

665. Cavennes, W. F. The development of the EEG expression of sleep in the monkey. EEG Clin. Neurophysiol., 13:493-94, 1961. 28

666. Cedercreutz, C. Hypnotic treatment of 70 enuretics. Ann. Paediat. Fenn. (Helsinki), 2:56-61, 1956. 284, 335

667. Cestan, P., et Sendrail. L'insomnie dans l'encéphalite léthargique. Sud Méd. Chir., 58:85-89, 1926. 244

668. Chafetz, M. E., and J. Cadilhac. A new procedure for a study of barbiturate effect and evoked potentials in the EEG. EEG Clin. Neurophysiol., 6:565-72, 1954. 296

669. Chalfen, S. S. Zur Frage der Sekretion des nuechternen Magens. Arch. Verdauungskr., 44:250-57, 1928. 54

670. _____. Die Sekretion des Magens waehrend der Nacht. Arch. Verdauungskr., 47:106-9, 1930. 54

671. Chambers, E. R. Paralysis of divergence in encephalitis lethargica. Brit. J. Ophthal., 8:417-18, 1924. 245

672. Chandler, J. F. High blood pressure as a cause or factor in insomnia. J. Missouri Med. Ass., 17:330, 1920.

673. Chandler, S. B. Shakespeare and sleep. Bull. Hist. Med. (Baltimore), 29:255-60, 1955. 4

674. Chant, N., and W. Blatz. A study of sleeping habits of children. Genet. Psychol. Monogr., 4:13-43, 1928. 117, 307

675. Chapman, R. McC. Control of sleeplessness. Am. J. Psychiat., 3:491-500, 1923-24. 286

676. Chastaing, M. La cohérence des rêves. J. Psychol. Norm. Path. (Paris), 41:359-73, 1948. 101

677. Chatfield, P. O., A. F. Battista, C. P. Lyman, and J. P. Garcia. Effects of cooling on nerve conduction in a hibernator (golden hamster) and non-hibernator (albino rat). Am. J. Physiol., 155:179-85, 1948. 327

678. _____, and C. P. Lyman. Circulatory changes during process of arousal in the hibernating hamster. Am. J. Physiol., 163:566-74, 1950. 323, 327, 328

679. _____, and _____. Subcortical electrical activity in the golden hamster during arousal from hibernation. EEG Clin. Neurophysiol., 6:403-8, 1954. 326

680. _____, _____, and D. P. Purpura. The effects of temperature on the spontaneous and induced electrical activity in the cerebral cortex of the golden hamster. EEG Clin. Neurophysiol., 3:225-30, 1951. 326
Chatfield, P. O., co-author: 2594-96.

681. Chatrian, G. E., and W. P. Chapman. Electrographic study of the amygdaloid region with implanted electrodes in patients with temporal lobe epilepsy. In: Electrical Studies of the Unanesthetized Brain, E. R. Ramey and D. S. O'Doherty, Eds., New York: P. B. Hoeber, 1960, Chapter 18, pp. 351-68. 260

682. Chauchard, P. Recherches sur les mécanismes du sommeil. Rev. Sci. (Paris), 80:424-30, 1942. 14, 73, 348

683. _____. Les résultats de l'analyse chronaximétrique des états de sommeil. Presse Méd., 52:228-29, 1944. 14, 73, 348

684. _____. La régulation centrale des fonctions nerveuses et le pro-

blème du sommeil. J. Psychol. Norm. Path., 39:204-19, 1946. <u>14</u>, <u>73</u>, <u>348</u>

685. _____. Le Sommeil et les Etats de Sommeil. Paris: Flammarion, 1947. Pp. 283. <u>14</u>, <u>73</u>, <u>348</u>, <u>349</u>

686. _____. Recherches électrophysiologiques sur le déterminisme des états de sommeil. Anesth. Analg. (Paris), 7:1-10, 1950. <u>348</u>

687. Chaudhry, A. P., F. Halberg, and J. J. Bittner. Mitoses in pinna and interscapular epidermis of mice in relation to physiologic 24-hour periodicity. Fed. Proc., 15:34, 1956. <u>169</u>

688. _____, _____, C. E. Keenan, R. N. Harner, and J. J. Bittner. Daily rhythms in rectal temperature and in epithelial mitoses of hamster pinna and pouch. J. Appl. Physiol., 12:221-24, 1958. <u>169</u>

689. Cheney, R. H. Reaction time behavior after caffeine and coffee consumption. J. Exp. Psychol., 19:357-69, 1936. <u>299</u>

690. Chernish, S. M., C. M. Gruber, Jr., and K. G. Kohlstaed. Obtaining data by telephone. A clinical evaluation of hypnotic drugs. Proc. Soc. Exp. Biol. Med., 93:162-64, 1956. <u>295</u>

691. Chertok, L. Sommeil hypnotique prolongé. In: La Cure de Sommeil, 1954 (3021), pp. 57-70. <u>335</u>

692. _____, and P. Kramarz. Hypnosis, sleep and electro-encephalography. J. Nerv. Ment. Dis., 128:227-38, 1959. <u>330</u>

693. Chideckel, M. Sleep, Your Life's One Third. New York: Saravan House, 1939. Pp. xiii + 183. <u>312</u>

694. Chieffi, A., e L. Rosselli del Turco. Variazioni individuali nel bambino della curva glicemica e della curva lipemica in rapporto alla funzione del sonno. Riv. Clin. Med., 38:208-24, 1937. <u>34</u>

695. Chiles, W. D. The effects of sleep deprivation on performance of a complex mental task. USAF WADC Tech. Note, 1955, No. 55-423, v. Pp. 13. <u>226</u>
Chiles, W. D., co-author: 13, 1904, 2222.

696. Chodoff, P. Sleep paralysis with report of two cases. J. Nerv. Ment. Dis., 100:278-81, 1944. <u>236</u>

697. Chow, K. L., W. C. Dement, and S. A. Mitchell, Jr. Effects of lesions of the rostral thalamus on brain waves and behavior in cats.

EEG Clin. Neurophysiol., 11: 107-20, 1959. <u>210</u>
Chow, K. L., co-author: 383.

698. Christake, A. Conditioned emotional stimuli and arousal from sleep. Am. Psychologist, 12:405, 1957. <u>29</u>

699. Christenson, J. A., Jr. Dynamics in hypnotic induction. Psychiatry, 12:37-54, 1949. <u>336</u>

700. Chrysanthis, K. The length and depth of sleep. Acta Med. Orient., 5:152-55, 1946. <u>99</u>

701. Chuche, C. Hygiène de l'insomnie. Ann. Hyg. Publ., 25:142-44, 1947.

702. Chweitzer, A., E. Geblewicz, et W. Liberson. Action de la mescaline sur les ondes alpha (rythme de Berger) chez l'homme. C. R. Soc. Biol., 124:1296-99, 1937. <u>303</u>

703. Cier, J.-F. Physiologie de la substance réticulée du tronc cérébral. Lyon Méd., 195:281-90, 1956.

704. Cipiccia, D. Studi sul letargo. IX. Influenza dei gas-attivi (CO_2) ed inerti (H) su alcuni anfibi (Bufo vulgaris e viridis, Rana esculenta, Triton taeniatus) allo stato di letargo, di risveglia e di veglia. Ann. Fac. Med. Chir. Fac. Med. Vet., 28:183-218, 1926. <u>324</u>

705. Claparède, E. Esquisse d'une théorie biologique du sommeil. Arch. Psychol., 4:245-349, 1905. <u>349</u>

706. _____. La question du sommeil. Année Psychol., 18:419-59, 1912. <u>349</u>, <u>362</u>

707. _____. Discussion du rapport de Jean Lhermitte et Auguste Tournay: le sommeil normal et pathologique. Rev. Neurol., I:835-37, 1927. <u>328</u>, <u>349</u>

708. _____. Opinions et travaux divers relatifs à la théorie biologique du sommeil et de l'hystérie. Arch. Psychol., 21:113-74, 1928. <u>74</u>, <u>349</u>, <u>362</u>

709. _____. Le sommeil et la veille. J. Psychol. (Paris), 26:433-93, 1929. <u>349</u>, <u>362</u>

710. _____. Le sommeil et la veille. In: Nouveau Traité de Psychologie, par Georges Dumas. Paris: Librairie Félix Alcan, 1934, pp. 455-522. <u>349</u>

711. Clardy, E. R., and B. C. Hill. Sleep disorders in institutionalized disturbed children and de-

linquent boys. Nervous Child, 8: 50-53, 1949. 281, 284, 285

712. Clark, B., and N. Warren. The effect of loss of sleep on visual tests. Am. J. Optom., 16:80-95, 1939. 226

713. _____, and _____. A photographic study of reading during a sixty-five-hour vigil. J. Educ. Psychol., 31:383-90, 1940. 225
Clark, B., co-author: 1508, 1509, 4122.

714. Clark, S. L., and J. W. Ward. Electroencephalogram of different cortical regions of normal and anesthetized cats. J. Neurophysiol., 8:99-112, 1945. 296

715. Clark, W. E. L., and M. Meyer. Anatomical relationships between the cerebral cortex and the hypothalamus. Brit. Med. Bull., 6:341-45, 1950. 211

716. Claude, H., et H. Baruk. Les crises de catalepsie: leur diagnostic avec le sommeil pathologique, leur rapports avec l'hystérie et la catatonie. Encéphale, 23:373, 1928.

717. _____, _____, et R. Porak. Sommeil cataleptique et mise en train psychomotrice volontaire. Etude psychologique au moyen de l'ergographe de Mosso. Encéphale, 27: 665-83, 1932.

718. _____, S. de Sèze, et Tardieu. Syndrome de Gélineau: narcolepsie. Cataplexie. Action thérapeutique du sulfate de phényl-amino-propane et de l'éphédrine. Rev. Neurol., 73:126-31, 1941. 238, 239

719. Clavière, J. La rapidité de la pensée dans le rêve. Rev. Philos., 43: 507-12, 1897. 100

720. Clerici, A. Sonnambulismo. Gazz. Osp., 51:361-63, 1930. 282

721. Cloetta, M. Gedanken und Tatsachen ueber die biochemischen Grundlagen des Wachens und Schlafens. Festschr. Emil C. Barell, I:18-31. Basel: F. Reinhardt & Co., 1936. 35, 353

722. _____, und H. Fischer. Ueber die Wirkung der Kationen Ca, Mg, Sr, Ba, K und Na bei intracerebraler Injektion. Beitrag zur Genese von Schlaf und Erregung. Arch. exp. Path. Pharmakol., 158:254-81, 1930. 201

723. _____, _____, und M. R. van der Loeff. Die Biochemie von Schlaf und Erregung mit besonderer Beruecksichtung der Bedeutung der Kationen. Arch. exp. Path. Pharmakol., 174:589-675, 1934. 35, 201

724. Cobb, S. Photic driving as a cause of clinical seizures in epileptic patients. Arch. Neurol. Psychiat., 58:70-71, 1947. 259

725. _____, W. W. Sargant, and R. S. Schwab. Simultaneous respiratory and electroencephalographic recording in cases of petit mal. Arch. Neurol. Psychiat., 42:1189-91, 1939. 259

726. Cobb, W., and D. Hill. EEG in subacute progressive encephalitis. Brain, 73:392-404, 1950. 244

727. Coghill, G. E., and R. W. Watkins. Perodicity in the development of the threshold of tactile stimulation in Amblystoma. J. Comp. Neurol., 78:91-111, 1943. 365

728. Cohen, E. L. Length and depth of sleep. Lancet, II:830-31, 1944. 119, 312

729. _____. Acne and sleep. Brit. J. Dermatol., 57:147-51, 1945. 121

730. _____. Duración y profundidad del sueño. Rev. Neurol. Buenos Aires, 11:64-69, 1946. 99

731. Cohen, H. The treatment of narcolepsy with ephedrine. Lancet, 223(II):335-37, 1932. 300

732. Cohen, I., and E. C. Dodds. Twenty-four hour observations on the metabolism of normal and starving subjects. J. Physiol. (London), 59:259-70, 1924. 167

733. Cohen, S. Sleep regulation with Thalidomide. Am. J. Psychiat., 116:1030-31, 1960. 294

734. Cohn, R. Direct current recordings of eyeball movements in neurologic practice. Neurology, 7:684-88, 1957.

735. _____, and B. A. Cruvant. Relation of narcolepsy to the epilepsies. A clinical-electroencephalographic study. Arch. Neurol. Psychiat., 51:163-70, 1944. 237

736. _____, and S. Katzenelbogen. Electroencephalographic changes induced by intravenous sodium amytal. Proc. Soc. Exp. Biol. Med., 49:560-63, 1942. 296

737. Coirault, R. L'insomnie. Cah. Laennec, 19:37-43, 1959. 274

738. _____. L'insomnie, maladie du siècle? Hyg. Ment., 48:160-81,

1959; also Gaz. Hôp., 131:583-94, 1959.

739. Coleman, P. D., F. E. Gray, and K. Watanabe. EEG amplitude and reaction time during sleep. J. Appl. Physiol., 14:397-400, 1959. 29

740. _____, _____, _____, and D. Arey. Electroencephalographic correlates of reaction time during sleep. Q. Res. Eng. Center, Natick, Mass., Tech. Rep., March 1957. Pp. 14. 29

741. Collard, J. Arguments d'ordre structural et existentiel en faveur de la cure de sommeil dans les névroses. Acta Neurol. Psychiat. Belg., 58:959-71, 1958. 207
Collard, J., co-author: 061.

742. Collins, E. H. Localization of an experimental hypothalamic and midbrain syndrome simulating sleep. J. Comp. Neurol. 100:661-97, 1954. 206

743. Collins, H. A. Ephedrine in the treatment of narcolepsy. Ann. Int. Med., 5:1289-95, 1932. 300

744. Collins, J. Insomnia; How To Combat It. New York: Appleton & Co., 1930. Pp. 130. 275, 294

745. Collip, J. B. Effect of sleep upon alkali reserve of the plasma. J. Biol. Chem., 41:473-74, 1920. 33, 34, 51

746. Colucci, G. Il glutatione del'encefalo nel sonno sperimentale. Riv. Neurol., 6:716-24, 1933; also Riv. Pat. Nerv. Ment., 43:534-40, 1934. 297

747. Comelade, P., J. Cadilhac, and P. Passouant. Temporal epilepsy and narcoleptic attacks. EEG Clin. Neurophysiol., 13:487-88, 1961. 237, 238

748. Contreiras, A. (Portug.) Hygiene of Sleep. Lisboa: Gaz. dos Caminhos de Ferro, 1939. Pp. 27.

749. Coodley, A. Psychodynamic factors in narcolepsy and cataplexy. Psychiat. Q., 22:696-717, 1948. 237, 239

750. Cook, T. W. A case of abnormal reproduction during sleep. J. Abnorm. Soc. Psychol., 29:465-70, 1935.

751. Cooper, Z. K. Mitotic rhythm in human epidermis. J. Investig. Dermatol., 2:289-300, 1939. 169

752. Cooperman, N. R. Calcium and protein changes in serum during sleep and rest without sleep. Am. J. Physiol., 116:531-34, 1936. 36

753. _____, F. J. Mullin, and N. Kleitman. Studies on the physiology of sleep. XI. Further observations on the effects of prolonged sleeplessness. Am. J. Physiol., 107:589-93, 1934. 220, 223
Cooperman, N. R., co-author: 2193, 2200, 2943, 2944.

754. Copelman, L. S. Tumeur hypophysaire et hypersomnie. Rev. Path. Comp., 50:419-20, 1950. 270

755. _____, et M. Atanasiu. Tumeur pituitaire et narcolepsie. Rev. Path. Comp., 50:540-41, 1950. 237

756. Coraboeuf, E., G. Galand, et Y. M. Gargouil. Influence d'inhalations d'air chaud sur l'état vigile chez l'homme. C. R. Soc. Biol., 153:1579-80, 1959. 197

757. Cordeau, J. P., and M. Mancia. Evidence for the existence of an electroencephalographic synchronization mechanism originating in the lower brain stem. EEG Clin. Neurophysiol., 11: 551-64, 1959. 212

758. Coriat, I. H. The nature of sleep. J. Abnorm. Psychol., 6:329-67, 1912. 196, 337

759. _____. The evolution of sleep and hypnosis. J. Abnorm. Psychol., 7:94-98, 1912. 338

760. Corn-Becker, F., L. Welch, and F. Fisichelli. Conditioning factors underlying hypnosis. J. Abnorm. Soc. Psychol., 44:212-22, 1949. 336

761. Cornil, L., H. Gastaut, et J. Corriol. Appréciation du degré de conscience au cours des paroxysmes épileptiques, "Petit Mal." Rev. Neurol., 84:149-51, 1951. 259

762. Corson, S. A., T. Koppanyi, and A. E. Vivino. Studies on barbiturates: XXVIII. Effect of succinate and fumarate in experimental barbiturate poisoning. Curr. Res. Anesth., 24:177-92, 1945. 297

763. Costa, N. Ueber eine seltene Schlaferscheinung. Z. ges. Neurol., 93:336-49, 1924; also, Zur Psychpathologie des Schlafes. Dsche med. Wschr., 50:1086, 1924. 285, 335

764. Courbon, P. La nuit et le sommeil à l'asile d'aliénés. Rev. Neurol., I:869-73, 1927. 286

765. Coursin, D. B. Intramuscular paraldehyde for artificial sleep. EEG Clin. Neurophysiol., 5:305-8; 317, 1953. 294

766. Courtin, W. Die Beziehungen der Enuresis nocturna zum Schlafe. Arch. Kinderheilk., 73:40-49, 1923.

767. Coutière, H. Sommeil. Biol. Méd. (Paris), 22:269-312, 1932.

768. Cowan, N. R. Sleep behavior in the aged. Health Bull. (Edinburgh), 14:7-9, 1956. 285

769. Cox, G. H., and E. Marley. The estimation of motility during rest or sleep. J. Neurol. Neurosurg. Psychiat., 22(I):57-60, 1959.

770. Cox, L. B. Tumors of base of brain: their relation to pathologic sleep and other changes in conscious state. Med. J. Australia, 24(I):742-52, 1937. 265

771. Craig, D. R. An investigation of basic skin resistance levels during sleep under differing conditions. Psychol. Bull., 34:559, 1937. 311

772. Crasilneck, H. B., and J. A. Hall. Physiological changes associated with hypnosis: a review of the literature. Internat. J. Clin. Exp. Hypn., 7:9-50, 1959. 329
Crasilneck, H. B., co-author: 2742.

773. Creak, E. M. A case of narcolepsy. Lancet, 223 (II):514-15, 1932.

774. Cremerius, J., und R. Jung. Ueber die Veraenderungen des Elektroencephalogramms nach Elektroschockbehandlung. Nervenarzt, 18: 193-205, 1947.

775. Crémieux, A., Legree, et Porro. Sur quelques cas de rythmies du sommeil. Pédiatrie, 39:445-50, 1950. 285

776. Cress, C. H., and E. L. Gibbs. Electroencephalographic asymmetry during sleep. Dis. Nerv. Syst., 9:327-29, 1948.

777. Creutzfeldt, O., and R. Jung. Neuronal discharge in the cat's motor cortex during sleep and arousal. In: A CIBA Found. Symposium on the Nature of Sleep, 1961 (4270), pp. 131-70. 212
Creutzfeldt, O., co-author: 2055.

778. Crichton-Miller, H. Insomnia— An Outline for the Practitioner. London: Edward Arnold & Co., 1930. Pp. 172. 294

779. Crile, G. W. Studies in exhaustion. Arch. Surg., 2:196-220, 1921. 217

780. Crinis, M. de. Ueber Schlaf und Schlafmittel. Wien. klin. Wschr., 55:141-45, 1942. 294

781. Critchley, M. Disorders of nocturnal sleep in narcoleptics. J. Roy. Nav. Med. Serv., 26:238-48, 1940. 234

782. _____. Sleeplessness. Pharmaceut. J. (London), 107:231-32, 1948. 274

783. _____. Sleep as a neurological problem. Brit. Med. J., II:152-53, 1954. 71, 79

784. _____. The pre-dormitum. Rev. Neurol., 93:101-6, 1955. 71, 79, 285

785. _____, and H. L. Hoffman. The syndrome of periodic somnolence and morbid hunger (Kleine-Levin syndrome). Brit. Med. J., I:137-39, 1942. 267

786. Crofton, J. W. Abnormalities of sleep. J. Roy. Army Med. Corps, 80:314-20, 1943. 234

787. Crohm, W. H. Zusammenstellung von Mitteln gegen Kopfschmerzen, Schlaflosigkeit, Stuhlverstopfung. Med. Klin., 26:1755-57, 1930. 294

788. Crooks, J., and I. P. C. Murray. The sleeping pulse rate in thyrotoxicosis. Scot. Med. J., 3: 120-22, 1958. 42

789. Crosby, G. J. V. Insomnia and Disordered Sleep. London: Cassell & Co., 1935. Pp. 95. 114, 312

790. Crosby, W. H., and W. Dameshek. Paroxysmal nocturnal hemoglobinuria. Blood, 5:822-42, 1950. 39

791. Crosnier, R. Resistance au sommeil. [Amélioration de la vision.] Ann. Hyg. (Paris), 27:122-29, 1949.

792. Cross, G. K. Sleep disturbances in infancy and childhood. South African Med. J., 6:3-8, 1932.

793. Crouch, E. L. Narcolepsy. Med. Bull. Vet. Admin., 6:371-77, 1930.

794. Crozier, W. J. The distribution of temperature characteristics for biological processes; critical increments for heart rates. J. Gen. Physiol., 9:531-46, 1926. 159

795. Cruchet, R. Sur deux cas de tics convulsifs du cou persistant pendant le sommeil. Rev. Neurol., 14:293-99, 1906. 285

796. Cruden, W. V. A study of wake—

an approach to the problems of insomnia. Lancet, I:579-81, 1957. 4, 274, 362

797. _____. Sleep and wake. Brit. J. Clin. Sci., 14:475-79, 1960.

798. Cubberley, A. J. The effects of tensions of the body surface upon the normal dream. Brit. J. Psychol., 13:243-65, 1923. 106

799. Cullen, G., and I. P. Earle. Studies of the acid-base condition of blood. II. Physiological changes in acid-base condition throughout the day. J. Biol. Chem., 83: 545-59, 1929. 162

800. Curtis, D. Learn While You Sleep; The Theory and Practice of Sleep-Learning. New York: Libra Publ., 1960. Pp. 126.

801. Curtis. Q. F. Diurnal variation in the free activity of sheep and pig. Proc. Soc. Exp. Biol. Med., 35: 566-67, 1937. 149

802. Cushing, H. Counteractive effect of tribromethanol (avertin) on the stimulatory response to pituitrin injected in the ventricle. Proc. Nat. Acad. Sci., 17:248-53, 1931. 297

803. _____, and E. Goetsch. Hibernation and the pituitary body. J. Exp. Med., 22:25-47, 1915. 325

804. Cushny, A. R. Discussion on insomnia. Edinb. Med. J., 30:98-110, 1923. 294

805. Cuthbertson, D. P., and J. A. C. Knox. The effects of analeptics on the fatigued subject. J. Physiol. (London), 106:42-58, 1947. 301

806. Cutting, W. C. Coexistence of obesity and narcolepsy. Stanford Med. Bull., 2:172-75, 1944. 237

807. Czerny, A. Physiologische Untersuchungen ueber den Schlaf. Jahrb. Kinderheilk., 33:1-29, 1891.

808. _____. Zur Kenntnis des physiologischen Schlafes. Jahrb. Kinderheilk., 41:337-42, 1896. 46, 108

809. Daddi, L. Sulle alterazioni degli elementi del sistema nervoso centrale nell'insonnia sperimentale. Riv. Pat. Nerv. Ment., 3:1-12, 1898. 215

810. Dahl, A. Ueber den Einfluss des Schlafes auf das Wiedererkennen. Psychol. Forsch., 11:290-301, 1928. 125

811. Dale, P. W., and E. W. Busse. An elaboration of a distinctive EEG pattern found during drowsy states in children. Dis. Nerv. Syst., 12: 122-25, 1951; prelim. commun.,

EEG Clin. Neurophysiol., 2:226, 1950. 76

812. Dales, R. J. Afternoon sleep in a group of nursery-school children. J. Genet. Psychol., 58:161-80, 1941. 117

813. Dally, P. J. Basal and sleeping metabolic rates in psychiatric disorders. J. Ment. Sci., 104: 428-33, 1958. 55

814. Daly, D., E. Rodin, and P. White. Effects of photic stimulation in sleep: Preliminary observations. EEG Clin. Neurophysiol., 5:480-81, 1953. 257

815. _____, and R. E. Yoss. The electroencephalogram in narcolepsy. EEG Clin. Neurophysiol., 9:109-20; 168-69, 1957. 226, 238, 332
Daly, D. D., co-author: 3382, 4294-96.

816. Damasio, R., et V. Girard. Les modifications E.E.G. au cours du sommeil provoqué par un stéroïde anesthésique, le succinate sodique de 21 hydroxy-pregnandione (viadril). Rev. Neurol., 94:897, 1956. 296

817. Damstra, M. N. Telepathic mechanism in dreams. Psychiat. Q., 26:100-134, 1952. 103

818. Dana, C. L. Morbid somnolence and its relation to the endocrine glands. New York Med. J. Med. Rec., 89:1-5, 1916. 268, 348

819. Dandy, W. E. The location of the conscious center in the brain—the corpus striatum. Bull. Johns Hopkins Hosp., 79:34-58, 1946. 31, 273

820. Daniélopolu, D., et A. Carniol. Influence du sommeil sur la motilité de l'estomac chez l'homme. Arch. Mal. Appar. Dig., 13:201-4, 1923. 53

821. Daniels, L. E. Narcolepsy. Medicine, 13:1-122, 1934. 233, 234, 235, 236, 237, 241, 249, 272
Daniels, L. E., co-author: 973, 974.

822. Darrow, C. W. The behavior research photopolygraph. J. Gen. Psychol., 7:215-19, 1932. 18, 19

823. _____. The electroencephalogram and psychophysiological regulation in the brain. Am. J. Psychiat., 102:791-98, 1946.

824. _____. Psychological and psychophysiological significance of the electroencephalogram. Psychol. Rev., 54:157-68, 1947.

825. _____, C. E. Henry, M. Bren-

man, and M. Gill. Inter-area electroencephalographic relationships
affected by hypnosis: Preliminary
report. EEG Clin. Neurophysiol.,
2:231, 1950. 330

826. _____, _____, M. Gill, and M.
Brenman. Frontal-motor parallelism and motor-occipital in-
phase activity in hypnosis, drowsiness, and sleep. EEG Clin. Neurophysiol., 2:355, 1950. 75, 330
Darrow, C. W., co-author: 1273.

827. Das, B. B. Insomnia. Antiseptic,
39:174-84, 1942. 278

828. Das, J. P. A theory of hypnosis.
Internat. J. Clin. Exp. Hypn., 8:
69-77, 1959. 336

829. _____. Learning and recall under
hypnosis and in the wake state.
A.M.A. Arch. Gen. Psychiat., 4:
517-21, 1961. 332

830. Das, N. N., S. R. Dasgupta, and
G. Werner. The effect of chlorpromazine on the electrical activity
of the "cerveau isolé." Arch. exp.
Path. Pharmakol., 224:248-52,
1955. 301
Das, N. N., co-author: 179.

831. Dastre, A. Recherches sur les
variations diurnes de la sécrétion
biliaire. Arch. Physiol. Norm.
Path., 5ᵉ Ser., 2:800-809, 1890.
164

832. David, M., H. Hecaen, et J. Talai-
rach. Les troubles psychiques de
type expansif au cours des inter-
ventions sur la région du IIIe ventricule. Rev. Neurol., 78:541-60,
1946.

833. Davidoff, E. The relation of epilepsy to pathologic sleep. Nervous
Child, 8:54-62, 1949. 257

834. _____, and E. C. Reifenstein. The
stimulating action of benzedrine
sulfate. A comparative study of
the responses of normal persons
and of depressed patients. J. Am.
Med. Ass., 108:1770-76, 1937.
300

835. Davidoff, L. M. Studies in acromegaly. III. The anamnesia and
symptomatology in 100 cases. Endocrinology, 10:461-83, 1926. 269

836. Davidson, J. R., and E. Douglass.
Nocturnal enuresis: a special ap-
proach to treatment. Brit. Med.
J., I:1345-47, 1950. 285

837. Davis, D. H. S. Rhythmic activity
in the short-tailed vole, Microtus.
J. Animal Ecol., 2:232-39, 1933.
148, 172

838. Davis, E., M. Hayes, and B. H.

Kirman. Somnambulism. Lancet,
I:186, 1942. 282

839. Davis, H., and P. A. Davis. The
electrical activity of the brain:
its relation to physiological
states and to states of impaired
consciousness. Res. Publ. Ass.
Nerv. Ment. Dis., 19:50-80, 1939.
29

840. _____, _____, A. L. Loomis, E.
N. Harvey, and G. Hobart. Changes in human brain potentials during the onset of sleep. Science,
86:448-50, 1937. 75, 79

841. _____, _____, _____, _____, and
_____. Human brain potentials
during the onset of sleep. J. Neurophysiol., 1:24-38, 1938. 25, 75,
95

842. _____, _____, _____, _____, and
_____. Electrical reactions of
human brain to auditory stimulation during sleep. J. Neurophysiol., 2:500-514, 1939. 26

843. _____, _____, _____, _____, and
_____. Analysis of the electrical
response of the human brain to
auditory stimulation during sleep.
Am. J. Physiol., 126:P474-75,
1939. 26

844. _____, _____, _____, _____, and
_____. A search for changes in
direct-current potentials of the
head during sleep. J. Neurophysiol., 2:129-35, 1939. 32
Davis, H., co-author: 848, 1423,
3527.

845. Davis, L. W., and R. W. Husband.
A study of hypnotic susceptibility
in relation to personality traits.
J. Abnorm. Soc. Psychol., 26:
175-82, 1931. 335

846. Davis, P. A. Effects of acoustic
stimuli on the waking human
brain. J. Neurophysiol., 2:494-
99, 1939.

847. _____. Effect on the electroencephalogram of changing the blood
sugar level. Arch. Neurol. Psychiat., 49:186-94, 1944. 31

848. _____, F. A. Gibbs, H. Davis,
W. W. Jetter, and L. S. Trow-
bridge. The effects of alcohol
upon the electroencephalogram
(brain waves). Q. J. Stud. Alcohol, 1:626-37, 1941. 31
Davis, P. A., co-author: 839-44,
3527.

849. Davis, R. C., and J. R. Kantor.
Skin resistance during hypnotic
states. J. Gen. Psychol., 13:62-
81, 1935.

850. Davison, C. Psychological and psychodynamic aspects of disturbances in the sleep mechanism. Psychoanal. Q., 14:478-97, 1945. 286

851. _____, and E. L. Demuth. Disturbances in sleep mechanism (a clinicopathologic study). J. Nerv. Ment. Dis., 100:303-4, 1944. 266

852. _____, and _____. Disturbances in sleep mechanism (a clinicopathologic study). Trans. Am. Neurol. Ass., 70:173-74, 1944. 266

853. _____, and _____. Disturbances in sleep mechanism; a clinicopathologic study. Arch. Neurol. Psychiat., 53:79, 1945. 266

854. _____, and _____. Disturbances in sleep mechanism: a clinicopathologic study. I. Lesions at the cortical level. Arch. Neurol. Psychiat., 53:399-406, 1945. 266

855. _____, and _____. Disturbances in sleep mechanism. A clinicopathologic study. II. Lesions at the corticodiencephalic level. Arch. Neurol. Psychiat., 54:241-55, 1945. 266

856. _____, and _____. Disturbances in sleep mechanism: a clinicopathologic study. III. Lesions at the diencephalic level (hypothalamus). Arch. Neurol. Psychiat., 55:111-25, 1946. 266, 267

857. _____, and _____. Disturbances in the sleep mechanism; a clinicopathologic study; IV. Lesions at the mesencephalometencephalic level. Arch. Neurol. Psychiat., 55: 126-33, 1946. 266

858. _____, and _____. Disturbances in the sleep mechanism; a clinicopathologic study; V. Anatomic and neurophysiologic considerations. Arch. Neurol. Psychiat., 55:364-81, 1946. 271

859. Dawe, A. R., and P. R. Morrison. Characteristics of the hibernating heart. Am. Heart J., 49:367-84, 1955. 323, 326
Dawe, A. R., co-author: 2356.

860. Dawson, J. R., Jr. Cellular inclusions in cerebral lesions of lethargic encephalitis. Am. J. Path., 9:7-16, 1933. 245

861. Day, R. Effect of sleep on insensible perspiration in infants and children. Am. J. Dis. Child., 58: 82-91, 1939. 74

862. _____. Regulation of body temperature during sleep. Am. J. Dis. Child., 61:734-46, 1941. 74

863. Daynes, G. Shut the windows at night. Practitioner, 175:311-12, 1955.

864. Deane, H. W., and C. P. Lyman. Body temperature, thyroid and adrenal cortex of hamsters during cold exposure and hibernation, with comparison to rats. Endocrinology, 55:300-315, 1954.

865. De Beer, B. The effects of sodium succinate and sucrose diuresis upon pentobarbital anesthesia. J. Pharmacol. Exp. Therap., 88:366-72, 1946. 297

866. Debré, R., et A. Doumic. Le Sommeil de L'Enfant Avant Trois Ans. Paris: Presses Univ. de France, 1959. Pp. xii + 195. 278

867. De Caro, D. Modificazioni elettroencefalografiche provocate dalla LSD nell'uomo. Acta Neurol. (Napoli), 11:144-56, 1956. 303

868. _____. Effects of methedrine, dihydroergotamine and atropine on the electrical activity of the brain of rabbits. Adrenergic mechanism of alerting response of MDAS. In: Psychotropic Drugs, 1957 (1357), pp. 296-99. 304

869. Dechaume, J., et M. Jouvet. Etude séméiologique des troubles prolongés de la conscience. Ses bases physiopathologiques. Lyon Méd., 203:1401-20, 1960. 272
Dechaume, J., co-author: 2034.

870. Deely, D. C. Experimental evidence for a theory of hypnotic behavior: 1. "hypnotic color-blindness" without "hypnosis." Internat. J. Clin. Exp. Hypn., 9: 79-86, 1961. 332, 337

871. Deese, J. Some problems in the theory of vigilance. Psychol. Rev., 62:359-68, 1955.

872. Deglin, V. Ia. (Russ.) A study of sleep disturbances in schizophrenia. Zh. Vysshei Nerv. Deiat., 6:680-89, 1956. 288

873. Deighton, T. Physical factors in body temperature maintenance and heat elimination. Physiol. Rev., 13:427-65, 1933.

874. De Lacroix-Herpin, M. P. Cure de Sommeil dans les Hallucinations. Paris: Impr. R. Foulon, 1954, No. 248, Thèse. Pp. 60. 207

875. Delafresnaye, J. F., Ed. Brain Mechanisms and Consciousness. Springfield, Ill.: Charles C

Thomas, 1954. Pp. xv + 556. 30
876. Delange [Delange-Walter], M., P. Castan, J. Cadilhac, et P. Passouant. Etude E.E.G. des divers stades du sommeil de nuit chez l'enfant. Considérations sur le stade IV ou l'activité onirique. Rev. Neurol., 105:176-81, 1961; also EEG Clin. Neurophysiol., 14: 138, 1962. 26, 98, 102
877. Delay, J. Narcolepsie et hypoglycémie. Ann. Méd.-Psychol., 100 (II):375-79, 1942. 237, 256
878. _____. Conscience et diencéphale. Presse Méd., 55:681-82, 1947. 31
879. _____, et A. Corteel. Sur les troubles du sommeil, de la soif et de la diurèse au cours de la menstruation. Ann. Endocrinol., 6:47-48, 1945. 270
880. _____, P. Deniker, et Y. Tardieu. Hibernothérapie et cure de sommeil en thérapeutique psychiatrique et psycho-somatique. Presse Méd., 61:1165-66, 1953. 207
881. _____, F. Lhermitte, G. Verdeaux, et J. Verdeaux. Modifications de l'électrocorticogramme du lapin par le diéthylamide de l'acide d-lysergique (LSD 25). Rev. Neurol., 86:81-88, 1952. 303
882. _____, R. Suttel, et G. Verdeaux. Myoclonies du sommeil chez un épileptique. Action de l'amphétamine. Constatations électroencéphalographiques. Sem. Hôp. Paris, 23:1874-77, 1947. 257
883. Delbrück, H. Ein bemerkenswerter Fall von Schlaftrunkenheit. Dsche Z. ges. gerichtl. Med., 4: 369-73, 1924.
884. Delcourt-Bernard, et A. Mayer. Recherches sur le métabolisme de base. Ann. Physiol., 1:536-51, 552-79, 1925. 55
885. Delius, K. Eine kaum beobachtete Bedeutung des Traumes. Nervenarzt, 20:11-14, 1949. 106
886. Dell, P., et M. Bonvallet. Données expérimentales récentes sur la physiologie du sommeil (application à l'étude pharmacologique des amphétamines et de la chlorpromazine (largactil)). In: La Cure de Sommeil, 1954 (3021), pp. 23-36. 303
887. _____, and _____. The central action of adrenalin: pharmacological consequences. EEG Clin. Neurophysiol., 8:701-2, 1956. 213, 301, 303
888. _____, _____, et A. Hugelin. Tonus

sympathique, adrénaline et contrôle réticulaire de la motricité spinale. EEG Clin. Neurophysiol., 6:599-618, 1954. 214
889. _____, _____, and _____. Mechanisms of reticular deactivation. In: A CIBA Found. Symposium on the Nature of Sleep, 1961 (4270), pp. 86-102.
890. _____, et C. Kayser. Effet de la lumière sur la diurèse provoquée. J. Physiol. (Paris), 40: 165A-67A, 1948. 167
Dell, P., co-author: 407-9, 1005, 1761.
891. Dell'Acqua, G. Klinische Beobachtungen zur Pathologie des Hypophysenzwischenhirnsystems. Med. Klin., 39:459-61, 1943. 269
892. Delmas-Marsalet, P. Epilepsie et fonction hypnique. Essai de médications anti-hypniques. J. Méd. Bordeaux, 121:259-63, 1945. 259
893. _____, et J. Faure. Etude électroencéphalographique des épilepsies de structure morphéique. EEG Clin. Neurophysiol., 2:347, 1950. 259
894. Demant, E. Der Schlaf als Heilschlaf in der antiken und heutigen Medizin. Arch. phys. Therap. (Leipzig), 9:9-14, 1957. 206
895. DeMartino, M. F. Sex differences in the dreams of southern college students. J. Clin. Psychol., 9:199-201, 1953. 101
896. _____. Some characteristics of the manifest dream content of mental defectives. J. Clin. Psychol., 10:175-78, 1954. 103
897. _____. A review of literature on children's dreams. Psychiat. Q. Suppl., 29:90-101, 1955. 102
898. Dement, W. C. Dream recall and eye movements during sleep in schizophrenics and normals. J. Nerv. Ment. Dis., 122:263-69, 1955. 103, 288
899. _____. The occurrence of low voltage, fast electroencephalogram patterns during behavioral sleep in the cat. EEG Clin. Neurophysiol., 10:291-96, 1958. 26, 103, 212
900. _____. The effect of dream deprivation. Science, 131:1705-7; 132:1420-22, 1960. 105, 107, 224
901. _____, and N. Kleitman. Cyclic variations in EEG during sleep and their relation to eye movements, body motility, and dream-

ing. EEG Clin. Neurophysiol., 9: 673-90, 1957; prelim. commun., Fed. Proc., 14:37, 1955. <u>26</u>, <u>94</u>, <u>96</u>, <u>98</u>, <u>112</u>, <u>113</u>

902. _____, and _____. The relation of eye movements during sleep to dream activity: an objective method for the study of dreaming. J. Exp. Psychol., 53:339-46, 1957; prelim. commun., Fed. Proc., 15:46, 1956. <u>91</u>, <u>99</u>, <u>101</u>

903. _____, and E. A. Wolpert. Relationships in the manifest content of dreams occurring on the same night. J. Nerv. Ment. Dis., 126: 568-78, 1958. <u>101</u>

904. _____, and _____. The relation of eye movements, body motility, and external stimuli to dream content. J. Exp. Psychol., 55:543-53, 1958. <u>95</u>, <u>101</u>, <u>104</u>, <u>105</u>
Dement, W. C., co-author: 697.

905. Demidov, A. V., L. E. Kaplane, et A. B. Guenkina. L'état de la barrière hématoencéphalique dans les cas de trouble du rythme du sommeil et de la veille. I. Influence de la thyroïdine. Bull. Biol. Méd. Exp. U.R.S.S., 4:344-48, 1937. <u>218</u>
Demidov, A., co-author: 1043.

906. Demikhov, V. P. Experimental Transplantation of Vital Organs. New York: Consultants Bureau, 1962. Pp. x + 285. <u>354</u>

907. Demole, V. Catatonie expérimentale. Rev. Neurol., I:861-62, 1927. <u>253</u>

908. _____. Pharmakologisch-anatomische Untersuchungen zum Problem des Schlafes. Arch. exp. Path. Pharmakol., 120:229-58, 1927. <u>35</u>, <u>200</u>

909. _____. Pharmacodynamie et centres du sommeil (Mise en évidence des composantes anatomiques: végétative basilaire et corticale volitive). Cervello, 7:22-25, 1928; also Rev. Neurol., I:850-52, 1927.

910. Dempsey, E. W., and R. S. Morison. The production of rhythmically recurrent cortical potentials after localized thalamic stimulation. Am. J. Physiol., 135:293-300, 1942. <u>210</u>

911. _____, and _____. The electrical activity of a thalamocortical relay system. Am. J. Physiol., 138: 283-96, 1943. <u>210</u>
Dempsey, E. W., co-author: 2880, 2881.

912. De Moragas, J. Terror nocturno, pesadilla y somnambulismo. Rev. Españ. Pediat. (Zaragoza), 8:47-59, 1952.

913. Denier, A. EEG dans l'électroanesthésie. EEG Clin. Neurophysiol., 3:106, 1951. <u>298</u>

914. Denisova, M. P., and N. L. Figurin. (Russ.) Periodic phenomena in the sleep of children. Nov. Refl. Fiziol. Nerv. Syst., 2:338-45, 1926. <u>50</u>, <u>52</u>, <u>88</u>, <u>91</u>, <u>112</u>, <u>357</u>, <u>364</u>

915. Dennemark, H. G. Die medikamentoese Behandlung nervoeser Rhythmusstoerungen, insbesondere des "Dies inversus." Medizinische (Stuttgart), (25):1033-34, 1958. <u>294</u>

916. Dennis, W. Sidedness in sleeping position in two species. J. Genet. Psychol., 37:162. 1930. <u>10</u>

917. Derbyshire, A. J., B. Rempel, A. Forbes, and E. F. Lambert. The effect of anesthetics on action potentials in cerebral cortex of the cat. Am. J. Physiol., 116:577-96, 1936. <u>26</u>, <u>296</u>
Derbyshire, A. J., co-author: 3023.

918. Dercum, F. X. Profound somnolence or narcolepsy. J. Nerv. Ment. Dis., 40:185-87, 1913. <u>267</u>, <u>268</u>

919. Dereux, J. Cataplexie et narcolepsie. Apparition et disparition d'une affection médullaire pendant l'évolution du syndrome. Rev. Neurol., I:344-46, 1933. <u>280</u>

920. Deri, F. Neurotic disturbances of sleep (Symposium). Internat. J. Psycho-anal., 23:56-59, 1942. <u>276</u>, <u>286</u>

921. DeSanctis, S., and U. Neyroz. Experimental investigations concerning the depth of sleep. Psychol. Rev., 9:254-82, 1902. <u>100</u>

922. Desmedt, J.-E., et J. Schlag. Mise en évidence d'éléments cholinergiques dans la formation réticulée mésencéphalique. J. Physiol. (Paris), 49:136-38, 1957. <u>209</u>

923. Despert, J. L. Dreams in children of preschool age. In: The Psychoanalytic Study of the Child, New York: Internat. Univ. Press, 1949. Vol. 3/4:141-80. <u>102</u>

924. _____. Sleep in pre-school children: a preliminary study. Nervous Child, 8:8-27, 1949. <u>9</u>, <u>117</u>, <u>306</u>, <u>307</u>

925. Deutsch, E. The dream imagery of the blind. Psychoanal. Rev., 15: 288-93, 1928. 102

926. Devesa. An unpublished experience in the history of medicine: the examination of ailing man during his sleep. Santiago de Compostela, Spain: Author (?), 1945. Pp. 6.

927. Devic, A., et G. Morin. La région du ventricule moyen et le sommeil. J. Méd. Lyon, 9:357-60, 1928. 359

928. Devold, O., E. Barlinghaug, and J. E. Backer. (Norw.) Sleep disturbances during the season of darkness. Tskr. Norske Laegeforen. (Oslo), 77:836-37, 1957. 278

929. Dew, R., W. L. Klingman, and R. Leigh. An electroencephalographic study of 35 patients having nocturnal seizures. EEG Clin. Neurophysiol., 3:105, 1951. 259

930. Diamant, J., M. Dufek, J. Hoskovec, M. Krištof, V. Pekárek, B. Roth, and M. Velek. (Czech.) Electroencephalographic investigation of hypnosis. Ceskoslov. Psychiat., 55:185-95, 1959; also EEG Clin. Neurophysiol., 12:535, 1960. 330

931. Diamond, E. The Science of Dreams. Garden City, N.Y.: Doubleday & Co., 1962. Pp. 264. 99

932. Diaz-Guerrero, R., J. S. Gottlieb, and J. R. Knott. The sleep of patients with manic-depressive psychosis, depressive type. An electroencephalographic study. Psychosom. Med., 8:399-404, 1946. 29

933. Dide. Discussion du rapport de Jean Lhermitte et Auguste Tournay: le sommeil normal et pathologique. Rev. Neurol., I:860-61, 1927. 251

934. Dienst, C. Regulationsvorgaenge beim Schlaf und Schmerz. Klin. Wschr., 17:380-82, 1938.

935. _____, und B. Winter. Schlaf, Blutzucker und Saeurebasenaushalt. Z. klin. Med., 133:91-104, 1937. 34, 295, 353

936. Diez Blanco, A. El sueño y las funciones del alma; piensa el alma durante el sueño. Médicamenta (Madrid), 19:267-69, 1953.

937. Dikshit, B. B. Action of acetylcholine on the "sleep centre." J. Physiol. (London), 83:42P, 1934. 203, 357, 358

938. _____. The physiology of sleep. Lancet, 228(I):570, 1935. 203, 357, 358

939. Di Molfetta, N., e E. Mignani. Studio istochemico sul comportamento funzionale della corticale surrenale nella ipotermia da blocco farmacodinamico del sistema nervoso vegetativo e nella ibernazione naturale di Vesperugo noctula. Arch. Vecchi (Firenze), 22:1113-33, 1954.

940. Dimter, R. Ueber Schlaf und Schlafverlaengerung durch Quadro-Nox im Senium. Med. Klin., 30:940-41, 1934. 294

941. Di Raimondo, V. C., and P. H. Forsham. Some clinical implications of the spontaneous diurnal variation in adrenal cortical secretory activity. Am. J. Med., 21: 321-23, 1956.

942. Dische, Z., W. Fleischmann, und E. Trevani. Zur Frage des Zusammenhanges zwischen Winterschlaf und Hypoglykaemie. Pfluegers Arch., 227:235-38, 1931. 322

943. Ditman, K. S., and K. A. Blinn. Sleep levels in enuresis. Am. J. Psychiat., 111:913-20, 1955. 284 Ditman, K. S., co-author: 376

944. Dittborn, J. M., and V. Armengol. Expectation as a factor of sleep suggestibility. II. J. Psychol., 49:113-16, 1960. 197

945. _____, and _____. An operational definition of somnambulist hypnosis. J. Psychol., 49:117-21, 1960. 197, 335

946. _____, O. Guitierrez, and L. M. Godoy. Sleep suggestibility test. J. Psychol., 49:111-12, 1960. 197

947. _____, and M. V. Kline. An instrument for the measurement of sleep induction. J. Psychol., 46:277-78, 1958. 197

948. Dittmar, F. Die physikalische Behandlung der Schlafstoerungen. Med. Klin. (Berlin), 54:981-84, 1959. 278

949. Divry, P. Un cas de somnambulisme alcoolique. J. Neurol. Psychiat., 28:823-28, 1928. 283

950. _____. A propos de la catalepsie bulbocapnique. J. Neurol. Psychiat., 29:215-24, 1929. 253

951. _____, J. Bobon, et J. Collard. La lévomépromazine dans les cures de sommeil potentialisées et les cures neuroleptiques. Acta Neurol. Psychiat. Belg., 59:

325-36, 1959. 207

952. Dobbelstein, H. Gesunder Schlaf ohne Medikamente. Hennef/Sieg, Germany: Klefisch, 1951. Pp. 24. 274

953. Dobin, N. B., and E. C. Smith. Narcolepsy. Report of a case. Q. Bull. Northwest. Univ. Med. School, 29:114-19, 1955. 237

954. Dobreff, M., und T. Saprjanoff. Physiologische Tagesschwankungen in Liquor cerebrospinalis. Z. ges. exp. Med., 85:295-300, 1932. 166

955. Doe, R. P., E. B. Flink, and M. G. Goodsell [Flint]. Relationship of diurnal variation in 17-hydroxy-corticosteroid levels in blood and urine to eosinophils and electrolyte excretion. J. Clin. Endocrinol. Metab., 16:196-206, 1956; prelim. commun. 14:774-75, 1954. 167 Doe, R. P., co-author: 1212.

956. Doehner, W. Zur neurotischen Schlafsucht. Dsche med. Wschr., 80:1185-87, 1955. 271

957. Dogs, W. "Einschlafangst." Kasuistisches zur Therapie der Schlafstoerung. Med. Klin., 38(II): 848-50, 1942. 278, 335

958. Domino, E. F. A pharmacological analysis of the functional relationship between the brain stem arousal and diffuse thalamic projection systems. J. Pharmacol. Exp. Therap., 115:449-63, 1955. 362

959. Donato, R. A., and M. M. Strumia. An exact method for the chamber count of eosinophils in capillary blood and its application to the study of the diurnal cycle. Blood, 7:1020-29, 1952. 169

960. Dondey, M., et X. Machne. Notes préliminaires à propos de l'enregistrement de l'activité des neurones corticaux au cours de la réaction dite d'éveil chez le chat. Rev. Neurol., 93:485-86, 1955.

961. Dontcheff, L., et C. Kayser. La dépense d'énergie chez la marmotte en état d'hibernation. C. R. Soc. Biol., 119:565-68, 1935. 323, 324

962. _____, _____, et P. Reiss. Le rythme nycthéméral de la production de chaleur chez le pigeon et ses rapports avec l'excitabilité des centres thermorégulateurs. Ann. Physiol., 11:1185-1207, 1935. 138 Dontcheff, L., co-author: 571.

963. Dornblüth, O. Die Schlaflosigkeit und ihre Behandlung. Leipzig: Veit & Co., 1912. Pp. 92. 294

964. Dost, H. Zur Physiologie und Pharmakologie des Schlafes. I. Methodik der Schlafmittelpruefung an Voegeln. Arch. exp. Path. Pharmakol., 175:727-35, 1934. 295

965. _____. Zur Physiologie und Pharmakologie des Schlafes. II. Vegetative Gifte und ihre Schlafwirkung. Arch. exp. Path. Pharmakol., 176:478-85, 1934. 295

966. Douglas, D. M., and F. C. Mann. An experimental study of the rhythmic contractions in the small intestine of the dog. Am. J. Dig. Dis., 6:318-22, 1939. 55

967. Doupe, J., W. R. Miller, and W. K. Keller. Vasomotor reactions in the hypnotic state. J. Neurol. Psychiat., 2:97-106, 1939. 330, 332

968. Doust, J. W. L. Studies in the physiology of awareness: the incidence and content of dream patterns and their relationship to anoxia. J. Ment. Sci., 97:801-11, 1951.

969. _____. Studies on the physiology of awareness; oxymetric analysis of emotion and the differential planes of consciousness seen in hypnosis. J. Clin. Exp. Psychopath., 14:113-26, 1953. 330

970. _____, and R. A. Schneider. Studies on the physiology of awareness: anoxia and the levels of sleep. Brit. Med. J., I:449-55, 1952. 51

971. _____, and _____. Studies on the physiology of awareness: the effect of rhythmic sensory bombardment on emotions, blood oxygen saturation and the levels of consciousness. J. Ment. Sci., 98: 640-53, 1952. 51

972. Douthwaite, A. H. Sleep: A general medical problem. Brit. Med. J., II:152, 1954.

973. Doyle, J. B., and L. E. Daniels. Symptomatic treatment for narcolepsy. J. Am. Med. Ass., 96: 1370-72, 1931. 234, 238, 300

974. _____, and _____. Narcolepsy: results of treatment with ephedrine sulphate. J. Am. Med. Ass., 98:542-45, 1932. 238, 300

975. Doyle, M. R. Sleeping habits of in-

fants. Physiotherapy Rev., 25:74-75, 1945. <u>305</u>

976. Drăgănesco, S., et O. Sager. Ependymocytome kystique du troisième ventricule. Encéphale, 30:512-22, 1935. <u>264</u>
Drăgănesco, S., co-author: 2679.

977. Drake, F. R. Narcolepsy: Brief review and report of cases. Am. J. Med. Sci., 218:101-14, 1949. <u>234</u>

978. Dresel, K. Die Funktionen eines grosshirn- und striatumlosen Hundes. Klin. Wschr., 3:2231-33, 1924. <u>21</u>

979. Dresslar, F. B. Some influences which affect the rapidity of voluntary movements. Am. J. Psychol., 4:514-27, 1892. <u>150</u>

980. Dreyfus-Brisac, C., et C. Blanc. III. Aspects électroencéphalographiques de la maturation cérébrale pendant la première année de la vie. EEG Clin. Neurophysiol., Suppl. 6:432-40, 1955. <u>27</u>

981. _____, et _____. Electro-encéphalogramme et maturation cérébrale. Encéphale, 45:205-41, 1956. <u>27</u>

982. _____, _____, et P. Kramarz. La réactivité E.E.G. chez le jeune enfant. Rev. Neurol., 94:159, 1956. <u>27</u>

983. _____, _____, et _____. Etude électroencéphalographique du sommeil spontané de l'enfant atteint de convulsions avant trois ans. Rev. Neurol., 99:54-67, 1958. <u>27</u>

984. _____, et M. Monod. II. Veille, sommeil et réactivité chez le nouveau-né à terme. EEG Clin. Neurophysiol., Suppl. 6:425-31, 1955. <u>27</u>

985. _____, D. Samson, C. Blanc, et N. Monod. L'électroencéphalogramme de l'enfant normal de moins de 3 ans. Aspect fonctionel bio-électrique de la maturation nerveuse. Etudes Néo-Natales, 7:143-75, 1958. <u>27</u>

986. _____, _____, et N. Monod. Données sur l'électrogénèse cérébrale du nouveau-né à terme et du prématuré. Rev. Neurol., 94:160, 1956. <u>27</u>

987. _____, D. Samson-Dollfus, et S. Sainte-Anne-Dargassies. I. Veille, sommeil et réactivité sensorielle chez le prématuré. EEG Clin. Neurophysiol., Suppl. 6:418-24, 1955. <u>27</u>
Dreyfus-Brisac, C., co-author: 367, 1185, 3622.

988. Drogendijk, A. C. (Dutch) The nature of sleep. Geneesk. Gids, 23: 57-64, 1945; also Prensa Méd., 35: 1103-5, 1948; also Schweiz. med. Wschr., 79:100-103, 1949.

989. _____. (Dutch) The nature, cause, and purpose of sleep. Geneesk. Bl., 44:235-71, 1950.

990. Drohocki, Z. La respiration au cours de l'installation du sommeil et ses rapports avec l'électroencéphalogramme. C. R. Soc. Biol., 147:1226-28, 1953. <u>79</u>

991. _____. L'électroencéphalogramme quantitatif de l'homme au cours de l'installation du sommeil provoqué par le nembutal. Rev. Neurol., 96:475-89, 1957; also EEG Clin. Neurophysiol., 9:560-61, 1957. <u>296</u>

992. _____, et J. Drohocka. L'exploration électroencéphalographique de la localisation pharmacologique des narcotiques. C. R. Soc. Biol., 130:267-70, 1939. <u>295</u>

993. Droogleever Fortuyn, J. (Dutch) Consciousness and cerebral cortex. Ned. Tschr. Geneesk., 96: 990-94, 1952. <u>31</u>
Droogleever-Fortuyn, J., co-author: 1964.

994. Druckmann, A. Schlafsucht als Folge der Roentgenbestrahlung. Beitrag zur Strahlenempfindlichkeit des Gehirns. Strahlentherapie, 33:382-84, 1929. <u>268</u>, <u>294</u>

995. Dubois, F. S. Rhythms, cycles and periods in health and disease. Am. J. Psychiat., 116:114-19, 1959. <u>131</u>

996. Du Bois, P. H., and T. W. Forbes. Studies of catatonia. III. Bodily postures assumed while sleeping. Psychiat. Q., 8:546-52, 1934. <u>251</u>

997. Dubois, R. Variations des gaz du sang chez la marmotte pendant l'hibernation, en état de veille et en état de torpeur. C. R. Soc. Biol., 46:821-23, 1894. <u>322</u>

998. _____. Autonarcose carbonico-acétonémique ou sommeil hivernal de la marmotte. C. R. Soc. Biol., 47:149-50, 1895. <u>322</u>

999. _____. Le centre du sommeil. C. R. Soc. Biol., 53:229-30, 1901. <u>361</u>

1000. _____. Sommeil naturel par autonarcose carbonique provoqué expérimentalement. C. R. Soc. Biol., 53:231-32, 1901. <u>351</u>

1001. Dudley, G. A. Dreams; Their Meaning and Significance. London: Thorsons, 1956 [?]. Pp. xii + 108. <u>106</u>

1002. Duensing, F. Das Elektroencephalogramm bei Stoerungen der Bewusstseinslage. Befunde bei

Meningitiden und Hirntumoren mit Bemerkungen zur Pathophysiologie and Pathopsychologie der Bewusstseinstoerungen. Arch. Psychiat. Nervenkr., 183:71-114, 1949. 31

1003. Duffy, E. The psychological significance of the concept of "arousal" or "activation." Psychol. Rev., 64: 265-75, 1957. 209

1004. Dukes, C. Sleep in relation to education. J. Roy. Sanit. Inst., 26:41-44, 1905. 114, 117, 118, 305

1005. Dumont, S., et P. Dell. Facilitations spécifiques et non-spécifiques des réponses visuelles corticales. J. Physiol. (Paris), 50:261-64, 1950.
Dumont, S., co-author: 1859.

1006. Dumpert, V. Zur Kenntnis des Wesens und der physiologischen Bedeutung des Gaehnens. J. Psychol. Neurol., 27:82-95, 1921. 72

1007. Dunlap, K. Sleep and dreams. J. Abnorm. Soc. Psychol., 16:197-209, 1921. 107

1008. Dunlop, D. M. Sleep: Applied pharmacology. Brit. Med. J., II:151-52, 1954. 294

1009. Duran, P., M. Favier, P. Judeau, P. Juillet, et J. Gibert. Perturbations du tracé EEG dans l'énurésie. Rev. Neurol., 92:627-28, 1955. 284

1010. Durup, G. Les phénomènes hypnagogiques et l'invention. Année Psychol., 1932, pp. 94-105.

1011. Dutrey, J. Contribución al estudio de los accidentes nerviosos de la auroterapia. Síndrome insomníaco y ansioso. Rev. As. Méd. Argentina, 49:121-27, 1935. 277

1012. Duval, M. Hypothèse sur la physiologie des centres nerveux. Théorie histologique du sommeil. C. R. Soc. Biol., 47:74-76, 86-87, 1895. 343

1013. Dworkin, S., and W. H. Finney. Artificial hibernation in the woodchuck (Arctomys Monax). Am. J. Physiol., 80:75-81, 1927. 322

1014. Dyken, M., P. Grant, and P. White. Evaluation of electroencephalographic changes associated with chronic alcoholism. Dis. Nerv. Syst., 22:284-86, 1961. 31

1015. Dynes, J. B. An experimental study in hypnotic anesthesia. J. Abnorm. Soc. Psychol., 27:79-88, 1932.

1016. _____. Narcolepsy and cataplexy. Lahey Clin. Bull., 2:83-90, 1941. 238, 239

1017. _____. Cataplexy and its treatment.

J. Nerv. Ment. Dis., 98:48-55, 1943. 239

1018. _____. Objective method for distinguishing sleep from the hypnotic trance. Arch. Neurol. Psychiat., 57:84-93, 1947. 330

1019. _____, and K. H. Finley. The electroencephalograph as an aid in the study of narcolepsy. Arch. Neurol. Psychiat., 46:598-612, 1941. 238

1020. Eagles, J. B., A. M. Halliday, and J. W. T. Redfearn. The effect of fatigue on tremor. In: Fatigue, W. F. Floyd and A. T. Welford, Eds., London: Lewis, 1953, pp. 41-58. 226

1021. Eaton, L. M. Treatment of narcolepsy with desoxyephedrine hydrochloride. Proc. Staff Meet. Mayo Clin., 18:262-64, 1943. 238, 239

1022. Eaves, E. C., and M. M. Croll. The pituitary and hypothalamic region in chronic epidemic encephalitis. Brain, 53:56-75, 1930-31. 250

1023. Ebaugh, F. G. Sleep disorders in clinical practice. Calif. West. Med., 45:5-9, 128-32, 1936. 275, 294, 362
Ebaugh, F. G., co-author: 2721.

1024. Ebbecke, U. Physiologie des Schlafes. Handb. norm. path. Physiol., 17:563-90, 1926.

1025. _____. Schlaf als Affekt. Nervenarzt, 19:442-46, 1948. 362

1026. Eckerström, S. (Swed.) Insomnia at old people's homes and its treatment. Sven. Läkartidn., 51:70-73, 1954. 278

1027. Eckstein, A. Ueber die gesteigerte Erregbarkeit des Brechzentrums als Ursache des pylorospastischen Erbrechens und ihre Bekaempfung durch den Dauerschlaf. Z. Kinderheilk., 45:123-38, 1928. 206

1028. _____, und E. Rominger. Beitraege zur Physiologie und Pathologie der Atmung im Kindesalter. III. Ueber Schlafmittel im Saeuglingsalter und ihre Wirkung auf die Atmung. Arch. Kinderheilk, 70:1-22, 102-11, 1921. 294

1029. Eckstein, G. The sleep of canaries. Science, 92:577-78, 1940. 10

1030. Economo, C. von. Encephalitis lethargia. Wien. med. Wschr., 73:777-82, 835-38, 1113-17, 1243-49, 1334-38, 1923. 206, 243, 246, 262, 359

1031. _____. Ueber den Schlaf. Wien.

klin. Wschr., Sonderbeil., 1925.
Pp. 14. 206, 344, 359

1032. _____. Studien ueber den Schlaf.
Wien. med. Wschr., 76:91-92, 1926.
206

1033. _____. Die Pathologie des Schlafes.
Handb. norm. path. Physiol., 17:
591-610, 1926. 206, 246

1034. _____. Discussion du rapport de
Jean Lhermitte et Auguste Tournay.
Le sommeil normal et pathologique.
Rev. Neurol., I:837-41, 1927. 206,
295, 359

1035. _____. Théorie du sommeil. J. Neurol. Psychiat., 28:437-64, 1928.
206, 352

1036. _____. Schlaftheorie. Ergebn.
Physiol., 28:312-39, 1929. 206, 362

1037. _____. Sleep as a problem of localization. J. Nerv. Ment. Dis., 71:249-
59, 1930. 206

1038. _____. Das Schlafsteuerungszentrum. Scritti Med. in onore Gabbi,
I:117-31, 1930. 206, 362

1039. _____. Besteht im Zentralnerven-
system ein Zentrum das den Schlaf
reguliert? Wien. klin. Wschr., 44:
1603-4, 1932. 206, 362

1040. Edinger, L., und B. Fischer. Ein
Mensch ohne Grosshirn. Pfluegers
Arch., 152:535-61, 1913. 23

1041. Edwards, A. S. Effects of the loss
of 100 hours of sleep. Am. J. Psychol., 54:80-91, 1941. 225

1042. Eeman, L. E. How do You Sleep?
The Basis of Good Health. London:
Author-Partner Press, 1939. 2d ed.
Pp. xix + 82. 312

1043. Efimov, V., et A. Demidov. Change-
ment de rythme du sommeil et de
la veille chez les animaux sous
l'influence de la lumière et du son
d'après les actogrammes et l'enregistrement des mouvements des
paupières. Bull. Biol. Méd. Exp.
URSS, 7:392-96, 1939. 90

1044. _____, E. S. Lokshina, and L. B.
Utevskaia. (Russ.) Investigation
on the modifications of rhythm
of sleep and wakefulness in man
and animal; biological and physico-
chemical properties of the cerebrospinal fluid and blood of hypophys-
ectomized dogs; effect of light and
ultra-high frequency. Bull. Eksp.
Biol. Med., 14(2):54-60, 1942. 358

1045. _____, _____, and _____. (Russ.) II.
The changes of the rhythm of sleep
and wakefulness, of the biological
and physico-chemical properties of
the cerebrospinal fluid and blood
under the action of light and ultra-

high frequency in hypophysecto-
mized dogs. Bull. Eksp. Biol.
Med., 14(2):61-64, 1942. 356

1046. _____, _____, and _____. (Russ.)
III. Dissociation of the whole
sleep into sleep of the body and
sleep of the cerebral cortex under action of hypophyseal metabolites in animals. Bull. Eksp.
Biol. Med., 14(4): 28-33, 1942.
359

Efimov, V. V., co-author: 4049.

1047. Egdahl, R. H. Adrenal cortical
and medullary responses to
trauma in dogs with isolated pi-
tuitaries. Endocrinology, 66:200-
216, 1960. 356

1048. Eggan, D. The significance of
dreams for anthropological research. Am. Anthropol., 51:177-
98, 1949. 101

1049. _____. The manifest content of
dreams: a challenge to social
science. Am. Anthropol., 54:469-
85, 1952. 101

1050. Ehni, G. Numbness of hands at
night. J. Am. Med. Ass., 160:
922, 1956. 285

1051. Ehrenwald, J. Morning depression. Am. J. Psychother., 2:198-
214, 1948.

1052. Ehrström, C. Ueber Serumcal-
cium-Tageskurven. Acta Med.
Scand., Suppl., 59:97-103, 1934. 163

1053. Eiduson, B. T. Structural analysis of dreams: Clues to perceptual style. J. Abnorm. Soc. Psychol., 58:335-39, 1959. 101

1054. Eiff, A. W. von, E. M. Böckh, H.
Göpfert, F. Pfleiderer, und T.
Steffen. Die Bedeutung des Zeitbewusstseins fuer die 24 Stunden-
Rhythmen des erwachsenen Menschen. Z. ges. exp. Med., 120:
295-307, 1953. 158

1055. Eisentraut, M. Winterstarre,
Winterschlaf und Winterruhe.
Eine kurze biologische physiolo-
gische Studie. Monatsheft zool.
Mus., Berlin, 19:48-63, 1933.

1056. _____. Der Winterschlaf der Fle-
dermaeuse mit besonderer Beruecksichtung der Waermeregulation. Z. Morphol. Oekol., 29:
231-67, 1934. 324

1057. Eisler, M. J. Pleasure in sleep
and undisturbed capacity for sleep.
Internat. J. Psycho-anal., 3:30-42,
1922. 8

1058. Elder, J. H. Influence of assigned
hour for waking on sleep motility.
Psychol. Bull., 38:557-58, 1941.

1059. _____. A study of the ability to awaken at assigned hours. Psychol. Bull., 38:693, 1941. 127

1060. Eley, R. D. Neurologic conditions in infants and children. J. Pediat., 3:781-96, 1933. 235

1061. Elfvin, L.-G., T. Petrén, and A. Sollberger. Influence of some endogenous and exogenous factors on diurnal glycogen rhythm in chicken. Acta Anat., 25:286-309, 1955. 165

1062. Ellingson, R. J. Brain waves and problems of psychology. Psychol. Bull., 53:1-34, 1956. 362

1063. _____. Comments on Schmidt's "The reticular formation and behavioral wakefulness." Psychol. Bull., 54:76-78, 1957. 362

1064. _____. Comment on Kleitman's note. Psychol. Bull., 54:360, 1957. 362

1065. _____. Electroencephalograms of normal, full-term newborns immediately after birth with observations on arousal and visual evoked responses. EEG Clin. Neurophysiol., 10:31-50, 1958. 27

1066. _____. "Arousal" and evoked responses in EEGs of newborn. Proc. Fourth Internat. Congr. EEG Clin. Neurophysiol., Brussels, 1957. New York: Pergamon Press, 1959, pp. 57-60.

1067. _____, and D. B. Lindsley. Brain waves and cortical development in newborns and young infants. Am. Psychol., 4:248-49, 1949. 27

1068. _____, R. C. Wilcott, J. G. Sineps, and F. J. Dudek. EEG frequency-pattern variation and intelligence. EEG Clin. Neurophysiol., 9:657-60, 1957. 31

1069. Elliott, T. R., and F. M. R. Walshe. The Babinski or extensor form of plantar response in toxic states. Lancet, 208(I):65-68, 1925. 17, 267

1070. Elmadjian, F., and G. Pincus. Study of diurnal variations in circulating lymphocytes in normal and psychotic subjects. J. Clin. Endocrinol., 6:287-94, 1946. 162

1071. El-Maziny, A. R. Sleep and insomnia. J. Roy. Egypt. Med. Ass., 26:299-316, 1943. 95, 274

1072. Embden, G., und E. Grafe. Ueber den Einfluss der Muskelarbeit auf die Phosphorsaeureausscheidung. Z. physiol. Chem., 113:108-37, 1921.

1073. Emmons, W. H., and C. W. Simon. The non-recall of material presented during sleep. Am. J. Psychol., 69:76-81, 1956. 125
Emmons, W. H., co-author: 3706-9.

1074. Endres, G. Ueber Gesetzmaessigkeiten in der Beziehung zwischen der wahren Harnreaktion und der alveolaren CO_2 Spannung. Biochem. Z., 132:220-41, 1922. 64

1075. _____. Atmungsregulation und Blutreaktion im Schlaf. Biochem. Z., 142:53-67, 1923. 33, 51

1076. _____. Die physikalisch-chemische Regulation der Atmung bei winterschlafenden Hamstern. Verhandl. dsch. Gesellsch. inn. Med., 36:61-63, 1924. 322

1077. _____. Versuche zur Bestimmung der Schlaftiefe; der Begriff der Schlafmenge. Verhandl. phys.-med. Gesellsch., 54:133-40, 1930. 108

1078. _____. Neuere Untersuchungen ueber den Winterschlaf. Verhandl. phys.-med. Gesellsch., 55:172-81, 1930.

1079. _____. Schlafbilanzen. Verhandl. dsch. Gesellsch. inn. Med., 42:622-23, 1930. 108

1080. _____, und H. Lucke. Die Regulation des Blutzuckers und der Blutreaktion beim Menschen. III. Die Blutzuckerregulation bei Aenderungen der Blutreaktion. Z. ges. exp. Med., 45:669-81, 1925. 34

1081. _____, und W. von Frey. Ueber Schlaftiefe und Schlafmenge. Z. Biol., 90:70-80, 1930. 108, 313

1082. _____, B. H. C. Matthews, H. Taylor, and A. Dale. Observations on certain physiological processes of the marmot. Proc. Roy. Soc. London, Ser. B, 107:222-47, 1930. 322, 323, 324

1083. Engebretsen, R. Ueber den Schlaf. Med. Rev., Bergen, 51:289-304, 1934. 349, 362

1084. _____. Beitrag zur Lehre der nervoesen Schlafstoerungen. Med. Rev., Bergen, 52:501-13, 1935. 335

1085. Engel, G. L., J. Romano, E. B. Ferris, Jr., J. P. Webb, and C. D. Stevens. A simple method of determining frequency spectrums in the electroencephalogram. Observations on effects of physiological variations in dextrose, oxygen, posture and acid-base balance on the normal electroencephalogram. Arch. Neurol. Psychiat., 51:134-46, 1944. 31

1086. ____, and M. Rosenbaum. Delirium. III. Electroencephalographic changes associated with acute alcoholic intoxication. Arch. Neurol. Psychiat., 53:44-50, 1945. 31

1087. ____, J. P. Webb, and E. B. Ferris. Quantitative electroencephalographic studies of anoxia in humans; comparison with acute alcoholic intoxication and hypoglycemia. J. Clin. Investig., 24:691-97, 1945. 31
Engel, G. L., co-author: 3305, 3399.

1088. Engel, R., F. Halberg, and R. Gurly. The diurnal rhythm in EEG discharge and in circulating eosinophils in certain types of epilepsy. EEG Clin. Neurophysiol., 4:115-16, 1952. 260
Engel, R., co-author: 1588, 1589.

1089. Engelbach, W., and A. McMahon. Report of cases from the Engelbach Clinic. Endocrinology, 8: 109-14, 1924. 269

1090. Enke, W. Das Problem der Dauerschlafbehandlung in der Psychiatrie. Muench. med. Wschr., 76: 1961-62, 1929. 206

1091. Enomoto, T. F., and C. Ajmone-Marsan. Epileptic activation of single cortical neurones and their relationship with electroencephalographic discharges. EEG Clin. Neurophysiol., 11:199-218, 1959.

1092. Epstein, A. L. (Russ.) A sleep phenomenon in neuropathic and mental patients. Vrach. Delo, 10: 92-96, 1927. 286

1093. ____. (Russ.) Somato-biological sketches in psychiatry. Posture reflexes of sleep and their clinical significance. Soviet. Psikhonevrol., (5):5-16, 1934. 8

1094. ____. (Russ.) Problem of function of wakefulness in psychiatry. Problems Klin. Nevropatol. Psikhiat., Kharkov; Ukr. Psikhonevr. Akad., 1936, pp. 272-79. 362

1095. Epstein, J. A., and M. A. Lennox. Electroencephalographic study of experimental cerebro-vascular occlusion. EEG Clin. Neurophysiol., 1:491-502, 1949.

1096. Epstein, L. G., and A. S. Pipko. (Russ.) Effect of sleep on the gastric function of children. Vrach.

Delo, 19:67-72, 1936.

1097. Erickson, M. H. An experimental investigation of the possible anti-social use of hypnosis. Psychiatry, 2:391-414, 1939. 334

1098. ____. The induction of color blindness by a technique of hypnotic suggestion. J. Gen. Psychol., 20:61-89, 1939. 332

1099. ____. On the possible occurrence of a dream in an eight-month-old infant. Psychoanal. Q., 10:382-84, 1941. 102

1100. ____. Hypnotic investigation of psychosomatic phenomena; Psychomatic interrelationships studied by experimental hypnosis. Psychosom. Med., 5:51-58, 1943. 335

1101. ____. Hypnosis in medicine. Med. Clin. North Am., 28:639-52, 1944. 335

1102. ____, and E. M. Erickson. Concerning the nature and character of post-hypnotic behavior. J. Gen. Psychol., 24:95-133, 1941; also in: Modern Hypnosis, 1958 (2299), pp. 105-42. 333

1103. Erikson, H. Observations on the body temperature of Arctic ground squirrels (Citelus parryi) during hibernation. Acta Physiol. Scand., 36:79-81, 1956.

1104. Ernst, W. Ein neuer Weg zur Behandlung bestimmter Formen von Schlafstoerungen. Wien. klin. Wschr., 54:615, 1941. 286

1105. Errera, L. Note sur la théorie toxique du sommeil. C. R. Soc. Biol., 43:508, 1891. 352

1106. Erwin, D. An analytical study of children's sleep. J. Genet. Psychol., 45:199-226, 1934. 118, 187

1107. Escudero Ortuno, A. Aspectos clínicos del insomnio. Médicamenta (Madrid), 7 (No. 119):69-73, 1947. 274

1108. Essler, W. O., and G. E. Folk, Jr. Determination of physiological rhythms of unrestrained animals by radio telemetry. Nature, 190:90-91, 1961. 163

1109. Estabrook, G. H. The psychogalvanic reflex in hypnosis. J. Gen. Psychol., 3:150-57, 1930. 330

1110. Ethelberg, S. Sleep-paralysis or postdormitial chalastic fits in cortical lesions of frontal pole. Acta Psychiat. Neurol. Scand., Suppl. 108:121-30, 1956. 236, 237

1111. Euler, U. S. von, und A. G. Holmquist. Tagesrhythmik der Adre-

nalinsekretion und des Kohlenhy-
dratstoffwechsel beim Kaninchen
und Igel. Pfluegers Arch., 234:
210-24, 1934. 166

1112. Eunson, L. H. Hypnosis. Brit.
Med. J., II:353, 1942.

1113. Euzière, J., T. Passouant-Fontaine, P. Passouant, et H. Latour.
Etude électroencéphalographique
du sommeil spontané et provoqué
par le pentothal au cours de divers états pathologiques. J.
Physiol. (Paris), 41:167A-72A,
1949. 257

1114. Evans, G. Insomnia. St. Barthol.
Hosp. J., 43:55-58, 1935. 294,
312

1115. Evarts, E. V. Spontaneous and
evoked activity of single units in
visual cortex of cat during sleep
and waking. Fed. Proc., 19:290,
1960. 211

1116. _____. Effect of sleep and waking
on spontaneous and evoked discharges of single units in visual
cortex. Fed. Proc., 19:828-37,
1960. 32

1117. _____. Effects of sleep on photically evoked responses in man.
Fed. Proc., 20:332, 1961. 347

1118. _____. Effects of sleep and waking
on activity of single units in the
unrestrained cat. In: A CIBA
Found. Symposium on the Nature
of Sleep, 1961 (4270), pp. 171-82.
212, 213

1119. _____. Activity of neurons in visual cortex of cat during sleep with
low voltage fast EEG activity. Fed.
Proc., 21:351B, 1962. 32, 347

1120. _____, E. Bental, B. Bihari, and
P. R. Huttenlocher. Spontaneous
discharges of single neurons during sleep and waking. Science,
135:726-28, 1962. 32, 347

1121. _____, T. C. Fleming, and P. R.
Huttenlocher. Recovery cycle of
visual cortex of the awake and
sleeping cat. Am. J. Physiol., 199:
373-76, 1960. 212

1122. _____, and H. W. Magoun. Some
characteristics of cortical recruiting responses in unanesthetized cats. Science, 125:1147-48,
1957. 30, 210
Evarts, E. V., co-author: 1209.

1123. Everett, G. M., and J. E. P. Toman. Mode of action of Rauwolfia
alkaloids and motor activity. Biol.
Psychiat., 1:75-81, 1958. 302

1124. Ewen, J. H. Sleep and its relationship to schizophrenia. J. Neurol.

Psychopath., 14:247-51, 1934.
357, 358

1125. Ey, H. Brèves remarques histo-
riques sur les rapports des états
psychopathiques avec le rêve et
les états intermédiaires au sommeil et à la veille. Ann. Méd.-
psychol., 92(II):101-10, 1934.

1126. _____. Théorie de l'identité du
rêve et de la pensée délirante.
J. Psychol. Norm. Path., 40:347-
68, 1947. 106

1127. _____, P. Sivadon, H. Faure, R.
Amiel, et C. Igert. Les paroxysmes oniriques et anxieux au
cours et au décours de la cure
de sommeil. Vers une socialisa-
tion de la cure. Evolut. Psychiat.,
No. 4:753-68, 1954. 206

1128. Eysenck, H. J. Suggestibility and
hypnosis—an experimental analysis. Proc. Roy. Soc. Med., 36:
349-54, 1943. 335

1129. Fabing, H. D. Narcolepsy. I.
Combat experience of a soldier
with narcolepsy. Arch. Neurol.
Psychiat., 54:367-71, 1945.

1130. _____. Narcolepsy. II. Theory
of pathogenesis of narcolepsy-
cataplexy syndrome. Arch. Neurol. Psychiat., 55:353-63, 1946.
240

1131. Fabricant, N. D. Snoring. Practitioner, 187:378-80, 1961; also
J. Am. Med. Ass., 175:265, 1961.
50

1132. Façon, E., M. Steriade, et N.
Wertheim. Hypersomnie prolongée engendrée par des lésions bi-
latérales du système activateur
médial. Le syndrome thrombo-
tique de la bifurcation du tronc
basilaire. Rev. Neurol., 98:117-
33, 1958. 267

1133. Fagan, A. P. Insomnia as an early sign of brain abscess. Irish J.
Med. Sci., 6th Ser., pp. 712-13,
1945. 276

1134. Failla, E. Studio elettrocortico-
grafico nel coniglio sull'effetto
dei barbiturici, di alcune sostanze
psicotrope e dell'acetilcolina. Acta Neurol. (Napoli), 13:813-40,
1958. 209, 303, 304

1135. Falcon-Lesses, M., and S. H.
Proger. Psychogenic fever. New
Engl. J. Med., 203:1034-36, 1930.
145

1136. Faltz, P., C. Kayser, et J. Rouil-
lard. Sommeil et hydrémie. C. R.
Soc. Biol., 140:301-3, 1946. 204

1137. Fantus, B. Therapy of insomnia:

Cook County Hospital. J. Am. Med. Ass., 102:1846-48, 1934. 294

1138. Farber, L. H., and C. Fisher. An experimental approach to dream psychology through the use of hypnosis. Psychoanal. Q., 12:202-15, 1943. 335

1139. Farmer, E., and E. G. Chambers. Concerning the use of the psychogalvanic reflex in psychological experiments. Brit. J. Psychol., 15:237-54, 1925. 19, 158

1140. Farrow, E. P. A psychoanalytical method of getting to sleep. J. Neurol. Psychopath., 6:123-25, 1925. 312

1141. Fasanaro, G., e S. Piro. Studio biologico di un caso di narcolessia. Trattamento efficace con acido glutamico. Acta Neurol. (Napoli), 8:1071-82, 1953. 239, 240

1142. Fau, R. Etude E.E.G. des degrés de la vigilance au cours d'un coma traumatique très prolongé. Rev. Neurol., 94:818-23, 1956. 262, 267, 272

1143. Faure, J. Au sujet de l'activité de la base du cerveau au cours du sommeil normal et pathologique (dérivation basale). Rev. Neurol., 80:619-21, 1948. 238, 239
Faure, J., co-author: 893.

1144. Favale, E., A. Giussani, e G. F. Rossi. Induzione del sonno profondo nel gatto mediante stimolazione elettrica della sostanza reticolare del tronco encefalico. Boll. Soc. Ital. Biol. Sper., 37: 265-66, 1961. 204

1145. ———, C. Loeb, G. F. Rossi, and G. Sacco. EEG synchronization and behavioral signs of sleep following low frequency stimulation of the brain stem reticular formation. Arch. Ital. Biol., 99:1-22, 1961. 204
Favale, E., co-author: 1624-26, 3425.

1146. Fawcett, D. W., and C. P. Lyman. The effect of low environmental temperature on the composition of depot fat in relation to hibernation. J. Physiol. (London), 126: 235-47, 1954. 327

1147. Febel, F. Sleep. J. School Health, 22:172-78, 1952.

1148. Fedor, E. J., B. Fisher, and S. H. Lee. Rewarming following hypothermia of two to twelve hours. I. Cardiovascular effects. Ann. Surg., 147:515-30, 1958. 327

Fedor, E. J., co-author: 1189, 1198.

1149. Feinschmidt, O., und D. Ferdmann. Beitraege zur Biochemie des Winterschlafs. Ueber die chemischen Bestandteile des Gehirns [und des Blutes] winterschlafhaltender Tiere. Biochem. Z., 248:101-14, 1932. 322, 323, 324
Feinschmidt, O., co-author: 1154

1150. Feldman, G. Z. (Russ.) The influence of sleep deprivation on the electrical activity and other indicators of cerebral activity of animals. Fiziol. Zh. SSSR, 47: 169-77, 1961. 219

1151. Feldner, A. Zwerchfelltonus und Schlafstoerung. Wien. klin. Wschr., 46:1076-77, 1933. 11

1152. Fenichel, M. Electro-sleep in a chronic disturbed service. Dis. Nerv. Syst., 19 Monogr. Suppl., 1958, pp. 84-86. 299

1153. Fenichel, O. Symposium on neurotic disturbances of sleep. Internat. J. Psycho-anal., 23:49, 62-64, 1942. 286

1154. Ferdmann, D., und O. Feinschmidt. Der Winterschlaf. Ergebn. Biol., 8:1-74, 1932.
Ferdmann, D., co-author: 1149.

1155. Féré, C. De la fréquence des accès d'épilepsie suivant les heures. C. R. Soc. Biol., 40:740-42, 1888. 260

1156. Ferguson, D. J., M. B. Visscher, F. Halberg, and L. M. Levy. Effects of hypophysectomy on daily temperature variation in C_3H mice. Am. J. Physiol., 190:235-38, 1957. 172

1157. Fernberger, S. W. Unlearned behavior of the albino rat. Am. J. Psychol., 41:343-44, 1929. 10

1158. Ferrero, R. Electroencephalography in senile depression. Proc Fourth Internat. Congr. EEG Clin. Neurophysiol., Brussels, 1957. New York: Pergamon Press, 1959, p. 478. 28

1159. Ferriere, A. Psychologic types revealed by dreams. New Era (An Internat. Rev. New Educ.), 6:88-90, 1925. 102

1160. Ferrio, C. La localizzazione dei processi di coscienza. Arch. Psicol. Neurol. (Milano), 13:488-508, 1952. 31

1161. Fessard, A. E. Mechanisms of nervous integration and conscious experience. In: Brain Mechanisms and Consciousness, 1954 (875), pp. 200-236. 30 Fessard, A., co-author: 405.

1162. Feuchtinger, O. Dienzephal-hypophysaere Krankheitsbilder. Schlafsucht als dienzephal-hypophysaeres Symptom. (Bemerkungen zu dem Aufsatz von Dell'Acqua: "Klinische Beobachtungen zur Pathologie des Hypophysenzwischenhirnsystems." I. "Koma pituitarum.") Med. Klin., 39:709-10, 1943. 269

1163. Feudell, P. Physiologie und Pathologie des Schlafes. Arch. phys. Therap. (Leipzig), 9:1-9, 1957.

1164. Filimonov, I. N. (Russ.) On the nature and origin of sleep and sleeplike states. Arch. Klin. Eksp. Med., (7/8):15-31, 1923; abstr. Zbl. ges. Neurol. Psychiat., 39:198-99, 1924-25. 362

1165. Filippini, A. L'autista che si addormenta al volante. Policlinico (Sez. Prat.), 46:1396-97, 1939. 315

1166. Filliozat, J. Le sommeil et les rêves selon les médicins indiens et les physiologistes grecs. J. Psychol. Norm. Path., 40:326-46, 1947. 99

1167. Finckh, J. Die nervoese Schlaflosigkeit und ihre Behandlung. Muenchen: Aerztl. Rundschau, 1933. Pp. 50. 274

1168. ———. Die nervoese Schlaflosigkeit. Leipzig: Aerztl. Verlag, 1941. Pp. 46. 278

1169. Finesinger, J. E., M. A. B. Brazier, J. H. Tucci, and H. H. W. Miles. A study of levels of consciousness based on electroencephalographic data in pentothal anesthesia. Trans. Am. Neurol. Ass., 72:183-85, 1947. 297 Finesinger, J. E., co-author: 468, 3991.

1170. Fink, B. R. The stimulant effect of wakefulness on respiration: clinical aspécts. Brit. J. Anaesth., 33:97-101, 1961. 52

1171. ———. Influence of cerebral activity in wakefulness on regulation of respiration. J. Appl. Physiol., 16:15-20, 1961. 52

1172. Finley, C. S. Endocrine stimulation as affecting dream content. Arch. Neurol. Psychiat., 5:177-81, 1921. 105

1173. Finnie, W. J. Sleep. Med. World (London), 80:132-37, 1954.

1174. Fisch, A. Beitrag zur Behandlung der Schlaflosigkeit mit Pas siflorin. Wien. med. Wschr., 82:162-63, 1932. 294

1175. Fischer, H. Die Rolle des Calciums beim Zustandekommen von Narkose und Erregungszustaenden am rindenlosen und am voellig dezerebrierten Tier. Arch. exp. Path. Pharmakol., 138:169-89, 1928. 35 Fischer, H., co-author: 722, 723.

1176. Fischer, S. Zur Klinik und Physiopathologie der Narkolepsie. Muenchen: Inaug. Diss., 1953. Pp. 88.

1177. Fischer-Defoy, W. Schlafen und Traeumen. Stuttgart: Frank'sche Verlagshandlung, 1918. 8th ed. Pp. 91. 99

1178. Fischgold, H. La conscience et ses modifications. Système de références en E.E.G. clinique. First Internat. Congr. Neurol. Sci., Seconde Journée Commune. Brussels: Acta Med. Belg., 1957, pp. 181-213.

1179. ———, et F. Berthault. Electroencéphalographie de l'épilepsie du nouveau-né et du nourrisson. Etudes Néonatales, 2(2):59-79, 1953. 257

1180. ———, G. Capdevielle, et S. Scarpalezos. Le sommeil comme activateur de l'E.E.G. dans l'épilepsie de l'enfant. Sem. Hôp. Paris, 26:2638-41, 1950. 257

1181. ———, et G. C. Lairy-Bounes. Réaction d'arrêt et d'éveil dans les lésions du tronc cérébral et des hémisphères. Rev. Neurol., 87:603-4, 1952. 211

1182. ———, et P. Mathis. Obnubilations comas et stupeurs. Etudes électroencéphalographiques. EEG Clin. Neurophysiol. Suppl. 11:1-125, 1959.

1183. ———, and B. A. Schwartz. A clinical, electroencephalographic and polygraphic study of sleep in the human adult. In: A CIBA Found. Symposium on the Nature of Sleep, 1961 (4270), pp. 209-31.

1184. ———, et ———. Problèmes du sommeil de nuit en neurochirurgie. Excerp. Med., Internat. Congr. Ser. No. 37, 1961, pp. 48-49

1185. ———, ———, et C. Dreyfus-Brisac. Indicateur de l'état de présence et tracés électroencéphalographiques dans le sommeil nembutalique. EEG Clin. Neurophysiol., 11:23-33, 1959. 30, 296

1186. ____, H. Torrubia, P. Mathis, et G. Arfel-Capdevielle. Réactions E.E.G. d'éveil (arousal) dans le coma. Presse Méd., 63:1231-33, 1955. 30
Fischgold, H., co-author: 123, 259, 260, 1686, 2348, 2712, 3247, 3622, 3623, 3755, 3874.

1187. Fischle-Carl, H. Ein Beitrag zur Kasuistik Schlafgestoerter Kinder. Prax. Kinderpsychol. Kinderpsychiat., 4:37-40, 1955. 286

1188. Fishbein, M. Sleep, blessed sleep. Postgrad. Med. (Minneapolis), 10: 257, 1951.

1189. Fisher, B., C. Russ, E. Fedor, R. Wilde, R. Engstrom, J. Happel, and P. Prendergast. Experimental evaluation of prolonged hypothermia. Arch. Surg., 71:431-48, 1955. 327
Fisher, B., co-author: 1148, 1198.

1190. Fisher, C. Hypnosis in treatment of neuroses due to war and to other causes. War Med. (Chicago), 4: 565-76, 1943. 335

1191. ____. Studies on the nature of suggestion. I. Experimental induction of dreams by direct suggestion. J. Am. Psychoanal. Ass., 1: 222-55, 1953.

1192. ____. Studies on the nature of suggestion. II. The transference meaning of giving suggestions. J. Am. Psychoanal. Ass., 1:406-37, 1953. 104

1193. ____. Dreams and perceptions: the role of preconscious and primary modes of perception in dream formation. J. Am. Psychoanal. Ass., 2:389-445, 1954. 104

1194. ____. Dreams, images, and perception. A study of unconscious-preconscious relationships. J. Am. Psychoanal. Ass., 4:5-48, 1956. 104

1195. ____. A study of the preliminary stages of the construction of dreams and images. J. Am. Psychoanal. Ass., 5:5-60, 1957. 104

1196. ____. Subliminal and supraliminal influences on dreams. Am. J. Psychiat., 116:1009-17, 1960. 104

1197. ____, and I. H. Paul. The effect of subliminal visual stimulation on images and dreams: a validation study. J. Am. Psychoanal. Ass., 7:35-83, 1959.
Fisher, C., co-author: 1138.

1198. Fisher, E. R., E. J. Fedor, and B. Fisher. Pathologic and histochemical observations in experimental hypothermia. Arch. Surg., 75: 817-27, 1957. 327

1199. Fisher, K. C. Narcosis. Canad. Med. Ass. J., 47:414-21, 1942.
Fisher, K. C., co-author: 3149.

1200. Fisher, V. E. Hypnotic suggestion and the conditioned reflex. J. Exp. Psychol., 15:212-17, 1932. 332

1201. Fiske, C. H. Inorganic phosphate and acid excretion in post-absorptive period. J. Biol. Chem., 49:171-81, 1921. 66, 167

1202. Fleeson, W., B. C. Glueck, Jr., and F. Halberg. Persistence of daily rhythms in eosinophil count and rectal temperature during "regression" induced by intensive electroshock therapy. Physiologist, 1:28, 1957.

1203. Fleisch, A. Erregbarkeitsaenderung des Atmungszentrums durch Schlaf. Pfluegers Arch., 221:378-85, 1929. 52, 123

1204. Fleischmann, B. [and others], Schlaf und Winterschlaf. Wien. med. Wschr., 87:904-6, 1937.

1205. Fleischmann, W. Physiologie des Winterschlafs. Biol. Gen. (Wien), 7:621-30, 1931.

1206. ____. Leukopenie waehrend des Winterschlafs. Pfluegers Arch., 234:489-91, 1934. 323

1207. ____. Ueber den Winterschlaf. Wien. med. Wschr., II:904, 1937. 325
Fleischmann, W., co-author: 942.

1208. Fleming, A. Note on the induction of sleep and anaesthesia by compression of the carotids. Brit. For. Med.-Surg. Rev., 15:529-30, 1855. 241

1209. Fleming, T. C., P. R. Huttenlocher, and E. V. Evarts. Effect of sleep and arousal on the cortical response to lateral geniculate stimulation. Fed. Proc., 18: 46, 1959. 347
Fleming, T. C., co-author: 1121.

1210. Flemming, B. M. A study of the sleep of young children. J. Am. Ass. Univ. Women, 19:25-27, 1925. 115, 117, 307

1211. Fletcher, H. M. Diurnal somnolence and nocturnal wakefulness as manifestations of lethargic encephalitis. Brit. J. Child. Dis., 18:69-75, 1921. 247

1212. Flink, E. B., and R. P. Doe. Effect of sudden time displacement by air travel on synchronization of adrenal function. Proc. Soc. Exp. Biol. Med., 100:498-501, 1959. 174

1213. _____, and F. Halberg. Clinical studies on eosinophil rhythm. J. Clin. Endocrinol., 12:922, 1952. 169
Flink, E. B., co-author: 955, 1590, 1601.

1214. Fluck, P. H. So you can't sleep? Today's Health, 28:34-35, 1950. 312

1215. Foà, C. Sonno, ipersonno e insonnia. Rassegna Med., (3):109-21, 1932.

1216. Fodor, N. Motives of insomnia. J. Clin. Psychopath., 7:395-406, 1945. 275

1217. _____. The negative in dreams. Psychoanal. Q., 14:516-27, 1945. 106

1218. Foerster, O., H. Altenburger, und F. W. Kroll. Ueber die Beziehungen des vegetativen Nervensystems zur Sensibilitaet. Z. ges. Neurol. Psychiat., 121:139-85, 1929.

1219. Fog, M. Two cases of brain-stem lesions. A preliminary report. Acta Neurol. Psychiat. Scand., Suppl. 108:131-34, 1956. 209

1220. Fog. T. (Swed.) Modern viewpoints on functions of consciousness; a brief review of neuro-physiological and neuro-anatomical viewpoints on the basis of newer literature. Ugeskr. Laeger, 118: 915-23, 1956.

1221. Fois, A. The Electroencephalogram of the Normal Child. Springfield, Ill.: Thomas, 1961. Pp. xvi + 124. 28, 76

1222. _____, E. L. Gibbs, and F. A. Gibbs. "Flat" electroencephalograms in physiological decortication and hemispherectomy (recordings awake and asleep). EEG Clin. Neurophysiol., 7:130-34, 1955. 29

1223. _____, _____, and _____. Bilaterally independent sleep patterns in hydrocephalus. A.M.A. Arch. Neurol. Psychiat., 79:264-68, 1958. 29

1224. _____, and C. M. Rosenberg. The electroencephalogram in microcephaly. Neurology, 7:703-4, 1957.

1225. Folk, G. E., Jr. The effect of restricted feeding time on the diurnal rhythm of running activity in the white rat. Anat. Rec., 120:786-87, 1954. 173

1226. _____. Twenty-four hour rhythms of mammals in a cold environment. Am. Naturalist, 91:153-66, 1957.

1227. _____. Modification by light of 24-hour activity of white rats. Proc. Iowa Acad. Sci., 66:399-406, 1959. 172, 173

1228. _____. Modification by light and feeding of the 24-hour rhythm of activity in rodents. In: Rep. 5th Conf., Soc. Biol. Rhythm, 1961 (3747), p. 80. 172, 173

1229. _____, and R. R. Schellinger. The diurnal rhythm of body temperature in the hamster. Anat. Rec., 120:787, 1954. 138
Folk, G. E., Jr., co-author: 1108, 3945.

1230. Fomin, S. V. (Ukrain.) The ascorbic acid content of the Glis-Glis brain during hibernation. Ukrain.-Biochem. Z., 9:879-95, 1936. 324

1231. Fontaine, M. De l'hibernation naturelle à "l'hibernation expérimentale." Rev. Path. Gén. Comp., 53:53-64, 1953.

1232. Fontès, G., et A. Yovanovitch. Influence du sommeil sur l'élimination des principaux composés azotés. C. R. Soc. Biol., 88: 456-58, 1923. 65, 167

1233. _____, et _____. Influence de la lumière sur le métabolisme azoté. C. R. Soc. Biol., 93:269-70, 1925. 65

1234. Forbes, A. Dream scintillations. Psychosom. Med., 11:160-62, 1949. 100

1235. Forbes, A., and B. R. Morison. Cortical response to sensory stimulation under deep barbital narcosis. J. Neurophysiol., 2: 112-28, 1939. 297

1236. _____, and L. H. Ray. The conditions of survival of mammalian nerve trunks. Am. J. Physiol., 64:435-66, 1923. 327
Forbes, A., co-author: 917.

1237. Forbes, H. S., and H. G. Wolff. Cerebral circulation. Arch. Neurol. Psychiat., 19:1057-86, 1928. 47

1238. Forbes, T. W. Studies of catatonia. II. Central control of cerea flexibilitas. Psychiat. Q., 8:538-45, 1934. 252, 287

1239. _____, and Z. A. Piotrowski. Studies of catatonia. IV. Electrical skin resistance of catatonics during sleep. Psychiat. Q., 8:722-

26, 1934. 19, 252
Forbes, T. W., co-author: 996, 3931.

1240. Ford, F. R., and W. Muncie. Malignant tumor within the third ventricle. Arch. Neurol. Psychiat., 39:82-95, 1938. 264

1241. Ford, W. L., and C. L. Yeager. Changes in the electroencephalogram in subjects under hypnosis. Dis. Nerv. Syst., 9:190-92, 1948. 330, .335

1242. Forsgren, E. 24-Stunden-Variationen der Gallensekretion. Skand. Arch. Physiol., 59:217-25, 1930. 164

1243. _____. Ueber die Beziehungen zwischen Schlaf und Leberfunktion. Skand. Arch. Physiol., 60: 299-310, 1930. 200, 362

1244. _____. 24-Stunden Variationen des Reststickstoffes im Blute. Acta Med. Scand., 73:213-23, 1930. 162

1245. _____. Ueber Leberfunktion, Harnausscheidung und Wasserbelastungsproben. Acta Med. Scand., 76:285-315, 1931. 165

1246. _____. Rhythmicity of liver function and of internal metabolism. Acta Med. Scand. Suppl. 59:95-96, 1934. 54, 165

1247. _____. Ueber die Rhythmik der Leberfunktion, des Stoffwechsels, und des Schlafes. Svenska Läk.-Sällsk. Handl., 61:1-56, 1935. 165, 200

1248. _____. Die Rhythmik der Leberfunktion und des Stoffwechsels. Dsche med. Wschr., 64:743-44, 1938. 165

1249. Fortier, C. Dual control of adrenocorticotropin release. Endocrinology, 49:782-88, 1951. 356

1250. Fortune, R. F. Sleep and muscular work. The effect of sleep on the ability to perform muscular work. Austral. J. Psychol., 4:36-40, 1926. 121

1251. Foster, H. H. The necessity for a new standpoint in sleep theories. Am. J. Psychol., 12:145-77, 1901. 362

1252. Foster, J. C. Hours spent in sleep by young children. Proc. Ninth Internat. Congr. Psychol., 1929, pp. 168-69. 115, 118

1253. _____, F. L. Goodenough, and J. E. Anderson. The sleep of young children. J. Genet. Psychol., 35: 201-18, 1928. 118, 307

1254. Foulkes, W. D. Dream reports from different stages of sleep.

Ph.D. Diss., Univ. of Chicago, 1960; also J. Abnorm. Soc. Psychol., 65:14-25, 1962. 98, 99

1255. Fox, B. H., and J. S. Robbins. The retention of material presented during sleep. J. Exp. Psychol., 43:75-79, 1952. 125

1256. Fox, H. M., and S. Gifford. Psychological responses to ACTH and cortisone. A preliminary theoretical formulation. Psychosom. Med., 15:614-27, 1953. 303
Fox, H. M., co-author: 1771.

1257. Français, H., et L. Vernier. Etude anatomo-clinique d'un cas de tumeur du IIIe ventricule cérébral. Rev. Neurol., 35:921-25, 1919. 263

1258. Francioni, C. Sindromi mesencefaliche con manifestazioni di sonno patologico. Riv. Clin. Pediat., 15:505-49, 1917. 263

1259. Franck, B. J. L'hypnose et l'EEG. EEG Clin. Neurophysiol., 2:107, 1950. 330

1260. François, M. Contribution à l'étude du sens du temps. La température interne comme facteur de variation de l'appréciation subjective des durées. Année Psychol., 28:186-204, 1928. 158

1261. _____. Influence de la température interne sur notre appréciation du temps. C. R. Soc. Biol., 98:201-3, 1928. 158

1262. Franek, B., und R. Thren. Hirnelektrische Befunde bei gestuften aktiven Hypnoseuebungen. Arch. Psychiat. Nervenkr., 181: 360-69, 1948. 330

1263. Frank, C. Intorno alla mia scoperta di due nuclei di mesencefalo dell'uomo ed ulteriori studi sui nuclei oculomotori dei mammiferi. Arch. Gen. Neurol. Psichiat. Psicoanal., 11:1-40, 1930. 361

1264. Frank, G., R. Harner, J. Matthews, E. Johnson, and F. Halberg. Circadian periodicity and the human electroencephalogram. EEG. Clin. Neurophysiol., 13:822, 1961. 170

1265. Franklin, J. C., B. C. Schiele, J. Brozek, and A. Keys. Observations on human behavior in experimental starvation and rehabilitation. J. Clin. Psychol., 4: 28-45, 1948. 104

1266. Fraser, R., and B. E. Nordin. The basal metabolic rate during sleep. Lancet, I:532-33, 1955. 55

1267. Fraser-Harris, D. F. Sleep. Forum, 79:744-53, 881-90, 1928. 312, 361

1268. Frazier, C. H. Tumor involving the frontal lobe alone. Arch. Neurol. Psychiat., 35:525-71, 1936. 265

1269. Frederick, W. S. Physiological aspects of human fatigue. A.M.A. Arch. Indust. Health, 20:297-302, 1959. 225

1270. Freed, S. C. Study of a new sedative-hypnotic drug (3,3-diethyl-2, 4-dioxotetrahydropyridine). J. Lab. Clin. Med., 32:895-900, 1947. 294

1271. Freeman, G. L. Compensatory reinforcements of muscular tension subsequent to sleep loss. J. Exp. Psychol., 15:267-83, 1932. 228

1272. _____. Diurnal variations in performance and energy expenditure. Chicago: Northwestern Univ. Press, 1935. Pp. 27. 56, 228

1273. _____, and C. W. Darrow. Insensible perspiration and the galvanic skin reflex. Am. J. Physiol., 111:55-63, 1935. 19

1274. _____, and C. I. Hovland. Diurnal variations in performance and related physiological processes. Psychol. Bull., 31:777-99, 1934. 150, 161

1275. Freeman, W. Pathologic sleep. J. Am. Med. Ass., 91:67-70, 1928. 262, 344, 359, 362

1276. Freistadt, K. Zur Pharmakotherapie der Schlafstoerungen. Med. Klin., 26:1709-10, 1930. 294, 295

1277. French, J. D. Brain lesions associated with prolonged unconsciousness. A.M.A. Arch. Neurol. Psychiat., 68:727-40, 1952. 273

1278. _____. Some contributions of the physiological laboratory to problems of consciousness. First Internat. Congr. Neurol. Sci., Seconde Journée Commune. Brussels: Acta Med. Belg., 1957, pp. 97-109.

1279. _____. The reticular formation. Sci. Am., 196(5):54-60, 1957. 209

1280. _____, F. K. von Amerongen, and H. W. Magoun. An activating system in brain stem of monkey. A.M.A. Arch. Neurol. Psychiat., 68:577-90, 1952. 209

1281. _____, R. Hernández-Peón, and R. B. Livingston. Projections from cortex to cephalic brain stem (reticular formation) in monkey. J. Neurophysiol., 18:74-95, 1955. 209

1282. _____, and E. E. King. Mechanisms involved in the anesthetic state. Surgery, 38:228-38, 1955. 209, 297

1283. _____, R. B. Livingston, and R. Hernández-Peón. Cortical influences upon the arousal mechanism. Trans. Am. Neurol. Ass., 78:57-59, 1953. 209, 211

1284. _____, and H. W. Magoun. Effects of chronic lesions in central cephalic brain stem of monkeys. A.M.A. Arch. Neurol. Psychiat., 68:591-604, 1952. 209, 273

1285. _____, M. Verzeano, and H. W. Magoun. Contrasting features of corticopetal conduction in direct and indirect sensory systems. Trans. Am. Neurol. Ass., 77:44-47, 1952. 209

1286. _____, _____, and _____. An extralemniscal sensory system in the brain. A.M.A. Arch. Neurol. Psychiat., 69:505-18, 1953. 210

1287. _____, _____, and _____. A neural basis for the anesthetic state. A.M.A. Arch. Neurol. Psychiat., 69:519-29, 1953. 297, 298 French, J. D., co-author: 2542, 3646, 4187.

1288. French, T. M. The Integration of Behavior. II. The Integrative Process in Dreams. Chicago: Univ. of Chicago Press, 1954. Pp. xi + 367. 103

1289. Freud, S. Dream Psychology—Psychoanalysis for Beginners. New York: J. A. McCann Co., 1920. Pp. 237. 103, 106

1290. Fridman-Pogosova, A. V. (Russ.) Effect of medicinally induced sleep on protein metabolism of various organs and tissues. Doklady Akad. Nauk SSSR, 102:1227-29, 1955. 297

1291. Friede, R. Ueber zentral-humorale Schlafsteuerung. Acta Neuroveget. (Wien), 2:270-83, 1951. 353

1292. Friedemann, A. Klinische Studien ueber Schlaf und Schlafmittel. Dsche med. Wschr., 55:91-94, 1929. 360

1293. Friedenwald, J. On the influence of rest, exercise and sleep on gastric digestion. Am. Med., 1: 249-55, 1906. 54

1294. _____. Discussion on sleep. South. Med. J., 16:661-62, 1923.

1295. Friedlander, J. W., and T. R. Sar-

bin. The depth of hypnosis. J. Abnorm. Soc. Psychol., 33:453-75,
1938. 335

1296. Friedlander, W. J. Alterations of
basal ganglion tremor during
sleep. Neurology, 2:222-25, 1952.
13

1297. _____, and E. Rottger. The effect
of cortisone on the electroencephalogram. EEG Clin. Neurophysiol.,
3:311-13, 1951. 303

1298. Friedman, M. Hyperthermia as a
manifestation of stress. Res.
Publ. Ass. Nerv. Ment. Dis., 29:
433-44, 1950.

1299. Friedman, M. F. H., and J. C.
Armour. Gastric secretion in the
groundhog (Marmota monax) during hibernation. J. Cell. Comp.
Physiol., 8:201-11, 1936. 324

1300. Friedmann, K. Zur Therapie der
Schlafstoerungen. Wien. med.
Wschr., 84:697-99, 1934. 294

1301. Frobenius, K. Ueber die zeitliche
Orientierung im Schlaf und einige
Aufwachphaenomene. Z. Psychol.,
103:100-110, 1927. 126

1302. _____. Die Bedeutung von Schlaf-
versuchen fuer die Theorie des
Zeitbewusstseins. Arch. Psychiat.,
86:314, 1929. 126

1303. Fröderberg, H. (Swed.) A case of
narcolepsy with cataplexy. Hygiea
(Stockholm), 92:788-97, 1930. 267

1304. Froeschels, E. A peculiar intermediary state between waking and
sleep. J. Clin. Psychopath. Psychotherap., 7:825-33, 1946. 79

1305. _____. A peculiar intermediary
state between waking and sleeping.
Am. J. Psychotherap., 3:19-25,
1949. 79

1306. Froment, J., et A. Chaix. Tonus
statique et sommeil. Rev. Neurol.,
I:874-77, 1927. 12, 249

1307. Frommel, E. Recherches dans le
domaine du sommeil et de la thérapeutique de l'insomnie. Rev.
Méd. Suisse Rom., 67:799, 1947.

1308. _____. Le problème de la potentialisation des barbituriques par
un vagotonique. (Recherches sur
les synergies médicamenteuses
utiles et la physiologie du sommeil). Praxis, 38:675-77, 1949.
303

1309. _____, und I. T. Beck. Beitrag zur
Pathophysiologie der Schlaflosig-
keit beim Menschen, gewonnen an
Hand der "paradoxen" Wirkung
von Belladonna. Wien. med.
Wschr., 99:507-8, 1949. 278

1310. _____, _____, M. Favre, et F.
Vallette. Études dans le domaine
du sommeil. IV. Le taux de la
cholinestérase sérique de la
poule à l'état de veille et au
cours du sommeil physiologique.
Helvet. Physiol. Pharmacol.
Acta, 5:361-63, 1947. 35

1311. _____, A. Bischler, P. Gold, M.
Favre, et F. Vallette. Recherches dans le domaine du sommeil; I. De la potentialisation
de l'action des barbituriques
par la médication anticholines-
térasique. Helvet. Physiol. Pharmacol. Acta, 5:64-77, 1947. 303

1312. _____, _____, _____, _____, et
_____. Recherches dans le do-
maine du sommeil; II. De la potentialisation de l'action des barbituriques par la médication va-
gale (sels de choline, pilocarpine),
et accessoirement l'action de la
morphine et de la scopolamine
sur le sommeil dû aux malonylu-
rées. Helvet. Physiol. Pharmacol. Acta, 5:78-84, 1947. 303

1313. _____, M. Favre, et F. Vallette.
Recherches dans le domaine du
sommeil; III. Sympathicomimé-
tiques, sympathicolytiques, va-
golytiques et sommeil barbiturique. Helvet. Physiol. Pharmaco-
col. Acta, 5:85-90, 1947. 303

1314. _____, et C. Radouco-Thomas.
De la sensibilité des centres nerveux à la cholinergie. Centres du
sommeil. Arch. Internat. Pharmacodyn., 104:462-68, 1956. 303

1315. Frost, E. P. The characteristic
form assumed by dreams. Am.
J. Psychol., 24:410-13, 1913.
101

1316. _____. Dreams. Psychol. Bull.,
12:22-25, 1915; 15:12-15, 1918.
99

1317. Frumusan, P., et R. Gattan. Réflexions à propos de sept cas de
cure de sommeil dans la maladie
ulcérique. In: La Cure de Sommeil, 1954 (3021), pp. 190-202.
207

1318. Fuchs, A., and F. C. Wu. Sleep
with half-open eyes (physiological lagophthalmus). Am. J. Ophthal., 31:717-20, 1948. 11

1319. Fujisawa, K., and T. Obonai.
(Jap.) The psycho-physiological
studies of hypnotic sleep. Jap.
J. Psychol., 31:94-102, 1960. 337
Fujisawa, K., co-author: 3034.

1320. Fulton, J. F., and P. Bailey. Contribution to the study of tumors in the region of the third ventricle: their diagnosis and relation to pathological sleep. J. Nerv. Ment. Dis., 69:1-25, 145-64, 261-77, 1929. 263, 269

1321. Funderburk, W. H., and T. J. Case. The effect of atropine on cortical potentials. EEG Clin. Neurophysiol., 3:213-23, 1951. 304

1322. _____, and C. C. Pfeiffer. Effect of drugs on brain waves. Mod. Hosp., 75(9):104-10, 1950. 296

1323. Furchgott, E., and W. W. Willingham. The effect of sleep deprivation upon the threshold of taste. Am. J. Psychol., 69:111-12, 1956. 225

1324. Furniss, A. Sleep and its importance. Prescriber, 38:50-52, 1944. 307

1325. Furtado, D., and F. E. P. Valente. A case of narcolepsy with oneiric manifestations. J. Ment. Sci., 90:538-49, 1944. 234

1326. Fuster, B. EEG activation under natural or induced sleep. EEG Clin. Neurophysiol., Suppl. 4: 108-20, 1953. 296

1327. _____, C. Castells, and M. Etcheverry. Epileptic sleep terrors. Neurology, 4:531-40, 1954.

1328. _____, E. L. Gibbs, and F. A. Gibbs. Pentothal sleep as an aid to the diagnosis and localization of seizure discharges of the psychomotor type. Dis. Nerv. Syst., 9:199-202, 1948. 257
Fuster, B., co-author: 1418, 1421, 1426.

1329. Fuster, J. M. Effects of stimulation of brain stem on tachistoscopic perception. Science, 127: 150, 1958.

1330. Futer, D. S. (Russ.) Syndrome of a sleep disturbance with bulimia and polydipsia. Nevropat. Psikhiat., 9(10):68-72, 1940. 267

1331. Gaede. Schlaflosigkeit. Dsche med. Wschr., 67(II):1269-70, 1941. 274

1332. Gahagan, L. Sex differences in recall of stereotyped dreams, sleep-talking and sleep-walking. J. Genet. Psychol., 48:227-36, 1936.

1333. Gaito, J. A neurophysiological approach to thinking. Psychol. Rep., 4:323-32, 1958. 107

1334. Gakkel', L. B. (Russ.) Sleep,

Dreams, and Hypnosis. Leningrad: All-Union Soc. Dissem. Polit. Sci. Inform., 1955. Pp. 26.

1335. Galambos, R. Suppression of auditory nerve activity by stimulation of efferent fibers to cochlea. J. Neurophysiol., 19: 424-37, 1956.

1336. _____, G. Sheatz, and V. C. Vernier. Electrophysiological correlates of a conditioned response in cats. Science, 123:376-77, 1956.

1337. Galamini, A. Sulla curva termica giornaliera del ratto albino. Atti Acad. Naz. Lincei, 6:249-57, 1927. 148, 164

1338. Galant, J. S. Beitrag zur Psychopathologie des Traumlebens. Neopsychiatria, 3:1-6, 1937. 106

1339. _____, und J. Zimmer. Ueber hypnoreaktive und hypersomnische Zustaende bei jugendlichen Psychopathen. Kinderaerztl. Praxis, 6:97-101, 1935.

1340. Galbraith, T. T., and S. Simpson. Conditions influencing the diurnal wave in the temperature of the monkey. J. Physiol. (London), 30:20-22, Proc., 1903-4. 173

1341. Galkin, W. [V.] S. Die Schwankungen der Erregbarkeit der Nervenzelle und der epileptische Anfall. Z. ges. exp. Med., 81: 374-89, 1932.

1342. _____. (Russ.) On the importance of the receptors for the working of the higher divisions of the nervous system. Arkh. Biol. Nauk, 33(1-2): 27-55, 1933; also in: The Sleep Problem, 1954 (392), pp. 122-46.

1343. Gallavardin, M. L. Les malaises du premier sommeil. Lyon Méd., 138:587-95, 1926.

1344. Gallini, R. La cura del sonno nel trattamento dello stato di male asmatico. Sett. Med. (Firenze), 42:582-85, 1954. 207

1345. Galton, E. M. G. Note on the effect of sleep on glaucoma. Brit. J. Ophthal., 33:511-12, 1949.

1346. Gamper, E. Bau und Leistungen eines menschlichen Mittelhirnwesens (Arhinocephalie mit Encephalocele). Zugleich ein Beitrag zur Teratologie und Fasersystematik. Z. ges. Neurol. Psychiat., 102:154-235, 1926.

1347. _____. Bau und Leistungen eines menschlichen Mittelhirnwesens (Arhinocephalie mit Encephalocele). Zugleich ein Beitrag zur Teratologie und Fasersystematik. II. Klinischer Teil. Z. ges. Neurol. Psychiat., 104:49-120, 1926. 23

1348. _____. Schlaf, Delerium tremens, Korsakowsches Syndrom. Arch. Psychiat., 86:294-301, 1928; also Dsche Z. Nervenheilk., 102: 122-29, 1928. 362

1349. Ganado, W. The narcolepsy syndrome. Neurology, 8:487-96, 1958. 234, 235, 236, 282

1350. Gangloff, H. and M. Monnier. Electrographic aspects of an "arousal" or attention reaction induced in the unanesthetized rabbit by the presence of a human being. EEG Clin. Neurophysiol., 8:623-29, 1956. 210

1351. Ganry, C. H. J. La Cure de Sommeil en Psychiatrie. Paris: Thèse de Méd., 1953. Pp. 102. 207

1352. Gans, M. The interrelationship of sleep and migraine. Acta Med. Orient., 2(3):97-104, 1943. 113, 121

1353. _____. Sleep and third circulation; an attempt to solve the problem of sleep. J. Nerv. Ment. Dis., 103:473-83, 1946. 353

1354. _____. Der Schlaf und die dritte Zirkulation. Der Versuch einer Loesung des Schlafproblems. Schweiz. Arch. Neurol. Psychiat., 64:88-100, 1949. 353

1355. _____. I. Migraine as a form of neurasthenia. J. Nerv. Ment. Dis., 113:315-31, 1951.

1356. _____. II. Treating migraine by "sleep-rationing." J. Nerv. Ment. Dis., 113:405-29, 1951. 121

1357. Garattini, S., and V. Ghetti, Eds. Psychotropic Drugs. New York: Elsevier Publ. Co., 1957. Pp. xiv + 606.

1358. Garcia, J. A. Régulation hormonale du sommeil. Ann. Méd. Psychol., 108:452-65, 1950; also in Portug., Resenha Clín. Cient., 19:83-88, 1950. 356

1359. García Flores, J., y S. Madrigal Moreno. Tratamiento antialérgico del insomnio. Sugestiones (Mex.), 11, No. 123:56-61, 1945; also Medicina (Mex.), 25(II):414-18, 1945. 278

1360. Garma, A. The traumatic situation in the genesis of dreams. Internat. J. Psycho-anal., 27: 134-39, 1946. 104

1361. _____. Vicissitudes of the dream screen and the Isakower phenomenon. Psychoanal. Q., 24:369-82, 1955. 101

1362. Gartkiewicz, A. Contributions à la caratéristique du sommeil des lamellibranches. Rythme cardiaque et movements de l'épithélium ciliaire. Arch. Internat. Physiol., 26:229-36, 1926.

1363. Garvey, C. R. An experimental study of the sleep of preschool children. Proc. Ninth Internat. Congr. Psychol., 1929, pp. 176-77. 78, 89, 187

1364. _____. The Activity of Young Children during Sleep. Minneapolis: Univ. Minn. Press, 1939. Pp. x + 102. 89, 91, 112, 364

1365. Gastaut, H. Etude électrocorticographique de la réactivité des rythmes rolandiques. Rev. Neurol., 87:176-82, 1952.

1366. _____. The brain stem and cerebral electrogenesis in relation to consciousness. In: Brain Mechanisms and Consciousness, 1954 (875), pp. 249-83. 209

1367. _____, and J. Bert. Electroencephalographic detection of sleep induced by repetitive sensory stimuli. In: A CIBA Found. Symposium on the Nature of Sleep, 1961 (4270), pp. 260-71. 197

1368. _____, S. Ferrer, C. Castells, N. Lesèvre, et K. Luschnat. Action de la diéthylamide de l'acide d-lysergique (LSD 25) sur les fonctions psychiques et l'électroencéphalogramme. Confin. Neurol. (Basel), 13:102-20, 1953. 303

1369. _____, R. Naquet, R. Vigouroux, A. Roger, et M. Badier. Etude électrographique chez l'homme et chez l'animal des décharges épileptiques dites "psychomotrices." Rev. Neurol., 88:510-54, 1953. 258

1370. _____, A. Roger, et J. Roger. De l'intérêt de l'électroencéphalogramme dans les indications de la cure de sommeil. In: La Cure de Sommeil, 1954 (3021), pp. 37-56. 206

1371. _____, et B. Roth. A propos des manifestations électroencéphalographiques de 150 cas de narcolepsie avec ou sans cataplexie. Rev. Neurol., 97:388-93,

1957. 238, 241
Gastaut, H., co-author: 761,
2887, 2974, 3385, 4293.

1372. Gates, A. I. Diurnal variations
in memory and association.
Univ. Calif. Publ. Psychol., 1:
323-44, 1916. 119, 150, 158

1373. ____. Variations in efficiency
during the day together with
practice effects, sex differences
and correlations. Univ. Calif.
Publ. Psychol., 2:1-156, 1916.
150.

1374. Gaul, L. E. Time-lapse photography: Usefulness for investigation of normal sleeping patterns.
J. Indiana Med. Ass., 51:1675-
77, 1958. 89

1375. Gauthier, C., M. Parma, e A.
Zanchetti. Stimolazione di nuclei talamici a proiezione spe-
cifica e risveglio corticale. Boll.
Soc. Ital. Biol. Sper., 31:462-63,
1955.

1376. ____, ____, and ____. Effect
of electrocortical arousal upon
the development and configura-
tion of specific evoked potentials.
EEG Clin. Neurophysiol., 8:237-
44, 1956.

1377. Gayet. Affection encéphalique
(encéphalite diffuse probable).
Arch. Physiol. Norm. Path., 2ᵉ
Ser., 2:341-51, 1875. 243

1378. Gaylord, C., and H. C. Hodge.
Duration of sleep produced by
pentobarbital sodium in normal
and castrate female rats. Proc.
Soc. Exp. Biol. Med., 55:46-48,
1944.

1379. Geldard, F. A., and H. H. Manchester. Sleep motility in student
pilots. Psychol. Bull., 38:693-94,
1941. 86

1380. Gélineau, [J. B. E.] De la narcolepsie. Lancette Franç., Gaz.
Hôp., 53:626-28, 635-37, 1880.
233, 237

1381. Gelineo, S. Sur la thermogenèse
de l'hibernant lors du passage de
l'état de veille à l'état de torpeur.
C. R. Soc. Biol., 127:1360-61,
1938. 321

1382. Geller, I. M., and A. V. Chapek.
(Russ.) Portable device for the
study of human sleep by actography. Gig. Sanit. (Moskva),
21(2):60-61, 1956.

1383. Gellhorn, E. Experimental contribution to the duplicity theory
of consciousness and perception.
Pfluegers Arch., 255:75-92, 1952.

1384. ____. The hypothalamic-corti-
cal system in barbiturate anesthesia. Arch. Internat. Pharmacodyn., 93:434-42, 1953. 298

1385. ____. Physiological Foundations
of Neurology and Psychiatry.
Minneapolis: Univ. Minn. Press,
1953. Pp. xiii + 556. 241

1386. ____. Physiological processes
related to consciousness and perception. Brain, 77:401-15, 1954.
31

1387. ____. The physiological basis
of neuromuscular relaxation.
Arch. Int. Med., 102:392-99,
1958.

1388. ____. Prolegomena to a theory
of emotion. Perspect. Biol. Med.,
4:403-36, 1961.

1389. ____, and H. M. Ballin. Water
intoxication and the electroencephalogram. Am. J. Physiol.,
146:559-66, 1946. 259

1390. ____, and M. Bernhaut. Physiology of arousal reaction. Fed.
Proc., 10:48-49, 1951. 209

1391. ____, W. P. Koella, and H. M.
Ballin. Interaction on cerebral
cortex of acoustic or optic with
nociceptive impulses: the problem of consciousness. J. Neurophysiol., 17:14-21, 1954. 31
Gellhorn, E., co-author: 315,
1885, 2952.

1392. Gelma, E., et A. Hanns. Sur le
sommeil et les troubles psychiques dans l'encéphalite léthargique. Ann. Méd., 9:17-21,
1921. 244

1393. Gélyi, D. (Hungar.) On sleep.
Gyógyászat, (1):7-9, 1922; abstr.
Zbl. ges. Neurol. Psychiat., 28:
380, 1922. 356

1394. Genoese, G. Disturbi del sonno
nella malaria dei bambini. Pediatria, 40:965-74, 1932. 267

1395. Gentry, E. F., and C. A. Aldrich.
Rooting reflex in the newborn infant: incidence and effect on it of
sleep. Am. J. Dis. Child., 75:528-
39, 1948. 111

1396. Georgi, F. La thérapeutique des
troubles légers du sommeil: dif-
ficulté à s'endormir et réveil
prématuré à heure fixe. Schweiz.
med. Wschr., 72:1440-42, 1942.

1397. Geppert, T. V. Management of
nocturnal enuresis by conditioned
response. J. Am. Med. Ass., 152:
381-83, 1953. 285

1398. Gerard, M. W. Enuresis. A study
in etiology. Am. J. Orthopsychiat.,

9:48-58, 1939. 285

1399. Gerber, W. Ueber den Schlaf des Menschen und einen in der Praxis verwendbaren Schlafkontrollapparat. Muench. med. Wschr., 69: 1399-1400, 1922. 294

1400. _____. Kann man den Schlaf objectiv beobachten? Selbsttaetige, unbeeinflusste Kranken- und Schlafbeobachtung. Dsche med. Wschr., 79:1785-87, 1954.

1401. _____, und G. Rembold. Untersuchungen ueber die Wirkung einzelner Schlafmittel mit dem Schlafkontrollapparat. Muench. med. Wschr., 70:1386-88, 1923. 295

1402. Gerebtzoff, M. A. Recherches sur la projection corticale du labyrinthe. I. Des effets de la stimulation labyrinthique sur l'activité électrique de l'écorce cérébrale. Arch. Internat. Physiol., 50:59-99, 1940.

1403. _____. Etat fonctionnel de l'écorce cérébrale au cours de l'hypnose animale. Arch. Internat. Physiol., 51:365-78, 1941. 336

1404. Gero, J., and M. Háva. (Czech.) Depth of sleep and unconditioned interoception. Česk. Fysiol., 2: 416-21, 1953.

1405. Gerritzen, F. Liver diuresis. Acta Med. Scand., 89:101-23, 1936. 166

1406. _____. Der 24-Stunden Rhythmus der Chlorausscheidung. Pfluegers Arch., 238:483-88, 1937. 166, 167

1407. _____. Der 24-Stundenrhythmus in der Diurese. Dsche med. Wschr., 64:746-48, 1938. 166

1408. _____. The rhythmic function of the human liver. Acta Med. Scand., Suppl. 108:121-31, 1940. 166

1409. Gerstmann, J., und P. Schilder. Zur Frage der Katalepsie. Med. Klin., 17:193-94, 1921. 249

1410. Gerver, A. B. (Russ.) Pathologic-clinical observations of sleep disorders in diseases of the nervous system. Soviet Nevropat. Psikhiat. Psikhogig., 10:1649-72, 1936.

1411. Gesell, A., and C. Amatruda. The Embryology of Behavior. The Beginnings of the Human Mind. New York: Harper & Bros., 1945. Pp. xix + 289. 114, 115

1412. Gessler, H. Untersuchungen ueber die Waermeregulation. III. Die taeglichen Schwankungen der Koerpertemperatur. Pfluegers Arch., 207:390-95, 1925. 138

1413. Geyer, G., und E. Keibl. Die Pepsinogenausscheidung im Harn und ihre tagesrhythmischen Schwankungen. Wien. med. Wschr., 103:748-52, 1953. 164

1414. Geyer, H. Subcorticale Mechanismen bei schlafenden Zwillingen. Zbl. ges. Neurol. Psychiat., 87: 697, 1938. 17, 308, 359

1415. Ghosh, J. Insomnia and its treatment. Calcutta Med. J., 38:637-44, 1941. 274

1416. Giani. Del sonno e sue varietà. Liguria Med., (1):4-9; (2):33-37, 1922.

1417. Gibb, J. R. The relative effects of sleeping and waking periods on the retention of nonsense syllables. Psychol. Bull., 38:734, 1941. 124

1418. Gibbs, E. L., B. Fuster, and F. A. Gibbs. Peculiar low temporal localization of sleep-induced seizure discharges of psychomotor type. Arch. Neurol. Psychiat., 60:95-97, 1948. 258

1419. _____, and F. A. Gibbs. Diagnostic and localizing value of electroencephalographic studies in sleep. Res. Publ. Ass. Nerv. Ment. Dis., 26:366-76, 1947. 96, 256, 348

1420. _____, and _____. Electroencephalographic changes with age during sleep. EEG Clin. Neurophysiol., 2:355, 1950.

1421. _____, _____, and B. Fuster. Psychomotor epilepsy. Arch. Neurol. Psychiat., 60:331-39, 1948. 258

1422. _____, and F. M. Lorimer. Clinical correlates of exceedingly fast (30-40 per sec.) activity appearing chiefly in drowsiness. EEG Clin. Neurophysiol., 2:226, 1950. 76

Gibbs, E. L., co-author: 11, 776, 1222, 1223, 1328, 1424-29, 2428.

1423. Gibbs, F. A., H. Davis, and W. G. Lennox. The electro-encephalogram in epilepsy and in conditions of impaired consciousness. Arch. Neurol. Psychiat., 34: 1133-48, 1935. 256

1424. _____, and E. L. Gibbs. Routine Seconal sedation; a major aid to clinical electro-encephalography. EEG Clin. Neurophysiol., 1:245,

1949. 296
1425. _____, and _____. Atlas of Elec-troencephalography. I. Methodology and Normal Controls. Cambridge: Addison-Wesley Press, 1950. 2d ed. Pp. 324.

1426. _____, _____, and B. Fuster. Anterior temporal localization of sleep-induced seizure discharge of psychomotor type. Trans. Am. Neurol. Ass., 72:180-82, 1947. 258

1427. _____, _____, and W. G. Lennox. The cerebral blood flow during sleep in man. Brain, 58:44-48, 1935. 47

1428. _____, _____, and _____. Effect on the electroencephalogram of certain drugs which influence nervous activity. Arch. Int. Med., 60:154-66, 1937. 296

1429. _____, _____, and _____. Cerebral dysrhythmias of epilepsy. Arch. Neurol. Psychiat., 39:298-314, 1938. 296

1430. _____, and J. R. Knott. Growth of the electrical activity of the cortex. EEG Clin. Neurophysiol., 1: 223-29, 1949. 27, 28

1431. _____, and G. L. Maltby. Effect on the electrical activity of the cortex of certain depressant and stimulant drugs—barbiturates, morphine, caffeine, benzedrine, and adrenalin. J. Pharmacol. Exp. Therap., 78:1-10, 1943. 296, 299, 300, 303
Gibbs, F. A., co-author:11, 848, 1222, 1223, 1328, 1418-21, 2217, 2428, 2586, 2587.

1432. Gibson, R. B. The effects of transposition of the daily routine on the rhythm of temperature variation. Am. J. Med. Sci., 129: 1048-59, 1905. 173

1433. Giddings, G. Child's sleep—effect of certain foods and beverages on sleep motility. Am. J. Publ. Health, 24:609-14, 1934. 307

1434. _____. Normal sleep pattern for children. J. Am. Med. Ass., 102: 525-29, 1934. 89, 307

1435. _____. The effect of study and physical exercise on your child's sleep. Hygeia, 12:781-83, 1934. 90, 307

1436. _____. A study of child's sleep. South. Med. J., 27:312-18, 1934.

1437. _____. The effect of emotional disturbances on sleep. J. Med. Ass. Georgia, 25:351-57, 1936. 90, 307

1438. _____. Motility of school children during sleep. Am. J. Physiol., 127:480-85, 1939. 89

1439. Gidro-Frank, L., and M. K. Bowersbuch. A study of plantar response in hypnotic age regression. J. Nerv. Ment. Dis., 107: 443-58, 1948. 333
Gidro-Frank, L., co-author: 563.

1440. Gieseking, C. F., H. L. Williams, and A. Lubin. The effect of sleep deprivation upon information learning. Walter Reed Army Inst. Res., Sept. 1957. Pp. 6. 226

1441. _____, _____, and _____. A generalization of Bills' concept of "blocks" to performance lapses in reaction time during sleep loss. Walter Reed Army Inst. Res., Sept. 1958. Pp. 6. 226

1442. Gifford, S. Sleep, time, and the early ego. J. Am. Psychoanal. Ass., 8:5-42, 1960. 134, 366
Gifford, S., co-author: 1256.

1443. Gilbert-Dreyfus et L.-J. Frank. Cure de sommeil dans les troubles de la régulation pondérale. In: La Cure de Sommeil, 1954 (3021), pp. 212-15. 207

1444. Gill, A. W. Idiopathic and traumatic narcolepsy. Lancet, I: 474-76, 1941. 237

1445. Gill, M. M., and M. Brenman. Hypnosis and Allied States. New York: Internat. Univ. Press, 1959. Pp. 405. 336
Gill, M. M., co-author: 495, 825, 826.

1446. Gillespie, R. D. Sleep. Clin. J., 57:289-97, 301-10, 1928. 275, 362

1447. _____. Sleep and the Treatment of Its Disorders. London: Ballière, Tindall & Cox, 1929. Pp. 267. 275, 294, 362

1448. _____. Safeguarding sleep. Lancet, I:26-27, 1941.

1449. Gillon. Les rythmes du travail. Hyg. Ment. (Paris), 46:36-67, 1957. 316, 317

1450. Gilman, L. Insomnia and Its Relation to Dreams. Philadelphia: J. B. Lippincott Co., 1958. Pp. 237. 106, 275, 295

1451. Gilyarovski, V. A., N. M. Liventsev, Yu. E. Segal, and Z. A. Kirillova. (Russ.) Electrosleep; Clinical-Physiological Investigation. Moskva: Medgiz, 1953. Pp. 125. Summary in: The Sleep Problem, 1954 (392), pp. 405-22. 299

1452. Ginzberg, R. Sleep and sleep disturbances in geriatric psychiatry. J. Am. Geriat. Soc., 3:493-511, 1955. 285

1453. Giorgio, A. M. di. Comportamento di alcune reazioni labirintiche durante il sonno fisiologico (ricerche nei bambino). Boll. Soc. Ital. Biol. Sper., 10:951-53, 1935. 16, 358

1454. Gjessing, R. Beitraege zur Kenntnis der Pathophysiologie des katatonen Stupors. I. Ueber periodisch rezidivierenden katatonen Stupor mit kritischem Beginn und Abschluss. II. Ueber aperiodisch rezidivierend verlaufenden katatonen Stupor mit lytischem Beginn und Abschluss. Arch. Psychiat., 96:319-91, 393-473, 1932. 251

1455. ———. Beitraege zur Somatologie der periodischen Katatonie. VIII. Arch. Psychiat. Z. Neurol., 191: 297-326, 1953. 185

1456. Glass, L. B., and T. X. Barber. A note on hypnotic behavior, the definition of the situation and the placebo effect. J. Nerv. Ment. Dis., 132:539-41, 1961. 278, 337

1457. Glass, N. Eating, sleeping, and elimination habits in children attending day nurseries and children cared for at home by mothers. Am. J. Orthopsychiat., 19: 697-711, 1949. 307

1458. Glenn, C. G., and R. Knuth. Incidence of fourteen and six/sec positive spike discharges in routine sleeping EEG's. Dis. Nerv. Syst., 20:340-41, 1959. 29

1459. Gley, E., et C. Richet. Expériences sur la courbe horaire de l'urée et le dosage de l'azote total de l'urine. C. R. Soc. Biol., 39:377-85, 1887. 113

1460. Globus, J. H. Probable topographic relations of the sleep-regulating center. Arch. Neurol. Psychiat., 43:125-38, 1940. 266

1461. Gloning, K., und I. Sternbach. Ueber das Traeumen bei zerebralen Herdlaesionen. Wien. Z. Nervenheilk., 6:302-29, 1953. 103

1462. Gloor, P. Autonomic functions of the diencephalon: A summary of the experimental work of Prof. W. R. Hess. A.M.A. Arch. Neurol. Psychiat., 71:773-90, 1954. 358
Gloor, P., co-author: 1965.

1463. Glotfelty, J. S., and W. P. Wilson. Effects of tranquilizing drugs on reticular system activity in man. A preliminary report. North Carolina Med. J., 17:401-5, 1956. 302

1464. Godard, R. L'insomnie chez l'enfant. Bull. Méd. Paris, 46:183-84, 1932. 278, 294

1465. Gofferjé, F. Die Tagesschwankungen der Koerpertemperatur beim gesunden and beim kranken Saeugling. Jahrb. Kinderheilk., 68:129-90, 1908. 114, 138

1466. Goiffon, R. La narcolepsie digestive. Arch. Malad. Appar. Digestif, 9:95-102, 1916. 235, 237

1467. Gokhblit, I. I. (Russ.) On the electroencephalographic characteristics of the states of wakefulness and sleep in dogs at different ages. Bull. Eksp. Biol. Med., 46(7):30-35, 1958. 27

1468. Goldflam, S. Zur Lehre von den Hautreflexen an den Unterextremitaeten (insbesondere des Babinski'schen Reflexes). Neurol. Cbl., 22:1109-27, 1137-54, 1903. 17

1469. Goldie, L., and J. M. Green. Paradoxical blocking and arousal in the drowsy state. Nature, 187:952-53, 1960. 226, 238, 330, 331

1470. Goldschneider, A. Die nichtmedikamentoese Behandlung der Schlafstoerungen. Z. ges. phys. Therap., 45:247-65, 1933. 294

1471. Goldstein, N. P., and M. E. Giffin. Psychogenic hypersomnia. Am. J. Psychiat., 115:922-28, 1959. 271

1472. Goldwyn, J. The effect of hypnosis on basal metabolism. Arch. Int. Med., 45:109-14, 1930. 329, 330

1473. Gollwitzer-Meier, K., und C. Kroetz. Ueber den Blutchemismus im Schlaf. Biochem. Z., 154:82-89, 1924. 34, 35, 37

1474. Goltz, F. [L.] Der Hund ohne Grosshirn. Pfluegers Arch., 51: 570-614, 1892. 21

1475. Gonzáles Rincones, R. Explicación actual del sueño. Ritmo de Berger de las ondas cerebrales. Estudio de Liberson. Gac. Méd. Caracas, 53:83-89, 1945.

1476. González, J. de Jesús. Investigaciones acerca del estado de los reflejos durante el sueño. Crón. Méd.-Quir. Habana, 45: 285-92, 1919; abstr. J. Am. Med. Ass., 74:285, 1919. 15

1477. Good, T. S. Encephalitis lethargica. J. Ment. Sci., 71:225-35, 1925. 244

1478. Goode, G. B. Sleep paralysis. A.M.A. Arch. Neurol., 6:228-34, 1962. 236

1479. Goodenough, D. R., A. Shapiro, M. Holden, and L. Steinschriber. A comparison of "dreamers" and "nondreamers": eye movements, electroencephalograms, and recall of dreams. J. Abnorm. Soc. Psychol., 59:295-302, 1959. 98, 99
Goodenough, D. R., co-author: 3286.

1480. Goodhill, V., and D. B. Tyler. Experimental insomnia and auditory acuity. Arch. Otolaryngol., 46:221-24, 1947. 225

1481. Gootnik, A. Night cramps and quinine. Arch. Int. Med., 71:555-62, 1943. 285

1482. Gorbatsevitch, A. B. (Russ.) Conditioned-reflex technique for the production of natural and hypnotic sleep. Klin. Med. (Moskva), 33(9):64-65, 1955. 197

1483. Gordon, R. G. The treatment of insomnia and war dreams. Seale Hayne Neurol. Studies, 1:185-93, 1919. 294

1484. _____. The somnambulistic states. Seale Hayne Neurol. Studies, 1:322, 1920. 294

1485. _____. Insomnia. Bristol Med.-Chir. J., 49:147-56, 1932. 275, 294

1486. Gorer, P. A. Physiology of hibernation. Biol. Rev., 5:213-30, 1930.

1487. Goria, C., e B. Bonfante. Terapia dell'inversione del ritmo del sonno. Minerva Med. (Torino), 43:763, 1952. 294

1488. Gorriti, F. Mecanismo de los sueños. Sem. Méd. (Buenos Aires), 103:662-66, 1953. 99

1489. Gorton, B. E. The physiology of hypnosis: A review of the literature, I, II. Psychiat. Q., 23:317-43, 457-85, 1949. 336

1490. Goswell, G. Two cases of narcolepsy. Med. J. Australia, I:272-75, 1947. 238

1491. Gozzano, M., e S. Colombati. Osservazioni elettroencefalografiche in un caso di narcolessia. Riv. Neurol., 18:578-82, 1948. 237, 238

1492. Grabensberger, W. Untersuchungen ueber das Zeitgedaecht-nis der Ameisen und Termiten. Z. vergl. Physiol., 20:1-54, 1933. 175

1493. _____. Experimentelle Untersuchungen ueber das Zeitgedaechtnis von Bienen und Wespen nach Verfuetterung von Euchinin und Jodthyreoglobulin. Z. vergl. Physiol., 20:338-42, 1934. 175

1494. _____. Der Einfluss von Salicylsaeure, gelbem Phosphor und weissem Arsenik auf das Zeitgedaechtnis der Ameisen. Z. vergl. Physiol., 20:501-10, 1934. 175

1495. Graber, G. H. Psychoanalyse und Heilung eines nachtwandelnden Knabens. Zurich: Rascher, 1934. Pp. 67. 283

1496. Grabfield, G. P. Treatment of insomnia. Med. Clin. North Am., 19:1597-1601, 1936. 294

1497. _____, and E. G. Martin. Variations in the sensory threshold for faradic stimulation in normal human subjects. I. The diurnal rhythm. Am. J. Physiol., 31:300-308, 1913. 158

1498. Granda, A. M., and J. T. Hammack. Operant behavior during sleep. Science, 133:1485-86, 1961. 29
Granda, A. M., co-author: 4225.

1499. Grandjean, F. Ein Beitrag zur Behandlung der herzneurotischen Stoerungen und der Schlaflosigkeit Tuberkuloeser. Schweiz. med. Wschr., 65:1004-6, 1935. 294

1500. Grant, F. C., E. B. Spitz, H. A. Shenkin, C. F. Schmidt, and S. S. Kety. Cerebral blood flow and metabolism in idiopathic epilepsy. Trans. Am. Neurol. Ass., 72:82-86, 1947. 257

1501. Grant, W. W. Observations on sleep disturbances in pre-school children. Canad. Med. Ass. J., 77:444-50, 1957. 286

1502. Grassheim, K., und E. Wittkower. Ueber die suggestive Beeinflussbarkeit der spezifisch dynamischen Eiweisswirkung in Hypnose. Dsche med. Wschr., 1:141-43, 1931. 334

1503. Grastyán, E. The hippocampus and higher nervous activity. In: The Central Nervous System and Behavior, M. A. B. Brazier, Ed., Josiah Macy Found., 1959, pp. 119-205. 211, 212

1504. _____, T. Hasznos, K. Lissák,

L. Molnár, and Z. Ruzsonyi. Activation of the brain stem activating system by vegetative afferents. Acta Physiol. Acad. Sci. Hungar., 3:103-22, 1952. 358

1505. _____, and G. Karmos. A study of a possible "dreaming" mechanism in the cat. Acta Physiol. (Hungar.), 20:41-50, 1961. 103
Grastyán, E., co-author: 2082, 2538, 4047.

1506. Graveline, D. E., B. Balke, R. E. McKenzie, and B. Hartman. Psychobiologic effects of water-immersion-induced hypodynamics. Aerospace Med., 32:387-400, 1961. 120
Graveline, D. E., co-author: 2756.

1507. Graves, E. A. The effect of sleep upon retention. J. Exp. Psychol., 19:316-22, 1936. 125

1508. Graybiel, A., and B. Clark. Symptoms resulting from prolonged immersion in water: the problem of zero G asthenia. Aerospace Med., 32:181-96, 1961. 120

1509. _____, _____, and J. J. Zarriello. Observations on human subjects living in a "slow rotation room" for periods of two days. A.M.A. Arch. Neurol., 3:55-73, 1960. 197

1510. Green, E. H. Sleep and sleeplessness. Med. Bull. Vet. Admin., 8:140-45, 1932. 362

1511. Green, J. D., and A. A. Arduini. Hippocampal electrical activity in arousal. J. Neurophysiol., 17: 533-57, 1954. 211

1512. _____, and F. Morin. Hypothalamic electrical activity and hypothalamo-cortical relationships. Am. J. Physiol., 172:175-86, 1953.

1513. Greenblatt, M., and A. S. Rose. Electroencephalographic studies during fever induced by typhoid vaccine and malaria in patients with neurosyphilis. Am. J. Med. Sci., 207:512-19, 1944. 31
Greenblatt, M., co-author: 2517.

1514. Grewel, F. (Dutch) The Kleine-Levin syndrome: sleep periods with hunger. Ned. Tschr. Geneesk., 91:2894-98, 1947. 267

1515. Griffin, D. R., and J. H. Welsh. Activity rhythms in bats under constant external conditions. J. Mammal., 18:337-42, 1937. 172

1516. Griffith, C. R. An experimental study of the nature of sleep among athletes. Proc. Ninth Internat. Congr. Psychol., 1929, pp. 193-94. 87, 312

1517. Griffith, F., G. W. Puchern, K. A. Brownell, J. Klein, and M. Cormer. Studies in human physiology. II. Pulse rate and blood pressure. Am. J. Physiol., 88: 295-311, 1929. 55

1518. Griffiths, G. M., and J. T. Fox. Rhythm in epilepsy. Lancet, 235 (II):409-16, 1938. 260

1519. Grinker, R. R. Problems of consciousness: a review, an analysis, and a proposition. In: Problems of Consciousness, 1953 IV (4), pp. 11-46. 30

1520. _____, and H. Serota. Studies on corticothalamic relations in the cat and man. J. Neurophysiol., 1:573-89, 1938.

1521. Grobon, P. Le sommeil physiologique par l'extrait thalamique. J. Prat. (Paris), 63:631-33, 1949. 278

1522. Groethuysen, U. C., and R. G. Bickford. Study of the lambda-wave response of human beings. EEG Clin. Neurophysiol., 8:344-45, 1956.

1523. Grollman, A. Physiological variations in the cardiac output of man. XI. Pulse rate, blood pressure, oxygen consumption, arterio-venous oxygen difference and cardiac output of man during normal nocturnal sleep. Am. J. Physiol., 95:274-84, 1930. 40, 44, 56, 123

1524. Groos, K. Das Wesen und die Formen der Bewusstheit. Z. Psychol., 149:1-30, 1940.

1525. Grosch, H. Periodische und episodische Schlafzustaende mit endokriner, besonders hypophysaerer Dysfunktion. Allg. Z. Psychiat., 122:155-62, 1943. 269

1526. Gross, A. Sense of time in dreams. Psychoanal. Q., 18:466-70, 1949. 101

1527. Gross, G. K. Disorders of sleep in infancy and childhood. South Afr. Med. J., 6:3-8, 1932. 278

1528. Gross, M. The sleep of elementary school children. Lancet, 202(I):836-38, 1922. 307

1529. Grosscup, E. A. The value of rest and sleep. J. Educ. Sociol., 5:245-49, 1931. 307

1530. Grossman, A. J., R. C. Batterman, and P. Leifer. Comparative testing of daytime sedatives and hypnotic medications. Fed. Proc., 17:373, 1958. 294

1531. Grossman, C. Sensory stimulation during sleep. Observations on the EEG responses to auditory stimulation during sleep in patients with brain pathology (Preliminary Report). EEG Clin. Neurophysiol., 1:256, 487-90, 1949.

1532. _____, L. M. Golub, and J. K. Merlis. Influence of sleep on focal slow wave activity. (Correlation with epileptogenic and non-epileptogenic lesions.) EEG Clin. Neurophysiol., 4:195-200, 1952. 257
Grossman, C., co-author: 1702, 2782, 2783.

1533. Grossman, L. I., and B. M. Brickman. Comparison of diurnal and nocturnal pH values of saliva. J. Dent. Res., 16:179-82, 1937. 53, 163

1534. Grote, F. Zur Behandlung der Schlaflosigkeit. Untersuchungen ueber das neue Schlafmittel Medomin. Schweiz. med. Wschr., 23:1333-35, 1942. 294

1535. Grotjahn, M. Ueber Selbstbeobachtungen beim Erwachen. Z. ges. Neurol. Psychiat., 139:75-96, 1932. 123

1536. _____. Dream observations in a two-year-four-month-old baby. Psychoanal. Q., 7:507-13, 1938. 102

1537. _____. The process of awakening; contribution to ego psychology and the problem of sleep and dream. Psychoanal. Rev., 29:1-19, 1942. 123

1538. _____. Laughter in dreams. Psychoanal. Q., 14:221-27, 1945. 101

1539. Grünberger, F. Beobachtungen ueber das Sprechen aus dem Schlaf. Internat. Z. Individualpsychol., 5:384-88, 1927.

1540. Grueninger, U., and G. Scheurenberg. Studien ueber die Schlafmittelwirkung und Schlafmittelvertraeglichkeit im Kindesalter. III. Der Adalin- und Noctalgehalt des Kaninchensgehirns nach narkotischen Dosen. Z. ges. exp. Med., 107:529-31, 1940. 294

1541. Gruettner, R., und A. Bonkalo. Hirnbioelektrische Untersuchungen ueber die Wirkung des Pervitin und des Coffein bei Ermuedungszustaenden. Psychiat.-neu-

rol. Wschr., 42:243-48, 1940. 299

1542. _____, und _____. Ueber Ermuedung und Schlaf auf Grund hirnbioelektrischer Untersuchungen. Arch. Psychiat. Nervenkr., 111: 652-65, 1940. 26

1543. Gruhle, H. W. Der Schlaf der Altersstufen. Z. Altersforsch., 2:1-14, 1940.

1544. Grunewald, K. Reaction time for light and sound in neurotics with special reference to impaired wakefulness. Acta Psychiat. Neurol. Scand., 29:369-89, 1954. 272

1545. Gualtierotti, T., E. Martini, und A Marzorati. Untersuchungen ueber die Elektronarkose. Mit besonderer Beruecksichtung der aktiven elektrischen Erscheinungen des zentralen Nervensystems. Pfluegers Arch., 246:359-71, 1942. 298

1546. _____, _____, and _____. Electronarcosis. III. Inhibition of cortical electrical activity following local application of pulsed stimulus. J. Neurophysiol., 13: 5-8, 1950. 298
Gualtierotti, T., co-author: 2698, 2699.

1547. Gudden, H. Die physiologische und pathologische Schlaftrunkenheit. Arch. Psychiat., 40:989-1013, 1905. 122

1548. Guillain, G., P. Lechelle, et R. Garcin. La polyglobulie de certains syndromes hypophysaires et hypophyso-tubériens. C. R. Soc. Biol., 106:515-18, 1931. 237, 238

1549. _____, P. Mollaret, et G. Thoyer. Méningite syphilitique avec narcolepsie simulant l'encéphalite épidémique. Bull. Soc. Méd. Hôp. Paris, 46:334-36, 1930. 234

1550. Guillard, A. La Réactivité au cours du Sommeil Physiologique de l'Homme. Paris: Imprimerie R. Foulon, 1960. Pp. 126. 26, 86, 98

1551. _____, H. P. Cathala, and J. Calvet. The mechanogram recorded from the scalp and skin of the eyes during sensory stimulation in man while asleep. EEG Clin. Neurophysiol., 12:537, 1960; also Rev. Neurol., 102:318-20, 1960.
Guillard, A., co-author: 663.

1552. Guillemin, R. A re-evaluation of

acetyl-choline, adrenaline, nor-
adrenaline and histamine as possible mediators of the pituitary
adreno-corticotrophic activation
by stress. Endocrinology, 56:248-
55, 1955. 303

1553. _____, W. E. Dear, and R. A. Lie-
belt. Nychthemeral variations in
plasma free corticosteroid levels
of the rat. Proc. Soc. Exp. Biol.
Med., 101:394-95, 1959. 170

1554. Guilly, P. Formes cliniques et
traitement d'insomnie. Rev. Prat.,
4:1571-81, 1954. 275, 278
Guilly, P., co-author: 3247.

1555. Gujer, H. Der Einfluss von Schlaf,
Ruhe und verstaerkter Lungen-
ventilation auf das Pneumotacho-
gramm. Pfluegers Arch., 218:
698-707, 1928. 48

1556. Guliaev, P. I. (Russ.) Reflection
of parabiotic stages in the electrical processes of the cerebral
cortex of man in the course of
sleep. Fiziol. Zh. SSSR, 41:612-
19, 1955.

1557. _____. (Russ.) Reflection of the
dynamics of excitation and inhibition in the EEG of the sleeping
state. Fiziol. Zh. SSSR, 42:245-
52, 1956.

1558. _____. Phases of sleep and the
evolution of tidal excitability revealed in the E.E.G. patterns of
sleeping man. Sechenov Physiol.
J. USSR (Engl. ed.), 43:115-23,
1957.

1559. Gullota, S. Ipnotici e catatonia.
Atti Congr. Soc. Ital. Psichiat.,
20:765-68, 1935. 255

1560. Gunnarson, S., and K.-A. Melin.
The electroencephalogram in
enuresis. Acta Paediat., 40:496-
501, 1951. 284, 285

1561. Gutheil, E. A. The Language of
the Dream. New York: Macmillan, 1939. Pp. 286. 103

1562. Gutschmidt, J. Chemisch-phy-
siologische Untersuchungen
ueber die Abbaufaehigkeit des
Dormovits. Klin. Wschr., 19:
296-99, 1940. 294

1563. Guttmann, E. Aktogramme als
klinische Schlafkontrolle. Z. ges.
Neurol. Psychiat., 111:309-24,
1927. 294

1564. Gutwirth, S. W. How To Sleep
Well: The Cultivation of Natural
Rest. New York: Vantage Press,
1959. Pp. 97.

1565. Haas, A. Ueber Schlaftiefenmessungen. Psychol. Arb., 8:228-64,

1923. 113, 186

1566. Haberman, J. V. Sleep (normal
and abnormal) and the mechanism of sleep. New York Med.
J. Med. Rec., 101:265-72, 1922.

1567. Hackenberg, H. W. Ueber natuerlichen und kuenstlichen Schlaf.
Z. aerztl. Fortbild., 46:688-97,
1952.

1568. Hacker, F. Systematische
Traumbeobachtungen mit besonderer Beruecksichtung der
Gedanken. Arch. ges. Psychol.,
21:1-131, 1911. 100

1569. Hadfield, J. A. The influence of
hypnotic suggestion on inflammatory conditions. Lancet, II:
678-79, 1917. 331

1570. _____. The influence of suggestion on body temperature. Lancet, II:68-69, 1920. 337

1571. _____. Dreams and Nightmares.
London: Penguin Books, 1954.
Pp. xi + 244. 99, 280

1572. Hadley, H. G. Narcolepsy. Med.
Rec., 155:211-12, 1942; also J.
Nerv. Ment. Dis., 96:13-16,
1942. 234

1573. Hádlík, J. (Czech.) Employment
of reflex curative sleep. Cas.
Lék. Cesk., 93:967-71, 1954.

1574. Haeberlin, C. Lebensrhythmen
und Heilkunde. Entwurf einer
biozentrischen aerztlichen Betrachtung. Leipzig: Hippokrates-
Verlag, 1935. Pp. 74. 131

1575. Häberlin, P. Zur Lehre vom
Traum. Schweiz. Arch. Neurol.
Psychiat., 67:19-46, 1951. 99

1576. Haenel, H. Schlaf und Schlafzentrum. Med. Klin., 21:1258-61,
1925. 362

1577. _____. Eigenblut in der Behandlung der Schlaflosigkeit. Psychiat.-neurol. Wschr., 429-30,
1936. 294

1578. Hafer, E. C. Localization of an
experimental hypothalamic and
midbrain syndrome simulating
sleep. Ann Arbor, Michigan:
Univ. Microfilms, 1951. Pp. 63;
also Microfilm Abstr., 11:213-
14, 1951. 206

1579. Hagueneau, J. Les troubles du
sommeil. Rev. Crit. Path.
Thérap., 3:661-75, 1932.

1580. Haisch, E. Der Schlaf als ein
Trieb. Z. Psychotherap., 5:37-
42, 1955.

1581. Halberg, F. Some physiological
and clinical aspects of 24-hour
periodicity. J.-Lancet (Minneap-

olis), 73:20-32, 1953. 131, 172

1582. _____. Experimentelles zur Physiologie des Nebennieren-zyklus. Acta Med. Scand., Suppl. 307:117-18, 1955.

1583. _____. Physiologic 24-hour peri-odicity; General and procedural considerations with reference to the adrenal cycle. Z. Vitam.-Hormon-Fermentforsch., 10:225-96, 1959. 170, 172, 356

1584. _____. The 24-hour scale: a time dimension of adaptive functional organization. Perspect. Biol. Med., 3:491-527, 1960. 132

1585. _____, C. P. Barnum, R. H. Sil-ber, and J. J. Bittner. 24-hour rhythms at several levels of in-tegration in mice on different lighting regimens. Proc. Soc. Exp. Biol. Med., 97:897-900, 1958. 173

1586. _____, J. J. Bittner, R. J. Gully, P. G. Albrecht, and E. L. Brack-ney. 24-hour periodicity and au-diogenic convulsions in I mice of various ages. Proc. Soc. Exp. Biol. Med., 88:169-73, 1955. 159, 169

1587. _____, _____, und D. Smith. Be-lichtungswechsel und 24-Stunden-periodik von Mitosen im Hautepi-thel der Maus. Z. Vitam.-Hor-mon-Fermentforsch., 9:68-73, 1957. 173

1588. _____, R. Engel, E. Halberg, and R. J. Gully. Diurnal variations in amount of electroencephalograph-ic paroxysmal discharge and di-urnal eosinophil rhythm of epi-leptics on days with clinical sei-zures. Fed. Proc., 11:62, 1952. 170

1589. _____, _____, A. E. Treolar, and R. J. Gully. Endogenous eosino-penia in institutionalized patients with mental deficiency. A.M.A. Arch. Neurol. Psychiat., 69:462-69, 1953. 170

1590. _____, E. B. Flink, and M. B. Visscher. Alterations in diurnal rhythm in circulating eosinophil level in adrenal insufficiency. Am. J. Physiol., 167:791, 1951. 170

1591. _____, L. A. French, and R. J. Gully. 24-hour rhythms in rectal temperature and blood eosino-phils after hemidecortication in human subjects. J. Appl. Physiol., 12:381-84, 1958. 170

1592. _____, E. Halberg, C. P. Barnum, and J. J. Bittner. Physiologic 24-hour periodicity in human beings and mice, the lighting regimen and daily routine. In: Photoperiodism and Related Phe-nomena in Plants and Animals, Washington: Am. Ass. Advanc. Sci., 1959, pp. 803-78. 356

1593. _____, _____, and R. J. Gully. Ef-fect of modifications of the daily routine in healthy subjects and in patients with convulsive dis-order. Epilepsia, Ser. 3, 2:150, 1953. 174, 175

1594. _____, and R. B. Howard. 24-hour periodicity and experimen-tal medicine. Examples and inter-pretations. Postgrad. Med., 24: 349-58, 1958. 131

1595. _____, E. Jacobsen, G. Wads-worth, and J. J. Bittner. Audio-genic abnormality spectra, twen-ty-four hour periodicity, and lighting. Science, 128:657-58, 1958.

1596. _____, and I. H. Kaiser. Lack of physiologic eosinophil rhythm during advanced pregnancy of a patient with Addison's disease. Acta Endocrinol., 16:227-32, 1954. 170

1597. _____, L. Levy, and M. B. Vis-scher. Relation of 24-hour rhythm in body temperature to lighting conditions and to the adrenal. Fed. Proc., 12:59, 1953. 356

1598. _____, R. E. Peterson, and R. H. Silber. Phase relations of 24-hour periodicity in blood corti-costerone, mitosis in cortical adrenal parenchyma, and total body activity. Endocrinology, 64:222-30, 1959. 169

1599. _____, and R. A. Ulstrom. Morn-ing changes in number of circu-lating eosinophils in infants. Proc. Soc. Exp. Biol. Med., 80: 747-48, 1952. 170

1600. _____, and M. B. Visscher. Reg-ular diurnal physiological varia-tion in eosinophil levels in five stocks of mice. Proc. Soc. Exp. Biol. Med., 75:846-47, 1950. 169

1601. _____, _____, E. B. Flink, K. Berge, and F. Bock. Diurnal rhythmic changes in blood eosin-ophil levels in health and in cer-tain diseases. J.-Lancet (Minne-apolis), 71:312-19, 1951. 169, 170

1602. _____, H. A. Zander, M. W.

Houglum, and H. R. Mühlemann. Daily variations in tissue mitoses, blood eosinophils and rectal temperatures of rats. Am. J. Physiol., 177:361-66, 1954. 169
Halberg, F., co-author: 687, 688, 1088, 1156, 1202, 1213, 1264, 4065.

1603. Haldane, J. B. S., V. B. Wigglesworth, and C. E. Woodrow. Effect of reaction changes on human inorganic metabolism. Proc. Roy. Soc. London, Ser. B, 96:1-14, 1924. 34
Haldane, J. B. S., co-author: 426.

1604. Hall, B. The Gift of Sleep. New York: Moffat, Yard & Co., 1911. Pp. xiv + 305. 99, 100, 312

1605. Hall, C. Diagnosing personality by the analysis of dreams. J. Abnorm. Soc. Psychol., 42:68-79, 1947. 101

1606. _____. Three methods of analyzing dreams. Am. Psychol., 2:425, 1947. 101

1607. _____. Frequencies in certain categories of manifest content and their stability in a long dream series. Am. Psychol., 3:274, 1948. 101

1608. _____. Aggression and friendliness as expressed in the dreams of young adults. Am. Psychol., 5: 304, 1950. 101

1609. _____. What people dream about. Sci. Am., 184(5):60-63, 1951. 101, 102

1610. _____. The significance of the dream of being attacked. J. Personality, 24:168-80, 1955. 101

1611. _____. The Meaning of Dreams. New York: Dell Publ. Co., 1959. Pp. 256. 100, 101

1612. Hall, G., and G. B. Leroy. Posttraumatic narcolepsy. J. Am. Med. Ass., 106:431-34, 1936.

1613. Hallgren, B. Nocturnal enuresis in twins. Acta Psychiat. Neurol., 35:73-90, 1960. 284

1614. Hamar, N. Ueber Tagesschwankungen des Glucoseresorptionsvermoegens des Duenndarms. Pfluegers Arch., 244:164-70, 1940. 164

1615. Hamburger, C. Substitution of hypophysectomy by administration of chlorpromazine in the assay of corticotrophin. Acta Endocrinol., 20:383-90, 1955.

1616. Hamburger, F. Ueber Schlafstoerungen im Kindesalter. Muench. med. Wschr., 72:2021-23, 1925. 294

1617. _____. Ueber Schlafstoerungen bei Kindern. Erwiderung an Dr. Hartmann und Dr. F. Noltenius. Muench. med. Wschr., 74:284, 1927.

1618. Hamburger, W. W. The occurrence and meaning of dreams of food and eating. I. Typical food and eating dreams of four patients in analysis. Psychosom. Med., 20:1-16, 1958. 101

1619. Hamill, R. C. Insomnia. Med. Clin. North Am., 1:1409-15, 1918. 274, 294

1620. Hamilton, L. D., C. J. Gubler, G. E. Cartwright, and M. M. Wintrobe. Diurnal variation in the plasma iron level of man. Proc. Soc. Exp. Biol. Med., 75: 65-68, 1950. 163

1621. Hamoen, A. M. Signs of sleep in the EEG of waking patients. EEG Clin. Neurophysiol., 6:350-51, 1954. 30
Hamoen, A. M., co-author: 4239.

1622. Hanbery, J., and H. H. Jasper. Independence of diffuse thalamocortical projection system shown by specific nuclear destruction. J. Neurophysiol., 16:252-71, 1953; prelim. commun. Fed. Proc., 11:64, 1952. 210

1623. Happ, W. M., and K. D. Blackfan. Insomnia following acute encephalitis lethargica in children. J. Am. Med. Ass., 75:1337-39, 1920 246

1624. Hara, T., E. Favale, G. F. Rossi, e G. Sacco. Ricerche sull'attività elettrica cerebrale durante il sonno nel gatto. Riv. Neurol. (Napoli), 30:448-60, 1960; also EEG Clin. Neurophysiol., 13:130, 1961. 27

1625. _____, _____, _____, e _____. Ricerche sull'attività elettrica cerebrale nello stadio più profondo del sonno: depressione dei sistemi talamici e reticolari sincronizzanti. Boll. Soc. Ital. Biol. Sper., 36:1203-5, 1960. 212

1626. _____, _____, _____, e _____. Dati a favore dell'esistenza di un meccanismo inibitore desincronizzante l'elettroencefalogramma nello stadio più profondo di sonno. Boll. Soc. Ital. Biol. Sper., 36: 1205-7, 1960.
Hara, T., co-author: 3425.

1627. Hardcastle, D. N. A suggested approach to the problem of neuropsychiatry. J. Men.. Sci., 81:317-31, 1935.

1628. _____. Sleep, dreams and terrors. Lancet, 244(I):509, 1943.

1629. Harding, G. T., III, and T. Berg. Narcolepsy. Ohio State Med. J., 28:581-85, 1932. 238

1630. Harding, V. J., D. L. Selby, and A. R. Armstrong. Afternoon glycosuria. Biochem. J., 26:957-62, 1932. 166

1631. Harc, K., and W. A. Geohegan. Influence of frequency of stimulus upon response to hypothalamic stimulation. J. Neurophysiol., 4:266-73, 1941. 204

1632. Harker, J. E. Diurnal rhythms in the animal kingdom. Biol. Rev., 33:1-52, 1958. 132

1633. Harper, F. T. Narcolepsy. With report of 4 cases. N. Carolina Med. J., 6:96-98, 1945. 239

1634. Harreveld, A. van, und D. J. Kok. Ueber Elektronarkose. Acta Brev. Neerl., 3:45-46, 1933. 298

1635. _____, und _____. Ueber Elektronarkose und experimentelle Katatonie. Acta Brev. Neerl., 3: 106-8, 1933.

1636. _____, und _____. Ueber experimentelle Katalepsie durch sinusoidal Wechselstrom. Arch. Néerl. Physiol., 19:265-89, 1934. 254

1637. _____, et _____. A propos de la nature de la catalepsie expérimentale. Arch. Néerl. Physiol., 20:411-29, 1935. 254
Harreveld, A. van, co-author: 3941, 3942.

1638. Harriman, P. L. The dream of falling. J. Gen. Psychol., 20:229-33, 1939. 101

1639. Harrington, J. D., and R. M. Nardone. Hepatic function of the golden hamster after exposure to cold and during hibernation. Am. J. Physiol., 196:910-12, 1959. 324

1640. Harris, G. W. Electrical stimulation of the hypothalamus and the mechanism of neural control of the adenohypophysis. J. Physiol. (London), 107:418-29, 1948. 356

1641. _____. Neural control of the pituitary gland. Physiol. Rev., 28: 139-79, 1948. 356

1642. _____. Neural control of the pituitary gland: I. Neurohypophysis. Brit. Med. J., II:559-64, 1951. 356

1643. _____. Neural control of the pituitary gland: II. The adenohypophysis. With special reference to the secretion of A.C.T.H. Brit. Med. J., II:627-34, 1951. 356

1644. Harris, H. P., Jr. Some aspects of negativistic phenomena. South. Med. J., 45:70-74, 1952.

1645. Harris, I. [D.] Observations concerning typical anxiety dreams. Psychiatry, 11:301-9, 1948. 101

1646. _____. Characterological significance of the typical anxiety dreams. Psychiatry, 14:279-94, 1951. 101

1647. Harris, S. Epilepsy and narcolepsy associated with hyperinsulinism. J. Am. Med. Ass., 100:321-28, 1933. 256

1648. Harris, S. J. The effect of sleep loss on component movements of human motion. J. Appl. Psychol., 44:50-55, 1960. 225, 226

1649. Harris, W. Value of sleep. Practitioner, 122:18-20, 1929. 312

1650. Harrison, F. Somnolence produced by electrical currents in the brain. Arch. Neurol. Psychiat., 40:1274, 1938. 205

1651. _____. An attempt to produce sleep by diencephalic stimulation. J. Neurophysiol., 3:156-65, 1940. 204, 205

1652. _____. The hypothalamus and sleep. Res. Publ. Ass. Nerv. Ment. Dis., 20:635-56, 1940. 205

1653. Harrison, T. R., C. E. King, J. A. Calhoun, and W. G. Harrison. Congestive heart failure: Cheyne-Stokes respiration as the cause of paroxysmal dyspnea at the onset of sleep. Arch. Int. Med., 53:891-910, 1934. 33, 50, 51

1654. Hartley, D. Observations on Man. His Frame, his Duty, and his Expectations. Part I. London: J. Johnson, 1801. Pp. 512. 6

1655. Hartmann, A. Ueber Schlafstoerungen im Kindesalter. Muench. med. Wschr., 72:2229, 1925. 278

1656. Hartmann, E. von. Philosophy of the Unconscious. New York: Harcourt, Brace & Co., 1931. 3 vols. Vol. 2, pp. 28-44. 106

1657. Hartridge, H., and W. W. Smith. Sleep. Psyche, 2:57-63, 1921. 99

1658. Harvey, E. N., A. L. Loomis, and G. A. Hobart. Cerebral states during sleep as studied by human brain potentials. Sci. Monthly, 45:191-92, 1937; prelim. commun. Science, 85:443-44, 1937. 25

Harvey, E. N., co-author: 840-44, 2559-61.

1659. Hastings, A. B., and C. W. Eisele. Diurnal variations in the acid-base balance. Proc. Soc. Exp. Biol. Med., 43:308-12, 1940. 51

Hastings, A. B., co-author: 2597.

1660. Hathaway, S. R. Physiological Psychology. New York: D. Appleton-Century Co., 1942. Pp. xxi + 335. 31

1661. Hatlehol, R. Blood sugar studies. Acta Med. Scand., Suppl. 8:211-52, 1924. 165

1662. Hattingberg, H. Ueber die seelischen Ursachen der Schlaflosigkeit. Dsche med. Wschr., 61:1280-84, 1935. 294

1663. Hauffe, G. Die schlaffoerdernde Wirkung der Teilwasserbaeder. Therap. Gegenw., 73:248-52, 1932. 294

1664. Hauptmann, A. Zum Problem des Schlafes. Klin. Wschr., 10:2324-25, 1925.

1665. _____. Hypnosis. Bull. New Engl. Med. Center, 4:262-65, 1942. 336

1666. Hauty, G. T., and R. B. Payne. Behavioral and physiological consequences of 30 hours of sustained work. Am. Psychol., 12:405, 1957. 225

Hauty, G. T., co-author: 3801

1667. Hawkes, C. D., and M. Roark. Electroencephalographic diagnosis in children by means of sleep records. EEG Clin. Neurophysiol., 2:219, 1950. 257

1668. Hawkins, D. R., R. Pace, B. Pasternack, and M. G. Sandifer. A multivariant psychopharmacologic study in normals. Psychosom. Med., 23:1-17, 1961. 302

1669. _____, H. B. Puryear, C. D. Wallace, W. B. Deal, and E. S. Thomas. Basal skin resistance during sleep and "dreaming." Science, 136:321-22, 1962. 21, 98, 105, 110

1670. Hayashi, Y. (Jap.) On the sleeping hours of school children aged 6 to 20 years. Jido Jatshi (Child's J.), p. 296, 1925. 118, 186

1671. Heath, R. G., and R. Hodes. Induction of sleep by stimulation of the caudate nucleus in macaqus

rhesus and man. Trans. Am. Neurol. Ass., 77:204-10, 1952. 204

Heath, R. G., co-author: 1797, 2872.

1672. Hebb, D. O. The Organization of Behavior. A Neurological Theory. New York: John Wiley & Sons, 1949. Pp. xix + 335. 31

1673. _____. The problem of consciousness and introspection. In: Brain Mechanisms and Consciousness, 1954 (875), pp. 402-21. 31

1674. _____. Drives and the C.N.S. (conceptual nervous system). Psychol. Rev., 62:243-54, 1955. 31

1675. Hechst, B. Klinisch-anatomische Beitraege zur zentralen Regulation des Schlaf-Wachseins. Arch. Psychiat., 87:505-26, 1929. 265, 272, 360

1676. Hecker, C. H., and C. L. Carlisle. Benzedrine sulphate in catatonic stupors. Med. Bull. Vet. Admin., 12:224-27, 1937. 240, 300

1677. Hediger, [H.] Wie Tiere schlafen. Med. Klin. (Berlin), 54:938-46, 1959. 10

1678. Heerwagen, F. Statistische Untersuchungen ueber Traeume und Schlaf. Philos. Studien, 5:301-20, 1889.

1679. Heid, J. B. Thalamic lesions and coma. Bull. Los Angeles Neurol. Soc., 11:91-93, 1946. 273

1680. Heilbrunn, G. Fusion of the Isakower phenomenon with the dream screen. Psychoanal. Q., 22:200-204, 1953. 101

1681. Heilig, R., und H. Hoff. Schlafstudien. Klin. Wschr., 4:2194-98, 1925. 34, 35, 45

1682. Heimann, H. Hypnose und Schlaf. Mschr. Psychiat. Neurol. (Basel), 125:478-93, 1953. 337

1683. _____, und T. Spoerri. Elektroencephalographische Untersuchungen an Hypnotisierten. Mschr. Psychiat. Neurol. (Basel), 125:261-71, 1953. 330

1684. Heinbecker, P., and S. H. Bartley. The action of ether and nembutal on the nervous system. J. Neurophysiol., 3:219-35, 1940. 296

1685. Heinberg, C. J. A surgical procedure for the relief of snoring. Eye Ear Nose Throat Monthly (Chicago), 34:389, 395, 1955. 50

1686. Held, R., B.-A. Schwartz, et H.

Fischgold. Fausse insomnie; étude psychoanalytique et électroencéphalographique. Presse Méd., 67:141-43, 1959. 275

1687. Hellbruegge, T. Ueber Eigenheiten des kindlichen Schlafes. Med. Klin. (Berlin), 54(20):954-60, 1959. 131, 307

1688. _____. The development of circadian rhythms in infants. Cold Spring Harbor Symp. Quantit. Biol., 25:311-23, 1960. 131

1689. _____, und J. Lange. Ueber das Verhalten der Motilitaet in den fruehen kindlichen Entwicklungsstufen. Med. Klin. (Berlin), 54: 946-54, 1959.

1690. _____, _____, und J. Rutenfranz. Ueber die Entwicklung von tagesperiodischen Veraenderungen der Pulsfrequenz im Kindesalter. Z. Kinderheilk., 78:703-22, 1956. 163

1691. _____, _____, und _____. Schlafen und Wachen in der kindlichen Entwicklung. Beihefte Arch. Kinderheilk, Heft 39, 1959. Pp. 104. 117, 118, 307

1692. _____, und J. Rutenfranz. Schichtunterricht und Leistungbereitschaft. Muench. med. Wschr., 98:1713-18, 1956. 307
Hellbruegge, T., co-author: 3481, 3482.

1693. Hellebrandt, F. A., R. H. Tepper, H. Grant, and R. Catherwood. Nocturnal and diurnal variations in the acidity of the spontaneous secretion of gastric juice. Am. J. Digest. Dis. Nutrition, 3:477-81, 1936. 53, 54, 163

1694. Heller, A., J. A. Harvey, H. F. Hunt, and L. J. Roth. Effect of lesions in the septal forebrain of the rat on sleeping time under barbiturate. Science, 131:662-64, 1960. 297

1695. Hellmuth, F. H., und A. de Veer. Beziehungen zwischen Schlaf und Temperatur beim Menschen. Z. exp. Med., 98:41-48, 1936. 87, 310

1696. Helm, F. Die Dickdarmperistaltik im Schlafe. Med. Klin., 13: 1308-10, 1917. 55

1697. Helm, J. D., Jr., P. Kramer, R. M. MacDonald, and F. J. Ingelfinger. Changes in motility of the human small intestine during sleep. Gastroenterology, 10:135-37, 1948. 55

1698. Hemmingsen, A. M., and N. B.

Krarup. Rhythmic diurnal variations in the oestrous phenomena of the rat and their susceptibility to light and dark. Kgl. danske Vidensk. Biol. Meddelelser, 13(7):1-61, 1937. 175

1699. Henderson, V. E. On Bancroft's theory of anaesthesia, sleep and insanity. Am. J. Psychiat., 13: 313-19, 1933. 352

1700. _____. Sedatives and hypnotics. Bull. Acad. Med. Toronto, 9:256-60, 1936. 275, 294

1701. Henning, N., und L. Norpoth. Die Magensekretion waehrend des Schlafes. Dsch. Arch. klin. Med., 172:558-62, 1932. 54, 163

1702. Henriksen, G. F., O. Grossman, and J. K. Merlis. EEG observations in a case with thalamic syndrome. EEG Clin. Neurophysiol., 1:505-7, 1949. 76
Henriksen, G. F., co-author: 2782, 2783.

1703. Henry, C. E. Electroencephalographic individual differences and their constancy. I. During sleep. J. Exp. Psychol., 29:117-32, 1941.

1704. _____. Effect on the electroencephalogram of transorbital lobotomy. EEG Clin. Neurophysiol., 2:187-92, 1950.

1705. _____. The effect of Dormison on the electroencephalogram. EEG Clin. Neurophysiol., 5:321, 1953. 296

1706. _____, and W. B. Scoville. Suppression-burst activity from isolated cerebral cortex in man. EEG Clin. Neurophysiol., 4:1-22, 1952. 211
Henry, C. E., co-author: 825, 826, 2217, 2219, 4103.

1707. Henry, F. Cardiovascular effects of experimental insomnia. Am. J. Physiol., 138:65-70, 1942. 225

1708. Hernández-Peón, R., H. Brust-Carmona, E. Eckhaus, E. Lopez-Mendoza, and C. Alcocer-Cuarón. Functional role of the brain stem reticular system in salivary conditioned response. Fed. Proc., 15:91, 1956. 210

1709. _____, C. Guzmán-Flores, N. Alcaraz, and A. Fernández-Guardiola. Sensory transmission in visual pathway during "attention" in unanesthetized cats. Acta Neurol. Latinoam., 3:1-8, 1957. 210

1710. _____, and K.-E. Hagbarth. Interaction between afferent and cortically induced reticular responses. J. Neurophysiol., 18:44-55, 1955. 210, 211

1711. _____, M. Jouvet, and H. Scherrer. Auditory potentials at cochlear nucleus during acoustic habituation. Acta Neurol. Latinoam., 3:144-56, 1957. 210

1712. _____, A. Lavin, C. Alcocer-Cuarón, and J. P. Marcelin. Activity of the olfactory bulb during wakefulness and sleep. EEG Clin. Neurophysiol., 12:41-58, 1960. 204, 210

1713. _____, and H. Scherrer. Inhibitory influence of brain stem reticular formation upon synaptic transmission in trigeminal nucleus. Fed. Proc., 14:71, 1955. 209, 210

1714. _____, and _____. 'Habituation' to acoustic stimuli in cochlear nucleus. Fed. Proc., 14:71, 1955. 210

1715. _____, _____, and M. Jouvet. Modification of electrical activity in cochlear nucleus during "attention" in unanesthetized cats. Science, 123:331-32, 1956. 210
Hernández-Peón, R., co-author: 1281, 1283, 2542.

1716. Heron, W. The pathology of boredom. Sci. Am., 196(1):52-56, 1957. 31, 198
Heron, W., co-author: 326, 3634.

1717. Herring, V. V., and S. Brody. Diurnal metabolic and activity rhythms. Univ. Missouri Agric. Exp. Stat. Res. Bull., 274:1-30, 1938. 149

1718. Hersey, R. B. Seele und Gefuehl des Arbeiters. Leipzig: Konkordia, 1935. Pp. 171. 120, 185, 307

1719. Herter, K. Koerpertemperatur und Aktivitaet beim Igel. Z. vergl. Physiol., 20:511-44, 1934. 149, 321

1720. Herz, F. Selbstbeobachtung ueber freiwillige Schlafentziehung. Pfluegers Arch., 200:429-42, 1923. 224

1721. _____. (Dutch) On triphasic sleep in man. Ned. Tschr. Psychol., 1: 71-79, 1946.
Herz, F., co-author: 2276.

1722. Hess, L. Ueber natuerlichen und ueber krankhaften Schlaf. Klin. Wschr., 16:625-26, 1937.

1723. Hess, L. Differential diagnosis of physiological and pathological sleep. J. Nerv. Ment. Dis., 98:

474-77, 1943. 40

1724. Hess, R. Etude sur les potentiels du sommeil normal et pathologique dans l'électroencéphalogramme. EEG Clin. Neurophysiol., 2:108, 1950.

1725. _____. Bioelectrical and behavioural arousal with electrical stimulation of meso-diencephalic structures. EEG Clin. Neurophysiol., 6:528-29, 1954. 204

1726. _____. Die Narkolepsie. Med. Klin. (Berlin), 54:985-93, 1959. 237

1727. _____, K. Akert, et W. Koella. Les potentiels bioélectriques du cortex et du thalamus et leur altération par stimulation du centre hypnique chez le chat. Rev. Neurol., 83:537-44, 1950.

1728. _____, W. P. Koella, and K. Akert. Cortical and subcortical recordings in unanesthetized cats. EEG Clin. Neurophysiol., 4:370-71, 1952.

1729. _____, _____, and _____. Cortical and subcortical recordings in natural and artificially induced sleep in cats. EEG Clin. Neurophysiol., 5:75-90, 1953. 26
Hess, R., co-author: 33, 1758-60.

1730. Hess, S. M., P. A. Shore, and B. B. Brodie. Persistence of reserpine action after the disappearance of drug from brain: effect of serotonin. J. Pharmacol. Exp. Therap., 118:84-89, 1956. 302

1731. Hess, W. R. Ueber die Wechselbeziehungen zwischen psychischen und vegetativen Funktionen. Schweiz. Arch. Neurol. Psychiat., 15:260-77, 1924; 16:36-55, 285-306, 1925. 357

1732. _____. Stammganglien-Reizversuche. Ber. ges. Physiol., 42: 554-55, 1927. 204, 357

1733. _____. Hirnreizversuche ueber den Mechanismus des Schlafes. Arch. Psychiat., 86:287-92, 1929. 204, 357

1734. _____. Localisatorische Ergebnisse der Hirnreizversuche mit Schlafeffekt. Arch. Psychiat., 88: 813-16, 1929. 204, 357

1735. _____. Localisatorische Ergebnisse der Hirnreizversuche mit Schlafeffekt. Zbl. ges. Neurol. Psychiat., 54:325-26, 1929. 204, 357

1736. _____. The mechanism of sleep. Am. J. Physiol., 90:386-87, 1929. 204, 357

1737. _____. (Portug.) Results of experiments localizing cerebral stimulations causing sleep. Rev. Oto-Neuro-Oftal., 5:74, 1930. 204, 357

1738. _____. Die Funktionen des vegetativen Nervensystems. Klin. Wschr., 9:1009-12, 1930. 204, 357

1739. _____. Le sommeil. C. R. Soc. Biol., 107:1333-64, 1931. 204, 357

1740. _____. On the interrelationships between psychic and vegetative function. J. Nerv. Ment. Dis., 74:511-28, 645-53, 1931. 202, 204, 357

1741. _____. The autonomic nervous system. Lancet, 223(II):1199-1201, 1259-61, 1932. 204, 357

1742. _____. Der Schlaf. Klin. Wschr., 12:129-34, 1933. 204, 357

1743. _____. Beziehungen zwischen Winterschlaf und Aussentemperatur beim Siebenschlaefer. Z. vergl. Physiol., 26:529-36, 1939. 204, 357

1744. _____. Beitrag zur Technik des zentralen Reizversuches. Pfluegers Arch., 243:431-38, 1940. 204, 357

1745. _____. Hypothalamische Adynamie. Helvet. Physiol. Acta, 2:137-47, 1944. 204, 357

1746. _____. Das Schlafsyndrom als Folge diencephaler Reizung. Helvet. Physiol. Acta, 2:305-44, 1944. 204, 357

1747. _____. Vegetative Funktionen und Zwischenhirn. Helvet. Physiol. Acta, 5(Suppl. IV):5-65, 1947. 204, 357

1748. _____. Le sommeil comme une fonction physiologique. J. Physiol. (Paris), 41:61A-67A, 1949. 204, 357

1749. _____. Das Zwischenhirn—Syndrome, Lokalisationen, Funktionen. Basel: Benno Schwabe, 1949. Pp. 187. 204, 357

1750. _____. Diencephalon—Autonomic and Extrapyramidal Functions. New York: Grune & Stratton, 1954. Pp. xii + 79. 204, 357

1751. _____. The diencephalic sleep centre. In: Brain Mechanisms and Consciousness, 1954 (875), pp. 117-36. 204, 357, 358, 362

1752. _____. The Functional Organization of the Diencephalon. New York: Grune & Stratton, 1957. Pp. xii + 180. 204, 357

1753. Heucqueville, G. d', et C. Leclercq. Brome, inhibition, sommeil, hormones sédatives. Bull. Méd. (Paris), 51:35-39, 1937.

1754. Heus, H. von. Ueber die Pharmakologie und Toxikologie der Schlafmittel, insbesondere der Abkoemmlinge der Barbitursaeure. Med. Welt, 10:968-70, 1002-5, 1936.

1755. Heusner, A. P. Yawning and associated phenomena. Physiol. Rev. 26:156-68, 1946. 71

1756. Heuyer, G. Les troubles du sommeil chez l'enfant. J. Méd. Franç., 15:439-50, 1926; also Epinal: Imprim. Coopér., 1928. Pp. 70.

1757. _____, A. Rémond, R. Delarue. Activation de l'E.E.G. par le penthotal. Rev. Neurol., 80:642-45, 1948. 257

1758. Heyck, H., and R. Hess. EEG studies in narcolepsy. EEG Clin. Neurophysiol., 6:520, 1954. 238

1759. _____, and _____. Some results of clinical studies on narcolepsy. Schweiz. Arch. Neurol. Psychiat., 75:401-2, 1955. 238

1760. _____, und _____. Weitere Beitraege zur Klinik der Narkolepsie. Psychiat. Neurol. (Basel), 134:66-76, 1957. 237, 238

1761. Hiebel, G., M. Bonvallet, et P. Dell. Action de la chlorpromazine ("Largactil," 45 60 RP) au niveau du système nerveux central. Sem. Hôp., 30:2346-53, 1954. 214, 301

1762. _____, et C. Kayser. Recherches électrocardiographiques sur le réveil des hibernants. J. Physiol. (Paris), 42:606-12, 1950. 327 Hiebel, G., co-author: 407, 2113, 2117, 3397.

1763. Higgins, G. M., J. Berkson, and E. Flock. The diurnal cycle in the liver. I. Periodicity of the cycle with analysis of the chemical constituents involved. Am. J. Physiol., 102:673-82, 1932. 165

1764. _____, _____, and _____. The diurnal cycle in the liver of the white rat. II. Food, a factor in its determination. Am. J. Physiol., 105:177-86, 1933. 165

1765. Hildebrandt, F. W. Der Traum und seine Verwertung fuer's Leben. Leipzig: Gebrueder Senf, 1881. Pp. 60. 100

1766. Hildebrandt, G. Ueber tages-rhythmische Steuerung der Reagibilitaet; Untersuchungen ueber Tagesgang der akralen Wiedererwaermung. Arch. phys. Therap. (Leipzig), 9:292-303, 1957. 163

1767. Hildén, A., und K. S. Stenbäck. Zur Kenntnis der Tagesschwankungen der Koerpertemperatur bei den Voegeln. Skand. Arch. Physiol., 34:382-410, 1916. 173

1768. Hilgard, E. R., and D. G. Marquis. Conditioning and Learning. New York: Appleton-Century-Crofts, Inc., 1961. Revised by G. A. Kimble. Pp. ix + 590. 347

1769. Hill, D. Electroencephalography. In: Brain, R., and E. B. Strauss, Recent Advances in Neurology and Neuropsychiatry, London: Churchill, 1955, pp. 178-231. 31
Hill, D., co-author: 726.

1770. Hill, L. Arterial pressure in man while sleeping, resting, waking, bathing. J. Physiol. (London), 22: xxvi-xxix, 1898.

1771. Hill, S. R., F. C. Goetz, H. M. Fox, B. J. Murawski, L. J. Krakauer, R. W. Reifenstein, S. J. Gray, W. J. Reddy, S. H. Hedberg, J. R. St. Marc, and G. W. Thorn. Studies on adrenocortical and psychological response to stress in man. Arch. Int. Med., 97:269-98, 1956. 170

1772. _____, H. L. Halley, W. R. Starnes, and L. L. Hibbett. Studies on the diurnal pattern of urinary 17-hydroxycorticoid and 17-ketosteroid excretion in patients with rheumatoid arthritis. Ann. Rheumat. Dis., 15:69-71, 1956. 170

1773. Himwich, H. E. Psychopharmacologic drugs. Science, 127:59-72, 1958. 298, 301, 302

1774. _____. Tranquilizers, barbiturates, and the brain. J. Neuropsychiat., 3:279-94, 1962. 302, 304
Himwich, H. E., co-author: 1775, 1791, 3354-58.

1775. Himwich, W. E., E. Homburger, R. Maresca, and H. E. Himwich. Brain metabolism in man; unanesthetized and in pentothal narcosis. Am. J. Psychiat., 103:689-96, 1947. 297

1776. Hines, L. E. Peristalsis in a loop of small intestine. Arch. Int. Med., 38:536-43, 1926. 55

1777. Hinkle, L. E., and H. G. Wolff. Communist interrogation and indoctrination of "enemies of the state." A.M.A. Arch. Neurol. Psychiat., 76:115-74, 1956. 228

1778. Hinton, J. M., and E. Marley. The effects of meprobamate and pentobarbitone sodium on sleep and motility during sleep: A controlled trial with psychiatric patients. J. Neurol. Neurosurg. Psychiat. (London), 22: 137-40, 1959. 278

1779. Hirsch, E. Schlafsucht bei einem Thalamusherd. Zbl. ges. Neurol. Psychiat., 37:194, 1924. 266

1780. _____. Zur Frage der Schlafzentren im Zwischenhirn des Menschen. Med. Klin., 20:1322-24, 1924. 266, 360

1781. _____. Pathologische Schlafzustaende bei Herderkrankungen des Mittelhirns. Mschr. Psychiat., 63:113-29, 1927.

1782. _____. Zur Pathologie der Schlafzentren. Dsche Z. Nervenheilk., 102:143-44, 1928. 266

1783. Hirsch, L. Schlaflosigkeit, ihre Entstehung und Heilung. Hannover: Wilkens, 1931. Pp. 76. 275, 294, 349, 362

1784. Hirvonen, L. Temperature range of the spontaneous activity of the isolated hedgehog, hamster and rat auricle. Acta Physiol. Scand., 36:38-46, 1956. 327

1785. Ho, T., Y. R. Wang, T. A. N. Lin, and Y. F. Cheng. Predominance of electrocortical sleep patterns in the "encéphale isolé" cat and new evidence for a sleep center. Physiol. Bohemoslov., 9:85-92, 1960.

1786. Hoagland, H. The mechanism of tonic immobility ("animal hypnosis"). J. Gen. Psychol., 1:426-47, 1928. 336

1787. _____. The physiological control of judgments of duration: evidence for a chemical clock. J. Gen. Psychol., 9:267-87, 1933. 158, 159

1788. _____. Pacemakers of human brain waves in normals and in general paretics. Am. J. Physiol., 116:604-15, 1936; also Science, 83:84-85, 1936. 160

1789. _____. Brain mechanisms and brain wave frequencies. Am. J. Physiol., 123:102, 1938. 31, 160

1790. _____. Brain wave frequencies and brain chemistry. Arch. Neurol. Psychiat., 62:511-13,

1949. 31, 160

1791. _____, H. E. Himwich, E. Campbell, J. F. Fazekas, and Z. Hadidian. Effects of hypoglycemia and pentobarbital sodium on electrical activity of cerebral cortex and hypothalamus (dogs). J. Neurophysiol., 2:276-88, 1939. 31

1792. Hobbs, G. E., E. S. Goddard, and J. A. F. Stevenson. The diurnal cycle in blood eosinophils and body temperature. Canad. Med. Ass. J., 70:533-36, 1954. 169

1793. Hoche, A. Schlaflosigkeit. Dsche med. Wschr., 48:389-91, 1922. 294, 305

1794. _____. Der Traum. Handb. norm. path. Physiol., 17:622-42, 1026.

1795. Hochrein, M., J. Michelsen, und H. Becker. Schlaf, Schlaflosigkeit und koerperliche Arbeit in ihrem Einfluss auf den Blutchemismus. Die Erholungsphase. Pfluegers Arch., 226:244-54, 738-45, 1930-31.

1796. Hodes, R. Electrocortical synchronization (ECS) in cats from reduction of proprioceptive drive caused by a muscle relaxant (Flaxedil). Fed. Proc., 20:332, 1961. 205

1797. _____, R. G. Heath, and C. D. Hendley. Cortical and subcortical electrical activity in sleep. Trans. Am. Neurol. Ass., 77:201-3, 1952. 76

Hodes, R., co-author: 1671.

1798. Hoefer, P. F. A., and G. H. Glaser. Effects of pituitary adrenocorticotrophic hormone (ACTH) therapy. Electroencephalographic and neuropsychiatric changes in fifteen patients. J. Am. Med. Ass., 143:620-24, 1950. 303

1799. _____, E. S. Goldensohn, and L. Rosenkoetter. The diagnostic value of electroencephalograms in natural and drug-induced sleep. Trans. Am. Neurol. Ass., 80: 203-4, 1955. 296

1800. Hölzer, H. Der taegliche Mittagschlaf in seiner Bedeutung fuer die Entwicklung des Kindes, besonders im Schulkindes, im Rahmen des Schlafsolls. Z. aerztl. Fortbild., 50:26-30, 1956. 307

1801. _____. Physikalische Reize und Schlaf, aktive und passive Entwicklungsfaktoren beim Kind. Hippokrates (Stuttgart), 28:767-72, 1957. 307

1802. Hoff, F. Behandlung von Schlafstoerungen. Dsche med. Wschr., 68:375-78, 1942. 286

1803. _____. Das vegetative Nervensystem im Rahmen der gesamten vegetativen Steuerung. Dsche med. Wschr., 70:87-90, 1944. 358

1804. Hoff, H. Zusammenhang von Vestibularfunktion, Schlafstellung und Traumleben. Mschr. Psychiat., 71:366-72, 1929. 8

1805. _____. Schlaf und Winterschlaf. II. Teil. Wien. klin. Wschr., 2: 1223-25, 1248-50, 1936.

1806. _____. Schlaf. Wien. med. Wschr., 2:904-6, 1937. 8, 362

1807. _____. Diologie des Schlafes und Klinik der Schlafstoerung. Med. Klin. (Berlin), 54:961-64, 969, 1959. 286

1808. _____, und O. Pötzl. Ueber die labyrinthaeren Beziehungen von Flugsensationen und Flugtraeumen. Mschr. Psychiat. Neurol., 97:193-211, 1937. 101

Hoff, H., co-author: 1681.

1809. Hoffer, A. Induction of sleep by autonomic drugs. J. Nerv. Ment. Dis., 119:421-27, 1954. 203

1810. Hoffman, B. F., E. E. Suckling, C. McC. Brooks, E. H. Koenig, K. S. Coleman, and H. J. Treumann. Quantitative evaluation of sleep. J. Appl. Physiol., 8:361-68, 1956. 112

Hoffman, B. F., co-author: 524, 3863.

1811. Hoffman, C. E., R. T. Clark, Jr., and E. B. Brown, Jr. Blood oxygen saturations and duration of consciousness in anoxia at high altitudes. Am. J. Physiol., 145: 685-92, 1946. 31

1812. Hoffmann, R. W. Periodischer Tageswechsel und andere biologische Rhythmen bei den poikilothermen Tieren (Reptilien, Amphibien, Fische, Wirbellose). Handb. norm. path. Physiol., 17: 644-58, 1926. 132

1813. _____. Die reflektorischen Immobilisationszustaende im Tierreich. Handb. norm. path. Physiol., 17:690-714, 1926. 335, 338

1814. Hofmeister, M. Zur Frage des Mechanismus der narkoleptischen Attacke. Schweiz. Arch. Neurol. Psychiat., 62:96-112, 1948. 240

1815. Hofstadt, F. Ueber eine eigenartige Form von Schlafstoerung im Kindesalter als Spaetschaden nach Encephalitis lethargica. Muench. med. Wschr., 67:1400-1402, 1920. 246

1816. ____. Ueber Spaet- und Dauerschaeden nach Encephalitis epidemica im Kindesalter. Z. Kinderheilk., 29:272-305, 1921. 246

1817. Hollingworth, H. L. The influence of caffeine alkaloid on the quality and amount of sleep. Am. J. Psychol., 23:89-100, 1912. 119

1818. ____. Variations in efficiency during the working day. Psychol. Rev., 21:473-91, 1914. 150

1819. Holmgren, H. Studien ueber 24-Stundenrhythmische Variationen des Darm- Lungen- and Leberfetts. Acta Med. Scand., Suppl. 74, 1936. Pp. 202. 164

1820. Holmquist, A. G. Beitrage zur Kenntnis der 24-stuendigen Rhythmik der Leber. Z. mikr.-anat. Forsch., 25:30-43, 1931. 164

1821. ____. Ueber den Zusammenhang zwischen der Gallensekretion und der exocrinen Sekretion des Pancreas. Anat. Anz., 73:23-28, 1931. 54, 164

1822. ____. Der Zusammenhang zwischen dem Schlaf und dem Adrenalingehalt der Nebennieren. Skand. Arch. Physiol., 65:18-23, 1932. 57

1823. ____. Taegliche cyclische Schwankungen im Calciumgehalt des Blutes bei Menschen und Kaninchen. Z. ges. exp. Med., 93: 370-77, 1934. 162
Holmquist, A. G., co-author: 1111.

1824. Holt, M. P. Posture during sleep. Lancet, I:124, 1942. 9, 11

1825. Holtz, F., und C. Roggenbau. Zur Kenntnis des Bromspiegels: Bemerkungen zu den Veroeffentlichungen von H. Zondek, A. Bier und Mitarbeitern. Klin. Wschr., 12:1410-11, 1933. 57

1826. Holubář, J. (Czech.) Electroencephalographic studies on function of reticular formation in man. Českoslov. Physiol., 7(5):470-71, 1958. 209

1827. Holzer, P. E. Dream Phenomena. Minneapolis: Burgess Publ. Co., 1951. Pp. iii + 33. 99

1828. Hondelink, H. Expériences de sommeil sur des petits oiseaux. Arch. Néerl. Physiol., 16:292-95, 1931. 10, 294

1829. ____. Schlafmittelversuche an Finken. Arch. exp. Path. Pharmakol., 163:662-71, 1932. 294

1830. Hook, W. E. Effect of crude peanut oil extracts of brown fat on metabolism of white rat. Proc. Soc. Exp. Biol. Med., 45:37-40, 1940. 326

1831. Hopewell-Ash, E. Treatment of insomnia in nervous and mental diseases. Brit. J. Phys. Med., 9:39-41, 1934. 294

1832. Hopkins, H. Chemical studies in the epileptic syndrome. II. Nocturnal and diurnal rhythm in blood chemistry. Am. J. Psychiat., 92:75-88, 1935. 34, 259

1833. Horder, Lord. Use of narcotics in the treatment of nervous and mental patients. Brit. Med. J., II:619-21, 1934. 294

1834. Horowitz, Z. P., and M.-I. Chow. Desynchronized electroencephalogram in the deeply sleeping cat. Science, 134:945, 1961. 27, 212

1835. Horst, K., and W. L. Jenkins. The effect of caffeine, coffee and decaffeinated coffee upon blood pressure, pulse rate, and simple reaction time of men of various ages. J. Pharmacol. Exp. Therap., 53:385-400, 1935. 299

1836. Horst, L. van der, and H. de Jong. (Dutch) Comparative phenomenological investigation of cataleptic symptoms in human catatonia and in experimental bulbocapnine catatonia. Ned. Tschr. Geneesk., 76:3271-77, 1932. 252

1837. Horsten, G. P. M. Influence of body temperature on the EEG. Acta Brev. Neerl., 17:23-25, 1949. 327
Horsten, G. P. M., co-author: 662

1838. Horton, L. H. The illusion of levitation. I. A general presentation. J. Abnorm. Psychol., 13: 42-53, 1918. 101, 105

1839. ____. The illusion of levitation. II. Clinical aspects. J. Abnorm. Psychol., 13:119-27, 1918. 101, 105

1840. ____. Levitation dreams: their physiology. J. Abnorm. Psychol., 14:145-72, 1919. 101, 105

1841. ____. What drives the dream mechanism? Some questions raised by the inventorial analysis of dreams. J. Abnorm. Psychol., 15:224-58, 1920. 106

1842. ____. The mechanistic features

of the dream process. J. Abnorm.
Soc. Psychol., 16:168-96, 1921.
106

1843. Horvai, I. (Czech.) Sleep, Dreams,
Suggestion, and Hypnosis. Praha:
Statni Zdravotnicke Nakladatelstvi,
1958. 3rd ed. Pp. 51.

1844. Horwich, D. How To Stop Snoring.
New York: Exposition Press, 1951.
Pp. 80. 50

1845. Hosmer, G. W. The Nocturnal Ne-
gation. A Study of the Physiology
of Sleep. Portland, Maine: Smith
& Sale, 1914. Pp. 87.

1846. Howell, W. H. A contribution to
the physiology of sleep based upon plethysmographic experiments.
J. Exp. Med., 2:313-45, 1897. 46,
47, 109, 242

1847. Hoyt, W. G. The effect on learning of auditory material presented during sleep. Master's thesis,
George Washington Univ., Washington, D.C., 1953. Pp. 24. 125,
126

1848. Hubble, D. Enuresis. Brit. Med.
J., II:1108-11, 1950. 284

1849. Hubel, D. H. Single unit activity
in striate cortex of unrestrained
cats. J. Physiol. (London), 147:
226-38, 1959; prelim. commun.
Fed. Proc., 16:63, 1957. 211

1850. _____. Electrocorticograms in
cats during natural sleep. Arch.
Ital. Biol., 98:171-81, 1960. 27

1851. _____, and W. J. H. Nauta. Electrocorticograms of cats with
chronic lesions of the rostral
mesencephalic tegmentum. Fed.
Proc., 19:287, 1960. 212

1852. Hudson, T. J. The Law of Psychic
Phenomena. Chicago: A. C. Mc-
Clurg & Co., 1916. Pp. xvii + 409.
100

1853. Hübner, A. Die kriminalistische
Bedeutung des Schlafes. Arch.
Kriminol., 81:86-101, 1927.

1854. Hugelin, A. Etude comparée de
l'activation du système réticulaire activateur ascendant et du
système réticulaire facilitateur
descendant. C. R. Soc. Biol., 149:
1963-65, 1955. 209

1855. _____. Les bases physiologiques
de la vigilance. Encéphale, 45:
267-92, 1956.

1856. _____, et M. Bonvallet. Tonus
cortical et contrôle de la facilitation motrice d'origine réticulaire.
J. Physiol. (Paris), 49:1171-1200,
1957. 209

1857. _____, et _____. Etude expéri-

mentale des interrelations ré-
ticulo-corticales. Proposition
d'une théorie de l'asservisse-
ment réticulaire à un système
diffus cortical. J. Physiol. (Paris), 49:1201-23, 1957. 209

1858. _____, et _____. Effets moteurs
et corticaux d'origine réticulaire au cours des stimulations
somesthésiques. Rôle des inter-
actions cortico-réticulaires dans
le déterminisme du réveil. J.
Physiol. (Paris), 50:951-77,
1958. 211

1859. _____, S. Dumont, and N. Pail-
las. Tympanic muscles and control of auditory input during
arousal. Science, 131:1371-72,
1960.
Hugelin, A., co-author: 408, 409,
888, 889.

1860. Hug-Hellmuth, H. von. A Study
of the Mental Life of the Child.
Nerv. Ment. Dis. Monogr. Ser.,
No. 29, Washington, 1919. Pp.
viii + 154. 102

1861. Hughes, E. Seasonal Variation
in Man. London: H. K. Lewis &
Co., 1931. Pp. 126. 328

1862. Hughes, J. G., B. C. Davis, and
M. L. Brennan. Electroencepha-
lography of the newborn infant.
VI. Studies on premature infants.
Pediatrics, 7:707-12, 1951. 27

1863. _____, B. Ehemann, and U. A.
Brown. Electroencephalography
of the newborn; studies on normal, full term, sleeping infants.
Am. J. Dis. Child., 76:503-12,
1948. 27

1864. _____, _____, and F. S. Hill.
Electroencephalography of the
new-born; studies on normal,
full term infants while awake
and while drowsy. Am. J. Dis.
Child., 77:310-14, 1949. 27

1865. _____, F. S. Hill, C. R. Green,
and B. C. Davis. Electroencephalography of the newborn. V.
Brain potentials of babies born
of mothers given meperidine hydrochloride (demerol hydrochloride), vinbarbital sodium (delvi-
nal sodium) or morphine. Am. J.
Dis. Child., 79:996-1007, 1950.

1866. Hughes, L. Insomnia. Med. J.
Australia, II:330-32, 1944. 274

1867. _____, and S. E. Jones. Treatment of insomnia. Modern. Med.,
13:71-72, 1945. 274, 275

1868. Hull, C. L. Hypnosis and Suggestibility. New York: Appleton-Cen-

tury, 1933. Pp. 416.

1869. Humphrey, M. E., and O. L.
Zangwill. Cessation of dreaming
after brain injury. J. Neurol.
Neurosurg. Psychiat., 14:322-25,
1951. 103

1870. Humphreys, R. J., and W. Raab.
Response of circulating eosinophils to nor-epinephrine, epinephrine, and emotional stress in humans. Proc. Soc. Exp. Biol. Med.,
74:302-3, 1950. 170

1871. Humphris, F. H. Biophysical
treatment in some nervous disorders: II. Insomnia. Brit. J.
Phys. Med., 9:69-70, 1934. 294

1872. Hunt, E. L. Encephalitis lethargica. Trans. Sect. Nerv. Ment. Dis.
A.M.A., 1920, pp. 178-85. 244

1873. Hunter, H. The treatment of epilepsy. Dis. Nerv. Syst., 9:203-9,
1948. 258

1874. Hunter, J. Further observations
on subcortically induced epileptic
attacks in unanesthetized animals.
EEG Clin. Neurophysiol., 2:193-
201, 1950. 259

1875. _____, and H. H. Jasper. Effect of
thalamic stimulation in anaesthe-
tized animals. EEG Clin. Neurophysiol., 1:305-24, 1949. 204, 210,
211, 259
Hunter, J., co-author: 1908, 1966,
2796.

1876. Husband, R. W. The comparative
value of continuous versus interrupted sleep. J. Exp. Psychol.,
18:792-96, 1935. 313

1877. _____. Sleep, work and food habits in the tropics. J. Gen. Psychol., 15:210-11, 1936. 313

1878. _____. Sex differences in dream
content. J. Abnorm. Soc. Psychol., 30:513-21, 1936. 101
Husband, R. W., co-author: 845.

1879. Hussels, H. Ueber konstitutionell
gebundene tageszeitliche Schwankungen der alimentaeren Hyper-
glykaemie und Insulinempfindlich-
keit. Pfluegers Arch., 248:74-90,
1944. 166

1880. Hutchison, R. Treatment of insomnia. Brit. Med. J., II:775-76,
1925. 275, 294

1881. Huter, C. Der Wert von Ruhe und
Schlaf. Schwaig bei Nuernberg:
Kupfer, 1955. Pp. 36.

1882. Huttenlocher, P. R. Effects of
state of arousal on click responses
in the mesencephalic reticular formation. EEG Clin. Neurophysiol.,
12:819-27, 1960; prelim. commun.

Fed. Proc., 19:188-13, 1960.
209

1883. _____. Evoked and spontaneous
activity in single units of mesencephalic reticular formation
during sleep. EEG Clin. Neurophysiol., 13:304, 1961. 212, 213

1884. _____. Evoked and spontaneous
activity in single units of medial
brain stem during natural sleep
and waking. J. Neurophysiol.,
24:451-68, 1961. 212, 213, 347
Huttenlocher, P. R., co-author:
1120, 1121, 1209.

1885. Hyde, J., and E. Gellhorn. Influence of deafferentation on stimulation of motor cortex. Am. J.
Physiol., 156:311-16, 1949. 96,
209

1886. Hyland, H. H. Disturbances of
sleep and their treatment. Med.
Clin. North Am., March 1952,
pp. 539-55. 278

1887. Hylkema, E. A. (Dutch) A Contribution to Knowledge of Narcolepsy. Assen: van Gorcum,
1940. Pp. 183. 234

1888. Iakovleva, E. A. (Russ.) The
teachings of I. P. Pavlov on
sleep inhibition. Feldsher Akush.
(Moskva), No. 1:14-19, 1953. 344

1889. Iampietro, P. F., D. E. Bass,
and E. R. Buskirk. Diurnal oxygen consumption and rectal temperature of man during continuous cold exposure. J. Appl.
Physiol., 10:398-400, 1957. 138

1890. _____, E. R. Buskirk, D. E. Bass,
and B. E. Welch. Effect of food,
climate, and exercise on rectal
temperature during the day. J.
Appl. Physiol., 11:349-52, 1957.
138, 191
Iampietro, P. F., co-author:
2274, 2275.

1891. Ichihara, M. Sensations experienced in dreams of the blind, particularly sensations of smell.
Otolaryngology (Tokyo), 31:617-
18, 1959. 102

1892. Ichinose, N. Autonomic nerve
and brain wave. (Report 1). Type
of the autonomic nervous tension
and the brain wave. Folia Psychiat. Neurol. Jap., 2:205-13,
1947.

1893. _____. Electroencephalogram
during the fever period caused
through the injection of typhoid
vaccine. Folia Psychiat. Neurol.
Jap., 3:129-36, 1949; 4:108-14,
1950.

1894. Ignesti, C., e F. Burci. Il sonno artificiale prolungato mediante ipnotici nel trattamento degli stati ansiosi e confusionali dei vecchi. Sett. Med. (Firenze), 42: 147-51, 1954. 207

1895. Ikin, A. G., T. H. Pear, and R. H. Thouless. The psycho-galvanic phenomenon in dream analysis. Brit. J. Psychol., 15:23-44, 1924. 103

1896. Ilg, F. L., and L. B. Ames. Child Behaviour. New York: Harper & Bros., 1955. Pp. xi + 364. 117

1897. Illing, E. Schlaftrunkenheitdelikte bei Soldaten. Dsch. Militaerarzt, 6:617-22, 1941. 271

1898. Illingworth, R. S. Sleep problems in the first three years. J. Roy. Inst. Publ. Health, 15:191-94, 1952; also Brit. Med. J., I:722-28, 1951. 286

1899. Inaba, C. Experimentalstudien am Nervensystem; zur zentralen Localisation von Stoerungen des Wachzustandes. Z. ges. exp. Med., 55:164-82, 1927. 205
Inaba, C., co-author: 3766.

1900. Inghirami, G., e G. Mannironi. Aspetti elettroencefalografici della narcolessia. Rass. Stud. Psichiat., 46:314-28, 1957. 238

1901. Ingle, D. J. The functional inter-relationship of the anterior pituitary and the adrenal cortex. Ann. Int. Med., 35:652-72, 1951. 356

1902. Ingram, W. R. Brain stem mechanisms in behavior. EEG Clin. Neurophysiol., 4:397-406, 1952.

1903. _____, R. W. Barris, and S. W. Ranson. Catalepsy. Arch. Neurol. Psychiat., 35:1175-97, 1936. 254

1904. _____, J. R. Knott, and W. D. Chiles. Diencephalic-cortical relationships: an EEG demonstration. EEG Clin. Neurophysiol., 3: 384, 1951. 209

1905. _____, _____, and M. D. Wheatley. Electroencephalograms of cats with hypothalamic lesions. EEG Clin. Neurophysiol., 1:523, 1949. 209

1906. _____, _____, _____, and T. D. Summers. Physiological relationships between hypothalamus and cerebral cortex. EEG Clin. Neurophysiol., 3:37-58, 1951. 209
Ingram, W. R., co-author: 2220-23, 3269.

1907. Ingvar, D. H. Extraneural influences upon the electrical activity of the reticular activating system. Acta Physiol. Scand., 33:169-93, 1955.

1908. _____, and J. Hunter. Influence of visual cortex on light impulses in the brain stem of the unanesthetized cat. Acta Physiol. Scand., 33:194-218, 1955. 211

1909. _____, T. Krakau, and U. Söderberg. The cerebral blood flow during different EEG responses elicited by brain stem stimulation. EEG Clin. Neurophysiol., 9:371, 1957. 209

1910. _____, and U. Söderberg. A new method for measuring cerebral blood flow in relation to the electroencephalogram. EEG Clin. Neurophysiol., 8:403-12, 1956. 291

1911. _____, and _____. Cortical blood flow related to EEG patterns evoked by stimulation of the brain stem. Acta Physiol. Scand., 42:130-43, 1958. 209

1912. Ingvar, S. (Swed.) About Sleep. A Book for Insomniacs and for Those Who Sleep Well. Lund: Gleerup, 1949. Pp. 62.

1913. Irwin, O. C. The amount and nature of activities of newborn infants under constant external stimulating conditions during the first ten days of life. Genet. Psychol. Monogr., 8:1-92, 1930.

1914. _____. The amount of motility of seventy-three newborn infants. J. Comp. Psychol., 14:415-28, 1932. 88

1915. _____. The distribution of the amount of motility in young infants between two nursing periods. J. Comp. Psychol., 14:429-45, 1932. 88

1916. Isakower, O. Beitrag zur Pathophysiologie der Einschlafphaenomenen. Internat. Z. Psychoanal., 22:466-77, 1936.

1917. _____. A contribution to the patho-psychology of phenomena associated with falling asleep. Internat. J. Psycho-anal., 19: 331-45, 1938. 79

1918. _____. Spoken words in dreams. Psychoanal. Q., 23:1-6, 1954. 101

1919. Ischlondsky, N. The role of the cortex in consciousness as learned from conditioned reflex studies. J. Nerv. Ment. Dis., 116:440-53, 1952. 31

1920. Iselin, H. Physiologische Foerderung des Einschlafens. Schweiz.

med. Wschr., 64:153, 1934. 312

1921. Isenschmid, R. Physiologie der Waermeregulation. Handb. norm. path. Physiol., 17:3-85, 1926. 138

1922. Israel, L. Essai pour servir d'introduction à l'étude du sommeil chez les malades mentaux. Cah. Psychiat., No. 12:18-36, 1957. Israel, L., co-author: 2071.

1923. Issel, W. Ueber laryngeales Schnarchen. Aerztl. Wschr., 7: 779-80, 1952. 49

1924. Ivanov, V. Le traitement de certaines psychoses par le sommeil de longue durée et interrompu. Psychiat. Neurol., Basel, 136: 380-92, 1958. 207 Ivanov, V., co-author: 4089.

1925. Ivanov-Smolensky, A. G. (Russ.) Experimental and clinical investigations in the domain of protective inhibition and prolonged therapeutic sleep. Zh. Vysshei Nerv. Deiat., 1(3):347-61, 1951; also in: The Sleep Problem, 1954 (392), pp. 361-74. 206, 344

1926. Ivy, A. C., and J. G. Schnedorf. On the hypnotoxin theory of sleep. Am. J. Physiol., 119:342, 1937. 203, 216, 256 Ivy, A. C., co-author: 3580.

1927. Iwase, Y. Electrophysiological problems on induced sleep. Monogr. Ser., Res. Inst. Appl. Electricity, No. 5, Sapporo, 1955, pp. 101-30. 204

1928. _____, and K. Yanazume. On the sleep response induced electrically in cats. Jap. J. Physiol., 5:420-25, 1956. 204

1929. Izzo, J. L. Diurnal (24-hour) rhythm in diabetes mellitus. 1. Diurnal variation in levels of glucose in blood and urine. Proc. Am. Diab. Ass., 9:247-70, 1949. 165

1930. Jacarelli, E. I disturbi del sonno nelle lesioni del mesencefalo. Policlinico (Sez. Med.), 39:452-66, 1932. 359

1931. Jackson, D. D. An episode of sleepwalking. J. Am. Psychoanal. Ass., 2:503-8, 1954. 283

1932. Jackson, J. H. Remarks on the relations of different divisions of the central nervous system to one another and to parts of the body. Brit. Med. J., I:65-69, 1898.

1933. Jackson, M. M. An evaluation of sleep motility criteria. Psychol. Bull., 38:693, 1941. 42, 87

1934. _____. Anticipatory cardiac acceleration during sleep. Science, 96:564-65, 1942. 42, 87

1935. Jacobson, E. Electrical measurements of neuromuscular states during mental activities. III. Visual imagination and recollection. Am. J. Physiol., 95: 694-702, 1930. 93, 94

1936. _____. Progressive Relaxation. Chicago: Univ. Chicago Press, 1938. Pp. 494. 311

1937. _____. You Can Sleep Well. The A B C's of Restful Sleep for the Average Person. New York: Whittlesey House, 1938. Pp. xix + 269. 94

1938. _____. You Must Relax. New York: Whittlesey House, 1942. Pp. xix + 261. 312

1939. _____, and A. J. Carlson. The influence of relaxation upon the knee-jerk. Am. J. Physiol., 73: 324-28, 1925. 15

1940. Jähninchen, S. Ueber Schlaftiefenmessungen. Uebersicht und Versuche im Kindesalter. Wuerzburg: Inaug. Diss., 1955. Pp. 132. 257 Jaehninchen, S., co-author: 4261.

1941. Jagot, P., et P. Oudinot. L'Insomnie Vaincue—L'Art de s'endormir Aisément Malgré le Bruit, les Préoccupations ou la Douleur. Paris: Henri Dangles, 1928. Pp. 174; similar to 1954 edition (3073). 274

1942. Jahr, H. M. Why can't I sleep? Hygeia (Chicago), 26:708-9, 742-43, 1948. 274

1943. Janecke, A. Ein Fall von postenzephalitischer Schlafstoerung. Dsche med. Wschr., 46:1388-89, 1920. 247

1944. Janet, P. A case of sleep lasting five years with loss of sense of reality. Arch. Neurol. Psychiat., 6:467-75, 1921. 286

1945. _____. Further report on case of sleep lasting 5 years with loss of sense of reality. Arch. Neurol. Psychiat., 37:1222-24, 1937. 286

1946. Janichewski, A. La conception biologique du sommeil. Encéphale, 28:184-96, 1933. 362

1947. Jann, W. Die Bedeutung gewisser Hormone bei lethargischen Zustaenden und Winterschlaf: Hypnose bei Froeschen. Helvet. Med. Acta, 4:355-70, 1937.

1948. Janota, O. Symptomatische Behandlung der pathologischen

Schlafsucht, besonders der Narkolepsie. Med. Klin., 27:278-81,
1931. 238, 300

1949. Janz, D. "Nacht-" oder "Schlaf-"
epilepsien als Ausdruck einer
Verlaufsform epileptischer Erkrankungen. Nervenarzt, 24:361-
67, 1953. 260

1950. Janzen, E. Ueber Narkolepsie
(Gélineau-Redlich). Z. ges. Neurol. Psychiat., 104:800-812,
1926. 235

1951. Janzen, R. Hirnbioelektrische
Untersuchungen ueber den physiologischen Schlaf und den
Schlafanfall bei Kranken mit ge-
nuiner Narkolepsie. Dsche Z.
Nervenheilk. 149:93-106, 1939.
238

1952. ____, und G. Behnsen. Beitrag
zur Pathophysiologie des An-
fallsgeschehens, insbesondere
des kataplektischen Anfalls beim
Narkolepsiesyndrom. Klinische
und hirnbioelektrische Untersuchung. Arch. Psychiat. Nervenkr.,
111:178-89, 1940. 238

1953. ____, und A. E. Kornmueller.
Hirnbioelektrische Erscheinungen bei Aenderung der Bewusstseinslage. Dsche Z. Nerveheilk.,
149:74-92, 1939. 31

1954. Jarcho, L. W. Excitability of cortical afferent systems during
barbiturate anesthesia. J. Neurophysiol., 12:447-57, 1949. 297

1955. Jarkowski, J. Quelques réflexions
sur le sommeil. Rev. Neurol.,
I:862-66, 1927. 362

1956. Jasper, H. H. Cortical excitatory
state and variability in human
brain rhythms. Science, 83:259-
60, 1936.

1957. ____. Cortical excitatory state
and synchronism in the control
of bioelectric autonomous
rhythms. Cold Spring Harbor
Symp. Quant. Biol., 4:320-32,
1936.

1958. ____. Charting the sea of brain
waves. Science, 108:343-47,
1948.

1959. ____. Diffuse projection systems: The integrative action of
the thalamic reticular system.
EEG Clin. Neurophysiol., 1:405-
20, 1949. 210

1960. ____. Functional properties of
the thalamic reticular system.
In: Brain Mechanisms and Consciousness, 1954 (875), pp. 374-
401. 210, 211

1961. ____, and C. Ajmone-Marsan.
Thalamo-cortical integrating
mechanisms. Res. Publ. Ass.
Nerv. Ment. Dis., 30:493-512,
1952. 210

1962. ____, ____, and J. Stoll. Corticofugal projections to the
brain stem. A.M.A. Arch. Neurol. Psychiat., 67:155-71, 1952.
29, 210

1963. ____, and H. L. Andrews.
Electro-encephalography. III.
Normal differentiation of occipital and precentral regions in
man. Arch. Neurol. Psychiat.,
39:96-115, 1938. 160

1964. ____, and J. Droogleever-Fortuyn. Experimental studies on
the functional anatomy of petit
mal epilepsy. Res. Publ. Ass.
Nerv. Ment. Dis., 26:272-98,
1947. 258

1965. ____, P. Gloor, and B. Milner.
Higher functions of the nervous
system. Ann. Rev. Physiol., 18:
359-86, 1956.

1966. ____, J. Hunter, and R. Knighton. Experimental studies of
thalamo-cortical systems.
Trans. Am. Neurol. Ass., 73:
210-12, 1948. 210

1967. ____, and C.-L. Li. Microelec-
trode studies of 'spontaneous'
and evoked potentials of cerebral cortex. Fed. Proc., 12:73,
1953. 296

1968. ____, R. Naquet, and E. E.
King. Thalamocortical recruiting responses in sensory receiving areas in the cat. EEG
Clin. Neurophysiol., 7:99-114,
1955. 210

1969. ____, and C. Shagass. Conditioning the occipital alpha rhythm
in man. J. Exp. Psychol., 28:373-
88, 1941.
Jasper, H. H., co-author: 159,
1622, 1875, 2060, 2507, 2886,
3328, 3672.

1970. Jefferson, G. The nature of con-
cussion. Brit. Med. J., I:1-5,
1944.

1971. ____. Applied physiology of
sleep. Brit. Med. J., II:151, 1954.
362

1972. ____, and R. T. Johnson. The
cause of loss of consciousness in
posterior fossa compressions.
Folia Psychiat. (Amsterdam),
53:306-19, 1950. 267

1973. Jefferson, M. Altered consciousness associated with brain-stem

lesions. Brain, 75:55-67, 1952. 206

1974. Jekels, L. A bioanalytical contribution to the problem of sleep and wakefulness. Psychoanal. Q., 14:169-89, 1945. 362

1975. Jelliffe, S. E. Discussion of tumors of the third ventricle. Arch. Neurol. Psychiat., 20: 1403, 1928. 348
Jelliffe, S. E., co-author: 3027.

1976. Jenkins, J. G., and K. M. Dallenbach. Oblivescence during sleeping and waking. Am. J. Psychol., 35:605-12, 1924. 124

1977. Jenness, A. The facilitation of sleeping hypnosis by previous motor response in the waking state. Psychol. Bull., 30:580, 1933.

1978. _____. A comparative study of sleep and hypnosis by means of the electrocardiograph and the pneumograph. Psychol. Bull., 31:712, 1934. 49, 329, 330

1979. _____. Salivary secretion under hypnosis. Psychol. Bull., 33:746-47, 1936.

1980. _____, and R. C. Hackman. Salivary secretion during hypnosis. J. Exp. Psychol., 22:58-66, 1938.

1981. _____, and C. L. Wible. Respiration and heart action in sleep and hypnosis. J. Gen. Psychol., 16:197-222, 1937. 41, 329, 330
Jenness, A., co-author: 4199.

1982. Jenny, E. Tagesperiodische Einfluesse auf Geburt und Tod. Schweiz. med. Wschr., 14:15-17, 1933.

1983. Jéquier, M. Hallucinations hypnagogiques. Rev. Méd. Suisse Rom., 60:530-39, 1940. 79

1984. Jindrová, M., B. Roth, J. Stein, and M. Zuklínová. (Czech.) EEG studies of intrasellar tumours infiltrating or causing pressure on the meso-diencephalic region with special regard to sleep activity. Českoslov. Neurol., 23: 79-89, 1960. 206

1985. Jochims, J. Schlafsucht als Auftakt zur Menarchie. Arch. Kinderheilk., 147:156-58, 1953. 270

1986. Johansen, K., and J. Krog. Diurnal body temperature variations and hibernation in the birchmouse, Sicista betulina. Am. J. Physiol., 196:1200-1204, 1959.
Johansen, K., co-author: 59.

1987. Johansson, J. E. Ueber die Tagesschwankungen des Stoffwechsels und der Koerpertemperatur in nuechternem Zustaende und vollstaendiger Muskelruhe. Skand. Arch. Physiol., 8:85-142, 1898. 138

1988. Johnson, F. H. A study of the cause of brain waves. Fed. Proc., 19:189-5, 1960.

1989. Johnson, G. Ephedrine in narcolepsy. J. Nerv. Ment. Dis., 79: 652-55, 1934. 235

1990. Johnson, G. E. Hibernation of the 13-lined ground squirrel, Citellus tridecemlineatus (Mitchell). I. A comparison of the normal and hibernating states. J. Exp. Zool., 50:15-30, 1928.

1991. _____. III. The rise in respiration, heart beat and temperature in waking from hibernation. V. Food, light, confined air, precooling, castration, and fatness in relation to production of hibernation. Biol. Bull., 57:107-29, 1929; 59:114-27, 1930. 321

1992. _____. Hibernation in mammals. Q. Rev. Biol., 6:439-61, 1931.

1993. _____, and V. B. Hanawalt. Hibernation of the 13-lined ground squirrel, Citellus tridecemlineatus. IV. Influence of thyroxine, pituitrin, and desiccated thymus and thyroid on hibernation. Am. Naturalist, 64:272-84, 1930. 326

1994. Johnson, G. T. Sleep as a specialized function. J. Abnorm. Soc. Psychol., 18:88-96, 1923. 99, 113, 361

1995. Johnson, H. M. An essay toward an adequate explanation of sleep. Psychol. Bull., 23:141-42, 1926. 362

1996. _____. The measurement of sleep. Hosp. Progr., 8:361-63, 1927. 82

1997. _____. Is sleep a vicious habit? Harper's, November 1928, pp. 3-11. 78, 82

1998. _____. Rhythms and patterns of nocturnal motility. Proc. Ninth Internat. Congr. Psychol., 1929, pp. 238-39. 311

1999. _____. Reading 23. In: Readings in Experimental Psychology, W. L. Valentine, Ed., New York: Harper & Bros., 1931, pp. 241-91. 78, 82, 91, 110

2000. _____. Improvement of memory by sleep. Science, Suppl. No. 82, Dec. 15, 1935.

2001. _____, and T. H. Swan. Sleep. Psychol. Bull., 27:1-39, 1930.

2002. _____, _____, and G. E. Weigand. Sleep. Psychol. Bull., 23:482-503, 1926. 82

2003. _____, _____, and _____. In what position do healthy people sleep? J. Am. Med. Ass., 94:2058-62, 1930. 8, 82, 91, 310

2004. _____, and G. E. Weigand. Some recent experiments bearing on the problems of sleep. Psychol. Bull., 24:165-66, 1927. 82, 308

2005. Johnson, M. S. Activity and distribution of certain wild mice in relation to biotic communities. J. Mammal., 7:245-47, 1926. 172, 173, 175

2006. _____. Effect of continuous light on periodic spontaneous activity of white-footed mice (Peromyscus). J. Exp. Zool., 82:315-28, 1939. 172

2007. Johnston, R. L., and H. Washeim. Studies in gastric secretion. II. Gastric secretion in sleep. Am. J. Physiol., 70:247-53, 1924. 54, 330
Johnston, R. L., co-author: 2572.

2008. Jolowitz, E. Consciousness in dream and in hypnotic state. Am. J. Psychotherapy, 1:2-24, 1947. 333

2009. Jones, M. S. Recurrent attacks of prolonged sleep: case. J. Neurol. Psychopath., 16:130-39, 1935. 34, 271

2010. Jones, R. A., G. O. McDonald, and J. H. Last. Reversal of diurnal variation in renal function in cases of cirrhosis with ascites. J. Clin. Investig., 31:326-34, 1952. 174

2011. Jones, S. E. Insomnia. Med. J. Australia, II:332-35, 1944. 274
Jones, S. E., co-author: 1867.

2012. Jong, H. de. Ueber Bulbocapnine-Katalepsie. Klin. Wschr., I:684-85, 1922. 253

2013. _____. (Dutch) Experimental catatonia. Psychiat. Neurol. Bl., 33:481-86, 1929. 253
Jong, H. de, co-author: 239, 1836.

2014. Jongbloed, J. Experimentelle Katatonie durch Unterdruck. Arch. Néerl. Physiol., 19:538-53, 1934. 254

2015. _____. Anoxie et catatonie expérimentale. Arch. Néerl. Physiol., 21:144-61, 1936. 254

2016. Jorda, M. Les centres méso-diencéphaliques du sommeil. Algiers: Thèse, 1948. Pp. 109. 206 215
Jorda, M., co-author: 2644.

2017. Jores, A. Die Urineinschraenkung in der Nacht. Dsch. Arch. klin. Med., 175:244-53, 1933. 166

2018. _____. Tag- und Nachtwechsel in seiner Wirkung auf den Menschen. Klin. Wschr., 12:1538-40, 1933.

2019. _____. Ueber den Einfluss des Lichtes auf die 24-Stundenperioden des Menschen. Dsch. Arch. klin. Med., 176:544-49, 1934. 172, 174

2020. _____. Den 24-Stundenperioden des Menschen. Med. Klin., Ii 100-71, 1934. 54, 162, 165

2021. _____. Untersuchungen ueber die rhythmische Taetigkeit der menschlichen Leber. Die 24-Stundenvariationen des Blutbilirubins, des Harnurobilinogens und des Harnfarbwertes. Z. klin. Med., 129:62-69, 1935. 165

2022. _____. Physiologie und Pathologie der 24-Stunden-Rhythmik des Menschen. Ergeb. inn. Med. Kinderheilk., 48:574-629, 1935. 162, 172, 182

2023. _____. Das Problem der Tagesperiodik in der Biologie. Med. Klin., 31:1139-42, 1935.

2024. _____. Die Tagesrhythmen in ihrer Bedeutung fuer die Hormontherapie. Med. Welt, 10:1542-45, 1936. 138, 162

2025. _____. Die 24-Stunden-Periodik in der Biologie. Tabulae Biol., 14(I):77-109, 1937. 162

2026. _____. Endocrines und vegetatives System in ihrer Bedeutung fuer die Tagesperiodik. Dsche med. Wschr., 64:989-90, 1938. 356

2027. _____. Die Ursache der Rhythmik vom Gesichtspunkt des Menschen. Dsche med. Wschr., 64:995-96, 1938. 132

2028. _____, und H. Beck. Die Nykturie als zentral bedingte Funktionsstoerung des vegetativen Systems Dsche Z. Nervenheilk., 138:4-16, 1935. 166

2029. _____, und J. Frees. Die Tagesschwankungen der Schmerzempfindung. Dsche med. Wschr., 63:962-63, 1937. 158

2030. _____, und H. Strutz. Untersuchungen ueber die 24-Stunden-Rhythmik der Blutsenkung unter

normalen und pathologischen Bedingungen. Dsche med. Wschr.,
62:92-96, 1936. 162

2031. Joseph, H., and G. Zern. The
Emotional Problems of Children.
New York: Crown, 1954. Pp. ix +
310.

2032. Josephson, B., und H. Larsson.
Ueber die Periodizitaet der Gallensekretion bei einem Patienten
mit'Gallenfistel. Skand. Arch.
Physiol., 69:227-36, 1934. 164

2033. Jouvet, M. Telencephalic and
rhombencephalic sleep in the cat.
In: A CIBA Found. Symposium
on the Nature of Sleep, 1961
(4270), pp. 188-206. 13, 27, 112,
212, 367

2034. ____, J. Dechaume, et F. Michel. Etude des mécanismes du
sommeil physiologique. Lyon
Méd., 204:479-521, 1960. 212

2035. ____, et F. Michel. Recherches
sur l'activité électrique cérébrale au cours du sommeil. C.
R. Soc. Biol., 152:1167-70, 1958.
23, 212

2036. ____, et ____. Corrélations
électromyographiques du sommeil chez le chat décortiqué et
mésencéphalique chronique. C.
R. Soc. Biol., 153:422-25, 1959.
23, 212

2037. ____, et ____. Sur les voies
nerveuses responsables de l'activité rapide corticale au cours
du sommeil physiologique chez
le chat (phase paradoxale). C. R.
Soc. Biol., 154:995-98, 1960. 212

2038. ____, et ____. Nouvelles recherches sur les structures responsables de la "phase paradoxale" du sommeil. J. Physiol.
(Paris), 52:130-31, 1960. 212

2039. ____, et ____. II. Interprétation neurophysiologique des aspects E.E.G. du sommeil en
fonction de l'existence des deux
systèmes inhibiteurs différents.
Rev. Neurol., 102:310-11, 1960;
also EEG Clin. Neurophysiol.,
12:537, 1960. 212

2040. ____, et ____. Déclenchement
de la "phase paradoxale" du sommeil par stimulation du tronc cérébral chez le chat intact et mésencéphalique chronique. C. R.
Soc. Biol., 154:636-41, 1960. 212

2041. ____, et ____. Mise en évidence d'un "centre hypnique" au
niveau du rhombencéphale chez
le chat. C. R. Acad. Sci., 251:

1188-90, 1960. 212

2042. ____, ____, et J. Courjon. Sur
la mise en jeu de deux mécanismes à expression électro-encéphalographique différente au
cours du sommeil physiologique
chez le chat. C. R. Acad. Sci.,
248:3043-45, 1959. 212

2043. ____, ____, et ____. L'activité électrique du rhinencéphale
au cours du sommeil chez le
chat. C. R. Soc. Biol., 153:101-
5, 1959. 212

2044. ____, ____, et ____. Sur un
stade d'activité électrique cérébrale rapide au cours du sommeil physiologique. C. R. Soc.
Biol., 153:1024-28, 1959. 212

2045. ____, ____, et ____. Aspects
électroencéphaliques de deux
mécanismes inhibiteurs, télen-
céphalique et rhombencépha-
lique, entrant en jeu au cours
du sommeil. J. Physiol. (Paris),
51:490-92, 1959. 212

2046. ____ E.E.G., ____, et ____. I. Etude
E.E.G. du sommeil physiolo-
gique chez le chat intact, décortiqué et mésencéphalique chronique. Rev. Neurol., 102:309-10,
1960; also EEG Clin. Neurophysiol., 12:536, 1960. 13, 212

2047. ____, ____, et D. Mounier.
Analyse électroencéphalographique comparée du sommeil
physiologique chez le chat et
chez l'homme. Rev. Neurol.,
103:189-204, 1960. 26, 27, 212

2048. ____, et D. Mounier. Effets
des lésions de la formation réticulée pontique sur le sommeil
du chat. C. R. Soc. Biol., 154:
2301-5, 1960. 212

2049. ____, and ____. Neurophysiological mechanisms of the oneiric activity. Aerospace Med.,
32:236-37, 1961. 212

2050. ____, B. Pellin, et D. Mounier.
Etude polygraphique des différentes phases du sommeil au
cours des troubles de conscience
chroniques (comas prolongés).
Rev. Neurol., 105:181-86, 1961;
also EEG Clin. Neurophysiol.,
14:138, 1962. 212, 273
Jouvet, M., co-author: 869, 1711,
1715.

2051. Jundell, J. Ueber die nyktemera-
len Temperaturschwankungen
im ersten Lebensjahre des Menschen. Jahrb. Kinderheilk., 59:
521-619, 1904. 138

2052. Jung, R. Das Elektroencephalo-gramm und seine klinische Anwendung. I. Methodik der Ableitung, Registrierung und Deutung des EEG. II. Das EEG des Gesunden, seine Variationen und Veraenderungen und deren Bedeutung fuer das pathologische EEG. Nervenarzt, 12:569-91, 1939; 14:57-70, 104-17, 1941. 238

2053. _____. Correlation of bioelectrical and autonomic phenomena with alterations of consciousness and arousal in man. In: Brain Mechanisms and Consciousness, 1954 (875), pp. 310-44. 31

2054. _____. Tierexperimentelle Grundlagen und EEG-Untersuchungen bei Bewusstseinsveraenderungen des Menschen ohne neurologische Erkrankungen. First Internat. Congr. Neurol. Sci., Seconde Journée Commune, Brussels: Acta Med. Belg., 1957, pp. 148-79. 31

2055. _____, O. Creutzfeldt, und O.-J. Gruesser. Die Mikrophysiologie kortikaler Neurone und ihre Bedeutung fuer die Sinnes- und Hirnfunktionen. Dsche med. Wschr., 82:1050-59, 1957. 362
Jung, R., co-author: 774, 777.

2056. Junger, G. Der Traumrhythmus; Ergebnisse einer statistischen Untersuchung. Schweiz. Z. Psychol. Anwend., 14:297-308, 1955.

2057. Jus, A., and K. Jusowa. (Polish) The methodological principles of electroencephalographic investigations concerning the process of internal inhibition; (its retardation and passage into sleep). Neurol. Neurochir. Psychiat. Polska, 3:595-604, 1953. 344

2058. _____, and _____. (Polish) Electroencephalographic analysis of the processes of internal inhibition (delaying and transition into sleep). Neurol. Neurochir. Psychiat. Polska, 4:23-46, 1954. 344

2059. Kaada, B. R. (Norw.) The anatomical substratum of consciousness in the light of recent neurophysiological studies. Nord. Med., 47:845-57, 1952.

2060. _____, and H. Jasper. Respiratory responses to stimulation of temporal pole, insular and hippocampal and limbic gyri in man. A.M.A. Arch. Neurol. Psychiat., 68:609-19, 1952.

2061. Kahn, W. W. Sleep and sleep disturbances. J. Michigan Med. Soc., 15:366-69, 1916. 277, 362

2062. Kaine, H. D., H. S. Seltzer, and J. W. Conn. Mechanism of diurnal eosinophil rhythm in man. J. Lab. Clin. Med., 45:247-52, 1955. 169, 170

2063. Kajtor, F. Some anatomo-functional factors which may predispose to epileptic seizures occurring during sleep. EEG Clin. Neurophysiol., 13:400-410, 1961. 260

2064. _____, T. Nagy, und Gy. Velok. Ueber die Zusammenhaenge der Anfaelle im Schlaf und Wachzustand mit anatomisch-funktionellen Organisation des epileptogenen Herdes. Acta Med. Acad. Sci. Hungar., 12:239-54, 1958. 260

2065. Kalbian, V. Treatment of insomnia in left ventricular heart failure. J. Palestine Arab. Med. Ass., 1:180-83, 1946. 277

2066. Kalter, S., und C. Katzenstein. Ueber die Bedeutung des intermediaeren Alkohols fuer Schlaf und Narkose. Muench. med. Wschr., 79:793-94, 1932. 162, 353

2067. Kamensky, D. A. (Russ.) Effect of a short natural sleep on the restoration of conditioned reflex activity of the brain of the dog. Trudy Fiziol. Lab. Pavlova, 9: 417-25, 1940; also in: The Sleep Problem, 1954 (392), pp. 113-21. 198

2068. Kaminsky, S. D. (Russ.) Sleep and its curative role in the light of Pavlov's teachings on protective inhibition. Soviet. Med., 13(9):12-14, 1949. 206

2069. Kamiya, J. Behavioral, subjective, and physiological aspects of drowsiness and sleep. In: The Functions of Varied Experience, D. W. Fiske and S. R. Maddi, Eds., Homewood, Ill.: Dorsey Press, 1961, pp. 145-74. 21, 98, 282

2070. Kamman, G. R. Insomnia. Minnesota Med., 18:143-47, 1935. 307

2071. Kammerer, T., L. Israel, et P. Geissmann. Etude objective du sommeil chez lez malades mentaux. Présentation de la méthode et premiers résultats. Cah. Psychiat., No. 12:37-50, 1957. 86

2072. Kanner, L. The influence of rest, sleep and work on action of heart. Am. J. Med. Sci., 171: 331-40, 1926. 41

2073. _____. Child Psychiatry. Springfield, Ill.: Thomas, 1935. Pp. 527. 281

2074. Kant, O. Dreams of schizophrenic patients. J. Nerv. Ment. Dis., 95:335-47, 1942. 103

2075. Kanzer, M. G. The therapeutic use of dreams induced by hypnotic suggestion. Psychoanal. Q., 14:313-35, 1945. 335

2076. Kaplinsky, M. S. Anfaelle von kurzweiligen Einschlafen bei Transportfuehrern. Z. ges. Neurol. Psychiat., 147:101-8, 1933.

2077. _____, und E. D. Schulmann. Ueber die periodische Schlafsucht. Acta Med. Scand., 85:107-28, 1935. 270

2078. _____, und _____. Ueber die periodische Schlaefrigkeit und periodische Schlafanfaelle. Acta Med. Scand., 85:346-76, 1935.

2079. Karapetian, E. A. (Russ.) Role of protective sleep inhibition in narcolepsy and other forms of pathology of sleep. Trudy Inst. Fiziol. Pavlova, 1:381-93, 1952. 239, 241, 344
Karapetian, E. A., co-author: 74.

2080. Karger, P. Unsere heutigen Kenntnisse ueber den Schlaf. Fortschr. Med., 42:237-39, 1924. 88, 113

2081. _____. Ueber den Schlaf des Kindes. Abhandl. Kinderheilk. Grenzgebiet., 1925, pp. 1-50. 88, 89, 307

2082. Karmos, G., and E. Grastyán. An electrophysiological study of the sleep. EEG Clin. Neurophysiol., 12:933, 1960. 27, 211, 212
Karmos, G., co-author: 1505.

2083. Karnosh, L. J. The treatment of insomnia. J. Am. Med. Ass., 113:1322-26, 1939. 278

2084. Karplus, J. P., und A. Kreidl. Ueber Totalexstirpationen einer und beider Grosshirnhemisphaeren an Affen (Macacus rhesus). Arch. Anat. Physiol., 155-212, 1914. 23

2085. Kartun, P. Intérêt et difficultés de la cure de sommeil dans la maladie hypertensive essentielle. In: La Cure de Sommeil, 1954 (3021), pp. 137-48. 207

2086. Kasatkin, V. N. (Russ.) On the influence of stimuli, acting on a sleeping person, on the content of his dreams. Pop. Psikhol.,

4(4):58-59, 1958. 104

2087. Kasyanov, V. M. (Russ.) Sleep, Dreams, and Hypnosis in the Light of the Teaching of I. P. Pavlov. Moskva: Pravda, 1950. Pp. 37. 344

2088. Katan, M. Dream and psychosis: their relationship to hallucinating processes. Internat. J. Psycho-anal., 41:341-51, 1960. 106

2089. Katsch, G., und H. Pansdorf. Die Schlafbewegung des Blutdrucks. Muench. med. Wschr., 69:1715-18, 1922. 43, 44, 45, 109

2090. Katz, S. E., and C. Landis. Psychologic and physiologic phenomena during a prolonged vigil. Arch. Neurol. Psychiat., 34: 307-16, 1935. 225

2091. Katzenelbogen, S. The distribution of calcium between blood and cerebrospinal fluid in sleep induced by diallylbarbituric acid. Arch. Neurol. Psychiat., 27:154-58, 1932. 201

2092. _____. Calcium content of the brain and its distribution in various regions during diallybarbituric acid narcosis. Arch. Neurol. Psychiat., 28:405-12, 1932. 35, 201

2093. _____, and M. C. Meehan. The chemistry of the blood and the cerebrospinal fluid, with special reference to calcium, in the cataleptoid state induced by bulbocapnine. J. Pharmacol. Exp. Therap., 47:131-39, 1933. 254
Katzenelbogen, S., co-author: 736

2094. Kaye, G. Studies in the reaction of urine. Austral. J. Exp. Biol. Med., 6:187-214, 1929. 65, 167

2095. Kawakami, M., and C. H. Sawyer. Induction of behavioral and electroencephalographic changes in the rabbit by hormone administration or brain stimulation. Neuroendocrine correlates of changes in brain activity thresholds by sex steroids and pituitary hormones. Endocrinology, 65:631-43; 652-68, 1959. 209
Kawakami, M., co-author: 3531.

2096. Kayser, C. Echanges respiratoires des hibernants à l'état de sommeil hibernal. Ann. Physiol. Physicochim. Biol., 16:127-221, 1940. 323, 324

2097. _____. Essai d'analyse du mécanisme du sommeil hibernal.

Ann. Physiol. Physicochim. Biol., 16:313-72, 1940. 321

2098. _____. A propos de l'hiérarchisation des centres respiratoires bulbaires. Arch. Phys. Biol. (Paris), 15, Suppl. 51:4-6, 1941. 323

2099. _____. Le sommeil. J. Physiol. (Paris), 41:1A-53A, 1949.

2100. _____. Le sommeil hibernal. Biol. Rev., 25:255-82, 1950. 328

2101. _____. La léthargie hibernale des mammifères et le mécanisme de sa genèse. Mammalia, 14: 105-25, 1950. 321

2102. _____. Le sommeil. Strasbourg Méd., 2:366-81, 1951. 99

2103. _____. Les échanges respiratoires du Hamster doré (Mesocricetus auratus) en léthargie hivernale. C. R. Soc. Biol., 146: 929-32, 1952. 324

2104. _____. L'hibernation des mammifères. Année Biol., 29:109-50, 1953. 322

2105. _____. Recherches physiologiques sur l'hypothermie des mammifères et des hibernants. Arch. Anat. Histol. Embryol., 37:97-103, 1954. 327

2106. _____. Hibernation et hypothermie des mammifères. Acta Neuroveget. (Wien), 11:38-59, 1955. 327

2107. _____. Hibernation et hibernation artificielle. Rev. Path. Gén. (Paris), 55:704-29, 1955. 328

2108. _____. Le sommeil hivernal et les glandes surrénales. Etude faite sur le hamster ordinaire, Cricetus cricetus. C. R. Soc. Biol., 151:982-85, 1957. 325

2109. _____. Le sommeil hivernal, problème de thermorégulation. Rev. Canad. Biol., 16:303-89, 1957. 325, 326

2110. _____. Résistance à l'hypothermie profonde chez les mammifères hibernants et chez les mammifères homéothermes. C. R. Soc. Biol., 152:1198-201, 1958. 328

2111. _____. Les échanges respiratoires du hamster ordinaire (Cricetus cricetus) et du lérot (Eliomys quercinus) en hibernation. C. R. Soc. Biol., 153:167-70, 1959. 324

2112. _____, et M. Aron. Le cycle saisonnier des glandes endocrines chez les hibernants. Arch. Anat. Histol. Embryol.,

33:21-42, 1950. 325

2113. _____, et G. Hiebel. L'hibernation naturelle et artificielle des hibernants et l'hypothermie généralisée expérimentale du rat et de quelques hibernants. Presse Méd., 60:1699-702, 1952. 327

2114. _____, F. Lachiver, et M. L. Rietsch. La consommation d'oxygène et la fréquence cardiaque du lérot (Eliomys quercinus). C. R. Soc. Biol., 152:1810-12, 1958.

2115. _____, et A. Petrovic. Rôle du cortex surrénalien dans le mécanisme du sommeil hivernal. C. R. Soc. Biol., 152:519-22, 1958. 325

2116. _____, M.-L. Rietsch, et M.-A. Lucot. Les échanges respiratoires et la fréquence cardiaque des hibernants au cours du réveil de leur sommeil hivernal. Recherches physiologiques sur l'incrément thermique critique. Arch. Sci. Physiol. (Paris), 8: 155-93, 1954.

2117. _____, F. Rohmer, et G. Hiebel. L'E.E.G. de l'hibernant. Léthargie et réveil spontané du spermophile. Essai de reproduction de l'E.E.G. chez le spermophile réveilé et le rat blanc. Rev. Neurol., 84:570-78, 1951. 324
Kayser, C., co-author: 135, 328, 571, 572, 890, 961, 962, 1136, 1762, 2787, 3397.

2118. Kearney, J. A. Drowsiness. New York Med. J. Med. Rec., 119: 247-48, 1924.

2119. Keeser, E., und J. Keeser. Ueber die Lokalisation des Veronals, der Phenylaethyl- und Diallylbarbitursaeure im Gehirn. Arch. exp. Path. Pharmakol., 125:251-56, 1927. 295, 297

2120. _____, und _____. Ueber den Nachweis von Coffein, Morphin und Barbitursaeurederivaten im Gehirn (Beitrag zum Schlafproblem. II). Arch. exp. Path. Pharmakol., 127:230-35, 1928. 295, 361

2121. Keir, G. An experiment in mental testing during hypnosis. J. Ment. Sci., 91:346-52, 1945. 331

2122. Kellaway, P. The use of sedative-induced sleep as an aid to electroencephalographic diagnosis in children. J. Pediat., 37:

862-77, 1950; prelim. commun., EEG Clin. Neurophysiol., 2:361, 1950. 257

2123. _____. The interpretation of sleep tracings in infants and young children. EEG Clin. Neurophysiol., 3:103, 1951. 257

2124. _____. The development of sleep spindles and of arousal patterns in infants and their characteristics in normal and certain abnormal states. EEG Clin. Neurophysiol., 4:369, 1952. 29

2125. _____. The electroencephalogram in infancy and childhood. EEG Clin. Neurophysiol., Suppl. 4:211-12, 1953. 27, 28

2126. _____. Ontogenetic evolution of the electrical activity of the brain in man and in animals. First Internat. Congr. Neurol. Sci., Brussels: Acta Med. Belg., 1957, pp. 141-54. 27, 28, 76

2127. _____, and B. J. Fox. Electroencephalographic diagnosis of cerebral pathology in infants during sleep. I. Rationale, technique, and the characteristics of normal sleep in infants. J. Pediat., 41:262-87, 1952. 27

2128. Keller, H. Neuerscheinungen ueber Schlaf und Traum. Z. angew. Psychol., 41:517-18, 1932. 99

2129. Kelly, C. P. The Natural Way to Healthful Sleep. New York: Hawthorn Books, 1961. Pp. 223.

2130. Kelman, H. A new approach to dream interpretation. Am. J. Psychoanal., 4:89-107, 1944. 106

2131. Kelting, L. S. An investigation of the feeding, sleeping, crying and social behavior of infants. J. Exp. Educ., 3:97-106, 1934. 9

2132. Kennard, M. A. Electroencephalogram of decorticate monkeys. J. Neurophysiol., 6:233-42, 1943.

2133. _____. Effects on EEG of chronic lesions of basal ganglia, thalamus and hypothalamus of monkeys. J. Neurophysiol., 6:405-15, 1943.

2134. _____. The cingulate gyrus in relation to consciousness. J. Nerv. Ment. Dis., 121:34-39, 1955.

2135. _____. EEG changes occurring with drowsiness in emotionally disturbed children. EEG Clin. Neurophysiol., 13:305, 1961. 197, 272

2136. _____, A. E. Schwartzman, and

T. P. Millar. Sleep, consciousness, and alpha electroencephalographic rhythm. A.M.A. Arch. Neurol. Psychiat., 79:328-35, 1958.

2137. Kennedy, A. Brain structure and moral values. Advancement Sci., 7:53-56, 1950.

2138. Kennedy, F. Sleep. New York State J. Med., 36:1347-48, 1936. 312

Kennedy, F., co-author: 4281.

2139. Kennedy, J. L., R. M. Gottsdanker, J. C. Armington, and F. E. Gray. A new electroencephalogram associated with thinking. Science, 108:527-29, 1948.

2140. _____, and R. C. Travis. Prediction of speed of performance by muscle action potentials. Science, 105:410-11, 1947. 72, 197

2141. _____, and _____. Prediction and control of alertness. II. Continuous tracking. J. Comp. Physiol. Psychol., 41:203-10, 1948. 72, 197

Kennedy, J. L., co-author: 640, 641, 3968.

2142. Kerbikov, O. V. Treatment of mental disease by sleep. Lancet, I:744-45, 1955. 206

2143. Kernodle, C. E., Jr., H. C. Hill, and K. S. Grimson. Experimental technic for measuring mean systolic blood pressure during activity, rest, and natural sleep. Proc. Soc. Exp. Biol. Med., 55: 64-66, 1944. 42

2144. _____, _____, and _____. Effect of activity, rest, and natural sleep upon blood pressure of renal hypertensive dogs. Proc. Soc. Exp. Biol. Med., 63:335-36, 1946. 42

2145. Kerr, A. C. The effect of mental stress on the eosinophil leucocyte count in man. Q. J. Exp. Physiol., 41:18-24, 1956. 170

2146. Kershman, J. "The borderline of epilepsy"; a reconsideration. Arch. Neurol. Psychiat., 62: 551-59, 1949.

2147. Keschner, M. Presentation of a case of polycythemia with nervous symptoms. J. Nerv. Ment. Dis., 54:141-43, 1921. 277

2148. Kety, S. S. Consciousness and the metabolism of the brain. In: Problems of Consciousness, III, 1952 (4), pp. 11-75. 47, 51, 56, 272

2149. _____. Biochemical theories of schizophrenia. Science, 129: 1528-32, 1590-96, 1959. Kety, S. S., co-author: 1500, 2649, 4136.

2150. Key, B. J., and P. B. Bradley. The effects of drugs on conditioning and habituation to arousal stimuli in animals. Psychopharmacologica, 1:450-62, 1960; prelim. commun., Nature, 182: 1517-19, 1958. 301, 303 Key, B. J., co-author: 447, 448.

2151. Khait, M. B. (Russ.) On diencephalic insufficiency. Zh. Nevropat. Psikhiat., 24(4):16-23, 1931. 240

2152. Kikuchi, S. Verhalten der vegetativen Nerven im Schlaf. Verhandl. jap. Gesellsch. inn. Med., 23:1, 1926. 357

2153. Killam, K. F. Pharmacological influences upon evoked electrical activity in the brain. In: Psychotropic Drugs, 1957 (1357), pp. 244-51. 302 Killam, K. F., co-author: 3051.

2154. Kiloh, L. G., and J. W. Osselton. Clinical Electroencephalography. London: Butterworths, 1961. Pp. ix + 135. 28, 32

2155. _____, J. N. Walton, J. W. Osselton, and J. Farrell. On the significance of the sharp wave occurring at the vertex during the early stages of sleep. EEG Clin. Neurophysiol., 5:621, 1953. 257

2156. Kimmins, C. W. Children's Dreams. An Unexplored Land. London: George Allen & Unwin, 1937. Pp. 121. 102

2157. King, C. D. Electrometric studies of sleep. J. Gen. Psychol., 35:131-59, 1946. 32

2158. _____. Dream and the problem of consciousness. J. Gen. Psychol., 37:15-24, 1947. 106

2159. King, E. E., R. Naquet, and H. W. Magoun. Alterations in somatic afferent transmission through the thalamus by central mechanisms and barbiturates. J. Pharmacol. Exp. Therap., 119:48-63, 1957. 298 King, E. E., co-author: 1282, 1968.

2160. King, P. D. Hypnosis and schizophrenia. J. Nerv. Ment. Dis., 125:481-86, 1957. 336

2161. Kingman, R. The insomniac. New York Med. J. Med. Rec., 129: 683-87; 130:17-21, 1929. 274, 307

2162. Kirchhoff, H. W., und B. Fröhlich. Elektroencephalographische Untersuchungen ueber den Schlaf des Saeuglings. Arch. Psychiat. Nervenkr. (Berlin), 189:341-54, 1952. 27

2163. Kirikae, T., J. Wada, Y. Naoe, and O. Furuya. Clinico-physiological and bio-physiological studies of thalamus in man. Electrothalamographic studies. Folia Psychiat. Neurol. Jap., 7: 181-201, 1953. 210 Kirikae, T., co-author: 3047.

2164. Kirk, E. Untersuchungen ueber den Einfluss des normalen Schlafes auf die Temperatur der Fuesse. Skand. Arch. Physiol., 61:71-78, 1931. 62

2165. Kirstein, L. Suppression-burst activity during sleep. EEG Clin. Neurophysiol., 6:671-73, 1954. 29 Kirstein, L., co-author: 313.

2166. Kisselev, P. A., and F. P. Mayorov. (Russ.) Measuring motor chronaxie as a method for the study of somnial inhibition in man. Fiziol. Zh. SSSR, 27:290-98, 1939. 14

2167. _____, and _____. (Russ.) The phenomenon of equalization of the chronaxies of antagonists during sleep in man. Fiziol. Zh. SSSR, 27:299-308, 1939. 14

2168. _____, and _____. (Russ.) Alterations of motor chronaxie in the course of natural sleep in healthy human subjects. Fiziol. Zh. SSSR, 27:309-15, 1939. 14

2169. Kjos, K. (Norw.) Sleep disturbances as a school-hygiene problem in North Norway; an investigation of living habits and sleep-rate among school children in Tromsø. Tskr. Norske Laegeforen. (Oslo), 78:1241-45, 1958. 192

2170. Klar, E. Zur Kenntnis des Chemismus im Winterschlaf. Z. ges. exp. Med., 104:105-15, 1938. 323

2171. _____. Beitraege zur Biologie des Winterschlafes. Z. ges. exp. Med., 109:505-16, 1941. 326

2172. Klaue, R. Die bioelektrische Taetigkeit der Grosshirnrinde im normalen Schlaf und in der Narkose durch Schlafmittel. J. Psychol. Neurol., 47:510-31, 1937. 26, 295

2173. Klein, D. B. Experimental pro-

duction of dreams during hypnosis. Univ. Texas Bull., No. 3009,
1930. Pp. 71. 100, 334

2174. Kleinholz, L. H. Studies in the
pigmentary system of crustacea.
I. Color changes and diurnal
rhythm in Ligia baudiniana.
Biol. Bull., 72:24-36, 1937. 175

2175. Kleinsorge, H., K. Rösner, und
S. Dressler. Experimentelle Untersuchungen ueber den Elektro-
schlaf. Arch. phys. Therap.
(Leipzig), 9:20-24, 1957. 299

2176. Kleitman, N. The effects of prolonged sleeplessness on man.
Am. J. Physiol., 66:67-92, 1923.
5, 12, 15, 16, 17, 40, 44, 64, 65,
66, 167, 196, 220, 348

2177. ____. The effects of muscular
activity, rest and sleep on the
urinary excretion of phosphorus.
Am. J. Physiol., 74:225-37, 1925.
64, 66, 167, 168, 169

2178. ____. Studies on the physiology
of sleep. V. Some experiments on
puppies. Am. J. Physiol., 84:386-
95, 1927. 12, 15, 16, 195, 216

2179. ____. Sleep. Physiol. Rev., 9:
624-65, 1929. 5

2180. ____. The effect of continued
stimulation and of sleep upon
conditioned salivation. Am. J.
Physiol., 94:215-19, 1930. 198,
344

2181. ____. New methods for studying motility during sleep. Proc.
Soc. Exp. Biol. Med., 29:389-91,
1932. 83, 89

2182. ____. Diurnal variation in performance. Am. J. Physiol., 104:
449-56, 1933. 150

2183. ____. The modifiability of the
diurnal pigmentary rhythm in
isopods. Biol. Bull., 78:403-6,
1940. 175

2184. ____. A scientific solution of
the multiple shift problem. Min-
ing Congr. J., 29(I):15-16, 1943.
316, 317

2185. ____. The effect of motion pictures on body temperature. Science, 101:507-8; 102:430-31,
1945. 145

2186. ____. Biological rhythms and
cycles. Physiol. Rev., 29:1-30,
1949. 131, 172

2187. ____. The sleep-wakefulness
cycle in submarine personnel.
In: Human Factors in Undersea
Warfare. Washington: Nat. Res.
Council, 1949, pp. 329-41. 316

2188. ____. Mental hygiene of sleep

in children. Nerv. Child, 8:63-
66, 1949. 307

2189. ____. The sleep-wakefulness
cycle. In: Problems of Consciousness, I, 1950 (4), pp. 15-
60.

2190. ____. The role of the cerebral
cortex in the development and
maintenance of consciousness.
In: Problems of Consciousness,
V, 1954 (4), pp. 111-32. 30

2191. ____. Sleep, wakefulness, and
consciousness. Psychol. Bull.,
54:354-59, 1957. 4, 30

2192. ____, and N. Camille. Studies
on the physiology of sleep. VI.
Behavior of decorticated dogs.
Am. J. Physiol., 100:474-80,
1932. 22

2193. ____, N. R. Cooperman, and F.
J. Mullin. Motility and body
temperature during sleep. Am.
J. Physiol., 105:574-84, 1933.
59, 83, 89, 122, 187, 189

2194. ____, and A. Doktorsky. The
effect of the position of the body
and of sleep on rectal temperature in man. Am. J. Physiol.,
104:340-43, 1933. 58, 67

2195. ____, and T. G. Engelmann.
Diurnal cycle in activity and
body temperature of rabbits.
Fed. Proc., 6:143, 1947. 138,
149

2196. ____, and ____. Sleep characteristics of infants. J. Appl.
Physiol., 6:269-82, 1953; prelim. commun. Fed. Proc., 10:
73, 1951. 115, 133, 135, 137

2197. ____, and D. P. Jackson. Body
temperature and performance
under different routines. J.
Appl. Physiol., 3:309-28, 1950;
also Nav. Med. Res. Inst. (Bethesda, Maryland) Rep., Proj.
NM 004 005.01.02, 15 Feb. 1950.
Pp. 27. 157

2198. ____, and E. Kleitman. Effect
of non-twenty-four-hour routines of living on oral temperature and heart rate. J. Appl.
Physiol., 6:283-91, 1953; prelim. commun. Fed. Proc., 11:
83, 1952. 182

2199. ____, and H. Kleitman. The
sleep-wakefulness pattern in
the Arctic. Sci. Monthly, 76:
349-56, 1953. 192

2200. ____, F. J. Mullin, N. R. Coop-
erman, and S. Titelbaum. Sleep
Characteristics. Chicago: Univ.
Chicago Press, 1937. Pp. 86. 78,

90, 99, 119, 124, 185, 186, 187, 296, 308, 311, 312

2201. _____, and A. Ramsaroop. Body temperature and cutaneous sensitivity to tingling and pain. Fed. Proc., 5:56, 1946. 159, 196

2202. _____, and _____. Periodicity in body temperature and heart rate. Endocrinology, 43:1-20, 1948. 145, 163, 173, 174, 186

2203. _____, _____, and T. Engelmann. Variations in skin temperatures of the feet and hands and the onset of sleep. Fed. Proc., 7:66, 1948. 73

2204. _____, and J. S. Schreider. Diurnal variation in oculomotor performance. Année Psychol., 50: 201-15, 1951. 72, 158

2205. _____, S. Titelbaum, and P. Feiveson. The effect of body temperature on reaction time. Am. J. Physiol., 121:495-501, 1938. 153

2206. _____, _____, and H. Hoffmann. The establishment of the diurnal temperature cycle. Am. J. Physiol., 119:48-54, 1937; prelim. commun. Am. J. Physiol., 113: 82, 1935. 138, 144 Kleitman, N., co-author: 148-50, 366, 753, 901, 902, 2400, 2942-44, 3287.

2207. Klemperer, E., und M. Weissmann. Beitrag zur somatischen Reaktionsweise Hypnotisierter. Mschr. Psychiat. Neurol., 71: 356-65, 1929. 330

2208. Kletzkin, M., and F. M. Berger. Effect of meprobamate on limbic system of the brain. Proc. Soc. Exp. Biol. Med., 100:681-83, 1959. 302

2209. Klewitz, F. Der Puls im Schlaf. Dsch. Arch. klin. Med., 112:38-55, 1913. 41

2210. _____. Der Mechanismus der Herzaktion im Schlafe. Dsch. Arch. klin. Med., 130:212-20, 1919. 41

2211. Kline, M. V. Hypnotic retrogression: a neurophysiological theory of age regression and progression. J. Clin. Exp. Hypn., 1:21-28, 1953. 333 Kline, M. V., co-author: 947.

2212. Kliorin, A. I. (Russ.) On physiological sleep and its disturbances in infants. In: The Sleep Problem, 1954 (392), pp. 196-201. 88

2213. Kloek, J. Light and the diencephalon; a comparative biological treatise. Folia Psychiat. Neurol.

Neurochir. Neerl., 57:411-28, 1954. 356

2214. Klopp, H. W., und H. Selbach. Ueber die Gueltigkeit der Ausgangswertregel beim Epileptiker. Dsche Z. Nervenheilk, 167: 130-42, 1951. 257

2215. Knapp, A. Die epileptischen Daemmerzustaende. Arch. Psychiat. Nervenkr., 111:322-40, 1940. 31

2216. Knapp, P. H. Sensory impressions in dreams. Psychoanal. Q., 25:325-47, 1956. 102

2217. Knott, J. R., F. A. Gibbs, and C. E. Henry. Fourier transforms of electroencephalogram during sleep. J. Exp. Psychol., 31:465-77, 1942.

2218. _____, R. Hayne, and H. R. Meyers. Physiology of sleep: wave characteristics and temporal relations of human electroencephalograms simultaneously recorded from the thalamus, the corpus striatum, and the surface of the scalp. Arch. Neurol. Psychiat., 63:526-27, 1950.

2219. _____, C. E. Henry, and J. M. Hadley. Brain potentials during sleep: A comparative study of the dominant and non-dominant alpha groups. J. Exp. Psychol., 24:157-68, 1939. 28

2220. _____, and W. R. Ingram. EEG in cats with thalamic, hypothalamic and mesencephalic lesions. EEG Clin. Neurophysiol., 3:373-74, 1951. 210

2221. _____, and _____. The EEGs of cats with thalamic lesions. EEG Clin. Neurophysiol., 3:379, 1951. 210

2222. _____, _____, and W. D. Chiles. Effects of subcortical lesions on cortical electroencephalogram in cats. A.M.A. Arch. Neurol. Psychiat., 73:203-15, 1955.

2223. _____, _____, M. D. Wheatley, and T. D. Summers. Hypothalamic influence on cortical activity. EEG Clin. Neurophysiol., 3: 102, 1951. 206 Knott, J. R., co-author: 932, 1430, 1904-6, 3000.

2224. Koch, E. Ueber den depressorischen Gefaessreflex beim Karotisdruckversuch am Menschen. Muench. med. Wschr., 71:704-5, 1924. 241

2225. _____. Die Irradiation der pres-

soreceptorischen Kreislaufre-
flexe. Klin. Wschr., 11:225-27,
1932. 241

2226. Köhler, F. Hygiene des Schlafes.
Fortschr. Med., 50:309-10, 1932.
294, 307

2227. Koella, W. P., and H. M. Ballin.
The influence of environmental
and body temperature on the electroencephalogram in the anesthetized cat. Arch. Internat. Physiol.,
62:369-80, 1954. 160, 327
Koella, W. P., co-author: 33,
1391, 1727-29, 2971.

2228. Kohlschütter, E. Messungen der
Festigkeit des Schlafes. Z. ra-
tion. Med., 17:209-53, 1862. 108,
313

2229. Kolder, H. Verhalten von Koerpertemperatur und Schlafdauer
bei verschiedener Raumtemperatur. Z. Biol. (Berlin), 109:185-
91, 1957.

2230. _____. Extrarenale und renale
Wasserabgabe im Schlaf bei 37°
C. Raumtemperatur und Flues-
sigkeitzufuhr. Z. Biol. (Berlin),
109:192-96, 1957.

2231. Kolle, K., und M. Mikorey. Kuenst-
licher Winterschlaf in der Psychiatrie. Dsche med. Wschr., 78:
1723-24, 1953. 207

2232. Kolodny, A. The symptomatology
of tumors of the temporal lobe.
Brain, 51:385-417, 1928. 265

2233. Komarov, F. I. (Russ.) On the
secretory activity of the digestive glands during sleep. Klin.
Med. (Moskva), 29(9):45-51,
1951; also in: The Sleep Problem, 1954 (392), pp. 332-40. 54

2234. _____. (Russ.) Secretory Activity
of the Digestive Glands in Man
during Sleep. Leningrad: Medgiz,
1953. Pp. 81. 54

2235. Koppanyi, T., and J. M. Dille.
Remarks on the distribution of
barbiturates in the brain. J.
Pharmacol. Exp. Therap., 54:84-
86, 1935. 295

2236. _____, _____, and A. Krop. Distribution of barbiturates in the
brain. J. Pharmacol. Exp. Therap., 52:121-28, 1934. 295, 297
Koppanyi, T., co-author: 762.

2237. Koranyi, E. K., and H. E. Lehmann. Experimental sleep deprivation in schizophrenic patients.
A.M.A. Arch. Gen. Psychiat., 2:
534-44, 1960. 226

2238. Kornmüller, A. E. Die bioelek-
trischen Erscheinungen architek-

tonischer Felder der Grosshirnrinde. Biol. Rev., 10:383-422,
1935. 27
Kornmüller, A. E., co-author:
1953.

2239. Kornetsky, C. Effects of meprobamate, phenobarbital, and
dextro-amphetamine on reaction
time and learning in man. J.
Pharmacol. Exp. Therap., 123:
216-19, 1958. 302

2240. _____, A. F. Mirsky, E. K. Kessler, and J. E. Dorff. The effects
of dextro-amphetamine on behavioral deficits produced by
sleep loss in humans. J. Pharmacol. Exp. Therap., 127:46-50,
1959. 301

2241. Korotkin, I. I. (Russ.) The effect
of word-stimuli as conditioned
inhibitors in wakefulness and in
the hypnotic state. Trudy Inst.
Fiziol. Pavlova, 1:345-55, 1952.
336

2242. _____, and N. A. Kryshova.
(Russ.) Changes in motor chronaxie during sleep in infants. Fiziol. Zh. SSSR, 29:127-34, 1940.
14

2243. _____, and _____. (Russ.) Changes
in motor chronaxie in infants during sleep; II. Changes in motor
chronaxie in infants at the age of
two weeks to two months. Fiziol.
Zh. SSSR, 31:312-16, 1945. 14

2244. _____, and M. M. Suslova. (Russ.)
Study of higher nervous activity
of man in the somnambulistic
phase of hypnosis. Zh. Vysshei
Nerv. Deiat., 1:617-22, 1951. 336

2245. Kosenko, Z. (Russ.) Sleep and
Dreams. Moskva: "Young Guard,"
1944. Pp. 25.

2246. Koslowsky, S. Zum Schlafproblem. Fortschr. Med., 42:144-
45, 1924. 360

2247. Kosmarskaia, E. N., and V. R.
Purin. (Russ.) Changes in cerebral and body temperatures during drug-induced sleep. Fiziol.
Zh. SSSR, 43:40-45, 1957. 63

2248. Koster, S. (Dutch) A case of recurring hypersomnia as a residual symptom of encephalitis lethargica. Ned. Tschr. Geneesk.,
78:883-87, 1934. 249, 362

2249. Koster, S. Experimental investigation of the character of hypnosis. J. Clin. Exp. Hypn., 2:42-
54, 1954. 337

2250. Kosuge, T. Changes in the human sweating during sleep. J.

Orient. Med., 25:109-10, 1936. 18

2251. Kotlyarevsky, L. I. (Russ.) A study of neurodynamics of children. Arkh. Biol. Nauk, 42(1-2): 63-75, 1936; also in: The Sleep Problem, 1954 (392), pp. 202-16. 72, 78

2252. Kotsovsky, D. A. La significacion du sommeil et de la croisance pour la biologie de la vieillesse. Riv. Biol., 11:360-64, 1929. 305

2253. _____. El sueño y la vejez. Rev. Criminol. Psiquiat. Méd. Leg., 16:92-96, 1929. 362

2254. _____. Schlaf als Verjuengung. Hippokrates, 21:689-92, 1950.

2255. Kourétas, D., et P. Scouras. Sur un trouble particulier du sommeil: le cauchemar. Encéphale, 27:622-27, 1932. 280

2256. Kovàcs, L. Rassegna critica e considerazioni sul centro e meccanismo del sonno. Giorn. Psichiat. Neuropat., 60:344-84, 1932.

2257. _____. Ancora sul sonno. Giorn. Psichiat. Neuropat., 61:385-88, 1933. 355

2258. Krabbe, E., and G. Magnussen. On narcolepsy. I. Familial narcolepsy. Acta Psychiat. Neurol., 17:149-73, 1942. 234, 242

2259. Krakau, C. E. T., and G. E. Nyman. On the effect of artificial fever on the alpha activity in man. Acta Physiol. Scand., 29: 281-92, 1953. 31

2260. Krakora, B. (Czech.) The electroencephalogram whilst falling asleep, during sleep, and in hypnosis. Neurol. Psychiat. Česk. (Praha), 16:141-54, 1953. 330

2261. Krantz, J. C., Jr. Management of insomnia and restlessness—a pharmacologic viewpoint. Connecticut Med., 22:608-10, 1958. 278

2262. Krapivkin, A., and F. Paschenko. (Russ.) Two cases of hysterical sleep. Soviet. Nevropat. Psikhiat. Psikhogig., 5:401-5, 1932.

2263. Krasnjanskij, L. M. Die Tagesschwankungen des Blutzuckergehalts beim Menschen. Biochem. Z., 205:180-85, 1929. 166

2264. Krasnogorski, N. Der Schlaf und die Hemmung. Mschr. Kinderheilk., 25:372-89, 1923. 197

2265. _____. (Russ.) Sleep and inhibition in children. (Physiological

mechanism of sleep.) In: The Sleep Problem, 1954 (392), pp. 169-80. 197

2266. Kratin, Iu. G. Some aspects of the cortical analysis as reflected in the electroencephalogram of man. Sech. Physiol. J. USSR (Engl. Ed.), 43:123-33, 1957. 359

2267. Kraus, W. M., and O. C. Perkins. A syndrome of the cerebral origins of the visceral nervous system. Arch. Neurol. Psychiat., 18:249-62, 1927. 269

2268. Krauss, R. F. The electroencephalogram in normal infants and children. EEG Clin. Neurophysiol., 5:463, 1953. 27

2269. Krausse, H. Die moderne Methodik der Schlaftiefenmessung. Eine experimentelle Pruefung. Erlangen: Diss., 1935. Pp. 27. 51, 52, 87

2270. Krayevsky, Ia. M. (Russ.) Changes in the activity of the cerebral cortex in connection with the protective sleep inhibition in patients with cortical-subcortical lesions. Trudy Inst. Fiziol. Pavlova, 1:394-405, 1952. 207

2271. Kreider, M. B. Effects of sleep deprivation on body temperatures. Fed. Proc., 20:214, 1961. 173, 226

2272. _____, and E. R. Buskirk. Supplemental feeding and thermal comfort during sleep in the cold. J. Appl. Physiol., 11:339-43, 1957. 62

2273. _____, _____, and D. E. Bass. Oxygen consumption and body temperature during the night. J. Appl. Physiol., 12:361-66, 1958. 62

2274. _____, and P. F. Iampietro. Oxygen consumption and body temperature during sleep in cold environments. J. Appl. Physiol., 14:765-67, 1959; prelim. commun. Fed. Proc., 18:84, 1959. 56, 62

2275. _____, _____, E. R. Buskirk, and D. E. Bass. Effect of continuous cold exposure on nocturnal body temperatures of man. J. Appl. Physiol., 14:43-45, 1959; prelim. commun. Fed. Proc., 17:90, 1958. 62

2276. Kreidl, A., und F. Herz. Der Schlaf des Menschen bei Fernbleiben von Gesichts und Ge-

hoerseindruecken: ueber den Schlaf der Mindersinnigen. Pfluegers Arch., 203:459-71, 1924. 74
Kreidl, A., co-author: 2084.

2277. Kremen, I. Dream Reports and Rapid Eye Movements: An Appraisal. Thesis Summary, Harvard Univ., 1961. Pp. 6. 98

2278. Kremer, M., R. W. Gilliatt, J. S. R. Golding, and T. G. Wilson. Acroparaesthesiae in the carpal-tunnel syndrome. Lancet, II:590-95, 1953. 285

2279. Krieger, H. P., I. H. Wagman, and M. B. Bender. Eye movements and the state of consciousness. Trans. Am. Neurol. Ass., 81st Meet., 1956, pp. 112-14; also J. Neurophysiol., 21:224-30, 1958. 102

2280. Kriegman, G., and H. B. Wright. Brief psychotherapy with enuretics in the army. Am. J. Psychiat., 104:254-58, 1947. 284

2281. Kris, C. Diurnal variation in periorbitally measured eye potential level. EEG Clin. Neurophysiol., 9:382, 1957. 93, 159

2282. _____. Vision: Electro-Oculography. In: Medical Physics, O. Glasser, Ed., Chicago: Year Book Publ., 1960, Vol. III, pp. 692-700. 93

2283. Krisch, H. Weitere Beitraege zur Pathophysiologie der epileptischen motorischen Varianten und der migraenoesen Hirnstammsyndrome (Kombination mit Chorea, Schlafsucht). Z. ges. Neurol. Psychiat., 98:80-92, 1925. 256

2284. Kristiansen, K., and G. Courtois. Rhythmic activity from isolated cerebral cortex. EEG. Clin. Neurophysiol., 1:265-72, 1949. 211

2285. Kroetz, C. Ueber einige stoffliche Erscheinungen bei verlaengertem Schlafentzug. I. Der Saeurebasenaushalt. Blut- und Harnreaktion, Wasser- und Salzbestand des Serums. Z. ges, exp. Med., 52:770-78, 1926. 65, 224

2286. _____. Der 24-Stunden-Rhythmus der Kreislaufregulation. Acta Med. Scand., Suppl. 108:234-40, 1940. 163
Kroetz, C., co-author: 1473.

2287. Kroll, F. W. Ueber das Vorkommen von uebertragbaren schlaferzeugenden Stoffen im Hirn Schlafender Tiere. Z. ges. Neu-

rol. Psychiat., 146:208-18, 1933. 203, 352

2288. _____. Gibt es einen humoralen Schlafstoff im Schlafhirn? Dsche med. Wschr., 77:879-80, 1952. 352
Kroll, F. W., co-author: 1218.

2289. Krueger, E. G., and H. L. Wayne. Clinical and electroencephalographic effects of prefrontal lobotomy and topectomy in chronic psychoses. A.M.A. Arch. Neurol. Psychiat., 67:661-71, 1952.

2290. Krupp, P., M. Monnier, und S. Stille. Topischer Einfluss des Coffein auf das Gehirn. Arch. exp. Path. Pharmakol., 235:381-84, 1959. 299

2291. Kryshova, N. A. (Russ.) Changes in motor chronaxie in infants during sleep; III. Changes in motor chronaxie in infants at age of one to ten days. Fiziol. Zh. SSSR, 31:317-23, 1945. 14
Kryshova, N. A., co-author: 2242, 2243.

2292. Kubie, L. S. Instincts and homoeostasis. Psychosom. Med., 10:15-30, 1948.

2293. _____. Psychiatric and psychoanalytic considerations of the problem of consciousness. In: Brain Mechanisms and Consciousness, 1954 (875), pp. 444-69. 30

2294. _____, and S. Margolin. A physiological method for the induction of states of partial sleep, and securing free association and early memories in such states. Trans. Am. Neurol. Ass., 68: 136-39, 1942. 197

2295. _____, and _____. An apparatus for the use of breath sounds as a hypnagogic stimulus. Am. J. Psychiat., 100:610, 1944. 197

2296. _____, and _____. The process of hypnotism and the nature of the hypnotic state. Am. J. Psychiat., 100:611-22, 1944. 336
Kubie, L. S., co-author: 271.

2297. Kugel, M. A. Hypnotika und Diurese. Studien ueber die Wasser- und Kochsalzausscheidung im Schlaf mit und ohne Hypophysenwirkung. Arch. exp. Path. Pharmakol., 142:166-88, 1929. 297

2298. Kuhlenbeck, H. Brain and consciousness; some prolegomena to an approach of the problem. Confinia Neurol. (Basel), 17 (Suppl.):1-344, 1957. 31, 107

2299. Kuhn, L., and S. Russo, Eds. Modern Hypnosis. Hollywood, Calif.: Wilshire Book Co., 1958. 2nd Ed. Pp. 349. 336

2300. Kukuev, L. A., and V. A. Abovian. (Russ.) Critical remarks on certain views of localization of consciousness (Brain, 1953). Zh. Nevropat. Psikhiat. (Moskva), 54:362-63, 1954. 31

2301. Kunkel, O. Enuresis und Enkopresis eines Dreizehnjaehrigen geheilt durch psychotherapeutische Behandlung der Mutter. Z. Psychotherap. med. Psychol., 8:236-39, 1958. 284

2302. Kuno, Y. The significance of sweating in man. Lancet, 218(I): 912-15, 1930. 18

2303. _____. Human Perspiration. Springfield, Ill.: Thomas, 1956. Pp. xv + 416. 18

2304. _____, and K. Ikeuchi. On the perspiration by the human skin. J. Biophys., 2:cxxii-cxxiv, 1927. 18

2305. Kunz, A.-M. Ueber die Narkolepsie als diencephales Problem. Muenchen: Inaug. Diss., 1951. Pp. 42. 237

2306. Kunze, J. Die Veraenderung der Hydrogenionkonzentration des Blutes waehrend des Schlafes. Z. ges. exp. Med., 59:248-51, 1928. 33

2307. Kupalov, P. S. (Russ.) The functional mosaic in the skin area of the cerebral cortex and its influence on the limitation of sleep. Fiziol. Zh., 9:147, 1926. 197

2308. _____. (Russ.) On irradiation of internal inhibition and its passage into sleep. In: The Sleep Problem, 1954 (392), pp. 154-57. 197

2309. _____. (Russ.) Consciousness and higher nervous activity. Vest. Akad. Med. Nauk, SSSR, 13(12): 3-6, 1958.

2310. Kupper, H. I. Psychic concomitants of wartime injuries. Psychosom. Med., 7:15-21, 1945. 333

2311. _____. Some aspects of the dream in psychosomatic disease. Psychosom. Med., 9:310-19, 1947. 106

2312. Kyriaco-Roques, A. Etude sur les Narcolepsies. Paris: Maloine, 1930. Pp. 195. 269, 272
Kyriaco, A., co-author: 2501.

2313. Laache, S. Ueber Schlaf und Schlafstoerungen. Stuttgart: F. Enke, 1913. Pp. 60. 286

2314. Labauge, R., J. Cadilhac, and P. Passouant. Electroencephalographic study during sleep of unilateral cerebral atrophies in children. EEG Clin. Neurophysiol., 6:164, 1954.
Labauge, R., co-author: 3103.

2315. Labbé, M., P. L. Violle, et E. Azérad. Action de la rétropituitrine sur la diurèse chez l'homme en état de sommeil. C. R. Soc. Biol., 94:848-49, 1926.

2316. Laborit, H. Les déconnecteurs végétatifs et l'hibernation provoquée du point de vue pharmacologique, chirurgical et médical. Rev. Path. Gén. Comp., 53:65-74, 1953. 328

2317. _____, et P. Huguenard. L'hibernation artificielle par moyens pharmacodynamiques et physiques. Presse Méd., 59:1329, 1951. 328

2318. La Cassie, R. Une forme rare d'insomnie. Aspects cliniques des troubles du sommeil de la malade post-opératoire. Presse Méd., 44:1892-94, 1936. 276

2319. Ladame, C. Du sommeil et de quelques-unes de ses modalités chez les aliénés. Schweiz. Arch. Neurol. Psychiat., 13:371-90, 1923. 119, 286

2320. Ladd, G. T. Contribution to the psychology of visual dreams. Mind, 1:299-304, 1892. 94

2321. Lafon, R., P. Passouant, et J. Minvielle. Etude électro-encéphalographique du sommeil des schizophrènes hébéphréno-catatoniques. Comparaison avec le tracé de repos et l'activation cardiazolique. Ann. Méd.-Psychol., 113(II):258-68, 1955.

2322. Lafora, G. R. Narcolepsia esencial y narcolepsia sintomática o letárgica (observaciones personales). Arch. Neurobiol., 7:49-63, 1927. 233

2323. _____, e J. Sanz. Sul sonno sperimentale prodotto da un'azione su la regione del diencefalo e del III. ventricolo. Cervello, 11: 86, 1932. 202

2324. Laget, P., R. Laplane, et R. Salbreux. Etude de l'action de la chlorpromazine sur l'électroencéphalogramme du nourrisson. Presse Méd., 66:395-97, 1958. 301

2325. Lagrandcourt, C. J. M.-A. Une Indication Majeure de la Cure de

Sommeil: L'hypertension Artérielle. Paris: D. P. Taib, 1955.
Pp. 45. 207

2326. Laidlaw, J. C., D. Jenkins, W. J.
Reddy, and T. Jakobson. The diurnal variation in adrenocortical
secretion. J. Clin. Investig., 33:
950, 1954. 170
Laidlaw, J. C., co-author: 3934.

2327. Laing, A. M. The Sleep Book; An
Anthology for the Pillow. London:
F. Muller, 1948. Pp. 150.

2328. Laird, D. A. Effects of loss of
sleep on mental work. Indust.
Psychol., 1:427-28, 1926. 228

2329. _____. One third of life is sleep.
Hygeia (Chicago), 9:535-38, 1931.

2330. _____. The role of diet in sleep
and fatigue with special reference
to the carbohydrates. Med. Rev.
Rev., 37:14-26, 1931.

2331. _____. A survey of the sleep habits of 509 men of distinction. Am.
Med., 26:271-75, 1931. 120

2332. _____. Practical consideration
about sleep of hospital patient.
Trans. Am. Hosp. Ass., 35:380-
87, 1933. 312

2333. _____. Fatigue: public enemy
number one: what it is and how
to fight it. Am. J. Nursing, 33(II):
835-41, 1933.

2334. _____. Calcium metabolism and
the quality of sleep. New York
Med. J. Med. Rec., 138:396-98,
1933.

2335. _____. Diaries of earlier generations in the study of sleep. Science, 80:382, 1934.

2336. _____. Seasonal changes in calcium metabolism and quality of
sleep. New York Med. J. Med.
Rec., 139:65-67, 1934. 187

2337. _____. The quality of American
sleep. New York Med. J. Med.
Rec., 139:169-70, 1934. 312

2338. _____. Did you sleep well? Rev.
Rev., 91:23, 1935. 86, 312

2339. _____. Bladder pressure and disturbed sleep. New York Med. J.
Med. Rec., 141:78-80, 1935. 87

2340. _____. Types of sleepers: normal and abnormal. New York
Med. J. Med. Rec., 142:13-15,
1935. 86

2341. _____. How To Sleep and Rest
Better. New York: Funk & Wag-
nalls, 1937. Pp. 83. 312

2342. _____. Sleeplessness and what
to do about it. Today's Health,
35(8):18-19, 42-43, 1957. 275

2343. _____. Helping the ears to go to

sleep. Hosp. Management, 83(2):
52-54, 70, 1957. 312

2344. _____, and H. Drexel. Experiments with foods and sleep. J.
Am. Diet. Ass., 10:89-99, 1934.
81, 87, 307, 309

2345. _____, and E. C. Laird. Sound
Ways to Sound Sleep. New York:
McGraw-Hill, 1959. Pp. vii +
190. 79

2346. _____, and W. Wheeler. What it
costs to lose sleep. Indust. Psychol., 1:694-96, 1926. 228
Laird, D. A., co-author: 3842.

2347. Lairy, G. C. Organisation de l'é-
lectroencéphalogramme normal
et pathologique. Aspect clinique.
Rev. Neurol., 94:749-801, 1956.
26

2348. Lairy-Bounes, G. C., et H.
Fischgold. Réactions EEG dif-
fuses aux stimulations psycho-
sensorielles: intérêt clinique.
EEG Clin. Neurophysiol., 5:343-
62, 1953. 211

2349. _____, J. Garcia-Badaracco, et
M. B. Dell. Epilepsie et troubles
de la vigilance. Encéphale, 42:
170-92, 1953. 259

2350. _____, M. Parma, et A. Zanchetti. Modifications pendant la réaction d'arrêt de Berger de l'activité convulsive produite par
l'application locale de strychnine
sur le cortex cérébral du lapin.
EEG Clin. Neurophysiol., 4:495-
502, 1952.
Lairy-Bounes, G. C., co-author:
119, 298, 1181.

2351. Lamarche, A., A. Roussel, et
M-me Rosendorf. Comparaisons
des résultats obtenus par la cure
de sommeil, la cure de somnolence, et la cure à la chlorpromazine seule et à dose élevée.
Résultats de quelques électro-
encéphalogrammes de contrôle.
Encéphale, 45:884-90, 1956. 206

2352. Lambranzi, R. Sulla profondità
del sonno. Riv. Sper. Freniat.,
26:828-30, 1900. 108

2353. Lambros, V. S. The use of reserpine in certain neurological disorders: organic convulsive states,
enuresis, and head injuries. Ann.
New York Acad. Sci., 61:211-14,
1955. 257, 284, 302

2354. Lamson, P. D., and M. E. Greig.
Blocking by Benodaine of the potassium effect of return to sleep
on awakening from barbiturate
anesthesia. J. Pharmacol. Exp.

Therap., 108:362-63, 1953. 303

2355. _____, _____, and B. H. Robbins. The potentiating effect of glucose and its metabolic products on barbiturate anesthesia. Science, 110:690-91, 1949; also Fed. Proc., 9:293-94, 1950. 297

2356. Landau, B. R., and A. R. Dawe. Respiration in the hibernation of the 13-lined ground squirrel. Am. J. Physiol., 194:75-82, 1958. 323

2357. Landau, J., and S. Feldman. Diminished endogenous morning eosinopenia in blind subjects. Acta Endocrinol., 15:53-60, 1954. 170

2358. Landauer, K. Handlungen des Schlafenden. Z. ges. Neurol. Psychiat., 39:329-51, 1918.

2359. Landis, C. Changes in the blood pressure during sleep as determined by the Erlanger method. Am. J. Physiol., 73:551-55, 1925. 43, 44

2360. _____. Electrical phenomena of the body during sleep. Am. J. Physiol., 81:6-19, 1927. 19, 87, 110
Landis, C., co-author: 2090.

2361. Langdon-Down, M., and W. R. Brain. Time of day in relation to convulsions in epilepsy. Lancet, 216(I):1029-32, 1929. 260, 261

2362. Lange, H., und J. Schloss. Ueber das Verhalten des Blutzuckers in der Nacht und in den Morgenstunden. Arch. exp. Path. Pharmakol., 39:274-89, 1929. 165

2363. Lange, J. F. Ueber die Entwicklung einer Tagesperiodik verschiedener Koerperfunktionen unter besonderer Beruecksichtung der Pulsfrequenz, der Schlaf-Wachverteilung und der Koerpertemperatur. Muenchen: UNI-Druck, 1957. Pp. 80. 41, 138, 163
Lange, J. F., co-author: 1689-91.

2364. Langelüddeke, A. Delikte in Schlafzustaenden. Nervenarzt, 26:28-30, 1955. 271

2365. Langworthy, O. R., and B. J. Betz. Narcolepsy as a type of response to emotional conflicts. Psychosom. Med., 6:211-26, 1944. 239

2366. Lansing, R. W., E. Schwartz, and D. B. Lindsley. Reaction time and EEG activation under alerted and nonalerted conditions. J. Exp. Psychol., 58:1-7, 1959.

2367. Lapicque, L. Hypothèse cellulaire pour l'origine de la conscience psychologique. C. R. Acad. Sci., 234:1109-12, 1952. 31

2368. _____. Sur la conscience psychologique considérée comme intégrale d'éléments cellulaires de conscience. C. R. Acad. Sci., 234:1511-14, 1952. 31

2369. Lardy, H. A., R. G. Hansen, and P. H. Phillips. Ineffectiveness of sodium succinate in control of duration of barbiturate anesthesia. Proc. Soc. Exp. Biol., Med., 55:277-78, 1944. 297

2370. Larsson, L.-E. The relation between the startle reaction and the non-specific EEG response to sudden stimuli with a discussion on the mechanism of arousal. EEG Clin. Neurophysiol., 8: 631-44, 1956.

2371. Lasch, C. H., und H. V. Billich. Die taeglichen Schwankungen der Erythrocytenzahlen, zugleich ein Beitrag zur Frage der Blutwasserbestimmung. Z. ges. exp. Med., 48:651-57, 1926. 162

2372. Lashley, K. S. The behavioristic interpretation of consciousness. Psychol. Rev., 30:237-72, 329-53, 1923. 31

2373. Laslett, H. R. An experiment on the effects of loss of sleep. J. Exp. Psychol., 7:45-58, 1924. 224

2374. _____. Experiments on the effects of the loss of sleep. J. Exp. Psychol., 11:370-96, 1928. 224
Laslett, H. R., co-author: 2819.

2375. Lauber, H., und R. Pannhorst. Ueber psychische Beeinflussung des Herz-Minuten-Volumens. Z. klin. Med., 114:111-19, 1930. 331

2376. Laudenheimer, R. Psychopatische Schlafsucht. Ein Beitrag zur Physiologie depressiver Zustaende. Z. ges. Neurol. Psychiat., 109:341-53, 1927. 270

2377. _____. Ueber Schlafstoerungen. Therap. Gegenw., 71:337-41, 1930. 294

2378. _____. Ueber Verkuerzung und Verlegung der Schlafzeit: aerztliche Bemerkungen zu der Mitteilung von Stöckmann. Muench. med. Wschr., 80:538, 1933. 307

2379. Laughlin, H. P. The dissociative reactions: dissociation, double personality, depersonalization, amnesia, fugue states, somnam-

bulism, and hypnosis. Med. Ann.
District of Columbia, 22:541-51,
578, 1953. 283

2380. _____. Research on sleep deprivation and exhaustion; an invita-
tion to further observation and
study. Internat. Rec. Med. Gen.
Pract. Clin., 166:305-10, 1953.
228

2381. Laurell, H. (Norw.) Neurological
and rhythm-biological viewpoints
of the ulcer problem. Nord. Med.,
23:1473-82, 1944. 316

2382. Lauterer, Z. (Czech.) The effect
of caffeine on noctambulism and
certain other morbid symptoms
dependent on sleep. Časop. Lék.
Česk., 70:340-45, 1931.

2383. Law, E. J. How soundly do birds
sleep? Condor, 28:51, 1926.

2384. Lawson, R. W. Blinking and
sleep. Nature, 165:81-82, 1950.
79, 90

2385. Lay, W. A. Ueber das Morgen-
und Abendlernen. Z. Erforsch.
Behandl. jugendl. Schwachsinns,
5:285-92, 1912. 124, 161

2386. Leahy, S. R., and I. J. Sands.
Mental disorders in children following epidemic encephalitis. J.
Am. Med. Ass., 76:373-77, 1921.
247

2387. Leak, W. N. Posture during
sleep. Lancet, I:26, 1942. 9, 11

2388. Leake, C., J. A. Grab, and M. J.
Senn. Studies in exhaustion due
to lack of sleep. II. Symptomatology in rabbits. Am. J. Physiol.,
92:127-30, 1927. 217

2389. Learoyd, C. G. The mechanism
of sleep. Practitioner, 164:261-
69, 1950.

2390. Leathes, J. B. On diurnal and
nocturnal variations in the excretion of uric acid. J. Physiol.
(London), 35:125-30, 1906. 65
Leathes, J. B., co-author: 511.

2391. Le Beau, J. Localisation cérébrale de la conscience. Rev.
Canad. Biol., 1:134-56, 1942.
344, 359

2392. Lebensohn, J. E. The eye and
sleep. Arch. Ophthalmol., 25:
401-11, 1941. 72

2393. Lechelle, Alajouanine, et Théve-
nard. Deux cas de tumeur du
lobe frontal à forme somnolente.
Bull. Mém. Soc. Méd. Hôp. Paris,
49:1347-52, 1925. 265, 266
Lechelle, P., co-author: 1548.

2394. Leclerc, H. La phytothérapie
dans le traitement de l'insomnie. J. Méd. Chir. Prat., 101:
870-80, 1930. 294

2395. Lecomte, R. Hypersomnie
Rythmée par les Règles. Paris:
Impr. R. Foulon, 1945. (Thèse)
Pp. 37. 270

2396. LeCron, L. M., Ed. Experimental Hypnosis. New York: Macmillan & Co., 1952. Pp. xviii +
483. 336

2397. _____, and J. Bordeaux. Hypnotism Today. New York: Grune
& Stratton, 1947. Pp. ix + 278.
336

2398. Leduc, S. Production du sommeil et de l'anesthésie générale
et locale par les courants électriques. C. R. Acad. Sci., 135:
199-200, 1902. 298

2399. _____. Production du sommeil
et de l'anesthésie générale par
les courants électriques. C. R.
Acad. Sci., 135:878-79, 1902.
298

2400. Lee, M. A. M., and N. Kleitman.
Attempts to demonstrate functional changes in the nervous
system during experimental insomnia. Am. J. Physiol., 67:
141-52, 1923. 15, 151, 220

2401. Legendre, R. Varicosités des
dendrites, étudiées par les mé-
thodes neurofibrillaires. C. R.
Soc. Biol., 62:257-59, 1907.
215, 343

2402. _____. The physiology of sleep.
Rep. Smithsonian Inst., 12:587-
602, 1911. 215, 349, 352

2403. _____, et H. Piéron. Les rapports entre les conditions physiologiques et les modifications
histologiques des cellules cérébrales dans l'insomnie expérimentale. C. R. Soc. Biol., 62:
312-14, 1907. 215, 352

2404. _____, et _____. Retour à l'état
normal des cellules nerveuses
après les modifications provoquées par l'insomnie expérimentale. C. R. Soc. Biol., 62:1007-8,
1907. 215, 352

2405. _____, et _____. Distribution des
altérations cellulaires du système nerveux dans l'insomnie expérimentale. C. R. Soc. Biol.,
64:1102-4, 1908. 215, 352

2406. _____, et _____. Réfutation expérimentale des théories dites
"osmotiques" du sommeil. C. R.
Soc. Biol., 68:962-64, 1910. 215,
352

2407. _____, et _____. La théorie de

l'autonarcose carbonique comme cause du sommeil et les données expérimentales. C. R. Soc.
Biol., 68:1014-15, 1910. 215,
351, 352

2408. _____, et _____. Le problème des
facteurs du sommeil. Résultats
d'injections vasculaires et intra-
cérébrales de liquides insomniques. C. R. Soc. Biol., 68:1077-
79, 1910. 203, 215, 352

2409. _____, et _____. Des résultats
histophysiologiques de l'injection
intra-occipito-atlantoïedienne de
liquides insomniques. C. R. Soc.
Biol., 68:1108-9, 1910. 203, 215,
352

2410. _____, et _____. Du développe-
ment, au cours de l'insomnie ou
périmentale, de propriétés hyp-
notoxiques des humeurs en relation avec le besoin croissant de
sommeil. C. R. Soc. Biol., 70:
190-92, 1911. 203, 215, 352

2411. _____, et _____. De la propriété
hypnotoxique des humeurs développée au cours d'une veille prolongée. C. R. Soc. Biol., 72:210-
12, 1912. 203, 215, 352

2412. _____, et _____. Destruction par
oxydation de la propriété hypnotoxique des humeurs développée
au cours d'une veille prolongée.
C. R. Soc. Biol., 72:274-75, 1912.
203, 215, 352

2413. _____, et _____. Recherches sur
le besoin de sommeil consécutif
à une veille prolongée. Z. allg.
Physiol., 14:235-62, 1912. 203,
215, 352

2414. LeGrand, A. Recherches expérimentales sur la durée des rêves
au moyen d'injections de bro-
mure d'acétylcholine. J. Physiol.
(Paris), 41:203A, 1949. 100

2415. Le Guillant, L. Problèmes thé-
oriques de la cure de sommeil.
In: La Cure de Sommeil, 1954
(3021), pp. 3-12. 206

2416. Lehmann, G. Tagesrhythmik und
Leistungsbereitschaft. Acta Med.
Scand., Suppl. 278:108-9, 1953. 158

2417. _____, und H. F. Michaelis. Adrenalin und Arbeit. IV. Adrenalin
und Leistungsfaehigkeit. Arbeitsphysiologie, 12:305-12, 1943.

2418. Lehmkuhl, R. A. (Russ.) Comparison of sleep and wakefulness
in normal and decerebrated
birds. Fiziol. Zh., 19:622-31,
1935. 173

2419. _____. Vergleichung von Schlaf

und Wachen bei normalen und
enthirnten Voegeln. Bull. Biol.
Méd. Exp. URSS, 1:366-67, 1936.
173

2420. Lehrman, N. S. Creativity, consciousness and revelation. Dis.
Nerv. Syst., 21:431-39, 499-504,
1960. 30

2421. Lehrmann, S. R., and E. J.
Weiss. Schizophrenia in cryptogenic narcolepsy. Psychiat. Q.,
17:135-43, 1943. 237

2422. Leiderman, H., J. H. Mendelson,
D. Wexler, and P. Solomon.
Sensory deprivation: clinical
aspects. Arch. Int. Med., 101:
389-96, 1958.
Leiderman, H., co-author: 3753,
4182.

2423. Leksell, L. Clinical recording
of eye movements. Acta Chir.
Scand., 82:262-70, 1939. 93

2424. Lemere, F. The significance of
individual differences in the
Berger rhythm. Brain, 59:366-
75, 1936. 28

2425. Lenk, E. Blutdruck und Hypnose.
Dsche med. Wschr., 46:1080,
1920. 329

2426. Lennox, M. A., and J. Coolidge.
Electroencephalographic changes
after prefrontal lobotomy, with
particular reference to the effect
of lobotomy on sleep spindles.
Arch. Neurol. Psychiat., 62:150-
61, 1949. 210

2427. _____, T. C. Ruch, and B. Guter-
man. The effect of Benzedrine
on the post-electroshock EEG.
EEG Clin. Neurophysiol., 3:63-
69, 1951. 300
Lennox, M. A., co-author: 1095,
2429.

2428. Lennox, W. G., F. A. Gibbs, and
E. L. Gibbs. Effect on the electro-encephalogram of drugs and
conditions which influence seizures. Arch. Neurol. Psychiat.,
36:1236-45, 1936. 257

2429. _____, and M. A. Lennox. Epilepsy and Related Disorders.
Boston: Little, Brown, 1960. 2
vols. Pp. xxv + 1168.
Lennox, W. G., co-author: 1423,
1427-29.

2430. Lenow, W. A. Ueber die Bildung
von bedingten Spurreflexen bei
Kindern. Pfluegers Arch., 214:
305-19, 1926. 197

2431. Leonhard, K. Partielle Schlafzustaende mit Halluzinationen
bei postenzephalitischem Parkin-

sonismus. Z. ges. Neurol. Psychiat., 131:234-47, 1930. 249

2432. _____. Eingenartige Tagesschwankungen des Zustandbildes bei Parkinsonismus. Z. ges. Neurol. Psychiat., 134:76-82, 1931.

2433. _____. Gesetze und Sinn des Traeumens; zugleich eine Kritik der Traumdeutung und ein Einblick in das Wirken des Unterbewusstseins. Stuttgart: Georg Thieme Verlag, 1951. 2nd ed. Pp. 146. 99

2434. Léopold-Lévi. Sommeil, normal et pathologique et glandes endocrines. Monde Méd., Paris, 39: 85-98, 1929. 269

2435. _____. Le lever matutinal précoce. Bull. Mém. Soc. Méd. Paris, 1932, pp. 117-21. 161, 308

2436. Lépine, R. Théorie mécanique de la paralysie hystérique, du somnambulisme, du sommeil naturel et de la distraction. C. R. Soc. Biol., 47:85-86, 1895. 343

2437. Leriche, R. Le syndrome du défilé costo-claviculaire; l'insomnie par douleur des bras dans d'horizontale. Presse Méd., 49 (II):825-26, 1941. 285

2438. Leroy, R., et G. Verdeaux. Crises comitiales avec sommeil postcritique. Activation de l'EEG par hyperpnée et le sommeil. Rev. Neurol., 82:558-59, 1950; prelim. commun. EEG Clin. Neurophysiol., 2:348, 1950. 257

2439. Leshan, L. The breaking of a habit by suggestion during sleep. J. Abnorm. Soc. Psychol., 37: 406-8, 1942. 125, 126

2440. Lesniowski, S. Schlafanfaelle und schlafaehnliche Zustaende. Abstr., Zbl. ges. Neurol. Psychiat., 53:818, 1929. 359

2441. Lester, D. Continuous measurement of the depth of sleep. Science, 127:1340-41, 1958. 113

2442. _____. A new method for the determination of the effectiveness of sleep-inducing agents in human. Comprehens. Psychiat., 1: 301-7, 1960. 295

2443. Leuba, C., and D. Bateman. Learning during sleep. Am. J. Psychol., 65:301-2, 1952. 125

2444. Levin, M. Narcolepsy and other varieties of morbid somnolence. Arch. Neurol. Psychiat., 22:1172-1200, 1929. 239

2445. _____. The pathogenesis of narcolepsy, with consideration of sleep-paralysis and localized sleep. J. Neurol. Psychopath., 14:1-14, 1933. 239

2446. _____. Military aspects of narcolepsy with remarks on the pathogenesis of narcolepsy and on fatigue. J. Neurol. Psychopath., 14:124-31, 1933. 239

2447. _____. "Crowding" of inhibition and of excitation. J. Neurol. Psychopath., 14:345-48, 1934. 239

2448. _____. Narcolepsy and the machine age; the recent increase in the incidence of narcolepsy. J. Neurol. Psychopath., 15:60-64, 1934. 239, 344

2449. _____. Role of cerebral cortex in narcolepsy. J. Neurol. Psychopath., 15:236-41, 1935. 239

2450. _____. Periodic somnolence and morbid hunger. Brain, 59:494-503, 1936. 267

2451. _____. Mental symptoms in narcolepsy. Forgetfulness and learning difficulty as manifestations of excessive inhibition of the highest cerebral centers. Am. J. Psychiat., 98:673-75, 1942.

2452. _____. Diplopia in narcolepsy. Arch. Ophthal., 29:942-55, 1943. 236

2453. _____. Military aspects of narcolepsy. War Med., 6:162-65, 1944; also: The sentinel asleep on post. Dis. Nerv. Syst., 12:15-18, 1951.

2454. _____. "Delay" (Pavlov) in human physiology. Sleepiness on delayed response to stimuli. Am. J. Psychiat., 102:483-85, 1946. 344

2455. _____. Narcolepsy. Cycloped. Med. Surg., Specialt., Davis Co., Philadelphia, 9:451-59, 1951. 240, 344

2456. _____. Diurnal rhythm in epilepsy. Am. J. Psychiat., 113:243-45, 1956. 237, 260

2457. _____. Premature waking and post-dormitial paralysis. J. Nerv. Ment. Dis., 125:140-41, 1957. 236

2458. _____. Hallucination: a problem in neurophysiology. J. Nerv. Ment. Dis., 125:308-11, 1957.

2459. _____. Aggression, guilt and cataplexy. Am. J. Psychiat., 116:133-36, 1959. 236

2460. _____. Sleep, cataplexy, and fa-

tigue as manifestations of Pavlovian inhibition. Am. J. Psychotherap., 15:122-37, 1961. 344

2461. Levin, P. M. Dormison as a hypnotic in clinical electroencephalography. EEG Clin. Neurophysiol., 5:129, 1953. 296

2462. Levin, S. (Russ.) Characteristics
of conditioned reflex activity in
hypnotic states in children. Fiziol. Zh., 17:196-205, 1934.
332

2463. Levine, M. Psychogalvanic reaction to painful stimuli in hypnotic
and hysterical anesthesia. Bull.
Johns Hopkins Hosp., 46:331-39,
1930. 331

2464. _____. Electrical skin resistance
during hypnosis. Arch. Neurol.
Psychiat., 24:937-42, 1930. 330

2465. Levinson, L. Narcolepsy. Tufts
Med. J., 9:46-50, 1942. 234

2466. Levinson, L., J. H. Welsh, and
A. A. Abramowitz. Effect of hypophysectomy on diurnal rhythm
of spontaneous activity in the rat.
Endocrinology, 29:41-46, 1941.
172

2467. Levy, E. Z., V. H. Thaler, and
G. E. Ruff. New technique for re-
cording skin resistance changes.
Science, 128:33-34, 1958. 21, 110

2468. Levy, F. M., et G. Conge. Action
de la lumière sur l'éosinophilie
sanguine chez l'homme. C. R.
Soc. Biol., 147:586-89, 1953. 170

2469. Levy, J. Les hypersomnies. Sem.
Hôp. (Paris), 24:3044-49, 1948.
272

2470. Lewin, B. D. Sleep, the mouth,
and the dream screen. Psychoanal. Q., 15:419-34, 1946. 101

2471. _____. Inferences from the dream
screen. Internat. J. Psycho-anal.,
29:224-31, 1948. 101

2472. _____. Mania and sleep. Psychoanal. Q., 18:419-33, 1949. 101

2473. _____. Reconsideration of the
dream screen. Psychoanal. Q.,
22:174-99, 1953. 101

2474. _____. Clinical hints from dream
studies. A.M.A. Arch. Neurol.
Psychiat., 74:224-25, 1955. 101

2475. Lewis, H. E., and J. P. Master-
ton. Sleep and wakefulness in the
Arctic. Lancet, I:1262-66, 1957.
192

2476. Lewis, J. H., and T. R. Sarbin.
Studies in psychosomatics. I.
The influence of hypnotic stimulation on gastric hunger contractions. Psychosom. Med., 5:125-

31, 1943. 331

2477. Lewis, P. R., and M. C. Lobban.
Persistence of a 24 hr pattern
of diuresis in human subjects
living on a 22 hr day. J. Physiol.
(London), 125:34P-35P, 1954.
182

2478. _____, and _____. The effects of
prolonged periods of life on abnormal time routines upon excretory rhythms in human subjects. Q. J. Exp. Physiol. (London), 42:356-71, 1957. 182

2479. _____, and _____. Dissociation
of diurnal rhythms in human
subjects living on abnormal
time routines. Q. J. Exp. Physiol. (London), 42:371-86, 1957.
182

2480. _____, and _____. The effects
of exercise on diurnal excretory
rhythms in man. J. Physiol.
(London), 143:8P-9P, 1958. 182

2481. _____, _____, and T. I. Shaw.
Patterns of urine flow in human
subjects during a prolonged period of life on a 22-hour day. J.
Physiol. (London), 133:659-69:
1956.

2482. Lewy, E. Ueber das Gaehnen. Z.
ges. Neurol. Psychiat., 72:161-
74, 1921. 72

2483. Ley, A. Discussion du rapport
de Jean Lhermitte et Auguste
Tournay: le sommeil normal et
pathologique. Rev. Neurol., I:
873-74, 1927. 349

2484. Leyser, E. Schlaf und Stupor. J.
Psychol. Neurol., 30:257-69,
1923-24. 361

2485. Lhermitte, J. Données anatomo-
physiologiques récentes sur le
centre du sommeil. Encéphale,
22:357-60, 1927. 240

2486. _____. Le sommeil et les narcolepsies. Progr. Méd., I:962-75,
1930. 233

2487. _____. Le Sommeil. Paris: Ar-
mand Colin, 1931. Pp. 211. 359

2488. _____. La cataplexie, équivalent
nomatique de la narcolepsie.
Médicine, 18:133-41, 1937.

2489. _____. Désordre de la fonction
hypnique et hallucinations. Ann.
Méd.-Psychol., I:1-14, 1938.

2490. _____. Macrogénitosomie précoce, hallucinations et narcolepsie
dans un cas d'encéphalite épidémique. Rev. Neurol., 69:65-68,
1938. 250

2491. _____. Les Rêves. Paris: Presses Univ. de France, 1941. Pp.

127. 99

2492. _____. Hypersomnie périodique et menstruation. Progr. Méd., 70:68, 71-72, 75, 1942. 270

2493. _____. Le sommeil et ses altérations morbides. J. Sci. Méd. Lille, 69:616-24, 1951. 286

2494. _____. Les rêves, le somnambulisme, l'hypnose et l'insomnie. Rev. Prat. (Paris), 4:1563-69, 1954.

2495. _____. Des dissociations des états de conscience provoquées par des lésions localisées de l'encéphale. Rev. Neurol., 93: 233-40, 1955.

2496. _____, J. Bollack, et Delabos. Syndrome infundibulo-mésocéphalique, influence inverse de la fonction lombaire sur l'hypersomnie et la polyurie. Rev. Neurol. II:672-77, 1932. 269

2497. _____, et E. Dubois. Crises d'hypersomnie prolongée rythmées par les règles chez une jeune fille. Rev. Neurol., 73:608-9, 1941. 270

2498. _____, et A. Gauthier. La cataplexie et ses composantes somatiques et psychiques; l'onirisme hallucinatoire cataplectique. Ann. Méd., 42:50-68, 1937. 236, 240, 359

2499. _____, Hécaen, et Bineau. Un nouveau cas d'hypersomnie prolongée rythmée par les règles. Rev. Neurol., 75:299, 1943. 270

2500. _____, et R. Huguenin. Narcolepsie et onirisme avec somniloquie. Rev. Neurol., I:219-22, 1934.

2501. _____, et A. Kyriaco. Hypersomnie périodique régulièrement rythmée par les règles dans un cas de tumeur basilaire du cerveau. Rev. Neurol., II:715-21, 1929. 269

2502. _____, et E. Peyre. La narcolepsie-cataplexie, symptôme révélateur et unique de l'érythrémie occulte. Rev. Neurol., I:286-90, 1930. 234, 238

2503. _____, et Rouquès. Narcolepsie en apparence idiopathique, en réalité, séquelle d'encéphalite fruste. Rev. Neurol., I:849-50, 1927.

2504. _____, et J. Sigwald. Hypnagogisme, hallucinose et hallucinations. Rev. Neurol., 73:225-38, 1941. 79

2505. _____, et A. Tournay. Rapport sur le sommeil normal et pathologique. Rev. Neurol., I:751-822, 1927. 240, 362

2506. _____, P. Vallery-Radot, Delafontaine, et Miget. Sur quelques variétés de narcolepsie; le problème de la narcolepsie épileptique. Rev. Neurol., II:565-72, 1932. 256

2507. Li, C.-L., H. H. Jasper, and L. R. Henderson. The effect of arousal mechanisms on various forms of abnormality in the electroencephalogram. EEG Clin. Neurophysiol., 4:369, 513-26, 1952. 257

2508. Liberson, W. T. Functional electroencephalography in mental disorders. Dis. Nerv. Syst., 5:357-64, 1944.

2509. _____. Problem of sleep and mental disease. Digest Neurol. Psychiat., 13:93-108, 1945. 31

2510. _____. Prolonged hypnotic states with "local signs" induced in guinea pigs. Science, 108:40-41, 1948. 336

2511. _____. Contribution to the study of localization of EEG patterns during drowsiness and sleep. EEG Clin. Neurophysiol., 1:256, 1949.

2512. _____, and K. Akert. Hippocampal seizure states in guinea pig. EEG Clin. Neurophysiol., 7:211-22, 1955. 259
Liberson, W., co-author: 702.

2513. Lichtenstein, B. W., and A. H. Rosenblum. Sleep paralysis. J. Nerv. Ment. Dis., 95:153-55, 1942. 236
Lichtenstein, B. W., co-author: 4314.

2514. Licklider, J. C. R., and M. E. Bunch. Effects of enforced wakefulness upon the growth and the maze-learning performance of white rats. J. Comp. Psychol., 39:339-50, 1946. 218, 366
Licklider, J. R., co-author: 565.

2515. Liddell, H. S., O. D. Anderson, and W. T. James. An examination of Pavlov's theory of internal inhibition. Am. J. Physiol., 90:430-31, 1929. 347

2516. Lignac, G. O. E. Kann die pathologische Schlaefrigkeit auch als Herdsymptom aufgefasst werden? Klin. Wschr., 58:410-13, 1921. 265, 348

2517. Lin, T.-Y., M. M. Healy, M. F. Finn, and M. Greenblatt. EEG changes during fever produced by inductothermy (fever cabinet) in patients with neurosyphilis. EEG Clin. Neurophysiol., 5:

217-24, 1953. 31

2518. Lindhard, J. Investigations into the conditions governing the temperature of the body. Denmark Expedition to North Shore of Greenland, No. 1. Copenhagen, 1910, pp. 75-175. 178

2519. Lindig, P. Ueber Temperatur und Schlaf. Dsche med. Wschr., 48:765-67, 1922. 200, 203

2520. Lindner, R. M. Hypnoanalysis in the treatment of psychopathic characters. J. Am. Med. Ass., 127:1012, 1945. 335

2521. _____. Hypnoanalysis in a case of hysterical somnambulism. Psychoanal. Rev., 32:325-39, 1945. 335

2522. Lindsay, J. A. Nightmares. Brit. J. Med. Psychol., 27:224-34, 1954.

2523. Lindsley, D. B. Brain potentials in children and adults. Science, 84:354, 1936. 27, 28

2524. _____. Electrical potentials of the brain in children and adults. J. Gen. Psychol., 19:285-306, 1938. 27, 28, 29

2525. _____. A longitudinal study of the occipital alpha rhythm in normal children; frequency and amplitude standards. J. Genet. Psychol., 55:197-213, 1939. 27, 28

2526. _____. Psychological phenomena and the electroencephalogram. EEG Clin. Neurophysiol., 4:443-56, 1952. 30

2527. _____. Psychological aspects of consciousness. Clin. Neurosurg., 3:175-86, 1955. 30

2528. _____. Attention, consciousness, sleep and wakefulness. In: Handbook of Physiology, III. Neurophysiology, Washington, D.C., Am. Physiol. Soc., 1960. Pp. 1553-93. 30, 209, 210, 241

2529. _____, J. Bowden, and H. W. Magoun. The effect of subcortical lesions upon the electroencephalogram. Am. Psychol., 4:233-34, 1949.

2530. _____, _____, and _____. Effect upon the EEG of acute injury to the brain stem activating system. EEG Clin. Neurophysiol., 1:475-86, 1949.

2531. _____, L. H. Schreiner, W. B. Knowles, and H. W. Magoun. Behavioral and EEG changes following chronic brain stem lesions in the cat. EEG Clin. Neurophysiol., 2:483-98, 1950; prelim. commun.

Fed. Proc., 9:78, 1950. 206, 208
Lindsley, D. B., co-author: 1067, 2366, 4052.

2532. Lindsley, O. R. Operant behavior during sleep: a measure of depth of sleep. Science, 126:1290-91, 1957.

2533. Linn, L. Psychological implications of the "activating system." Am. J. Psychiat., 110:61-65, 1953. 209, 362

2534. _____. Color in dreaming. J. Am. Psychoanal. Ass., 2:462-65, 1954. 102

2535. Linschoten, J. Ueber das Einschlafen. I. Einschlafen und Erleben. II. Einschlafen und Tun. Psychol. Beitr., 2:70-97; 266-98, 1956. 79

2536. Lion, E. G. Mechanism of narcolepsy: physiology of autonomic neuro-endocrine system of 12 narcoleptics compared to 12 normals. J. Nerv. Ment. Dis., 85:424-37, 1937. 240

2537. Lisi, L. de. Su di un fenomeno motorio costante del sonno normale: le mioclonie ipniche fisiologiche. I. Descrizione. Riv. Pat. Nerv., 39:481-96, 1932. 74, 123

2538. Lissák, K., E. Grastyán, A. Czanaky, F. Kékesi, and G. Vereby. A study of hippocampal function in the waking and sleeping animal with chronically implanted electrodes. Acta Physiol. Pharmacol. Neerl., 6:451-59, 1957. 211
Lissák, K., co-author: 1504.

2539. Litwer, H. (Dutch) On the physiology of sleep. Ned. Tschr. Geneesk., 60:1541-57, 1916. 200, 352

2540. _____. Sur la physiologie du sommeil: contribution critique et expérimentale. Arch. Néerl. Physiol., 1:425-45, 1917. 200, 352

2541. Livingston, R. B. The cerebral cortex and consciousness. Clin. Neurosurg., 3:192-202, 1957. 31

2542. _____, R. Hernández-Peón, and J. D. French. Corticofugal projections to brain stem activating system. Fed. Proc., 12:89-90, 1953. 211
Livingston, R. B., co-author: 16, 1281, 1283.

2543. Lobban, M. C. Excretory rhythms in indigenous Arctic peoples. J. Physiol. (London), 143:69P, 1958. 191

2544. _____. The entrainment of cir-
cadian rhythms in man. Cold
Spring Harbor Symp. Quantit.
Biol., 25:325-32, 1960. 182

2545. _____, and H. W. Simpson. Diurnal excretory rhythms in man at
high latitudes. J. Physiol. (London), 155:64P-65P, 1961. 167
Lobban, M. C., co-author: 2477-
81.

2546. Locher, H. Ueber den Schlaf und
die Traeume, das Nachtwandeln
und die Visionen. Zuerich: S.
Hoehr, 1853. Pp. 53.

2547. Locke, W., and A. A. Bailey.
Narcolepsy: Report of an unusual
case. Proc. Staff Meet. Mayo
Clin., 15:491-93, 1940. 234

2548. Loeb, C. Electroencephalographic changes during the state of
coma. EEG Clin. Neurophysiol.,
10:589-606, 1958. 273

2549. _____, G. Massazza, e G. Stac-
chini. Effeti del risveglio sulla
risposta corticale da stimolo di-
retto. Riv. Neurol. (Napoli), 30:
442-48, 1960.

2550. _____, and G. Poggio. Electroencephalograms in a case with
ponto-mesencephalic haemorrhage. EEG Clin. Neurophysiol.,
5:295-96, 1953. 273
Loeb, C., co-author: 1145.

2551. Loewenstein, R. M. A posttraumatic dream. Psychoanal. Q.,
18:449-54, 1949. 103

2552. Lombard, W. P. The variations
of the normal knee-jerk, and
their relation to the activity of
the central nervous system. Am.
J. Psychol., 1:5-71, 1887, 74,
150

2553. London, L. S. The meaning of the
dream. J. Nerv. Ment. Dis., 75:
40-47, 1932. 106

2554. Longet, F. A. Traité de Physiologie. Paris: Libr. V. Masson,
1860. Vol. II. Pp. 948. 361

2555. Longo, V. G. Effects of scopolamine and atropine on electroencephalographic and behavioral
reactions due to hypothalamic
stimulations. J. Pharmacol. Exp.
Therap., 116:198-208, 1956. 209,
303

2556. _____, and B. Silvestrini. Effects
of adrenergic and cholinergic
drugs injected by intra-carotid
route on electrical activity of the
brain. Proc. Soc. Exp. Biol. Med.,
95:43-47, 1957. 303

2557. _____, et _____. Contribution à
l'étude des rapports entre le
potentiel réticulaire évoqué,
l'état d'anesthésie et l'activité
électrique cérébrale. EEG Clin.
Neurophysiol., 10:111-20, 1958.
298

2558. Longson, D., and J. N. Mills.
Excess carbon dioxide and
morning urine. J. Physiol.
(London), 118:6P, 1952. 65

2559. Loomis, A. L., E. N. Harvey,
and G. A. Hobart. Electrical potentials of the human brain. J.
Exp. Psychol., 19:249-79, 1936;
prelim. commun. Science, 81:
597-98, 1935; 82:198-200, 1935;
83:239-41, 1936. 25, 330, 331

2560. _____, _____, and _____. Cerebral states during sleep as
studied by human brain potentials. J. Exp. Psychol., 21:127-
44, 1937. 25, 26, 95

2561. _____, _____, and _____. Distribution of disturbance-patterns
in the human electroencephalogram, with special reference to
sleep. J. Neurophysiol., 1:413-
30, 1938. 25
Loomis, A. L., co-author: 840-
44, 1658.

2562. Loon, J. H. van. (Dutch) Some
psychological aspects of shiftwork. Mens Onderneming, 12:
357-65, 1958. 317

2563. _____. The diurnal rhythm of
body temperature in nightwork-
ers. Acta Physiol. Pharmacol.
Neerl., 8:302, 1959. 316

2564. Lorenzi, G. B. de. L'igiene del
sonno. Giorn. Reale Soc. Ital.
Igiene, 52:370-80, 1930. 312

2565. Loucks, R. B. The conditioning
of salivary and striped muscle
responses to faradization of
cortical sensory elements, and
the action of sleep upon such
mechanisms. J. Comp. Psychol.,
25:315-32, 1938. 362

2566. Louttit, C. M. Clinical Psychology. New York: Harper's, 1936.
Pp. xx + 695. 114

2567. Loveland, N. T., and M. T.
Singer. Projective test assessment of the effects of sleep deprivation. J. Project. Techniques,
23:323-34, 1959. 228

2568. Lovell, G. D., and J. B. Morgan. Physiological and motor responses to a regularly recurring
sound: a study in monotony. J.
Exp. Psychol., 30:435-51, 1942.
72, 196

2569. Low, A. A. Sabotaging Sleep. Recovery Publication No. 10. Chicago: Recovery, Inc., 1945. Pp. 11.

2570. Lubin, A., and H. L. Williams. Sleep loss, tremor, and the conceptual reticular formation. Perceptual Motor Skills, 9:237-38, 1959. 209, 225
Lubin, A., co-author: 1440, 1441, 2889, 2957, 4225-27.

2571. Luborsky, L., and H. Shevrin. Dreams and day-residues: a study of Poetzl observation. Bull. Menninger Clin., 20:135-48, 1956. 104
Luborsky, L., co-author: 3679.

2572. Luckhardt, A. B., and R. L. Johnston. The psychic secretion of gastric juice under hypnosis. Am. J. Physiol., 70:174-82, 1924. 54
Luckhardt, A. B., co-author: 2945.

2573. Luederitz, B. Untersuchungen ueber die Rhythmik der Koerpertemperatur. I. Koerpertemperatur und Urinausscheidung bei Kranken mit Fluessigkeitretention. Dsch. Arch. klin. Med., 196: 123-34, 1949. 64, 174

2574. ____. Ueber Stoerungen im Schlaf-Wachrhythmus. Acta Med. Scand., 152, Suppl. 307:191, 1955. 113

2575. Luksch, A. Ueber das "Schlafzentrum." Z. ges. Neurol. Psychiat., 93:83-94, 1924. 266, 360

2576. Lundervold, A. Electroencephalographic changes in a case of acute cerebral anoxia unconscious for about three years. EEG Clin. Neurophysiol., 6:311-15, 1954. 29

2577. ____. Discussion after Electroencephalographical expression of altered consciousness by H. Fischgold and R. Jung. First Internat. Congr. Neurol. Sci., Seconde Journée Commune. Brussels, Acta Med. Belg., 1957, pp. 214-18. 29

2578. ____, T. Hauge, and A. C. Loken. Unusual EEG in unconscious patient with brain stem atrophy. EEG Clin. Neurophysiol., 8:665-70, 1956. 273

2579. Lundholm, H., and H. Loewenbach. Hypnosis and the alpha activity of the electroencephalogram. Charact. Personal., 11: 145-49, 1942. 330

Lundholm, H., co-author: 4194, 4195.

2580. Lunedi, A., e E. Liesch. Ulcera gastro-duodenale, policitemia essenziale, sindrome adiposogenitale di Froelich in vari membri di una stessa famiglia. Riv. Clin. Med., 36:485-554, 1935. 268

2581. Lungwitz, H. Ueber neurotische Dysgrypnie. Psychiat.-neurol. Wschr., 42:95-98, 1940. 286

2582. Lush, J. L. "Nervous goats," J. Hered., 21:243-47, 1930. 255

2583. Lussheimer, P. Landmarks in the studies of dream-interpretation during the past half century. Am. J. Psychoanal., 7:36-44, 1947. 103

2584. Lust, F. Ueber die Beeinflussung der postenzephalitischen Schlafstoerung durch temperatursteigende Mittel. Dsche med. Wschr., 47:1545-47, 1921. 200, 203

2585. Lustig, E. Cura degli accessi di sonno. Policlinico (Sez. Prat.), 43:467, 1936.

2586. Lyketsos, G., L. Belinson, and F. A. Gibbs. Sleep recordings on psychotic patients with and without psychomotor seizures. EEG Clin. Neurophysiol., 4:379, 1952. 29

2587. ____, ____, and ____. Electroencephalograms of nonepileptic psychotic patients awake and asleep. A.M.A. Arch. Neurol. Psychiat., 69:707-12, 1953. 29

2588. Lyman, C. P. The oxygen consumption and temperature regulation of hibernating hamsters. J. Exp. Zool., 109:55-78, 1948. 324

2589. ____. Effect of increased CO_2 on respiration and heart rate of hibernating hamsters and ground squirrels. Am. J. Physiol., 167: 638-43, 1951. 323

2590. ____. Activity, food consumption and hoarding in hibernators. J. Mammal., 35:545-52, 1954. 321

2591. ____. Oxygen consumption, body temperature and heart rate of woodchucks entering hibernation. Am. J. Physiol., 194:83-91, 1958. 321

2592. ____. Hibernation in mammals. Circulation, 24:434-45, 1961. 328

2593. ____, and D. C. Blinks. The effect of temperature on the isolated hearts of closely related hibernators and non-hibernators. J. Cell. Comp. Physiol., 54:53-63, 1959. 323, 327

2594. ____, and P. O. Chatfield. Mechanisms of arousal in the hibernating hamster. J. Exp. Zool., 114:491-516, 1950. 326

2595. ____, and ____. Hibernation and cortical electrical activity in the woodchuck (Marmota monac). Science, 117:533-34, 1953. 324

2596. ____, and ____. Physiology of hibernation in mammals. Physiol. Rev., 35:403-25, 1955. 321, 328

2597. ____, and A. B. Hastings. Total CO_2, plasma pH, and pCO_2 of hamsters and ground squirrels during hibernation. Am. J. Physiol., 167:633-37, 1951. 323

2598. ____, and E. H. Leduc. Changes in blood sugar and tissue glycogen in the hamster during arousal from hibernation. J. Cell. Comp. Physiol., 41:471-92, 1953. 327
Lyman, C. P., co-author: 677-80, 864, 1146.

2599. Lyman, R. A., Jr. The blood sugar concentration in active and hibernating ground squirrels. J. Mammal., 24:467-74, 1943. 322

2600. Lynes, T. E. A cortical recruiting response elicited by low frequency stimulation of the mesencephalic reticular formation. Fed. Proc., 19:293, 1960. 210

2601. Maccone, L. L'insonnia nervosa nei bambini. Prat. Pediat., 13: 172-77, 1935. 294

2602. MacCurdy, J. T. The psychology and treatment of insomnia in fatigue and allied states. J. Abnorm. Psychol., 15:45, 1920. 276

2603. Macdonald, M. Sleeping and waking. Mind, 62:202-15, 1953. 106

2604. Macé de Lépinay, C.-E. Le nombre des insomniaques a-t-il augmenté du fait de la guerre ? Gaz. Méd. France, 53:239-40, 1946. 274

2605. Machne, X., I. Calma, and H. W. Magoun. Unit activity of cerebral cephalic brain stem in EEG arousal. J. Neurophysiol., 18: 547-58, 1955. 209
Machne, X., co-author: 960, 3066.

2606. Mackwood, J. Periodic somno-

lence and morbid hunger. Brit. Med. J., I:235, 1942. 267

2607. Maclay, J. A. Sleep and proper and improper methods of sleeping in relation to health and disease. J. Med. Soc. New Jersey, 14:144-47, 1917. 81, 312

2608. MacLean, K. S. Sleep and insomnia. Guy's Hosp. Gaz., 63: 175-81, 1949. 274, 362

2609. MacMahon, C. Posture during sleep. Lancet, I:242, 1942. 9, 11

2610. Macnish, R. The Philosophy of Sleep. New York: D. Appleton & Co., 1834. Pp. viii + 296. 310, 312

2611. MacWilliam, J. A. Some applications of physiology to medicine. III. Blood pressure and heart action in sleep and dreams: their relation to hemorrhages, angina and sudden death. Brit. Med. J., II:1196-1200, 1923. 44

2612. ____. Blood pressures in man, normal and pathologic. Physiol. Rev., 5:303-32, 1925. 44

2613. Maeder, A. E. The Dream Problem. Nerv. Ment. Dis. Monogr. No. 22, 1916. Pp. 43.

2614. Mädelä, S., E. Näätänen, and U. K. Rinne. The response of the adrenal cortex to psychic stress after meprobamate treatment. Acta Endocrinol., 32:1-7, 1959. 302

2615. Maenchen, A. Neurotic disturbances of sleep. Internat. J. Psycho-anal., 23:59-62, 1942. 286

2616. Magnes, J., G. Moruzzi, and O. Pompeiano. Electroencephalogram-synchronizing structures in the lower brain stem. In: A CIBA Found. Symposium on the Nature of Sleep, 1961 (4270), pp. 57-78. 212, 362

2617. ____, ____, and ____. Synchronization of EEG produced by low-frequency electrical stimulation of the region of the solitary tract. Arch. Ital. Biol., 99:33-67, 1961. 212

2618. Magni, F., G. Moruzzi, G. F. Rossi, e A. Zanchetti. Attivazione elettroencefalografica prodotta per mezzo di inattivazione temporanea delle parti caudali del tronco dell'encefalo. Riv. Neurol. (Napoli), 29:129-32, 1959. 212

2619. ____, ____, ____, and ____. EEG arousal following inactivation of the lower brain stem by selective injection of barbiturate into the vertebral circulation. Arch. Ital. Biol., 97:33-46, 1959. 362
Magni, F., co-author: 252, 253.

2620. Magnussen, G. Eighteen cases of epilepsy with fits in relation to sleep. Acta Psychiat. Neurol., 11:289-321, 1936. 260

2621. ____. Vasomotorische Veraenderungen in den Extremitaeten in Verhaeltnis zu Schlaf und Schlafbereitschaft. Acta Psychiat. Neurol., 14:39-54, 1939. 72

2622. ____. On narcolepsy. II. Studies on diurnal variations in the skin temperatures in narcoleptics. Acta Psychiat. Neurol., 18:457-85, 1943. 72, 79, 240

2623. ____. Studies on the Respiration during Sleep. A Contribution to the Physiology of the Sleep Function. London: H. K. Lewis, 1944. Pp. 276. 48, 49, 50, 51, 52, 72, 79, 109

2624. ____. (Danish) Sleep and Sleep Disturbances. Copenhagen: Forlaget for vidensk. Litter., 1946. Pp. 101. 72, 286

2625. ____. (Danish) The sleep function and sleep disturbances. Mskr. Pract. Laegegern. 27:309-46, 1949; also Ment. Hyg., 37:89-118, 1953. 72, 286
Magnussen, G., co-author: 2258.

2626. Magoun, H. W. Caudal and cephalic influences of the brain stem reticular formation. Physiol. Rev., 30:459-74, 1950. 209

2627. ____. An ascending reticular activating system in the brain stem. A.M.A. Arch. Neurol. Psychiat., 67:145-54, 1952. 209

2628. ____. The ascending reticular activating system. Res. Publ. Ass. Res. Nerv. Ment. Dis., 30:480-92, 1952. 209

2629. ____. Physiological interrelationships between cortex and subcortical structures. EEG Clin. Neurophysiol., Suppl. 4: 163-67, 1953. 209

2630. ____. The ascending reticular system and wakefulness. In: Brain Mechanisms and Consciousness, 1954 (875), pp. 1-20. 209, 210

2631. ____. Brain stem influences on consciousness. Clin. Neurosurg., 3:186-92, 1955. 209

2632. ____. The Waking Brain. Springfield, Ill.: Thomas, 1958. Pp. viii + 138. 209, 362
Magoun, H. W., co-author: 1122, 1280, 1284-87, 2159, 2529-31, 2605, 2900, 3270, 3329, 3788, 3789, 4052.

2633. Mahoney, W., and D. Sheehan. The pituitary-hypothalamic mechanism: experimental occlusion of the pituitary stalk. Brain, 59:61-74, 1936.

2634. Mai, H., E. Schuetz, und H.-H. Mueller. Ueber das Elektroencephalogramm von Fruehgeburten. Z. Kinderheilk., 69:251-61, 1951. 27

2635. Main, R. J. Alterations of alveolar CO_2 in man accompanying postural change. Am. J. Physiol., 118:435-40, 1937. 51

2636. Maizelis, M. R. (Russ.) Importance of a stereotype of eating, muscular activity and sleeping in the regulation of physiological functions. Zh. Vysshei Nerv. Deiat., 9(6):845-50, 1959.

2637. Malamud, W., and F. E. Linder. Dreams and their relationship to recent impressions. Arch. Neurol. Psychiat., 25:1081-99, 1931. 104

2638. Malcolm, N. Dreaming and skepticism. Philos. Rev., 65: 14-37, 1956. 106

2639. ____. Dreaming. New York: Humanities Press, 1959. Pp. vii + 128. 106

2640. Maliniak, S. Observations sur la mobilité dans le sommeil. Arch. Psychol., 24:177-226, 1934. 86, 87, 296

2641. Malmo, R. B., and W. W. Surwillo. Sleep Deprivation: Changes in Performance and Physiological Indicants of Activation. Psychol. Monogr., 74, No. 15 (Whole No. 502), 1960. Pp. 24. 225, 229

2642. Manacéine, M. de. Quelques observations expérimentales sur l'influence de l'insomnie absolue. Arch. Ital. Biol., 21:322-25, 1894. 215

2643. ____. Sleep: Its Physiology, Pathology, Hygiene, and Psychology. London: Walter Scott, 1897. Pp. vii + 341. 99, 305, 306, 310, 312

2644. Manceau, A., et M. Jorda. Les centres mésodiencéphaliques du sommeil. Sem. Hôp., 24:3193-

3202, 1948. 206

2645. Mancia, M., M. Meulders, et G.
Santibañez. Synchronisation de
l'électroencéphalogramme provoquée par la stimulation visu-
elle répétitive chez le chat "mé-
diopontin prétrigéminal." Arch.
Internat. Physiol., 67:661-70,
1959. 212

2646. _____, _____, and _____. Changes
of photically evoked potentials in
the visual pathway of the cerveau
isolé cat. Arch. Ital. Biol., 97:
378-98, 1959. 210

2647. _____, _____, and _____. Changes
of photically evoked potentials in
the visual pathway of the midpontine pretrigeminal cat. Arch.
Ital. Biol., 97:399-413, 1959. 210
Mancia, M., co-author: 521, 522,
757.

2648. Mangold, E. Schlaf und Schlafaehnliche Zustaende bei Menschen und Tieren. Berlin: Parey,
1929. Pp. 20.

2649. Mangold, R., L. Sokoloff, E. Con-
ner, J. Kleinerman, P.-O. G.
Therman, and S. S. Kety. The effects of sleep and lack of sleep
on cerebral circulation and metabolism of normal young men.
J. Clin. Investig., 34:1092-1100,
1955. 39, 47, 342

2650. Mann, L. The relation of Rorschach indices of extraversion-
introversion to certain dream dimensions. J. Clin. Psychol., 11:
80-81, 1955. 101

2651. Manoia, A. R. La vita sessuale
ed il sonno. Rassegna Studi
Sess. Eugen., 4:383-90, 1924.
276

2652. Mansfeld, G. Narcose et Sommeil. Lausanne: Roth, 1947. Pp.
35; also Narkose und Schlaf,
Wien. klin. Wschr., 60:796-801,
1948.

2653. Mansbach, M. Ueber den Einfluss
von Schlaflagen auf die Entstehung von Kieferanomalien. Z.
Stomatol., 29:1331-59, 1931. 11,
306

2654. _____. Ueber den Einfluss von
Schlaflagen auf die Entstehung
von Kieferanomalien. Z. Stomatol., 30:1364-66, 1932. 11

2655. Mantegazza, P. Della temperatura delle orine in diverse ore
del giorno e in diversi climi.
Gazz. Med. Ital. Lombard., 21:
209-12, 1862; also (in French)
Rev. Méd. Belge, 15:14, 1863. 138

2656. Mantegazzini, P., K. Poeck, and
G. Santibañez. The action of adrenaline and nor-adrenaline on
the cortical electrical activity
of the "encéphale isolé" cat.
Arch. Ital. Biol., 97:222-42,
1959; prelim. commun. Pfluegers Arch., 270:14-15, 1959.
303

2657. Manual, E. The modern hypnotics. Antiseptic, 44:215-21, 1947.
278

2658. Marburg, O. Schlaftheorien und
Hirnrindenfunktion. Wien. klin.
Wschr., 39:1076-77, 1926.

2659. Marchand, H. Cholestérine et
sommeil. C. R. Soc. Biol., 72:
615-16, 1912. 351

2660. Marchand, H. Ueber die Her-
beifuehrung des bedingt-reflec-
torischen Schlafes ohne Medikamente. Dsch. Gesundhwes.,
9:1255-56, 1954. 206

2661. Marchand, L., et J. Ajuriaguer-
ra. Le rire comme cause dé-
terminante des accidents épileptiques. Ann. Méd.-Psychol.
(Paris), 99:325-28, 1941. 256

2662. Marchini, E., R. Tagliacozzo,
e R. Vizioli. Epilessia e stato
di coscienza. Riv. Neurol. (Napoli), 27:410-12, 1957. 259

2663. Marck, H. La Cure de Sommeil.
Paris: Impr. R. Foulon, 1953.
(Thèse) Pp. 79. 206

2664. Marcus, H., und E. Sahlgren.
Untersuchungen ueber die Einwirkung der hypnotischen Suggestion auf die Funktion des vegetativen Systems. Muench.
med. Wschr., 72:381-82, 1925.
334

2665. Marcus, J. H. Importance of
sleep in infancy and early childhood. J. Med. Soc. New Jersey,
20:127-28, 1923. 114, 305

2666. Mare, W. de la. Behold, This
Dreamer! Of Reverie, Night,
Sleep, Dream, Love-Dreams,
Nightmare, Death, the Uncon-
scious, the Imagination, Divina-
tion, the Artist, and Kindred
Subjects. New York: Knopf,
1939. Pp. viii + 694.

2667. Marenina, A. I. (Russ.) Investigation of the dynamics of sleep
in man by measuring electrical
resistance of skin surface.
Trudy Inst. Fiziol. Pavlova, 1:
316-19, 1952; also in: The Sleep
Problem, 1954 (392), pp. 256-
59. 330

2668. _____. (Russ.) Investigation of the dynamics of sleep by measuring skin potentials. Trudy Inst. Fiziol. Pavlova, 1:320-24, 1952; also in: The Sleep Problem, 1954 (392), pp. 260-64.

2669. _____. (Russ.) Electroencephalographic investigation of natural and hypnotic sleep in man. Trudy Inst. Fiziol. Pavlova, 1:325-32, 1952; also in: The Sleep Problem, 1954 (392), pp. 265-72. 330

2670. _____. (Russ.) Investigation of the somnambulistic phase of hypnosis by means of electroencephalography. Trudy Inst. Fiziol. Pavlova, 1:333-38, 1952. 330

2671. _____. (Russ.) Investigations of sleep of narcoleptics by means of electroencephalography. Zh. Vysshei Nerv. Deiat., 2:219-23, 1952. 239, 330

2672. _____. (Russ.) Further investigation of the dynamics of cerebral potentials in various phases of hypnosis in man. Fiziol. Zh. SSSR, 41:742-47, 1955. 330

2673. _____. (Russ.) Cerebral potential changes in various phases of hypnosis in man. Trudy Inst. Fiziol. Pavlova, 5:299-306, 1956. 330

2674. Margolin, S., P. Perlman, F. Villani, and T. H. McGavack. A new class of hypnotics: unsaturated carbinols. Science, 114: 384-85, 1951. 294
Margolin, S., co-author: 2294-96.

2675. Margulies, M. Hypnose als Hilfsmittel psychiatrischer Begutachtung. Aerztl. sachverst. Z., 37: 371-73, 1931.

2676. Maria, G. Ricerche elettroencefalografiche nel pavor nocturnus. Cervello, 32:101-12, 1956. 281

2677. Mariani, C. Ricerche sul comportamento del glutatione nel sonno sperimentale. Boll. Soc. Ital. Biol. Sper., 4:865-67, 1929. 297

2678. Marinacci, A. A., and R. P. Sedwick. Electroencephalographic findings in an (an)encephalic monster. EEG Clin. Neurophysiol., 2:221, 1950. 29

2679. Marinesco, G., S. Drăgănesco, O. Sager, et A. Kreindler. Recherches anatomo-cliniques sur la localisation de la fonction du sommeil. Rev. Neurol., II:481-97, 1929. 263, 266

2680. _____, A. Kreindler, ed E. Cohen. Corea acuta e catalessia. Rifor-

ma Med., 46:1191-94, 1930. 255

2681. _____, O. Sager, et A. Kreindler. Recherches expérimentales sur le mécanisme du sommeil. Bull. Acad. Méd. Paris, 99:752-56, 1928. 202, 205

2682. _____, _____, y _____. Investigaciones experimentales sobre el mecanismo del sueño. Rev. Méd. Rosario (Argentina), 18: 371-74, 1928. 202, 205

2683. _____, _____, und _____. Experimentelle Untersuchungen zum Problem des Schlafmechanismus. Z. Neurol., 119:277-306, 1929. 202, 205

2684. _____, _____, und _____. Beitraege zu einer allgemeinen Theorie des Schlafes. Z. ges. Neurol. Psychiat., 122:23-47, 1929. 360

2685. _____, _____, et _____. Etudes électro-encéphalographiques: le sommeil naturel et le sommeil hypnotique. Bull. Acad. Méd. Paris, 117:273-76, 1937. 344, 359

2686. _____, _____, et _____. Etudes électroencéphalographiques: Le sommeil et le coma. (Septième note). Bull. Acad. Méd. Roumanie, 2:454-58, 1937. 273

2687. Markov, D. (Russ.) On the clinic of hypophyseal diseases (hypophyseal infantilism) in relation to the doctrine of the sleep center. Sovrem. Psikhonevrol., 1(5):58-62, 1925. 269

2688. Mármol Plaza, D. Contribución de la electroencéfalografía al studio de la narcolepsia y de la cataplejía. Clin. Laborat. (Zaragoza), 62:106-12, 1956. 234

2689. Marquis, D. P. A study of activity and postures in infants' sleep. J. Genet. Psychol., 42: 51-69, 1933. 9, 90

2690. _____. Learning in the neonate: The modification of behavior under three feeding schedules. J. Exp. Psychol., 29:263-82, 1941. 133
Marquis, D. P., co-author: 3320.

2691. Marsh, H. D. The Diurnal Course of Efficiency. Columbia Univ. Contrib. Philos. Psychol., 14:1-99, 1906. 150

2692. Martelli, G. Osservazioni elettroencefalografiche su un caso di narcolessia. Giorn. Psichiat. Neuropat. (Ferrara), 86:221-30, 1958. 237

2693. Martin, C. A. L'insomnie. Laval Méd., 13:492-506, 1948. 238, 274

2694. Martin, E. G., G. H. Bigelow, and G. B. Wilbur. Variations in the sensory threshold for faradic stimulation in normal human subjects. II. The nocturnal variation. Am. J. Physiol., 33:415-22, 1914. 158
Martin, E. G., co-author: 1497.

2695. Martin, J. P. Consciousness and its disturbances considered from the neurological aspect. Lancet, 257:1-6, 48-53, 1949. 31, 361

2696. Martin, P., et P. Cossa. Réaction d'éveil et décharge comitiale. EEG Clin. Neurophysiol., 4:238, 1952. 257

2697. Martin, W. W. Consciousness as organismic physiological functioning. Psychol. Rev., 54:99-115, 1947. 31

2698. Martini, E., T. Gualtierotti, und A. Marzorati. Die Rueckenmark-elektronarkose. Pfluegers Arch., 246:585-96, 1943. 298

2699. _____, _____, and _____. Electronarcosis. II. Inhibition of electrical activity of cerebral cortex following application of pulsed stimulus to diencephalon. J. Neurophysiol., 13:1-4, 1950. 298
Martini, E., co-author: 1545, 1546.

2700. Martini, F. La terapia del sonno nella pratica psichiatrica. Riv. Pat. Nerv. Ment., 77:549-50, 1956. 207

2701. Marvaud, A. Le Sommeil et l'Insomnie; Etude Physiologique, Clinique et Thérapeutique. Paris: J. B. Ballière & Fils, 1881. Pp. 137. 274, 294

2702. Masci, B. Movimenti rotatori del capo durante il sonno. Policlinico (Sez. Prat.), 24:925-29, 1917. 285

2703. Maslova, N. P. (Russ.) Change in the electroencephalogram in neurotics (neurasthenics) in the state of wakefulness, sleep, and awakening. Zh. Vysshei Nerv. Deiat., 8:517-23, 1958. 113

2704. Mason, A. A. Discussion on hypnotism in general practice. The scope of hypnotism. Practitioner, 180:598-99, 1958. 335

2705. Mason, E. D., and F. G. Benedict. The effect of sleep on human basal metabolism, with particular reference to South Indian women. Am. J. Physiol., 108:377-83, 1934. 55

2706. Mason, J. W. Some aspects of the central nervous system regulation of ACTH secretion. J. Clin. Endocrinol., 16:914, 1956. 170

2707. Mason-Browne, N. L. Alterations of consciousness: tumor of the reticular activating system. A.M.A. Arch. Neurol. Psychiat., 76:380-87, 1956. 209

2708. Maspes, P. L. Sindrome narcolessica-onirica d'origine diencefalica. Riv. Pat. Nerv., 41:137-62, 1933.

2709. Massaroti, V. Sonno e Insonnia: Cause, Consigli, Rimedi. Milano: Ediz. Giovanni Bolla, 1950. Pp. 207. 274, 275, 278

2710. Mathers, A. T. Sleep and its disorders. Northwest Med., 33: 115, 171, 1934.

2711. Mathieu-Pierre-Weil, C. Sichere, et J. van Peteghem. Cures de sommeil et maladies rhumatismales. In: La Cure de Sommeil, 1954 (3021), pp. 216-20. 207

2712. Mathis, P., et H. Fischgold. Inconscience et insomnie prolongées. Rev. Neurol., 94:816-18, 1956. 11, 273
Mathis, P., co-author: 1182, 1186.

2713. Matzkevich, A. N. (Russ.) The problem of the effect of experimental sleep—hypnotic state—upon the higher nervous functions. Psikhoterapia, 14:173-89, 1930. 334
Matzkevich, A. N., co-author: 3213.

2714. Maurer, L. Serumeisen—Tageskurven bei Kindern. Z. Kinderheilk., 70:527-34, 1952. 163

2715. Maurer, S., H. O. Wiles, E. W. Schoeffel, and M. L. Fischer. Effect of l-cevitamic acid on insomnia. Illinois Med. J., 74: 84-85, 1938. 294

2716. Maury, A. Sommeil et les Rêves; Etudes Psychologiques sur ces Phénomènes et les Divers Etats qui s'y Rattachent. Paris: Didier & Cie, 1878. Pp. 476.

2717. Mauthner, L. Pathologie und Physiologie des Schlafes. Wien. klin. Wschr., 3:445-46, 1890. 206, 243, 250, 262, 347, 359

2718. Max, L. W. Action current responses in deaf-mutes during sleep, sensory stimulation and dreams. J. Comp. Psychol., 19: 469-86, 1935. <u>12</u>, <u>16</u>, <u>74</u>, <u>100</u>

2719. _____. Action-current responses in the deaf during awakening, kinesthetic imagery and abstract thinking. J. Comp. Psychol., 24: 301-44, 1937. <u>123</u>

2720. May, E. Un cas de crises de sommeil d'origine anaphylactique. Bull. Mém. Soc. Méd. Hôp. Paris, 47:704-5, 1923. <u>268</u>

2721. May, P. R. A., and F. G. Ebaugh. Use of hypnotics in aging and senile patients. J. Am. Med. Ass., 152:801-5, 1953. <u>278</u>

2722. Mayer, C. Physiologisches und Pathologisches ueber das Gaehnen. Z. Biol., 73:101-14, 1921. <u>72</u>

2723. Mayer-Gross, W. Zur Struktur des Einschlaferlebens. Arch. Psychiat., 86:313, 1929. <u>79</u>

2724. _____, and F. Berliner. Observations in hypoglycaemia: IV. Body temperature and coma. J. Ment. Sci., 88:419-27, 1942.

2725. Mayo, J. G. Sleep and rest and their relation to the autonomic nervous system. Proc. Staff Meet. Mayo Clin., 5:27, 1930. <u>45</u>

2726. Mayon-White, R. M. Sleep-walking. Practitioner, 175:215-18, 1955. <u>283</u>, <u>286</u>, <u>289</u>

2727. Mayorov, F. P. (Russ.) Studies in the dynamics of sleep and transitory states in man by the chronaximetric method. Arkh. Biol. Nauk, 54:165-73, 1939. <u>14</u>

2728. _____. (Russ.) On the phases of sleep. Fiziol. Zh. SSSR, 34:421-30, 1948; also in: The Sleep Problem, 1954 (392), pp. 216-25. <u>14</u>, <u>330</u>

2729. _____. (Russ.) Physiological characteristics of the somnambulistic phase of hypnosis. Fiziol. Zh. SSSR, 36:649-52, 1950. <u>330</u>

2730. _____. (Russ.) Physiological Theory of Dreams. Nervous Mechanism of Dreams. Moskva-Leningrad: Iz'd. Akad. Nauk SSSR, 1951. Pp. 132. <u>100</u>

2731. _____. (Russ.) The theory of nervous traces. In: The Sleep Problem, 1954 (392), pp. 294-99. <u>106</u>

2732. _____, and M. I. Sandomirsky. (Russ.) Transitory states and types of nervous system. In: The Sleep Problem, 1954 (392), pp. 226-36. <u>78</u>
Mayorov, F. P., co-author:

2166-68.

2733. Mazer, M. An experimental study of the hypnotic dream. Psychiatry, 14:265-77, 1951. <u>334</u>

2734. Mazurkiewicz, J. L'état de sommeil et de veille au cours du cycle vital de l'homme. Rev. Neurol., 65:913-14, 1936.

2735. Mazzella, H., E. Garcia-Austt, and R. Garcia-Mullin. Carotid sinus and EEG. EEG Clin. Neurophysiol., 8:155, 1956. <u>213</u>, <u>241</u>

2736. McBirnie, J. E., F. G. Pearson, G. A. Trusler, H. H. Karachi, and W. G. Bigelow. Physiologic studies of the groundhog (Marmota monax). Canad. J. Med. Sci., 31:421-30, 1953. <u>322</u>, <u>323</u>

2737. McClendon, S. J. Management of nocturnal enuresis in childhood. Arch. Pediat., 75:101-5, 1958. <u>284</u>, <u>302</u>

2738. McCluskie, J. A. Children who spend too long in bed. Lancet, II:302-3, 1946. <u>307</u>

2739. McCord, F. Report of hypnotically induced dreams and conflicts. J. Personal. (Durham), 14:268-80, 1946. <u>333</u>

2740. McCordock, H. A., W. Collier, and S. H. Gray. Pathologic changes of St. Louis type of acute encephalitis. J. Am. Med. Ass., 103:822-24, 1934. <u>245</u>

2741. McCormick, W. J. Vitamin B$_1$ in relation to fatigue, sleep and narcosis. A new concept of the physiology of sleep. Med. Rec., 151:282-83, 1940. <u>353</u>

2742. McCranie, E. J., H. B. Crasilneck, and H. R. Teter. The electro-encephalogram in hypnotic age regression. Psychiat. Q., 29:85-88, 1955. <u>333</u>

2743. McCray, D. W. To sleep or not to sleep. Hygeia (Chicago), 18: 680-82, 732, 773-75, 837, 1940. <u>114</u>

2744. McCurdy, H. G. The history of dream theory. Psychol. Rev., 53:225-33, 1946. <u>99</u>

2745. _____. Consciousness and the galvanometer. Psychol. Rev., 57:322-27, 1950. <u>31</u>

2746. McDonagh, J. O. The problem as seen by the general practitioner. Brit. Med. J., II:152, 1954. <u>277</u>

2747. McDonald, D. A. The physiology of sleep. Lancet, I:1071, 1951.

2748. McDonald, R. H. Narcolepsy and cataplexy; report of two cases. Cleveland Clin. Q., 11:79-82, 1944. 237

2749. McDonald, R. K., F. T. Evans, V. K. Weise, and R. W. Patrick. Effect of morphine on adrenocorticotrophin in man. Fed. Proc., 17:109, 1958.

2750. McDonnell, J. Sleep posture: its implications. Brit. J. Phys. Med., 9:46-52, 1946. 9

2751. _____. Sleep posture; costo-vertebral manipulations. Rheumatism (London), 4:238-39, 1948.

2752. McFarland, R. A., and R. C. Moore. Human factors in highway safety. New Engl. J. Med., 256: 792-99, 1957. 315

2753. McGlade, H. B. The relationship between gastric motility, muscular twitching during sleep and dreaming. Am. J. Digest. Dis., 9: 137-40, 1942. 54, 87, 105

2754. McGovern, B. E. Somnolence associated with pituitary cachexia. Endocrinology, 16:402-6, 1932. 269

2755. McKendree, C. A., and L. Feinier. Somnolence: its occurrence and significance in cerebral neoplasms. Arch. Neurol. Psychiat., 17:44-56, 1927. 265

2756. McKenzie, R. E., B. Hartman, and D. E. Graveline. An exploratory study of sleep characteristics in a hypodynamic environment. USAF School Aviat. Med., Brooks AFB, Report 60-68, Oct. 1960. Pp. 8. 98
McKenzie, R. E., co-author: 1506.

2757. McLardy, T. Diffuse thalamic projection to cortex: an anatomical critique. EEG Clin. Neurophysiol., 3:183-88, 1951. 210

2758. McLauchlan, G. P. Sleep in children of school age. Med. Officer, 91:261-63, 1954. 118

2759. Mead, S., and E. S. Roush. A study of the effect of hypnotic suggestion on physiologic performance. Arch. Phys. Med., 30:700-706, 1949. 331

2760. Meares, A. A working hypothesis as to the nature of hypnosis. A.M.A. Arch. Neurol. Psychiat., 77:549-55, 1957. 336

2761. Medina, F. (Portug.) The importance of the reticular system in the neurophysiology of consciousness. Gaz. Méd. Portug. (Lisboa), 10:411-17, 1957. 31

2762. Meer, S. J. Authoritarian attitudes and dreams. J. Abnorm. Soc. Psychol., 51:74-78, 1955. 101

2763. Megroz, R. L. Dreams in childhood. Contemp. Rev., 153:458-65, 1938. 106

2764. Mehes, J. Studien ueber den Scopolaminschlaf und seine Verstaerkung durch Morphium. Arch. exp. Path. Pharmakol., 142:309-22, 1929. 297

2765. Meignant, P. Sommeil et réflectivité conditionelle. Encéphale, 28:197-230, 1933.

2766. Melin, K.-A. (Norw.) Cerebral activity in the newborn. Nord. Med., 46:1268-69, 1951. 27

2767. _____. The EEG in infancy and childhood. EEG Clin. Neurophysiol., Suppl. 4:205-11, 1953.
Melin, K.-A., co-author: 1560.

2768. Mellette, H. C., B. K. Hutt, S. I. Askovitz, and S. M. Horvath. Diurnal variations in body temperature. J. Appl. Physiol., 3: 665-75, 1951. 145

2769. Mendelson, J. H., L. Siger, and P. Solomon. Psychiatric observations on congenital and acquired deafness: Symbolic and perceptual processes in dreams. Am. J. Psychiat., 116:883-88, 1960. 102
Mendelson, J., co-author: 2422, 3752, 4182.

2770. Mendicini, A. La respirazione nella melancolia durante il sonno. Studio sperimentale di psicofisiologia. Arch. Gen. Neurol. Psichiat. Psicoanal., 1:194-232, 1920. 49

2771. Menninger-Lerchenthal, E. Periodische Traeume. Wien. Z. Nervenheilk, 10:121-26, 1954. 105

2772. Menzel, W. Der 24-Stunden-Rhythmus des menschlichen Blutkreislaufes. Ergebn. inn. Med. Kinderheilk., 61:1-53, 1942. 163

2773. _____. Zur Physiologie und Pathologie des Nacht- und Schichtarbeiters. Arbeitsphysiologie, 14:304-18, 1950. 316

2774. _____. Wellenlaenge und Phasenlage der menschlichen Nierenrhythmik mit Analysen nach dem Blumeschen Verfahren. Z. ges. exp. Med., 116:237-64, 1950. 167

2775. _____. Schlaf und innere Medi-

zin. Med. Welt, 20:583-87, 1951.
316

2776. _____. Ueber den heutigen Stand
der Rhythmenlehre in bezug auf
die Medizin. Z. Altersforsch.,
6:26-37, 104-21, 1952. 167

2777. _____. Langwellige Organperio-
dik im Rahmen von Regulationsvorgaenge. Verhandl. Dsch. Gesell. inn. Med., 59:399-402, 1953.
167

2778. _____. Perioden menschlicher
Koerperfunktionen in Diagnose
und Therapie. Medizinische, No.
43:1521-26, 1956. 167

2779. _____, J. Blume, und E. Lua. Untersuchungen zur Nierenrhythmik. III. Die Rhythmik der Kranken Niere. Σ. ges. exp. Med.,
120:396-410, 1953. 167

2780. _____, _____, und F.-F. v.
Schroeder. Klassifizierung klinischer Verlaeufe durch Perio-
denanalyse. Z. klin. Med., 155:
249-68, 1958. 167

2781. _____, R. Timm, und G. Herrn-
ring. Ueber den diagnostischen
Wert der Tag-Nacht-Schwankun-
gen des erhoehten Blutdrucks.
Verhandl. Dsch. Gesell. Kreis-
laufforsch., 15:256-60, 1949. 163

2782. Merlis, J. K., C. Grossman, and
G. F. Henriksen. Comparative
effectiveness of sleep and Metra-
zol-activated electroencephalography. EEG Clin. Neurophysiol.,
3:71-78, 1951. 257

2783. _____, G. F. Henriksen, and C.
Grossman. Sleep, metrazol, and
auditory stimulation techniques
in electroencephalography. J.
Nerv. Ment. Dis., 112:76-78,
1950. 257
Merlis, J. K., co-author: 1532,
1702, 4103.

2784. Merzbacher, L. Untersuchungen
an winterschlafenden Fleder-
maeusen. I. Das Verhalten des
Centralnervensystems im Winter-
schlafe und waehrend des Erwachens aus demselben. Pfluegers
Arch., 97:569-77, 1903. 324

2785. Mesel, E., and F. F. Ledford, Jr.
The electroencephalogram during
hypnotic age regression (to infancy) in epileptic patients. A.M.A.
Arch. Neurol., 1:516-21, 1959. 333

2786. Metz, B., et P. Andlauer. Le
rythme nycthéméral de la température chez l'homme. C. R. Soc.
Biol., 143:1234-36, 1949. 138

2787. _____, et C. Kayser. Réactions
thermorégulatrices immédiates
du pigeon au cours du nycthémère. J. Physiol. (Paris), 40:
262A-64A, 1948.

2788. _____, et J. Schwartz. Etudes
des variations de la température rectale, du débit urinaire
et de l'excrétion urinaire des
17-cétostéroïdes chez l'homme
au cours du nycthémère. C. R.
Soc. Biol., 143:1237-39, 1949.
166, 167

2789. _____, D. Sigwalt, et M. F.
Mours-Laroche. Effets combi-
nés du travail et de la chaleur
sur le rythme nycthéméral des
mouvements d'eau chez l'homme normal. C. R. Soc. Biol.,
152:1191-93, 1958. 166
Metz, B., co-author: 65, 4246.

2790. Meunier, P., et R. Masselon.
Les Rêves et leur Interprétation; Essai de Psychologie Mor-
bide. Paris: Bloud & Cie., 1910.
Pp. 211. 99

2791. Meunier, R. Une théorie psychologique du sommeil. Bull.
Inst. Gén. Psychol., 29:50-61,
1929.

2792. Meyer, E. Ueber organische
Nervenerkrankungen im Gefolge
von Grippe. Arch. Psychiat., 62:
598-626, 1921. 267, 361

2793. _____. Das Schlafproblem, Prophylaxe und Behandlung der
Schlaflosigkeit bei Nerven-
schwachen. Klin. Wschr., 13:
1339, 1364, 1934. 274

2794. Meyer, H. Altes und Neues ueber Schlaf und Narkose. Wien.
klin. Wschr., 1:757-59, 1937.

2795. _____, und E. P. Pick. Hypnotica. Handb. norm. path. Physiol.,
17:611-21, 1926.

2796. Meyer, J. S., and J. Hunter. Behavior deficits following chronic
diencephalic lesions. Neurology,
2:112-30, 1952. 206
Meyer, J. S., co-author: 262.

2797. Meyers, F., E. D. Cook, and R.
C. Page. A clinical study of
hypnotics. Effect on gross sleep
movements, length of sleep,
blood pressure, respiratory rate,
and pulse rate. New York State
J. Med., 40:12-19, 1940. 87

2798. Meyers, R. Dandy's striatal theory of "the center of consciousness": surgical evidence and
logical analysis indicating its
improbability. Trans. Am. Neurol. Ass., 75:44-49, 1950; also

A.M.A. Arch. Neurol. Psychiat.,
65:659-71, 1951. 31, 273

2799. _____. Problems in consciousness and coma; traditional modes
of approach and a proposed re-
vision. Clin. Neurosurg., 3:166-
75, 1955. 31, 273

2800. Meyerson, A. The sleeping and
waking mechanisms: a theory of
the depressions and their treatment. J. Nerv. Ment. Dis., 105:
598-606, 1947. 274, 278

2801. Meyerson, I. Remarques pour
une théorie du rêve; observations sur le cauchemar. J. Psychol., 34:135-50, 1937. 99, 107

2802. Michaels, J. J., and S. E. Goodman. The incidence of enuresis
and the age of cessation in one
thousand neuro-psychiatric patients: with a discussion of the
relationship between enuresis
and delinquency. Am. J. Orthopsychiat., 9:59-71, 1939. 284

2803. Michels, R. Die Behandlung
chronischer Schlaflosigkeit mit
medikamentoesen Kuren (Lubro-
kalenkuren). Therap. Gegenw.,
72:256-60, 1931. 294

2804. Michelson, E. Untersuchungen
ueber die Tiefe des Schlafes.
Psychol. Arbeiten, 2:84-117,
1897. 108

2805. Miculicich, M. Ueber den heuti-
gen Stand der Schlaffrage und
Schlafforschung. Zagreb: M.
Prestini, 1928. Pp. 27. 362

2806. Middlemiss, J. E. Treatment by
hypnosis. Brit. Med. J., II:588-
89, 1942. 335

2807. Middleton, W. C. Nocturnal
dreams. Sci. Monthly, 37:460-64,
1933. 99

2808. _____. The frequency with which
a group of unselected college
students experience colored
dreaming and colored hearing.
J. Gen. Psychol., 27:221-29,
1942. 99, 102

2809. Migeon, C. J., A. B. French, L.
T. Samuels, and J. Z. Bowers.
Plasma 17-hydroxycorticosteroid
level and leucocyte values in the
rhesus monkey, including normal
variation and the effect of ACTH.
Am. J. Physiol., 182:462-68,
1955. 169, 170

2810. _____, F. H. Tyler, J. P. Mahoney, A. A. Florentin, H. Castle, E. L. Bliss, and L. T. Samuels. The diurnal variation of
plasma levels and urinary excre-

tion of 17-hydroxycorticoster-
oids in normal subjects, night
workers and blind subjects.
J. Clin. Endocrinol. Metab., 16:
622-33, 1956. 174
Migeon, C., co-author: 4000.

2811. Mihaleva, O. A., E. A. Moisseeff,
and A. V. Tonkih (Tonkikh).
(Russ.) Sleep produced by electrical stimulation of subcortical
ganglia. Fiziol. Zh. SSSR, 26:
389-93, 1939. 204

2812. Mikhailova, N. V. (Russ.) The
influence of the central nervous
system on the adrenocortico-
tropic function of the anterior
lobe of the hypophysis. Probl.
Endokrinol. (Moskva), 1:59-64,
1955. 356

2813. Mikheev, V. E. (Russ.) On the
anatomical aspects of the sleep
problem. Zh. Nevropat. Psikhiat.,
24(3):75-82, 1931.

2814. Mikiten, T. M., P. H. Niebyl,
and C. D. Hendley. EEG desynchronization during behavioral
sleep associated with spike discharges from the thalamus of
the cat. Fed. Proc., 20:327,
1961.

2815. Miles, W. R. Eye movements
during profound sleepiness.
Proc. Ninth Internat. Congr.
Psychol., 1929, pp. 308-9. 72

2816. _____. Horizontal eye movements at the onset of sleep.
Psychol. Rev., 36:122-41, 1929.
72, 225

2817. _____. Sleeping with your eyes
open. Sci. Am., 140:489-92,
1929. 72

2818. _____. Duration of sleep and the
insensible perspiration. Proc.
Soc. Exp. Biol. Med., 26:577-80,
1929. 56

2819. _____, and H. R. Laslett. Eye
movement and visual fixation
during profound sleepiness.
Psychol. Rev., 38:1-13, 1931.
224, 361

2820. Miller, E. Insomnia and Other
Disturbances of Sleep. London:
John Bale, Sons and Danielson,
1935. Pp. 88. 274, 278, 286

2821. Miller, H. R., and E. A. Spiegel.
Sleep induced by subthalamic
lesions with the hypothalamus
intact. Proc. Soc. Exp. Biol.
Med., 43:300-302, 1940. 206

2822. Miller, J. G. Unconsciousness.
New York: John Wiley & Sons,
1942. Pp. ix + 329. 31

Miller, J. G., co-author: 3805.

2823. Miller, M. Changes in the response to electric shock produced by varying muscular conditions. J. Exp. Psychol., 9:26-44, 1926. 76, 196

2824. Miller, M. M. Low sodium chloride intake in the treatment of insomnia and tension states. J. Am. Med. Ass., 129:262-66, 1945. 278

2825. Millet, J. A. P. Insomnia. Its Causes and Treatment. New York: Greenberg, 1938. Pp. 195. 274

2826. ———. How Did You Sleep Last Night? The Causes and Treatment of Insomnia. Kingswood, Surrey, Engl.: The World's Work, 1946. Pp. ix + 135. 274

2827. Mills, J. N. Diurnal rhythm in urine flow. J. Physiol. (London), 113:528-36, 1951; prelim. commun. 112:53P, 1950. 175

2828. ———. Changes in alveolar carbon dioxide tension by night and during sleep. J. Physiol. (London), 122:66-80, 1953. 51

2829. ———. All around the clock—a renal discourse. Manchester Univ. Med. School Gaz., 37:177-81, 1958. 174

2830. ———, and S. W. Stanbury. Persistent 24-hour renal excretory rhythm on a 12-hour cycle of activity. J. Physiol. (London), 117: 22-37, 1952; prelim. commun. 115:18P-19P, 1951. 175

2831. ———, and ———. A reciprocal relationship between K+ and H+ excretion in the diurnal excretory rhythm in man. Clin. Sci., 13:177-86, 1954. 167

2832. ———, and ———. Rhythmic diurnal variations in the behaviour of the human renal tubule. Acta Med. Scand., Suppl. 307:95-96, 1955. 167

2833. ———, and S. Thomas. Diurnal excretory rhythms in a subject changing from night to day work. J. Physiol. (London), 137:65P-66P, 1957. 174

2834. ———, ———, and P. A. Yates. Reappearance of renal excretory rhythm after forced disruption. J. Physiol. (London), 125:466-74, 1954; prelim. commun. 121:14P-15P, 1953. 173

Mills, J. N., co-author: 2558.

2835. Mingazzini, G. Klinischer und anatomisch-pathologischer Beitrag zum Studium der Encephalitis epidemica (lethargica). Z. ges. Neurol. Psychiat., 63:199-244, 1921. 243, 247

2836. Minkowski, E. Les voies d'accès au conscient (la conscience et l'inconscient). Evolut. Psychiat. (Paris), No. 3:383-405, 1949. 31

2837. Mintz, A. Y. (Russ.) Narcolepsy, cataplexy, and diencephalic epilepsy. Zh. Nevropat. Psikhiat., 58:410-17, 1958. 237

2838. Mirsky, A. F., and P. V. Cardon, Jr. A comparison of the behavioral and physiological changes accompanying sleep deprivation and chlorpromazine administration in man. EEG Clin. Neurophysiol., 14:1-10, 1962. 227, 302

Mirsky, A. F., co-author: 2240.

2839. Mirzoyants, N. S. (Russ.) Bioelectrical activity of the cerebral cortex in children of an early age and in initial phases of natural sleep. Zh. Vysshei Nerv. Deiat., 11:432-37, 1961. 27

2840. Mishchenko, M. N. (Russ.) On changes in higher nervous activity during experimental and natural sleep in humans. Eksp. Med., (4):59-69, 1935. 73

2841. ———. (Russ.) On changes in the motor spheres during experimental and natural sleep. Eksp. Med., (4):77-86, 1935. 73

2842. ———. (Russ.) On correlations between the hypnotic state and experimental sleep in man. Eksp. Med., (7/8):175-87, 1935. 337

2843. ———. (Russ.) Requirements for inducing experimental sleep in humans. Eksp. Med., (8):57-63, 65-66, 1936.

2844. Missriegler, A. On the psychogenesis of narcolepsy: report of a case cured by psychoanalysis. J. Nerv. Ment. Dis., 93:141-62, 1941. 237, 239

2845. Mitchell, M. B. Retroactive inhibition and hypnosis. J. Gen. Psychol., 7:343-59, 1932. 332

2846. Mitnick, L. L., and J. C. Armington. Alpha rhythm during sleep deprivation and recovery. Am. Psychol., 12:405-6, 1957. 226

Mitnick, L. L., co-author: 129.

2847. Miyagi, O. (Jap.) The hypnagogic neologisms. Jap. J. Exp. Psychol., 4:109-11, 1937. 79

2848. _____. (Jap.) Sleep. Jap. J. Exp. Psychol., 4:211-54, 1937.

2849. Modlin, H. C. Military aspects of narcolepsy. Milit. Surgeon, 98:329-37, 1946. 234

2850. _____. Ulcers, phobias, and narcolepsy. Bull. Menninger Clin., 12:203-9, 1948. 237

2851. _____, and W. deM. Scriver. Recovery from refractory diabetes insipidus associated with narcolepsy. Ann. Int. Med., 35:710-17, 1951. 238

2852. Møller, E., and I. Ostenfeld. Studies on the cerebral carotid sinus syndrome and the physiological basis of consciousness. Acta Psychiat. Neurol., 24:59-80, 1949. 241

2853. Möllerström, J. Periodicity in the carbohydrate metabolism. Acta Med. Scand., Suppl. 50:250-57, 1932. 166

2854. Möllmann, M. Ueber den Einfluss von Schlaflage und Bewegung bei Schwangeren auf die Kindeslage. Bonn: P. Kubens, 1933. Pp. 32.

2855. Moenninghoff, O., und F. Piesbergen. Messungen ueber die Tiefe des Schlafes. Z. Biol., 19: 114-28, 1883. 108

2856. Mörchen, F. Die Schlafmittelfrage. Dsche med. Wschr., 60: 798-800, 1934. 294

2857. Moers-Messmer, H. v. Traeume mit der gleichzeitigen Erkenntnis des Traumzustandes. Arch. ges. Psychol., 102:291-318, 1938. 101

2858. Moiseev, E. A., and A. B. Tonkikh. (Russ.) The role of the sympathetic nervous system in the phenomena of sleep in the course of electrical stimulation of subcortical nuclei. Fiziol. Zh. SSSR, 26:394-99, 1939. Moiseev (Moisseeff), E. A., co-author: 2811.

2859. Molfino, F. I disturbi del sonno di origine endocrina. Rinasc. Med., 10:307-8, 1933. 357

2860. Molitor,'H., und E. P. Pick. Verstaerkte Schlafwirkung durch gleichzeitige Beeinflussung verschiedener Hirnteile. Arch. exp. Path. Pharmakol., 115:318-27, 1926. 295, 297

2861. Mollica, A. Assenza di reazione elettroencefalografica di risveglio per stimolazione elettrica

corticale nel gatto "cervello isolato." Arch. Sci. Biol., 40:179-91, 1956; prelim. commun. Boll. Soc. Ital. Biol. Sper., 31:249-50, 1955. 211

2862. _____. Absence de réaction électroencéphalographique d'éveil par stimulation électrique corticale chez le chat "cerveau isolé." Arch. Ital. Biol., 96:216-30, 1958. 211

2863. _____, A. Roger, G. F. Rossi, e A. Zirondoli. Effetti di stimolazioni elettriche corticali sul sonno del gatto "encefalo isolato" gasserectomizzato. Boll. Soc. Ital. Biol. Sper., 31:1219-20, 1955. 212
Mollica, A., co-author: 449, 3550.

2864. Monnier, M. Contribution histopathologique à l'étude de la narcolepsie et du tremblement avec rigidité musculaire. Tubercule du lobe frontal avec lésions diencéphaliques juxtaventriculaires et lésions des corps striés. Rev. Neurol., II:130-45, 1935. 264

2865. _____. Les manifestations électriques corticales du sommeil provoqué par stimulation du centre somnogène chez le chat. Helvet. Physiol. Acta, 8:C7-C9, 1950; prelim. commun. EEG Clin. Neurophysiol., 2:352, 1950. 204

2866. _____. Action de la stimulation électrique du centre somnogène sur l'électrocorticogramme chez le chat (réactions hypniques et réactions d'éveil). Rev. Neurol., 83:561-63, 1950; also EEG Clin. Neurophysiol., 3:106, 1951. 204

2867. _____. Experimental work on sleep and other variations of consciousness. In: Problems of Consciousness, III, 1952 (4), pp. 107-56. 362

2868. _____. Topic action of psychotropic drugs on the electrical activity of cortex, rhinencephalon and mesodiencephalon (excitement, tranquillization, sedation and sleep). In: Psychotropic Drugs, 1957 (1357), pp. 216-34. 302, 358

2869. _____, A. Falbriard, et H. Laue. L'action de l'hormone adréno-corticotrope (ACTH) sur l'activité électrique du cerveau. Rev. Méd. Suisse Rom., 73:511-20, 1953.

2870. _____, und H. Willi. Die integrative Taetigkeit des Nervensystems beim normalen Saeugling und beim bulbo-spinalen Anencephalen (Rautenhirnwesen). Ann. Paediat., 169:289-308, 1947. 23

Monnier, M., co-author: 1350, 2290, 3947.

2871. Monro, A. B. Electro-narcosis in the treatment of schizophrenia. J. Ment. Sci., 96:254-64, 1950. 298

2872. Monroe, R. R., R. G. Heath, W. A. Mickle, and W. Miller. A comparison of cortical and subcortical brain waves in normal, barbiturate, reserpine, and chlorpromazine sleep. Ann. New York Acad. Sci. 61:56-71, 1955. 302

2873. Montorsi, W., P. Pietri, e A. Peracchia. Simposio sul sonno. Atti Soc. Lombarda Sci. Med.-Biol., Suppl. 13, 1958. Pp. 208.

2874. Moore, D. The use of sleep therapy in psychiatric treatments. Med. J. Australia, I:9-11, 1958. 207

2875. Moore, J. E. Some psychological aspects of yawning. J. Gen. Psychol., 27:289-94, 1942. 72

2876. Moore, L. M., M. Jenkins, and L. Barker. Relation of number of hours of sleep to muscular efficiency. Am. J. Physiol., 59: 471, 1922. 121

2877. Moore, M. Recurrent nightmares: a simple procedure for psychotherapy. Milit. Surgeon, 97:282-85, 1945. 281

2878. Moore, T., and L. E. Ucko. Night waking in early infancy. Arch. Dis. Childh., 32:333-42, 1957. 133

2879. Morishita, T., H. Iwai, K. Kadowaki, A. Koizumi, N. Hanazono, and Y. Shimoda. The electroencephalographic study on the endocrine diseases. Diseases of thyroid gland. Proc. VI Ann. Meet. Jap. EEG Soc., 1957, pp. 90-91.

2880. Morison, R. S., and E. W. Dempsey. A study of thalamo-cortical relations. Am. J. Physiol., 135: 281-92, 1942. 210

2881. _____, and _____. Mechanism of thalamocortical augmentation and repetition. Am. J. Physiol., 138: 297-308, 1943. 210

2882. _____, K. H. Finley, and G. N. Lothrop. Spontaneous electrical activity of thalamus and other forebrain structures. J. Neurophysiol., 6:243-54, 1943. 210

Morison, R. S., co-author: 910, 911.

2883. Morocutti, C. Sindrome narcocataplettica da focolaio epilettogeno temporale profondo. Riv. Neurol. (Napoli), 27:461-66, 1957. 237, 238

2884. _____, e R. Vizioli. Epilessia e stato di coscienza: le sincronie delta posteriori. Riv. Neurol. (Napoli), 27:438-40, 1957. 259

2885. Morrell, F. Electroencephalographic studies of conditioned learning. In: The Central Nervous System and Behavior, M. A. B. Brazier, Ed., Josiah Macy Found., 1958, pp. 306-74. 210

2886. _____, and H. H. Jasper. Electrographic studies of the formation of temporary connections in the brain. EEG Clin. Neurophysiol., 8:201-15, 1956.

2887. _____, R. Naquet, and H. Gastaut. Evolution of some electrical signs of conditioning. I. Normal cat and rabbit. J. Neurophysiol., 20:574-87, 1957. 72

2888. Morris, G. O., and M. T. Singer. Sleep deprivation. Transactional and subjective observations. A.M.A. Arch. Gen. Psychiat., 5: 453-61, 1961. 228

2889. _____, H. L. Williams, and A. Lubin. Misperception and disorientation during sleep deprivation. A.M.A. Arch. Gen. Psychiat., 2:247-54, 1960. 228

2890. Morsier, G. de. Les amnésies transitoires. Conception neurologique des états dits: somnambulisme naturel, état second, automatisme comitial ambulatoire. Encéphale, 26:18-41, 1931. 283, 284

2891. Moruzzi, G. Il contenuto in bromo del sangue durante il sonno. Boll. Soc. Ital. Biol. Sper., 11: 728-30, 1936. 57

2892. _____. Influence of brain stem reticular formation on cortical electrical activity. EEG Clin. Neurophysiol., 1:519, 1949. 209

2893. _____. La reazione di arresto di Berger e il problema fisiologico del sonno. Ricerca Sci., 20:491-95, 1950. 209

2894. _____. Il meccanismo fisiologico del sonno. Minerva Med. (Torino), 43(I):730-34, 1952. 209, 362

2895. ____. L'attività dei neuroni corticali durante il sonno e durante la reazione elettroencefalografica di risveglio. Ricerca Sci., 22: 1165-73, 1952. 209, 212

2896. ____. Il risveglio della corteccia cerebrale. Medicina, 2:577-96, 1952. 209, 211

2897. ____. The physiological properties of the brain stem reticular system. In: Brain Mechanisms and Consciousness, 1954 (875), pp. 21-53. 209

2898. ____. The functional significance of the ascending reticular system. Arch. Ital. Biol., 96:17-28, 1958. 209

2899. ____. Synchronizing influences of the brain stem and the inhibitory mechanisms, underlying the production of sleep by sensory stimulation. EEG Clin. Neurophysiol., Suppl. 13:231-56, 1960. 212, 362

2900. ____, and H. W. Magoun. Brain stem reticular formation and activation of the EEG. EEG Clin. Neurophysiol., 1:455-73, 1949; 2:110, 1950. 208

2901. ____, M. Palestini, G. F. Rossi, e A. Zanchetti. Comportamento e quadro elettroencefalografico nel gatto dopo lesioni, complete o parziali, della sostanza reticolare mesencefalica. Boll. Soc. Ital. Biol. Sper., 32:958-59, 1956.

2902. ____, G. F. Rossi, e A. Zanchetti. Recenti contributi alla fisiologia del sonno. Atti Soc. Lombarda Sci. Med. Biol., 31 (Suppl.):14-25, 1958. 362
Moruzzi, G., co-author: 120, 121, 254, 255, 521, 522, 2616-19, 3550, 4196, 4307.

2903. Moseley, H. G. Medical history of the Berlin Airlift. U.S. Armed Forces Med. J., 1:1249-63, 1950. 316, 317

2904. Mosinger, M. Anatomie de l'hypothalamus et du sous-thalamus élargi (Cyto-architectonie, voies de conduction, histo-physiologie). Schweiz. Arch. Neurol., 65:135-86, 1950. 209, 356

2905. Moss, C. S. Dream symbols and disguises. Etc., Rev. Gen. Semant., 14:267-73, 1957. 106

2906. Mosso, A. Sui rapporti della respirazione addominale e toracica nell'uomo. Arch. Sci. Med. (Torino), 2:433-64, 1878. 48, 49

2907. Mosso, U. Recherches sur l'inversion des oscillations diurnes de la température chez l'homme normal. Arch. Ital. Biol., 8:177-85, 1887. 173

2908. Mott, F. Sleep, sleeplessness and sleepiness. Lancet, 207 (II): 1161-65, 1924. 47

2909. Mowrer, O. H., and W. M. Mowrer. Enuresis—A method for its study and treatment. Am. J. Orthopsychiat., 8:436-59, 1938. 285

2910. ____, T. C. Ruch, and N. E. Miller. The corneo-retinal potential difference as the basis of the galavanometric method of recording eye movements. Am. J. Physiol., 114:423-28, 1936. 93

2911. Moyer, W. The Witchery of Sleep. New York: Ostermoor & Co., 1903. Pp. 205.

2912. Mühlmann, M. Ueber die Ursache der taeglichen Schwankung der Koerpertemperatur. Pflugers Arch., 69:613-31, 1898.

2913. Müller, C. Die Messung des Blutdrucks am Schlafenden als klinische Methode speziell bei der gutartigen (primaeren) Hypertonie und der Glomerulonephritis. Acta Med. Scand., 55: 381-442, 1921. 43, 44, 45

2914. ____. Die Schlafbewegungen des Blutdrucks (Bemerkungen zu den Artikel von Katsch und Pansdorf in Muench. med. Wschr., No. 50, 1922). Muench. med. Wschr., 70:180-81, 1923.

2915. ____. Die Messung des Blutdrucks am Schlafenden als klinische Methode. Acta Med. Scand., 55:381-485, 1921. 43, 45, 297

2916. Mueller, E. Selbstbehandlung der Schlaflosigkeit. Psychiat. neurol. Wschr., 45:151-52, 1943. 278, 335

2917. Müller, L. R. Ueber Ermuedung und ueber Muedigkeit, ueber Schlaf und ueber Erholung. Dsche med. Wschr., 61:613-19, 1935. 362

2918. ____. Ueber das Einschlafen, ueber den Schlaf und ueber das Aufwachen. Muench. med. Wschr., 84:681-86, 1937; also Psychiat. Neurol. Jap., 41:746-51, 1937. 353

2919. ____. Ueber die physikalisch-chemischen Vorgaenge, welche dem Einschlafen, dem Schlaf und dem Aufwachen zugrunde liegen. Verhandl. dsch. Gesellsch. inn. Med., 49:194-97, 1937. 353

2920. _____. Ueber Ermuedung und ueber Erholung. Klin. Wschr., 18(I): 113-18, 1939.

2921. _____. Ueber bioelektrische Vorgaenge im Grosshirn waehrend des Wachens und des Schlafes. Klin. Wschr., 18:1589-92, 1939. 113

2922. _____. Ueber den Schlaftraum. Dsche med. Wschr., 66(I):293-96, 1940. 99

2923. _____. Ueber das Aufwachen, das Bewusstsein und ueber Weltanschauung. Dsche med. Wschr., 67(I):156-58, 186-87, 1941. 31

2924. _____. Ueber die Ursachen der Schlafbewusstlosigkeit. Dsche med. Wschr., 69(I):336-40, 1943. 274

2925. _____. Ueber die erholende Kraft des Schlafes. Muench. med. Wschr., 90:165-68, 1943.

2926. _____. Ueber den Schlaf. Berlin-Muenchen: Urban & Schwarzenberg, 1948. 2nd ed. Pp. 180. 286

2927. _____. Ueber den Energiewechsel zwischen dem Wachen und Schlafen. Dsche med. Wschr., 73:592-94, 1948.

2928. _____. Studien ueber den Schlaf. Acta Med. Scand., 134:1-5, 1949. 353

2929. _____. Die Beziehungen des Traumes zum Gedaechtnis. Dsche med. Wschr., 76:695-98, 1951. 99

2930. _____. Ueber das Traumleben. Dsche med. Wschr., 77:591-94, 1952. 99

2931. _____. Zur Physiologie der Traeume; zusammenfassende Traumstudien. Muench. med. Wschr., 95:893-97, 1953. 99

2932. _____. Offene Fragen in der Lehre von der Physiologie des Schlafes. Muench. med. Wschr., 95:1193-94, 1953. 353

2933. _____. Zusammenfassung und kritische Verwertung von Traumstudien. Dsche med. Wschr., 80: 614-17, 1955. 100

2934. _____. Was berichtet das Gedaechtnis von den Traeumen der letzten Nacht? Medizinische, No. 41:1477-79, 1956. 99

2935. _____. Ueber die nervoesen Vorgaenge, die waehrend des Schla-

fes und waehrend des Traumes sich abspielen. Muench. med. Wschr., 98:393-95, 1956.

2936. Mueller, M., und H. Giersberg. Ueber den Einfluss der inneren Sekretion auf die tagesperiodische Aktivitaet der weissen Maus. Z. vergl. Physiol., 40: 454-72, 1957. 172

2937. Mueller, S. C., and G. F. Brown. Hourly rhythms in blood pressure in persons with normal and elevated pressures. Ann. Int. Med., 3:1190-1200, 1930. 163

2938. Müller, W. Schlafmittelmissbrauch und natuerliche Schlafmittel. Hospitalis (Zuerich), 23: 110-11, 1953. 278

2939. Münzer, F. T. Ueber hypnagoghalluzinatorische Erlebnisse bei Narkolepsie: ein Beitrag zur Frage der subcortical-ausgeloesten Halluzinationen und des pathophysiologischen Mechanismus des narkoleptischen Syndroms. Arch. Psychiat., 102: 349-71, 1934. 239

2940. Muggia, A. Sonno e sonniferi nell'età infantile. Igiene Vita, 15:617-19, 1932.

2941. Mullin, F. J. Development of the diurnal temperature and motility patterns in a baby. Am. J. Physiol., 126:P589, 1939. 142

2942. _____, and N. Kleitman. Variations in threshold of auditory stimuli necessary to awaken the sleeper. Am. J. Physiol., 123: 477-81, 1938. 76, 79

2943. _____, _____, and N. R. Cooperman. The effect of alcohol and caffein on motility and body temperature during sleep. Am. J. Physiol., 106:478-87, 1933. 61, 87

2944. _____, _____, and _____. Changes in irritability to auditory stimuli during sleep. J. Exp. Psychol., 21:88-96, 1937. 76, 79, 111, 198

2945. _____, and A. B. Luckhardt. Effects of certain drugs on cutaneous and tactile sensitivity. Arch. Internat. Pharmacodyn., 55:112-24, 1937. 223
Mullin, F. J., co-author: 753, 2193, 2200.

2946. Mulvany, B. Insomnia. Med. J. Australia, I:598-601, 1959. 274

2947. Muncie, W. Insomnia in clinic psychiatric practice. Bull. Johns Hopkins Hosp., 55:131-

53, 1934. 287, 312
Muncie, W., co-author: 1240.

2948. Mundy-Castle, A. C., L. A. Hurst, D. M. Beerstecher, and T. Prinsloo. The electroencephalogram in the senile psychoses. EEG Clin. Neurophysiol., 6:245-52, 1954. 28

2949. Murawski, B. J., and J. Crabbe. Effect of sleep deprivation on plasma 17-hydroxycorticosteroids. J. Appl. Physiol., 15:280-82, 1960. 170, 226
Murawski, B. J., co-author: 1771.

2950. Murphy, G. Parálisis del sueño. Prensa Méd. Argent., 34:2061-64, 1947. 236

2951. Murphy, J. P. Electroencephalography in lobotomy. Digest Neurol. Psychiat., 17:419-20, 1949.

2952. _____, and E. Gellhorn. The influence of hypothalamic stimulation on cortically induced movements and on action potentials of the cortex. J. Neurophysiol., 8: 341-64, 1945.

2953. Murphy, W. F. Narcolepsy. A review and presentation of seven cases. Am. J. Psychiat., 98:334-39, 1941. 234, 236

2954. Murray, E. J. Conflict and repression during sleep deprivation. J. Abnorm. Soc. Psychol., 59:95-101, 1959. 228, 350

2955. _____, E. H. Schein, K. T. Erikson, W. F. Hill, and M. Cohen. The effects of sleep deprivation on social behavior. J. Soc. Psychol., 49:229-36, 1959. 228

2956. _____, and H. L. Williams. Sleepiness ratings and body temperature during sleep deprivation. Walter Reed Army Inst. Res. Rep., 1957. Pp. 17. 225, 226

2957. _____, _____, and A. Lubin. Body temperature and psychological ratings during sleep deprivation. J. Exp. Psychol., 56:271-73, 1958. 158, 173, 225, 226, 227

2958. Musaph, H. Researches into the so-called animal magnetism or mesmerism. Folia Psychiat. Neurol. Neerl., 52:264-84, 1949. 337

2959. Mussio-Fournier, J. C., J. C. Barsantini, et S. Barbieri. Hyperostose frontale, obésité, narcolepsie et oedèmes mous des membres inférieurs. Rev. Neurol., 79:413-19, 1947. 237

2960. _____, and R. A. Larrosa Helguera. Postencephalitic narco-

lepsy and cataplexy; muscles and motor nerves inexcitability during the attack of cataplexy. J. Nerv. Ment. Dis., 80:159-62, 1934. 250

2961. Myers, G. C. The Land of Nod; Training Child to Sleep Well. Chicago: Child Develop. Found., 1934. Pp. 12. 307

2962. Myers, J. W. Narcolepsy (case report). Southwest. Med., 24: 372-73, 1940. 237

2963. Myerson, A. Social conditioning of visceral activities during sleep. II. Section on sleep and fatigue. New Engl. J. Med., 211: 189-93, 1934. 308

2964. _____. The sleeping and waking mechanisms: A theory of the depressions and their treatment. J. Nerv. Ment. Dis., 105:598-606, 1947. 278

2965. Nachmansohn, D. Zur Frage des Schlafzentrums. Eine Betrachtung der Theorien ueber Entstehung des Schlafes. Z. ges. Neurol. Psychiat., 107:342-401, 1927. 347

2966. _____. Die Entstehung des Schlafes. Med. Klin., 24:1192-95, 1928.

2967. Nachmansohn, M. Wesen und Theorie der Hypnose. Zbl. Psychotherap., 4:537-58, 1931. 334, 337

2968. _____. Zur Biologie des Traumes. Allg. Z. Psychiat., 95:133-44, 1931. 106

2969. Naesgaard, S. (Norw.) Our consciousness. Nord. Psychol., 3: 46-53, 1951. 31

2970. Nagy, M. Symptomatologie und Behandlung der Narkolepsie. Mschr. Psychiat. Neurol., 89: 286-306, 1934. 239

2971. Nakao, H., and W. P. Koella. Influence of nociceptive stimuli on evoked sub-cortical and cortical potentials in the cat. J. Neurophysiol., 19:187-95, 1956.

2972. Narbutovich, I. O. (Russ.) Possibility of inducing hypnotic sleep and dehypnotization in man by means of indifferent stimuli according to the conditioned reflex method. Arkh. Biol. Nauk, 34:1-14, 1934. 333

2973. Nathanson, M., and P. S. Bergman. Newer methods of evaluation of patients with altered states of consciousness. Med. Clin. North Am., 42:701-10, 1958.

2974. Natter, S., et H. Gastaut. L'aspect électroencéphalographique de la "cataplexie épileptique." Rev. Neurol., 82:525, 1950. 257

2975. Naumova, T. S. (Russ.) Of the so-called "activating system" of the brain stem (Review of the literature). Zh. Nevropat. Psikhiat., 56:668-75, 1956. 344

2976. Nauta, W. J. H. Hypothalamic regulation of sleep in rats. An experimental study. J. Neurophysiol., 9:285-316, 1946. 206

2977. _____. Hippocampal projections and related neural pathways to the mid-brain in the cat. Brain, 81:319-40, 1958. 213
Nauta, W. J. H., co-author: 1851.

2978. Necheles, H. Basal metabolism in Orientals. Am. J. Physiol., 91:661-63, 1930. 55

2979. _____, und C. T. Loo. Ueber den Stoffwechsel der Chinesen. IV. Ueber den niedrigen Grundumsatz und Methoden. Chinese J. Physiol., 6:201-24, 1932. 55

2980. Neisser. Fall von Schlafsucht und Hyperglobulia. Klin. Wschr., 45:1206-7, 1908. 267

2981. Nekhorocheff, I. L'électroencéphalogramme du sommeil chez l'enfant. Rev. Neurol. 82:487-95, 1950. 76

2982. _____. La valeur du sommeil en tant que méthode de sensibilisation E.E.G. chez l'enfant. Rev. Neurol., 83:570-75, 1950. 29

2983. _____. L'E.E.G. dans le sommeil spontané et le sommeil provoqué chez l'enfant. Rev. Neurol., 83:575-76, 1950. 29

2984. Nelson, H. (Pseud. of K. Kumpmann) Der Gesunde Schlaf. Stuttgart: Marquardt, 1937. Pp. 94. 312

2985. _____. Die Kunst des Schlafes. Stuttgart: Hippokrates-Verlag, 1941. 3rd ed. Pp. 128. 312

2986. Neri, V. Studi sperimentali sul meccanismo del sonno. Cervello, 13:301, 1934. 203, 354

2987. _____, Borgatti, Dagnini, et Scaglietti. Recherches expérimentales sur le mécanisme par lequel l'excitation d'infundibulum produit le sommeil. Riv. Neurol., 1:909-12, 1934. 203, 354

2988. Neufeld, A. H. Contributions to the biochemistry of bromine. I. Canad. J. Res., Sect. B, 14:160-94, 1936. 57

2989. Neuhold, K., M. Taeschler, und A. Cerletti. Beitrag zur zentralen Wirkung von LSD: Versuche ueber die Lokalisation von LSD-Effekten. Helvet. Physiol. Pharmacol. Acta, 15:1-7, 1957. 303

2990. Neumann, J. Ueber Beziehungen zwischen paroxysmaler Laehmung und "verzoegertem psychomotorischem Erwachen." Nervenarzt, 20:161-64, 1949.

2991. Nevsky, I., and J. Arkhangelskaia. (Russ.) The influence of hypnosis on the morphology of leucocytes. Nov. Refl. Fiziol. Nerv. Sistemy, 3:138-43, 1929. 330

2992. _____, and K. Zrjacick. (Russ.) The influence of hypnosis on muscular strength. Nov. Refl. Fiziol. Nerv. Sistemy, 3:480-84, 1929. 330, 331

2993. Nevsky, I. M., and S. L. Levin. (Russ.) On unconditioned and conditioned salivation during hypnosis in children. Kasan. Med. Zh., 28:343-51, 1932. 332

2994. Nevsky, M. P. (Russ.) Bioelectrical activity of the brain in hypnotic sleep. Zh. Nevropat. Psikhiat., 54:26-32, 1954. 330

2995. Newman, E. B. Forgetting of meaningful material during sleep and waking. Am. J. Psychol., 52:65-71, 1939. 124

2996. Newman, I. Neurone-mechanisms in sanity and insanity. J. Abnorm. Soc. Psychol., 25:424-35, 1941. 362

2997. Niazi, S. A., and F. J. Lewis. Profound hypothermia in the dog. Surg. Gynecol. Obst., 102:98-106, 1956. 328

2998. _____, and _____. Profound hypothermia in the monkey with recovery after long periods of cardiac standstill. J. Appl. Physiol., 10:137-38, 1957. 328

2999. _____, and _____. Profound hypothermia in man. Ann. Surg., 147:264-66, 1958.

3000. Nicholson, J. M., and J. R. Knott. Sleep EEGs in psychiatric patients. EEG Clin. Neurophysiol., 9:174-75, 1957.

3001. Nicoll, M. Dream Psychology. London: Oxford Univ. Press, 1920. Pp. 194. 99

3002. Niederland, W. G. The earliest dreams of a young child. Psychoanal. Stud. Child, 12:190-208, 1957. 102, 305

3003. Nielsen, J. M. Extreme encephalitic parkisonism with contractures which relax during the somnambulistic state. Bull. Los Angeles Neurol. Soc., 1:28-30, 1936. 283

3004. _____. Encephalitis with hypothalamic signs. Bull. Los Angeles Neurol. Soc., 10:80-81, 1945. 237, 276

3005. _____. Occipital lobes, dreams and psychosis. J. Nerv. Ment. Dis., 121:50-52, 1955. 103

3006. _____, and R. P. Sedgwick. Instincts and emotions in an anencephalous monster. J. Nerv. Ment. Dis., 110:387-94, 1949. 24

3007. _____, and G. N. Thompson. The Engrammes of Psychiatry. Springfield, Ill.: Thomas, 1947. Pp. xix + 509. 31
Nielsen, J. M., co-author: 3927.

3008. Nieman, E. A. The electroencephalogram in myxoedema coma: clinical and electroencephalographic study of three cases. Brit. Med. J., I:1204-8, 1959. 273

3009. _____. The electroencephalogram in congenital hypothyroidism: a study of 10 cases. J. Neurol. Neurosurg. Psychiat., 24:50-57, 1961. 32

3010. Niemi, M., S. Punakivi, and K. Saikku. Observations on the sleeping posture of man. Duodecim (Helsinki), 74:512-18, 1958. 9

3011. Nieuwenhuyzen, F. J. Etude sur la localisation des phénomènes cataleptiques chez le chat. Acta Brev. Neerl., 4:89, 1934. 253

3012. Niles, G. M. Relation of sleep to bodily nutrition. J. Am. Med. Ass., 79:2030, 1922. 55

3013. _____. A physiologic and philosophic study of the relation of sleep to bodily nutrition. South. Med. J., 16:659-63, 1923. 362

3014. Nitschke, A. Ueber die Beeinflussung des Winterschlafes durch bestrahltes Ergosterin. Z. ges. exp. Med., 82:227-35, 1932. 326

3015. _____, und E. Maier. Ueber das Vergiftungsbild nach Injektion von Extrakten auf lymphatischem Gewebe (P-Substanz) und seine Beziehung zum Winterschlaf. Z. ges. exp. Med., 82:215-26, 1932. 326

3016. Noble, D. A study of dreams in schizophrenia and allied states. Am. J. Psychiat., 107:612-16, 1951. 103

3017. Nobre de Melo, A. L. (Portug.) Human consciousness and animal consciousness: an attempt at comparative psychology. J. Brasil. Psiquiat., 1(13):33-43, 1952. 30

3018. _____. Sonambulismo epiléptico. Rev. Neuro-Psiquiat., 16:272-85, 1953. 256, 283

3019. Noll, V. H. A study of fatigue in 3-hour college ability tests. J. Appl. Psychol., 16:175-83, 1932. 158

3020. Noltenius, F. Ueber Schlafstoerungen. Muench. med. Wschr., 73:1654-55, 1926.

3021. Nora, G., et M. Sapir, Eds. La Cure de Sommeil. Paris: Masson & Cie, 1954. Pp. xi + 238. 206

3022. Norgate, R. H. Sleeplessness of encephalitis lethargica. Lancet, 207(II):782, 1924. 247

3023. Norkus, F. J., A. J. Derbyshire, P. J. Mills, and R. L. Carter. Frequency measure of the EEG. J. Acoust. Soc. Am., 32:1147-50, 1960. 113

3024. Norn, M. Ueber Schwankungen der Kalium-, Natrium- und Chlorid-Ausscheidung durch die Niere im Laufe des Tages. Skand. Arch. Physiol., 55:184-210, 1929. 65, 166, 167

3025. North, H. M. Sleep and sleeplessness. Med. J. Australia, 22:167-70, 1935. 294

3026. Northfield, W. Sound Sleep. Proved Methods of Attaining It. London: The Psychologist, 1937. Pp. 46. 312

3027. Notkin, J., and S. E. Jelliffe. The narcolepsies. Am. J. Psychiat., 3:733-37, 1934.

3028. Noyes, C. R. Economic Man in Relation to his Natural Environment. New York: Columbia Univ. Press, 1948. 2 vols.' Pp. xiv + 1443. 4, 362

3029. Nulsen, F. E., S. P. W. Black, and C. G. Drake. Inhibition and facilitation of motor activity by the anterior cerebellum. Fed. Proc., 7:86-87, 1948. 204

3030. Nyáry, A. von. Ueber die Wirkung der Diuretica im Chloreton- und Luminal-schlaf. Arch. exp. Path. Pharmakol., 162:565-74, 1931.

3031. Nygard, J. W. Cerebral circulation prevailing during sleep and hypnosis. J. Exp. Psychol., 24:

1-20, 1939; prelim. commun. Psychol. Bull., 34:727, 1937. 40, 46, 330

3032. Oatis, W. N. Why I confessed. Life, Sept. 21, 1953, pp. 131-42. 228

3033. Obarrio, J. M. El sueño y los estados depresivos. Sem. Méd., II: 1317-23, 1926.

3034. Obonai, T., K. Fujisawa, and K. Yamaoka. Electroencephalographic researches of hypnotic state. Proc. VI Ann. Meet. Jap. EEG Soc., 1957, pp. 50-51. 333
Obonai, T., co-author: 1319.

3035. Obrador, S. Effect of hypothalamic lesions on electrical activity of cerebral cortex. J. Neurophysiol., 6:81-84, 1943.

3036. Obrist, W. D. The electroencephalogram of normal aged adults. EEG Clin. Neurophysiol., 6:235-44, 1954. 28

3037. O'Connor, W. A. A case of periodic hypersomnia. Brit. J. Med. Psychol., 24:296-300, 1951. 271

3038. ———. Narcolepsy. Med. Illustr. (London), 6:270-75, 1952. 95, 238

3039. Odier, C. Le réveil-matin diencéphalique. Schweiz. Z. Psychol., 5:113-17, 1946. 127

3040. Oepen, H. Schlafanfaelle und Daemmerattacken. Beitrag zur Differenzialdiagnose der Narkolepsie und temporalen Epilepsie. Arch. Psychiat. Nervenkr., 200: 567-84, 1960.

3041. Østergaard, T. The excitability of the respiratory centre during sleep and during Evipan anaesthesia. Acta Physiol. Scand., 8: 1-15, 1944. 49, 50, 51

3042. Oettel, H. Ueber "Schlaf und Schlafmittel." Tung-Chi med. Mschr., 12:169-78, 215-19, 234-38, 1937; abstr. Z. ges. Neurol. Psychiat., 87:326-27, 1937. 294, 295

3043. Ogle, W. On the diurnal variations in the temperature of the human body in health. St. George's Hosp. Rep., 1:221-45, 1866. 138

3044. Ohkuma, T., und K. Tuyuno. Zum Problem der Schlafzentren. Folia Psychiat. Neurol. Jap., 1:346-54, 1935. 266

3045. Ohlmeyer, P., und H. Brilmayer. Periodische Vorgaenge im Schlaf. II. Pfluegers Arch., 249:50-55, 1947. 112

3046. ———, ———, und H. Huellstrung. Periodische Vorgaenge im Schlaf. Pfluegers Arch., 248: 559-60, 1944. 112

3047. Okamoto, Y., and T. Kirikae. Encephalographic studies on brain of foetus, of children of premature birth and new-born, together with a note on reactions of foetus brain upon drugs. Folia Psychiat. Neurol. Jap., 5:135-46, 1951. 27

3048. Okazaki, S. (Jap.) An experimental study of the lack of sleep. Shinkei Gaku Zatshi, 25:55-100, 1925; abstr. Psychol. Abstr., 2: 628, 1928. 215

3049. Okuma, T., Y. Shimazono, T. Fukuda, and H. Narabayashi. Cortical and subcortical recordings in non-anesthetized and anesthetized periods in man. EEG Clin. Neurophysiol., 6:269-86, 1954.
Okuma, T., co-author: 3681.

3050. Olden, C. Neurotic disturbances of sleep. Internat. J. Psychoanal., 23:52-56, 1942. 275, 286

3051. Olds, J., K. F. Killam, and P. Bach-y-Rita. Self-stimulation of the brain used as a screening method for tranquilizing drugs. Science, 124:265-66, 1956. 302

3052. Olnyanskaya, R. P. (Russ.) Gaseous exchange of schizophrenics during prolonged narcosis. In: The Sleep Problem, 1954 (392), pp. 423-30. 206, 286

3053. Olson, W. C. Child Development. Boston: D. C. Heath & Co., 1949. Pp. xiii + 417. 114, 117, 118

3054. Olszewski, J. The cytoarchitecture of the human reticular formation. In: Brain Mechanisms and Consciousness, 1954 (875), pp. 54-80. 209

3055. Omwake, K. T. Effect of varying periods of sleep on nervous stability. J. Appl. Psychol., 16: 623-32, 1932. 124, 153

3056. ———, and M. Loranz. Study of ability to wake at a specified time. J. Appl. Psychol., 17:468-74, 1933. 126, 311

3057. Onghia, F. d'. Dal Conscio all'Inconscio nella Veglia e nel Sonno. Rocca San Casciano: Cappelli, 1959. Pp. 126. 31

3058. Oppenheimer, Z. Zur Physiologie des Schlafes. Arch. Anat. Physiol. (Leipzig), pp. 68-102, 1902. 99

3059. Oppler, W. Electroencephalograms following deep coma insulin therapy. EEG Clin. Neurophysiol., 7:473, 1955.

3060. Orne, M. T. The mechanisms of
hypnotic age regression: an experimental study. J. Abnorm.
Soc. Psychol., 46:213-25, 1951.
333

3061. _____. Die Leistungsfaehigkeit
in Hypnose und im Wachzustand.
Psychol. Rundschau, 5:291-97,
1954.

3062. _____. The nature of hypnosis:
artifact and essence. J. Abnorm.
Soc. Psychol., 58:277-99, 1959.
335

3063. Orthner, H. Pathologische Anatomie der von Hypothalamus ausgeloesten Bewusstseinsstoerungen. First Internat. Congr. Neurol. Sci., Seconde Journée Commune. Brussels: Acta Med. Belg.,
1957, pp. 77-96. 272

3064. Osborne, C. A. The sleep of infancy as related to physical and
mental growth. Pedagog. Semin.,
19:1-47, 1912. 186, 305

3065. Osborne, W. A. Body temperature and periodicity. J. Physiol.
(London), 36:xxxix-xli, 1908. 174

3066. Ostfeld, A. M., X. Machne, and
K. R. Unna. The effects of atropine on the electroencephalogram
and behavior in man. J. Pharmacol. Exp. Therap., 128:265-72,
1960. 304

3067. Oswald, I. Sudden bodily jerks on
falling asleep. Brain, 82:92-103,
1959. 75 ·

3068. _____. Experimental studies of
rhythm, anxiety and cerebral vigilance. J. Ment. Sci., 105:269-94,
1959. 48, 75, 79

3069. _____. Deliberate re-hypnotiza-
tion after the patient's refusal.
J. Ment. Sci., 105:795-97, 1959.
335

3070. _____. Falling asleep open-eyed
during intense rhythmic stimulation. EEG Clin. Neurophysiol.,
12:544, 1960; also Brit. Med. J.,
I:1450-55, 1960. 197, 344

3071. _____, A. M. Taylor, and M.
Treisman. Discriminative responses to stimulation during
human sleep. Brain, 83:440-53,
1960; prelim. commun. EEG
Clin. Neurophysiol., 11:603, 1959.
29

Oswald, I., co-author: 303.

3072. Otto, H. Vom Recken, Strecken,

Gaehnen und Husten. Fortschr.
Med., 53:304-6, 1935. 123, 161

3073. Oudinot, P., et P.-C. Jagot.
L'Insomnie Vaincue. Paris: H.
Dangles, 1954. Pp. 176; includes
1928 edition (1941). 276, 278

3074. Ozeki, M. (Jap.) Theory of sleep
and cure of insomnia. Osaka Iji,
Shinshi, 7:904, 1936; abstr. Psychol. Abstr., 11:243, 1937. 294

3075. Page, J. D. An experimental
study of the day and night motility of normal and psychotic individuals. Arch. Psychol., 28:
1-40, 1935. 78, 86, 149, 252,
287, 295

3076. _____. The effect of barometric
pressure on nocturnal motility.
J. Genet. Psychol., 49:471-74,
1936. 186

3077. Pai, M. N. Sleep-walking and
sleep activities. J. Ment. Sci.,
92:756-65, 1946. 282, 283

3078. _____. Hypersomnia syndromes.
Brit. Med. J., I:522-24, 1950.
267, 271

3079. _____. Sleep and its disturbances.
Recent Progr. Psychiat., 2:587-
614, 1950. 274, 286

3080. Pakhomov, A. N. (Russ.) A new
method of measuring and recording muscle tonus, and its
application to the study of the
physiology of sleep in man. Fiziol. Zh. SSSR, 33:245-54, 1947;
also in: The Sleep Problem, 1954
(392), pp. 241-48. 13

3081. Pallis, C. A. Narcolepsy. Brit.
J. Clin. Pract., 11:17-20, 1957.
234

3082. Palmer, H. A. The value of continuous narcosis in the treatment
of mental disorder. J. Ment. Sci.,
83:636-78, 1937. 207

3083. _____. Narcolepsy. Brit. Med.
J., II:478, 1941. 237, 239

3084. Palmieri, V. M. Il centro nervoso per la regolazione del sonno. Riforma Med., 33(I):1266,
1931. 361

3085. Pampiglione, G. Some phenomena in the EEG during waking
and sleeping states. EEG Clin.
Neurophysiol., 5:622-23, 1953.

3086. _____. Alertness and sleep in
young pigs. EEG Clin. Neurophysiol., 13:827, 1961. 28

3087. _____, and B. Ackner. The effects of repeated stimuli upon
EEG and vaso-motor activity
during sleep in man. Brain, 81:
64-74, 1958. 47

Pampiglione, G., co-author: 8.

3088. Pankratov, M. A. (Russ.) Experimental sleep in monkeys. Trudy Inst. Fiziol. Pavlova, 1:213-21, 1952; also in: The Sleep Problem, 1954 (392), pp. 158-66. 197

3089. Papez, J. W. Central reticular path to intralaminar and reticular nuclei of thalamus for activating EEG related to consciousness. EEG Clin. Neurophysiol., 8:117-28, 1956. 210

3090. Papper, S., and J. D. Rosenbaum. Diurnal variation in the diuretic response to ingested water. J. Clin. Investig., 31:401-5, 1952. 167

3091. Parhon, C. I., et E. Tomorug. Acromégalie et hypersomnie, examen anatomopathologique. Bull. Soc. Roum. Endocrinol., 5:358-63, 1939. 270

3092. Parington, C. B. Narcoleptic syndrome. Vet. Bur. Med. Bull., 6:148-50, 1930.

3093. Parkin, A. Emergence of sleep during psycho-analysis. A clinical note. Internat. J. Psychoanal., 36:174-76, 1955.

3094. Parmeggiani, P. L. Hirnreizversuche mit Schlafeffekt aus subcorticalen Strukturen. Helvet. Physiol. Pharmacol. Acta, 16: C73-C76, 1958. 204

3095. Parmelee, A. H., Jr. Sleep patterns in infancy. A study of one infant from birth to eight months of age. Acta Pediat., 50:160-70, 1961. 114

3096. _____, H. R. Schulz, and M. A. Disbrow. Sleep patterns of the newborn. J. Pediat., 58:241-50, 1961. 114

3097. Parmenter, D. C., and R. C. Cheney. Case of encephalitis lethargica with markedly choked discs in which diagnosis of brain tumor was made: ocular changes in encephalitis lethargica. Boston Med. Surg. J., 190:928-30, 1924. 244

3098. Parsons, F. B. Posture during sleep. Lancet, 242 (I):91, 1942. 9

3099. Partridge, M. Pre-frontal Leucotomy; A Survey of 300 Cases Personally Followed over 1-1/2-3 Years. Springfield, Ill.: Thomas, 1950. Pp. vii + 496. 103

3100. Parturier, G., et R. Feldstein. La phytothérapie des troubles du sommeil chez les hépato-biliaires. Rev. Méd.-Chir. Mal. Foie, 8: 351-71, 1933. 276, 294

3101. Pascal, G. R. The effect of relaxation upon recall. Am. J. Psychol., 62:32-47, 1949.

3102. Passouant, P. Séméiologie électroencéphalographique du sommeil normal et pathologique. Rev. Neurol., 83:545-59, 1950. 257

3103. _____, J. Cadilhac, et R. Labauge. La localisation électroencéphalographique d'un foyer anatomique au cours du sommeil. Montpellier Méd., 45:581-97, 1954.

3104. _____, _____, et H. Latour. Renseignements apportés par la stimulation auditive au cours du sommeil des épileptiques. EEG Clin. Neurophysiol., 4:237, 1952. 257

3105. _____, _____, et T. Passouant-Fontaine. Influence, en cours de sommeil spontané, de la stimulation électrique réticulaire et des stimuli sensoriels sur les rythmes hippocampiques du chat. J. Physiol. (Paris), 47:715-18, 1955. 211

3106. _____, _____, et M. Philippot. Rythmicité du Petit Mal au cours du sommeil, décharges rythmiques généralisées et localisées. Rev. Neurol., 84:659-63, 1951. 257

3107. _____, N. Duc, and J. Minvielle. EEG study of sleep in a group of schizophrenics. EEG Clin. Neurophysiol., 13:488, 1961.

3108. _____, H. Latour, et J. Cadilhac. L'épilepsie morphéique. Ann. Méd.-Psychol., 109:526-40, 1951. 259

3109. _____, et J. Mirouze. L'EEG au cours des hémiplégies d'origine vasculaire. Modifications à l'état de veille et en cours de narcose (245 R. P. ou Nesdonal). EEG Clin. Neurophysiol., 2:348, 1950. 296

3110. _____, et J. Minvielle. L'influence de la région sino-carotidienne sur la conscience et l'état de veille. Etude électro-clinique. Montpellier Méd., 45:555-80, 1954.

3111. _____, et _____. Etude de la réaction d'éveil provoquée par l'infiltration péricarotidienne de novocaïne. Rev. Neurol., 90:140-52, 1954.

3112. _____, T. Passouant-Fontaine, et J. Cadilhac. Hippocampe et réaction d'éveil. C. R. Soc. Biol., 149: 164-66, 1955; also Hippocampe et comportement. Les modifications du comportement chez le chat après stimulation de l'hippocampe (projection de film). Rev. Neurol., 94:292-95, 1956. 211

3113. _____, et M. Philippot. Expression rythmique du petit mal au cours du sommeil. EEG Clin. Neurophysiol., 4:239, 1952.

3114. _____, R. S. Schwab, M. A. B. Brazier, and J. Casby. Activation of the EEG during sleep with regular repetitive sounds every 2 to 10 seconds. EEG Clin. Neurophysiol., 4:382-83, 1952. Passouant, P., co-author: 601, 747, 876, 1113, 2314, 2321, 3353, 3619.

3115. Patrick, G. T. W., and J. A. Gilbert. On the effects of loss of sleep. Psychol. Rev., 3:469-83, 1896. 219, 221, 226

3116. Patry, F. L. The relation of time of day, sleep and other factors to the incidence of epileptic seizures. Am. J. Psychiat., 10:789-813, 1931. 260

3117. Pattie, F. A., Jr. The genuineness of hypnotically produced anesthesia of the skin. Am. J. Psychol., 39:435-43, 1937. 332

3118. _____. The genuineness of unilateral deafness produced by hypnosis. Am. J. Psychol., 63:84-86, 1950. 332

3119. Paul, B. Lerne gut schlafen und bleibe gesund. Zuerich: O. Fuessli Verlag, 1950. Pp. 61. 312

3120. Paul-David, J., J.-L. Riehl, and K. R. Unna. Quantification of effects of depressant drugs on EEG activation response. J. Pharmacol. Exp. Therap., 129:69-74, 1960. 209, 303

3121. Pavlov, I. P. The identity of inhibition with sleep and hypnosis. Sci. Monthly, 17:603-8, 1923. 197, 337

3122. _____. (1) Die normale Taetigkeit und allgemeine Konstitution der Grosshirnrinde. (2) "Innere Hemmung" der bedingten Reize und der Schlaf—ein und derselbe Prozess. Skand. Arch. Physiol., 44:32-41, 42-58, 1923. 32, 197, 344

3123. _____. On the identity of inhibition—as a constant factor in the waking state—with hypnosis and sleep. Q. J. Exp. Physiol., Suppl. Vol., 1923, pp. 39-43. 336, 344

3124. _____. Conditioned Reflexes. An Investigation of the Physiological Activity of the Cerebral Cortex. New York: Oxford Univ. Press, 1927. Pp. 430. 197, 344

3125. _____. Essai de dégression d'un physiologiste dans le domaine de la psychiatrie. Arch. Internat. Pharmacodyn. Thérap., 38:222-27, 1930. 336, 344

3126. _____. (Russ.) The sleep problem. Feldsher Akush. (Moskva), No. 8:3-7, No. 9:3-7, No. 10:3-5, 1952. 106, 344

3127. _____. Drei Abhandlungen ueber die Taetigkeit der Grosshirnrinde aus den Jahren 1922, 1923, und 1925. Berlin: Verlag Volk u. Gesundheit, 1952. Pp. 40. 344

3128. _____. (Russ.) The sleep problem. In: The Sleep Problem, 1954 (392), pp. 57-68. 344, 345

3129. _____, and M. Petrova. (Russ.) On the physiology of the hypnotic state in dogs. Trudy Fiziol. Lab. Pavlova, 4:3-13, 1932. 336

3130. _____, and _____. A contribution to the physiology of the hypnotic state of dogs. Charact. Personal., 2:189-200, 1934. 336

3131. _____, et I. Voskressensky. Contribution à la physiologie du sommeil. C. R. Soc. Biol., 79: 1079-84, 1916. 73

3132. Pedersen, V. C. Insomnia from another point of view. New York Med. J. Med. Rec., 146:434-38, 1937. 275, 294

3133. Peillet, F. La Thérapeutique par le Sommeil dans la Perspective Pavlovienne. Lyon: Impr. de Trévoux, 1952. Pp. 99. 206

3134. Peiper, A. Untersuchungen ueber den galvanischen Hautreflex (psychogalvanischen Reflex) im Kindesalter. Jahrb. Kinderheilk., 107:139-50, 1924. 19, 331, 362

3135. _____. Ueber die Erregbarkeit des autonomen Nervensystems im Schlafe. Jahrb. Kinderheilk., 107:191-200, 1924. 16, 46

3136. _____. Ueber die Reizbarkeit im Schlafe. Med. Klin., 20:1559-60, 1924. 46

3137. _____. Das Gaehnen. Dsche med. Wschr., 58:693-94, 1932. 72

3138. _____. Erregung und Hemmung.

Jahrb. Kinderheilk., 143:143-52, 1934. 50

3139. _____. Der Schlaf des Kindes. Muench. med. Wschr., 85:1585-87, 1938.

3140. Peltier, L. F. Obstructive apnea in artificially hyperventilated subjects during sleep. J. Appl. Physiol., 5:614-18, 1953.

3141. Pembrey, M. S., and B. A. Nicol. Observations upon the deep and surface temperature of the human body. J. Physiol. (London), 23:386-406, 1898. 58

3142. Pen, R. N., and M. A. Jagarov. (Russ.) The formation of conditioned linkages during hypnotic sleep. Arkh. Biol. Nauk, 42:77-88, 1936. 332

3143. Penfield, W. The cerebral cortex in man. I. The cerebral cortex and consciousness. Arch. Neurol. Psychiat., 40:417-42, 1938. 30

3144. _____. Studies of the cerebral cortex of man. A review and an interpretation. In: Brain Mechanisms and Consciousness, 1954 (875), pp. 284-309. 30

3145. _____. The twenty-ninth Maudsley Lecture; The role of the temporal cortex in certain psychical phenomena. J. Ment. Sci., 101:451-65, 1955. 30

3146. _____. Consciousness and the centrencephalic organization. First Internat. Congr. Neurol. Sci., Seconde Journée Commune. Brussels: Acta Med. Belg., 1957, pp. 7-18. 30

3147. _____. Centrencephalic integrating system. Brain, 81:231-34, 1958. 30

3148. _____. L'état de conscience et l'organisation centrencéphalique. Laval Méd. (Quebec), 26:469-81, 1958. 31

3149. Pengelley, E. T., and K. C. Fisher. Onset and cessation of hibernation under constant temperature and light in the golden-mantled ground squirrel (Citellus lateralis). Nature, 180:1371-72, 1957. 321

3150. Penta, P. Deux cas de narcolepsie; recherches cliniques et biochimiques. Rev. Neurol., II,533, 1931. 238

3151. _____. L'azione dell'efedrina (cloridrato di fenilmetilamminopropanolo), quale farmaco diencefalico, sugli accessi narcolet-

tici totali e parziali. Boll. Soc. Ital. Biol. Sper., 6:1026-29, 1931. 295

3152. _____. Contributo clinico alla conoscenza del sonno e della sonnolenza accessuali. Minerva Med., 1:91-96, 1934.

3153. Pepino, A. T., and W. W. Bare. Insomnia in the aged. Delaware Med. J., 33:146-50, 1961. 278 Pepino, A. T., co-author: 218.

3154. Pepler, R. D. Warmth and lack of sleep: accuracy or activity reduced. J. Comp. Physiol. Psychol., 52:446-50, 1959. 226

3155. Perera, G. A., and R. W. Berliner. The relation of postural hemodilution to paroxysmal dyspnea. J. Clin. Investig., 22:25-28, 1943. 38

3156. Perget, G. La thérapeutique de l'insomnie chez les anxieux et les névropathes. Prat. Méd. Franç., 11:347-48, 1930. 294

3157. Peritz, G. Ueber Schlafstoerungen und ihre Behandlung. Therap. Gegenw., 74:433-36, 1933. 362

3158. Perkoff, G. T., K. Eik-Nes, C. A. Nugent, H. L. Fred, R. A. Nimer, L. Rush, L. T. Samuels, and F. H. Tyler. Studies of the diurnal variation of plasma 17-hydroxycorticosteroids in man. J. Clin. Endocrinol. Metab., 19:432-43, 1959. 35, 171, 174

3159. Perov, O. V. (Russ.) Seasonal influences on the speed of falling asleep in children of pre-school age. Pediatria (Moskva), (6):52-55, 1958. 78, 117

3160. Persky, H., H. J. Grosz, J. A. Norton, and M. McMurtry. Effect of hypnotically-induced anxiety on plasma hydrocortisone level of normal subjects. J. Clin. Endocrinol. Metab., 19:700-710, 1959. 331

3161. Peterson, D. B., J. W. Sumner, Jr., and G. A. Jones. Role of hypnosis in differentiation of epileptic from convulsive-like seizures. Am. J. Psychiat., 107:428-33, 1950. 335 Peterson, D. B., co-author: 3866.

3162. Petrén, T. Die 24-Stunden-Rhythmik des Leberglykogens bei Cavia cobaya nebst Studien ueber die Einwirkung der "chronischen" Muskelarbeit auf diese Rhythmik. Morphol. Jahresber., 83:256-67, 1939. 165

Petrén, T., co-author: 1061,
3747.

3163. Petrunkina, A. M., and M. L.
Petrunkin. (Russ.) On the conditions of sleep from magnesium
and bromide. Arkh. Biol. Nauk,
29:461-79, 1929. 295

3164. Petry, F. Zur "kleinen" Psychotherapie der Einschlafstoerung.
Dsche med. Wschr., 80:1094-96,
1955.

3165. Pette, H. Die epidemische Encephalitis in ihren Folgezustaenden.
Dsche Z. Nervenheilk., 76:1-70,
1923. 245

3166. _____. Zur Klinik und zur Anatomie der Schlafregulationszentren.
Dsche Z. Nervenheilk., 105:250-
75, 1928. 245, 246

3167. _____. Zur Anatomie und Pathologie der Schlafregulationszentren. Zbl. ges. Neurol. Psychiat.,
51:234-35, 1928-29. 360

3168. _____. Zur Anatomie und Pathologie der Schlafregulationszentren. Arch. Psychiat., 86:301,
1929. 360

3169. _____. Stoerungen des Schlaf-
Wach-Mechanismus als Symptom
organischer Gehirnerkrankungen:
zugleich ein Beitrag zur Lehre
von den Schlaf-Wach Regulations-
zentren. Klin. Wschr., 9:2329-33,
1930. 362

3170. Petzoldt, G. Schlafzeit und Ener-
giebedarf des Saeuglings in und
ausserhalb der Anstalt. Mschr.
Kinderheilk., 45:193-205, 1929.
115

3171. Petzold, H. Der medikamentose
Heilschlaf in der Behandlung Ma-
genkranker. Muench. med.
Wschr., 98:123-25, 1956. 207

3172. Petzsch, H. Winterschlaf und
Ueberwinterung des Hamsters.
Leipzig: Gebr. Gerhart, 1936.
Pp. 32. 321

3173. Pfannenstiel, W., und W. Doetzer.
Beobachtungen ueber den Einfluss
des fortgesetzten Schlafmangels
auf den Vitamin-C-Spiegel und
die keimfeindliche Kraft des
menschlichen Blutes. Z. Immun.-
forsch., 99:86-94, 1940.

3174. Pfanner, A. Disfunzione infundi-
bulo-ipofisaria e narcolessia.
Riv. Pat. Nerv., 35:80-84, 1930.

3175. Phalen, J. M. Get your sleep.
Milit. Surgeon, 110:362-63, 1952.
307

3176. Philip, A. P. W. An Inquiry into
the Nature of Sleep and Death.

London: Henry Renshaw, 1834.
Pp. xix + 254. 3

3177. Pick, E. P. Pharmakologie des
vegetativen Nervensystems.
Dsche Z. Nervenheilk., 106:238-
68, 304-19, 1928. 294, 295, 348
Pick, E. P., co-author: 2795,
2860.

3178. Pick, M. P. Infants' legs and
the sleeping position. Lancet,
II:1339-41, 1953. 9

3179. Pickenhain, L. Zur Pathophysiologie des Schlafes. Dsch. Gesundhwes., 10:162-68, 1955.

3180. Pieck, K. Halluzinosen nach
Schlafentzug—Ein kasuistischer
Beitrag. Allg. Z. Psychiat.,
124:432-43, 1949. 228

3181. Piehler, R. Ueber das Traum-
erleben Leukotomierter.
Nervenarzt, 21:517-21, 1950.
103

3182. Pierach, A. Die vegetative Ta-
gesrhythmik und ihre klinische
Bedeutung. Muench. med.
Wschr., 96:465-69, 1954. 312

3183. _____. Nachtarbeit und Schicht-
wechsel beim gesunden und
kranken Menschen. Acta Med.
Scand., Suppl. 307:159-66, 1955.
275, 316

3184. _____. Klinische Beobachtungen
ueber vegetative Regulationsstoerungen beim Einschlafen,
Aufwachen und waehrend des
Schlafes. Muench. med. Wschr.,
97:1560-62, 1955.

3185. Pierce, C. M., and H. H. Lipcon. Clinical relationship of
enuresis to sleep-walking and
epilepsy. A.M.A. Arch. Neurol.
Psychiat., 76:310-16, 1956. 256

3186. _____, and _____. Somnambulism. U.S. Armed Forces Med.
J., 7:1143-53, 1956. 283

3187. _____, and _____. Somnambulism: Electroencephalographic
studies and related findings.
U.S. Armed Forces Med. J., 7:
1419-26, 1956. 282, 283, 284

3188. _____, _____, J. H. McLary, and
H. F. Noble. Enuresis: Clinical,
laboratory, and electroencephalographic studies. U.S. Armed
Forces Med. J., 7:208-19, 1956.
282, 283, 284

3189. _____, _____, _____, and _____.
Enuresis: psychiatric interview
studies. U.S. Armed Forces
Med. J., 7:1265-80, 1956. 284

3190. _____, R. M. Whitman, J. W.
Maas, and M. L. Gay. Enuresis

and dreaming. A.M.A. Arch. Gen. Psychiat., 4:166-70, 1961. 98, 103, 284, 289

Pierce, C. M., co-author: 4198.

3191. Piéron, H. L'étude expérimental du sommeil normal. La méthode. C. R. Soc. Biol., 62:307-9, 1907. 215

3192. _____. Le Problème Physiologique du Sommeil. Paris: Masson & Cie., 1913. Pp. 520. 3, 14, 15, 33, 40, 42, 45, 58, 62, 63, 64, 138, 215, 243, 257, 341, 347, 351

3193. _____. Discussion du rapport de Jean Lhermitte et Auguste Tournay: le sommeil normal et pathologique. Rev. Neurol., I:830-32, 1927. 346, 352

3194. _____. Le phénomène de l'audition atonale dans le sommeil léger. Année Psychol., 52:393-95, 1952. 101

Piéron, H., co-author: 2403-13, 3959, 4041.

3195. Pietrusky, F. Das Verhalten der Augen im Schlafe. Klin. Augenheilk., 68:355-60, 1922. 11, 12, 16, 113

3196. Pilcz, A. Ueber Hypnose und deren therapeutische Anwendung. Wien. klin. Wschr., 38:280-81, 1925. 335, 337

3197. _____. Ueber Schlafmittel. Wien. klin. Wschr., 43:1377-80, 1930. 294

3198. Pilleri, G. Der pathologische Schlaf im Lichte der Lokalisationslehre und Neurophysiologie. Psychiat. Neurol. (Basel), 136: 36-58, 1958. 246

3199. Pilling, W. E., und H. Kirchner. Schlafstoerungen und ihre Behandlung. Dsche med. Wschr., 60:945-50, 1934. 294

3200. Pincher, C. Sleep: How To Get More of It. London: "Daily Express," 1954. Pp. 120. 312

3201. Pincus, G. A diurnal rhythm in the excretion of urinary ketosteroids by young men. J. Clin. Endocrinol., 3:195-99, 1943. 170

3202. _____. Studies of the role of the adrenal cortex in the stress of human subjects. Recent Progr. Hormone Res., 1:123-45, 1947. 170

Pincus, G., co-author: 1070.

3203. Pinelli, P. Sonno, Sogno, Ipnosi e Stati Patologici di Inibizione Cerebrale. Pavia: Renzo Cortina, 1959. Pp. 314. 272

3204. Pinotti, O., e L. Tanfani. Varia-

zioni circolatorie che accompagnano il sonno fisiologico. Arch. Fisiol., 40:335-47, 1940. 40, 74

3205. Pinschmidt, N. W., H. Ramsey, and H. B. Haag. Studies on antagonism of sodium succinate to barbiturate depression. J. Pharmacol. Exp. Therap., 83:45-52, 1945. 297

3206. Pintus, G., e A. Falqui. Sulla sede di origine delle "mioclonie ipniche fisiologiche." Riv. Neurol., 7:133-60, 1934. 74

3207. Pirenne, M. H. On physiology and consciousness. Brit. J. Psychol., 37:82-86, 1947. 30

3208. Pisa, M. Influenza del sonno sulle alterazioni dell'equilibrio acido-base nei malati di reni. Policlinico (Sez. Med.), 38:638-48, 1931.

3209. Pitfield, R. L. Capricious slumber. Med. Rec., 154:448-50, 1941.

3210. Pitts, G. C. A diurnal rhythm in the blood sugar of the white rat. Am. J. Physiol., 139:109-16, 1943. 166

3211. Planques, Baïsset, et M-me Grezes-Rueff. L'électro-encéphalographie du sommeil hypnotique. Toulouse Méd., 49:728, 1948. 330

3212. Platonow, K. I. Suggestion und Hypnose im Lichte der Lehre I. P. Pawlows. Z. aerztl. Fortbild., 47:1-8, 61-68, 1953. 336

3213. _____, and A. N. Matzkevich. (Russ.) Hypnosis and the nervous system under the influence of alcohol. Trudy Ukrain. Psikhonevr. Inst., 15:93-106, 1931. 332

3214. Plaut, A. Aspects of consciousness. Brit. J. Med. Psychol., 32:239-48, 1959. 30

3215. Pletscher, A., P. A. Shore, and B. B. Brodie. Serotonin as a mediator of reserpine action in brain. J. Pharmacol. Exp. Therap., 116:84-89, 1956. 302

3216. Ploog, D. Physiologie und Pathologie des Schlafes. Fortschr. Neurol. Psychiat., 21:16-56, 1953.

3217. _____. Ueber den Schlaf und seine Beziehungen zu endogenen Psychosen. Muench. med. Wschr., 95:897-900, 1953.

3218. _____. Ueber den Einfluss des Schlafes auf das Gedaechtnis

(Vorlaeufige Mitteilung). Nervenarzt, 28:277-78, 1957. 124

3219. Poetzl, O. Experimentell erregte
Traumbilder in ihren Beziehungen zum indirekten Sehen. Z. ges.
Neurol. Psychiat., 37:278-349,
1917. 104

3220. _____. Schlafzentrum und Traeume. Diskussionsbemerkungen.
Med. Klin., 22:1877-80, 1926. 359

3221. _____. Zur Topographie der
Schlafzentren. Mschr. Psychiat.
Neurol., 64:1-24, 1927. 359
Poetzl, O., co-author: 1808.

3222. Pol, B. van der. Biological
rhythms considered as relaxation oscillations. Acta Med.
Scand., Suppl. 108:76-88, 1940.
356

3223. Polimanti, O. Sopra la possibi-
lità di una inversione della temperatura giornaliera nell'uomo.
Z. allg. Physiol., 16:506-12,
1914. 174

3224. Pollock, L. J. Disorders of sleep.
Med. Clin. North Am., 13:1111-
20, 1930. 234, 244, 245

3225. Pompeiano, O., e J. E. Swett.
Sincronizzazione elettrica corticale prodotta da stimoli perife-
rici. Boll. Soc. Ital. Biol. Sper.,
37:432-35, 1961. 204
Pompeiano, O., co-author: 2616,
2617.

3226. Pond, D. A. Narcolepsy: a brief
critical review and study of eight
cases. J. Ment. Sci., 98:595-604,
1952. 237, 240

3227. _____. New physiological data
bearing on the problem of consciousness. Proc. Roy. Soc. Med.,
47, 775-78, 1954. 31

3228. Popov, A. K. (Russ.) On the question of studying sleep in man by
means of actography. Zh. Vysshei
Nerv. Deiat., 4:133-36, 1954.

3229. Popov, E. A. (Russ.) Delirium and
insomnia. Vrach. Delo, 17:141-
44, 1934. 275

3230. _____. (Russ.) The problem of the
theory of dreams in the light of
Pavlov's teachings. In: The Sleep
Problem, 1954 (392), pp. 273-81.
100, 344, 345

3231. Porak, R. La fréquence du pouls
radial suivant les changements
de position du corps humain. J.
Physiol. Path. Gén., 27:770-76,
1929. 163

3232. _____. Psychophysiologie de
l'homme. I. La détente du cycle
moteur. II. Le freinage des

rythmes d'après le thermomètre
clinique. III. Le démarrage des
rythmes d'après le thermomètre
clinique. Progr. Méd., (39):1617-
22; (40):1649-57; (41):1697-1702,
1930. 362
Porak, R., co-author: 717.

3233. Porter, R. W. Alterations in
electrical activity of the hypothalamus induced by stress
stimuli. Am. J. Physiol., 169:
629-37, 1952; prelim. commun.
Fed. Proc., 11:124-25, 1952. 170

3234. _____. Hypothalamic involvement in the pituitary-adrenocor-
tical response to stress stimuli.
Am. J. Physiol., 172:515-19,
1953. 170

3235. _____. The central nervous system and stress-induced eosinopenia. Recent Progr. Hormone
Res., 10:1-27, 1954. 170

3236. Poucel, J. Le sommeil naturel.
Pourquoi et comment dormir?
Marseille Méd., 71(I):489-532,
1934. 307

3237. Poulin, J. M. L'insomnie des
surmenés. Bull. Méd., Paris,
47:163-64, 1933. 276

3238. Powsner, E. R., and K. S. Lion.
Testing eye muscles. Electronics, 23(3):96-99, 1950. 93

3239. Preston, J. B. Effects of chlorpromazine on the central nervous system of cat: a possible
neural basis for action. J. Pharmacol. Exp. Therap., 118:100-
115, 1956. 301

3240. Pribram, B. O. Zur Frage des
Alterns. Destruktive Hypophyseo-
thyreoditis; pathologisches Alten
und pathologischer Schlaf. Arch.
path. Anat. Physiol., 264:498-
521, 1927.

3241. Prinzmetal, M., and W. Bloomberg. The use of benzedrine for
the treatment of narcolepsy. J.
Am. Med. Ass., 105:2051-54,
1935. 239, 300

3242. Probst, J. Y. Die Aktographie
als klinische Untersuchungs-
methode des Schlafes. Arch.
phys. Therap. (Leipzig), 9:25-
27, 1957.

3243. Proctor, L. D., J. A. (C.?)
Churchill, R. S. Knighton, and
J. Bebin. Changes in behavior
through stimulation of the reticular formation of the monkey.
Biol. Psychiat., 1:20-26, 1958.
72

3244. _____, R. S. Knighton, and J. A.

Churchill. Variations in consciousness produced by stimulating reticular formation of the monkey. Neurology, 7:193-203, 1957. 210

3245. _____, _____, J. Lukaszewski, and J. Bebin. Behavioral changes during hypothalamic and limbic stimulation in the monkey. Am. J. Psychiat., 117:511-18, 1960. 204

3246. Propper-Grashchenkov, N. I. (Russ.) On the question of a sleep center. Nevropat. Psikhiat., 12(1): 8-16, 1943. 362

3247. Puech, P., P. Guilly, H. Fischgold, et G. Bunes. Un cas d'anencéphalie hydrocéphalique. Etude électro-encéphalographique. Rev. Neurol., 79:116-24, 1947. 121

3248. Purpura, D. P. Further analysis of evoked "secondary discharge"; a study of reticulo-cortical relations. J. Neurophysiol., 18:246-60, 1955. 209

3249. _____. A neurohumoral mechanism of reticulo-cortical activation. Am. J. Physiol., 186:250-54, 1956. 209

3250. _____. Observations on the cortical mechanisms of EEG activation accompanying behavioral arousal. Science, 123:804, 1956. 343

Purpura, D. P., co-author: 680.

3251. Quilliam, J. P. The pharmacology of consciousness. Med. Press, 238:121-26, 1957. 294

3252. Rabinowitsch, W. Untersuchungen ueber die alveolare Kohlensaeurespannung bei natuerlichen Schlaf und bei Wirkung von Schlafmitteln. Z. ges. exp. Med., 66:284-90, 1929. 51

3253. Raboutet, J., G. Bousquet, E. Granotier, et R. Angiboust. Troubles du sommeil et du rythme de vie chez le personnel navigant effectuant des vols à longue distance. Méd. Aéronaut., 13:311-22, 1958. 315

3254. _____, N. Lesèvre, and A. Rémond. Involuntary falling asleep. Investigation of contributing factors. EEG Clin. Neurophysiol., 12:231, 1960. 78

3255. Racamier, P. C., L. Carretier, et C. Sens. Les lendemains de cure de sommeil. Evolut. Psychiat., 2:305-30, 1959. 206

3256. Rademaker, G. G. J., and C. Winkler. Annotations on the physi-

ology and the anatomy of a dog, living 38 days, without both hemispheres of the cerebrum and without cerebellum. Proc. Sect. Sci., Konkl. Akad. Wetensch., Amsterdam, 31:332-38, 1928. 22

3257. Radestock, P. Schlaf und Traum. Eine physiologisch-psychologische Untersuchung. Leipzig: Breitkopf und Haertel, 1879. Pp. x + 330. 106

3258. Raehlmann, E., und L. Witkowski. Ueber atypische Augenbewegungen. Arch. Physiol., pp. 454-71, 1877. 297

3259. Raginsky, B. B. Temporary cardiac arrest induced under hypnosis. Internat. J. Clin. Exp. Hypn., 7:53-58, 1959. 331

3260. Rahn, H., and F. Rosendale. Diurnal rhythm of melanophore hormone secretion in the Anolis pituitary. Proc. Soc. Exp. Biol. Med., 48:100-102, 1941. 172, 356

3261. Rakestraw, N. W., and F. O. Whittier. The effect of loss of sleep on the composition of the blood and urine. Proc. Soc. Exp. Biol. Med., 21:5-6, 1923. 224

3262. Ralston, B., and C. Ajmone-Marsan. Thalamic control of certain normal and abnormal cortical rhythms. EEG Clin. Neurophysiol., 8:559-82, 1956.

3263. Ramsey, G. V. Studies of dreaming. Psychol. Bull., 50:432-55, 1953. 99

3264. Ramsay, R. E. The under-rested child. Arch. Pediat., 42:816-20, 1925. 306

3265. Rankin, G. Broken sleep. Brit. Med. J., II:77-78, 1918. 294

3266. Ranson, S. W. The hypothalamus. Trans. Coll. Physicians, Philadelphia, Ser. 4, 2:222-42, 1934. 205, 362

3267. _____. Sleep. Sci. Monthly, 38: 473-76, 1934. 205

3268. _____. Somnolence caused by hypothalamic lesions in the monkey. Arch. Neurol. Psychiat., 41:1-23, 1939. 205

3269. _____, and W. R. Ingram. Catalepsy caused by lesions between the mammillary bodies and third nerve in the cat. Am. J. Physiol., 101:690-96, 1932. 254

3270. _____, H. Kabat, and H. W. Magoun. Autonomic response to electrical stimulation of hypo-

thalamus, preoptic region and
septum. Arch. Neurol. Psychiat.,
33:467-74, 1934. 204, 362
Ranson, S. W., co-author: 1903.

3271. Ranström, S. The hypothalamus
and sleep regulation. An experimental and morphological study.
Acta Path. Microbiol. Scand.,
Suppl. 70, 1947. Pp. 90. 206, 209,
362

3272. Rapaport, D. Consciousness: a
psychopathological and psychodynamic view. In: Problems of
Consciousness, II, 1951 (4), pp.
18-57. 31, 79

3273. Rapport, N. Pleasant dreams.
Psychiat. Q., Suppl. 22:309-17,
1948; also Am. Imago, 6:311-20,
1949. 100, 101

3274. Rasmussen, A. T. The hypophysis cerebri of the woodchuck
(Marmota monax) with special
reference to hibernation and in-
anition. Endocrinology, 5:33-64,
1921. 325
Rasmussen, A. T., co-author:
315.

3275. Raths, P. Untersuchungen ueber
die Blutzusammensetzung und
ihre Beziehungen zur vegetativen
Tonuslage beim Hamster (Cricetus cricetus L.). Ein Beitrag zur
Physiologie des Winterschlafs.
Z. Biol. (Berlin), 106:109-23,
1953. 323, 327

3276. _____. Die bioelektrische Hirn-
taetigkeit des Hamsters im Ver-
laufe des Erwachens aus Winterschlaf und Kaeltenarkose. Z. Biol.
(Berlin), 110:62-80, 1958. 326

3277. _____, und W. Schulze. Die Nebennieren des Goldhamsters im
Winterschlaf und bei anderen Ak-
tivitaetszustaenden. Z. Biol.
(Berlin), 109:233-43, 1957.

3278. Ratschow, M. Der Heilschlaf mit
Phenothiazin-Derivaten (Atosil
und Megaphen). Medizinische,
(42):1351-53, 1953. 206

3279. Rauschkolb, E. W., and G. L.
Farrell. Evidence for diencephalic regulation of aldosterone
secretion. Endocrinology, 59:
526-31, 1956. 356

3280. Ravaud, C. Le Métabolisme de
Sommeil. Paris: Dactylo-Sor-
bonne, 1956. Pp. 35. 55

3281. Ravenhill, A. Some results of an
investigation into hours of sleep
among children in the elementary schools of England. Internat.
Arch. Schulhyg., 5:9-25, 1908.

117, 118

3282. Ravina, A. Sommeil normal et
pathologique. Presse Méd., 36:
645-47, 1928. 344, 359

3283. Ravitz, L. J. Standing potential
correlates of hypnosis and narcosis. A.M.A. Arch. Neurol.
Psychiat., 65:413-36, 1951. 330

3284. Raybaud, A. Syndrome hypo-
physo-infundibulaire fruste,
avec insomnie: guérison après
traitement par l'extrait post-
hypophysaire. Rev. Oto-Neuro-
Ophthalm., 10:771-73, 1932. 294

3285. Read, C. S. Role of hypnotics in
mental disorders. Med. Press
(London), 217:11-14, 1947. 278

3286. Rechtschaffen, A., D. R. Goodenough, and A. Shapiro. Patterns
of sleep talking. A.M.A. Arch.
Gen. Psychiat., 7:418-26, 1962.
282
Rechtschaffen, A., co-author:
3985.

3287. Reed, C. I., and N. Kleitman.
The effect of sleep on respiration. Am. J. Physiol., 75:600-
608, 1926. 48, 49

3288. Reed, D. J., and R. H. Kellogg.
Changes in respiratory response
to CO_2 during natural sleep at
sea level and at altitude. J. Appl.
Physiol., 13:325-30, 1958. 51,
52

3289. Rees, L. Physiological concomitants of electronarcosis. J.
Ment. Sci., 95:162-70, 1949. 298

3290. _____. Electronarcosis in the
treatment of schizophrenia. J.
Ment. Sci., 95:625-37, 1949. 298

3291. Reese, M. A study of the effect
of daylight saving time upon the
sleep of young children. Child
Developm., 3:86-89, 1932. 306

3292. Regan, P. F., III, and A. N.
Browne-Mayers. Electroencephalography, frequency analysis,
and consciousness. A correlation during insulin-induced hypoglycemia. J. Nerv. Ment. Dis.,
124:142-47, 1956. 273

3293. Regelsberger, H. Ueber das
Zustandekommen des Schlafes.
Dsche med. Wschr., 53:1847-50,
1927. 362

3294. _____. Untersuchungen ueber
die Schlafkurve des Menschen.
Z. klin. Med., 107:674-92, 1928.
51, 295

3295. _____. Tagesrhythmik und Reak-
tionstypen des Polarizationswi-
derstandes der menschlichen

Haut. II. Ueber den Galvanismus der menschlichen Haut. Z. ges. exp. Med., 70:438-51, 1930. 158

3296. _____. Der Schlaf und das vegetative Nervensystem. In: L. R. Müller, Lebensnerven und Lebenstriebe. Berlin: Springer, 1931, pp. 483-94. 52

3297. _____. Zur Technik der Schlaftiefenmessung und Schlafmittel-Pruefung. Z. klin. Med., 126:395-404, 1934. 51, 110, 295

3298. _____. Die Veraenderungen des elektrischen Gleichstromwiderstandes im Schlaf. Ein Beitrag zur Innervationsfrage der Perspiratio insensibilis. Z. ges. Neurol. Psychiat., 174:66-79, 1942, 21

3299. _____. Ueber vegetative Korrelationen im Schlafe des Menschen. Z. ges. Neurol. Psychiat., 174: 727-39, 1942. 21, 52, 112

3300. _____. Das Elektrodermatogramm und seine Messung. Med. Klin., 44(I):817-25, 1949. 21

3301. _____, und B. Hain. Die automatische Registrierung des Elektrodermatogramms. Acta Neuroveget. (Wien), 13(I):112-24, 1955. 21

3302. Reh, T. Agrypnie avec agitation nocturne chez des enfants. Rev. Méd. Suisse Rom., 41:184, 1921.

3303. Reichelt, K. E. Ueber die Entstehungsweise der Schlafkrankheit nach Grippe (Encephalomyelitis epidemica). Z. ges. Neurol. Psychiat., 78:153-96, 1922. 248

3304. Reichert, K., und E. Woehlisch. Zur Methodik der Schlaftiefenmessung. II. Elektrodermatographie nach dem Verfahren von C. P. Richter. Klin. Wschr., 35: 1188-89, 1957. 112
Reichert, K., co-author: 4261.

3305. Reichsman, F., J. Cohen, J. Colwill, N. Davis, W. Kessler, C. R. Shardson, and G. L. Engel. Natural and histamine-induced gastric secretion during waking and sleeping states. Psychosom. Med., 22:14-23, 1960. 54

3306. Reinberg, A., et J. Ghata. Rythmes et Cycles Biologiques. Paris: Presses Univ. de France, 1957. Pp. 128. 131

3307. Reinert, A. Keine Schlaflosigkeit mehr! Gesunde Nerven! Hildesheim: August Lax, 19?? Pp. 20. (after 1951) 278

3308. Reinhard, J. F. Prolongation of hypnosis by epinephrine and insulin. Proc. Soc. Exp. Biol. Med., 58:210-11, 1945. 303

3309. Reisinger, L. Hypnose der Voegel. Biol. Zbl., 52:420-29, 1932. 336

3310. Reiter, M. Pharmakologische Betrachtung der Schlafmittel. Med. Klin., 54:973-77,1959. 294

3311. Rémond, A., and N. Lesèvre. The conditions of appearance and the statistical importance of the lambda waves in normal subjects. EEG Clin. Neurophysiol., 8:172, 1956.
Rémond, A., co-author: 1757, 3254.

3312. Ronbourn, E. T. Variation, diurnal and over longer periods of time, in blood haemoglobin, haematocrit, plasma protein, erythrocyte sedimentation rate, and blood chloride. J. Hyg., 45: 455-67, 1947. 38, 39, 162

3313. _____. Body temperature and pulse rate in boys and young men prior to sporting contests. A study of emotional hyperthermia: with a review of the literature. J. Psychosom. Res., 4: 149-75, 1960. 145

3314. _____, and P. F. Taylor. Body temperature studies. II. Rectal and oral indices of internal temperatures. Some theoretical and practical considerations. V Commonwealth Confer. on Clothing and General Stores, Canada, 1956. Pp. 29. 59, 145

3315. Renneker, R. Dream timing. Psychoanal. Q., 21:81-91, 1952. 100

3316. _____. Pre-sleep mechanisms of dream control. Psychoanal. Q., 21:528-36, 1952. 106

3317. Renner, A. Schlafmittel-therapie. Berlin: Springer, 1925. Pp. 125. 294

3318. Renold, A. E., T. B. Quigley, H. E. Kennard, and G. W. Thorn. Reaction of adrenal cortex to physical and emotional stress in college oarsmen. New Engl. J. Med., 244:754-57, 1951. 170

3319. Renshaw, S. Sleep motility as an index of motion picture influence. J. Educ. Sociol., 6:226-30, 1932. 89

3320. _____, V. L. Miller, and D. P. Marquis. Children's Sleep. New York: Macmillan, 1933. Pp. 242. 89, 307

3321. Renton, G. H., and H. Weil-
Malherbe. Adrenaline and nor-
adrenaline in human plasma
during natural sleep. J. Physiol.
(London), 131:170-75, 1956. 35

3322. Rentz, E. Zur Frage der Ein-
teilung der Schlafmittel in kor-
tikale und thalamische. Latv.
Biol. Biedr. Raksti, 6:157-62,
1936; abstr. Zbl. ges. Neurol.
Psychiat., 87:297, 1937. 295,
353

3323. Répond-Malévaz, A. Considérations psychologiques et psycho-
pathologiques sur le sommeil.
Schweiz. med. Wschr., 61:63-67,
1931.

3324. Rétif, E. Le sommeil dissocié.
Auto-observation. Rev. Neurol.,
I:880-82, 1927. 297, 360

3325. Reynard, M. C., and F. C. Dockeray. The comparison of temporal intervals in judging depth of
sleep in newborn infants. J.
Genet. Psychol., 55:103-20,
1939. 112

3326. Reynolds, M. M. Sleep of young
children in 24 hour nursery
school. Ment. Hyg., 19:602-9,
1935. 117

3327. ____, and H. Mallay. The sleep
of children in a 24 hour nursery
school. Psychol. Bull., 30:552,
1933; also J. Genet. Psychol.,
43:322-51, 1933. 305

3328. Rheinberger, M. B., and H. H.
Jasper. Electrical activity of the
cerebral cortex in the unanesthetized cat. Am. J. Physiol., 119:
186-96, 1937.

3329. Rhines, R., and H. W. Magoun.
Brain stem facilitation of cortical motor response. J. Neurophysiol., 9:219-29, 1946. 209

3330. Ricci, G. F. Cortical and hippocampal 'arousal' in response to
cortical stimulation in the rabbit. Am. J. Physiol., 183:655,
1955. 211

3331. Rice, H. Insomnia and the wet
sheet pack. Pac. Coast J. Nursing, 23:6-7, 1927. 294

3332. Rice, T. B. Gentle sleep: a third
lesson in relaxation by a re-
formed insomniac. Hygeia (Chicago), 9:461-63, 1931. 309

3333. Richards, L. S. I. Analysis and
Cause of the Existence of Mem-
ory. II. Analysis and Cause of
Consciousness and Sleep. Boston:
Author, 1920. Pp. 90.

3334. Richards, O. W. The dream liter-

ature. Psychol. Bull., 21:338-
46, 1924. 99

3335. Richards, T. W. The relationship between bodily and gastric
activity of newborn infants. I.
Correlation and influence of
time since feeding. II. Simultaneous variations in the bodily
and gastric activity of newborn
infants under long-continued
light stimulation. Human Biol.,
8:368-86, 1936. 133

3336. ____. The importance of hunger in the bodily activity of the
neonate. Psychol. Bull., 33:817-
35, 1936. 133

3337. Richter, C. P. The significance
of changes in the electrical resistance of the body during
sleep. Proc. Nat. Acad. Sci.,
12:214-22, 1926. 19, 110, 252

3338. ____. The electrical skin resistance. Diurnal and daily
variations in psychopathic and
normal persons. Arch. Neurol.
Psychiat., 19:488-508, 1928.

3339. ____. Pathologic sleep and
similar conditions studied by
the electrical skin resistance
method. Arch. Neurol. Psychiat., 21:363-75, 1929. 238,
244

3340. ____. Sleep produced by hypnotics studied by the electrical
skin resistance method. J. Pharmacol. Exp. Therap., 42:471-86:
1931. 295

3341. ____. Cyclic manifestations in
the sleep curves of psychotic
patients. Arch. Neurol. Psychiat., 31:149-51, 1934. 185, 287

3342. ____. Diurnal cycles of man and
animals. Science, 128:1147-48,
1958. 172

3343. ____, and A. S. Paterson. Bulbocapnine catalepsy and the
grasp reflex. J. Pharmacol.
Exp. Therap., 43:677-91, 1931.
253

3344. Richter, D., and R. M. C. Dawson. Brain metabolism in emotional excitement and in sleep.
Am. J. Physiol., 154:73-79, 1948.

3345. Richter, R. B., and E. F. Traut.
Chronic encephalitis. Pathological report of a case with protracted somnolence. Arch. Neurol. Psychiat., 44:848-66, 1940.
243

3346. Rieper, P. Zu viel Schlaf—zu
wenig Schlaf? Umschau, 38:575-
86, 1934. 161, 313

3347. Riesenman, F. R. Anxiety and tension in the pathogenesis of sleep disturbances. J. Clin. Psychopath., 11:82-84, 1950. 286

3348. Riess, L. Ueber ein neues vegetabilisches Sedativum, Passiflorin. Wien. med. Wschr., 82: 288-90, 1932. 294

3349. Rigden, B. G. Posture during sleep. Lancet, I:215, 1942. 11

3350. Righetti, R. Contributo clinico ed anatomo-patologico allo studio dei gliomi cerebrali. Riv. Pat. Nerv., 8:241-67, 1903. 262

3351. Rignano, E. A new theory of sleep and dreams. Mind, 29:313-22, 1920. 99, 362

3352. Rijlant, P. Etude chez la poule des activités toniques et contractiles du muscle strié pendant l'hypnose; le tonus musculaire chez un mammifère en état d'hypnose. C. R. Soc. Biol., 113: 417-21, 421-24, 1933. 336

3353. Rimbaud, L., P. Passouant, et J. Cadilhac. Participation de l'hippocampe à la régulation des états de veille et de sommeil. Rev. Neurol., 93:303-8, 1955. 211

3354. Rinaldi, F., and H. E. Himwich. A comparison of effects of reserpine and some barbiturates on the electrical activity of cortical and subcortical structures of the brain of rabbits. Ann. New York Acad. Sci., 61:27-35, 1955. 302

3355. _____, and _____. Alerting responses and actions of atropine and cholinergic drugs. A.M.A. Arch. Neurol. Psychiat., 73:387-95, 1955. 209, 303

3356. _____, and _____. Cholinergic mechanism involved in function of mesodiencephalic activating system. A.M.A. Arch. Neurol. Psychiat., 73:396-402, 1955. 209, 303

3357. _____, and _____. The site of action of antiparkinson drugs. Confinia Neurol., 15:209-24, 1955. 209, 303

3358. _____, and _____. Drugs affecting psychotic behavior and the function of the mesodiencephalic activating system. Dis. Nerv. Syst., 16:133-41, 1955. 301, 302

3359. Rioch, D. McK. Discussion of paper by W. R. Hess. In: Brain Mechanisms and Consciousness,

1954 (875), pp. 133-34. 199, 366 Rioch, D. McK., co-author: 3592.

3360. Ríos Sasiain, M. El color de las imágenes oníricas. Clín. y Labor., 42:169-71, 1946. 101

3361. Riser, Arlet, et Dardenne. Epilepsie par hypoglycémie paroxystique spontanée et à l'effort. Bull. Soc. Méd. Hôp. Paris, 62: 415-17, 1946. 256

3362. Riser, Canceil, et Gayral. Chorée prolongée et narcolepsie. Rev. Neurol., 75:148, 1943. 237

3363. Riser, et Dardenne. Narcolepsie et hypoglycémie permanente (action favorable de l'extrait hypophysaire et de l'électrochoc). Bull. Soc. Méd. Hôp. Paris, 62:413-15, 1946. 237, 256, 270

3364. Rivas Cherif, M. de. Un caso de insomnio de origen ocular. An. Soc. Mex. Oftalm., 17:1-8, 1942. 277

3365. Rizzo, E. M., e M. C. Cortesi. Narcolessia con onirismo e subnarcosi barbiturica. Rass. Stud. Psichiat., 39:307-24, 1950. 239

3366. Rizzolo, A. A study of 100 consecutively recorded dreams. Am. J. Psychol., 35:244-54, 1924. 100, 101

3367. Roasenda, G. Inversione del ritmo del sonno, con agitazione psicomotoria notturna. Policlinico (Sez. Prat.), 28:181-86, 1921. 247

3368. Robb, E. F. Enuresis. Minnesota Med., 30:91-96, 1947.

3369. Roberts, D. R. An electrophysiological theory of hypnosis. Internat. J. Clin. Exp. Hypn., 8: 43-55, 1960.

3370. Roberts, G. M., and L. A. Crandall, Jr. The role of the portal system in the regulation of circulating blood volume. Am. J. Physiol., 106:423-31, 1933. 37

3371. Roberts, K. E., and J. A. Schoellkopf. Eating, sleeping, and elimination practices of a group of two-and-one-half-year-old children. III. Sleeping practices. A.M.A. Am. J. Dis. Child., 82: 132-36, 1951. 307

3372. Robiczek, H. Die Kunst nach Belieben zu schlafen; ein Beitrag zur Theorie und Praxis der Atmungstherapie. Fortschr. Med., 51:212-13, 1933. 294

3373. Robin, E. D. Some interrelationships between sleep and disease.

A.M.A. Arch. Neurol. Psychiat.,
102:669-75, 1958. 39

3374. ____, R. D. Whaley, C. H.
Crump, and D. M. Travis. The
nature of the respiratory acidosis of sleep and of the respiratory alkalosis of hepatic coma.
J. Clin. Investig., 36:924, 1957.
51, 272

3375. ____, ____, ____, and ____.
Alveolar gas concentrations and
respiratory center sensitivity to
CO_2 during natural sleep. Fed.
Proc., 16:107-8, 1957. 51

3376. ____, ____, ____, and ____.
Alveolar gas tensions, pulmonary ventilation and blood pH
during physiologic sleep in normal subjects. J. Clin. Investig.,
37:981-89, 1958. 33, 49, 50, 51,
56

3377. Robin, I. G. Snoring. Proc. Roy.
Soc. Med., 41:151-53, 1948. 49,
50

3378. Robinson, E. S., and S. O. Herrmann. Effects of loss of sleep. I.
J. Exp. Psychol., 5:19-32, 1922.
219

3379. ____, and F. Richardson-Robinson. Effects of loss of sleep.
II. J. Exp. Psychol., 5:93-100,
1922. 220, 224

3380. Robinson, G. W. Sleep and its
disorders. J. Missouri Med. Ass.,
13:313-19, 1926. 274, 294, 362

3381. Rodale, J. I. Sleep and Rheumatism. Emmaus, Pa.: Rodale
Press, 1945. Pp. 32.

3382. Rodin, E. A., D. D. Daly, and R.
G. Bickford. Effects of photic
stimulation during sleep. A study
of normal subjects and epileptic
patients. Neurology, 5:149-59,
1955.

3383. ____, C. E. Frohman, and E. D.
Luby. The EEG in experimental
sleep deprivation. EEG Clin.
Neurophysiol., 13:310, 1961. 226
Rodin, E., co-author: 814.

3384. Roéland, C. L'air et le pouvoir
réparateur du sommeil. Rev.
Path: Comp. (Paris), 50:442-43,
805-7, 1950; 51:453, 1951.

3385. Roger, A., et H. Gastaut. Les
mécanismes neurophysiologiques
du conditionnement et leurs modifications sous l'effet des médi-
caments psychotropes. In: Psychotropic Drugs, 1957 (1357), pp.
252-70. 347

3386. ____, G. F. Rossi, e A. Zirondoli. Sull'importanza dei nervi

encefalici nei mantenimento
della veglia nel preparato "encefalo isolato." Boll. Soc. Ital.
Biol. Sper., 31:463-64, 1955.
212

3387. ____, ____, e ____. Effetti di
sezioni acute e croniche di nervi cranici sull'elettroencefalogramma del gatto "encefalo isolato." Boll. Soc. Ital. Biol. Sper.,
31:810-12, 1955. 212

3388. ____, ____, et ____. Le rôle
des afférences des nerfs crâni-
ens dans le maintien de l'état
vigile de la préparation "encéphale isolé." EEG Clin. Neurophysiol., 8:1-13, 1956. 212

3389. ____, E. N. Sokolov, et L. G.
Voronin. Le conditionnement
moteur à l'état de veille et pendant le sommeil. Etude électro-
encéphalique chez l'homme normal. Rev. Neurol., 96:460-69,
1957; also EEG Clin. Neurophysiol., 9:561-62, 1957.
Roger, A., co-author: 1369,
1370, 2863.

3390. Roger, H. Les sécousses nerveuses de l'endormissement.
Rev. Méd. Franç., 12:847-52,
1931. 74, 359

3391. ____. Le sommeil normal, la
fonction hypnique. Marseille
Méd., I:5-26, 27-37, 1931; also
Rev. Neurol., II:397, 1932. 359

3392. ____. Les Troubles du Sommeil—Hypersomnies, Insomnies,
Parasomnies. Paris: Masson &
Cie, 1932. Pp. 206. 275, 277,
280, 281, 282, 283, 289

3393. ____, Y. Poursines, et G. Pitot.
Spasmes des inférogyres avec
arrêt des mouvements volontai-
res des membres au cours d'un
Parkinson fruste avec épisode
hypersomnique tardif. Rev. Oto-
Neuro-Ophthalm., 9:510-13,
1931. 279

3394. ____, et J. Roger. La narcolepsie familiale. Marseille Méd.,
79:49-62, 1942.

3395. ____, et ____. Les hypersomnies. Rev. Prat. (Paris), 4:1533-
49, 1954. 272

3396. ____, et Vaissade. Méningite
tuberculeuse apyrétique de l'a-
dolescence avec inversion du
rythme du sommeil et paralysie
verticale du regard. Traitement.
Bull. Mém. Soc. Méd. Hôp. Paris, 49:1309-14, 1933. 279

3397. Rohmer, F., G. Hiebel, et C.

Kayser. Recherches sur le fonctionnement du système nerveux des hibernants. Les ondes cérébrales pendant le sommeil hibernal et le réveil. Etude sur le spermophile. C. R. Soc. Biol., 145:747-52, 1951. 323, 324, 326
Rohmer, F., co-author: 2117.

3398. Rokhlin, L. L. (Russ.) Sleep, Hypnosis, and Dreams in the Light of the Teachings of I. P. Pavlov. Moskva: All-Union Soc. Dissemin. Polit. Sci. Inform., 1952. Pp. 40. 344

3399. Romano, J., and G. L. Engel. Delirium; I. Electroencephalographic data. Arch. Neurol. Psychiat., 51:356-77, 1944. 32
Romano, J., co-author: 1085.

3400. Rominger, E. Zur Anwendung von Beruhigungs- und Schlafmitteln in der Kinderheilkunde. Klin. Wschr., 1:1949-54, 1922. 278, 294

3401. _____, und E. Krueger. Schlafwirkung vegetativer Gifte im Kindesalter. Klin. Wschr., 11(I):1096-97, 1932. 294
Rominger, E., co-author: 1028.

3402. Ronald, R. Hypersomnia associated with abnormal hunger: The Kleine-Levin syndrome. Brit. Med. J., II:326-27, 1946. 267

3403. Rondelli, U. Ematologia del sonno. Minerva Med., 1:825-28, 1931. 295

3404. Rorke, R. F. Disorders of sleep in childhood. Brit. Med. J., II:525, 1930.

3405. Rose, S., and D. Rabinov. Electrical anesthesia. Med. J. Australia, I:657-59, 1945. 298

3406. Rosenbach, O. Das Verhalten der Reflexe bei Schlafenden. Z. klin. Med., 1:358-74, 1880. 16

3407. Rosenbaum, J. D., B. C. Ferguson, R. K. Davis, and E. C. Rossmeisl. The influence of cortisone upon the diurnal rhythm of renal excretory function. J. Clin. Instig., 31:507-20, 1952. 167
Rosenbaum, J. D., co-author: 3090.

3408. Rosenberg, P., and J. M. Coon. Increase of hexobarbital sleeping time by certain anticholinesterases. Proc. Soc. Exp. Biol. Med., 98:650-52, 1958. 297

3409. Rosenbloom, J. The sleep of an insomnia sufferer as recorded by himself. Interstate Med. J., 25:451, 1918. 274

3410. Rosenblum, M. J., and A. J. Cummins. The effect of sleep and amytal on the motor activity of the human sigmoid colon. Gastroenterology, 27:445-50, 1954. 55

3411. Rosental, D., and V. Filipova. (Russ.) Excitability of the muscles of man during sleep and awakeness. Bull. Eksp. Biol. Med., Suppl. 1:138-41, 1957. 14

3412. Rosenthal, C. Ueber das verzoegerte psychomotorische Erwachen, seine Entstehung und seine nosologische Bedeutung. Arch. Psychiat., 81:159-71, 1927. 260

3413. _____. Ueber den normalen Schlaf des Menschen. Klin. Wschr., 6:1457-61, 1927. 328

3414. _____. Ueber das Auftreten von halluzinatorisch-kataplektischen Angstsyndrom, Wachanfaellen und aehnlichen Stoerungen bei Schizophrenen. Mschr. Psychiat. Neurol. (Basel), 102:11-38, 1939. 236

3415. Rosenthal, J. S. (Russ.) The passage of internal inhibition into sleep during the extinction of the investigatory reflex. Arkh. Biol. Nauk, 29:367-84, 1929; also in: The Sleep Problem, 1954 (392), pp. 100-112. 197

3416. Rosett, J. An apparatus for the induction of muscular relaxation and sleep. Arch. Neurol. Psychiat., 22:737-45, 1929. 311

3417. _____. Induction of sleep in epileptic persons. Arch. Neurol. Psychiat., 26:131-40, 1931.

3418. _____. The Mechanism of Thought, Imagery, and Hallucination. New York: Columbia Univ. Press, 1939. Pp. x + 289. 79

3419. Roskam, J. Un nouveau traitement de la narcolepsie-cataplexie. Acta Clin. Belg., 1:377-82, 1946. 239

3420. Rosman, N. P. Prolonged sleep therapy in the treatment of mental disorders. McGill Med. J., 27:45-52, 1958. 207

3421. Ross, T. A. An aspect of insomnia. Practitioner, 144:329-36, 1940. 274

3422. Rossi, G. F. Indipendenza dalle afferenze retiniche della miosi che si osserva durante il sonno prodotto dall'interruzione del tegmento mesencefalico. Boll. Soc. Ital. Biol. Sper., 29:313-14, 1953.

3423. _____. Ricerche sulla natura della miosi nel sonno e nella narcosi barbiturica. Arch. Sci. Biol., 41:46-56, 1957.

3424. _____, and A. Brodal. Corticofugal fibres to the brain-stem reticular formation. An experimental study in the cat. J. Anat., 90:42-62, 1956. 211

3425. _____, E. Favale, T. Hara, A. Giussani, and G. Sacco. Researches on the nervous mechanisms underlying deep sleep in the cat. Arch. Ital. Biol., 99: 270-92, 1961. 27, 212

3426. _____, e L. Steffanon. Facilitazione olfattiva delle risposte elettrocorticographiche e pupillari alla stimolazione elettrica dell'ipotalamo. Boll. Soc. Ital. Biol. Sper., 28:1344-45, 1952.

3427. _____, and A. Zanchetti. The brain stem reticular formation. Anatomy and physiology. Arch. Ital. Biol., 95:199-435, 1957. 209, 362

3428. _____, e A. Zirondoli. Sulle strutture anatomiche che permettono la veglia nel gatto "encefalo isolato." Boll. Soc. Ital. Biol. Sper., 30:494-95, 1954. 212

3429. _____, and _____. On the mechanism of the cortical desynchronization elicited by volatile anesthetics. EEG Clin. Neurophysiol., 7:383-90, 1955. 298
Rossi, G. F., co-author: 252-56, 518, 1144, 1145, 1624-26, 2618, 2619, 2863, 2901, 2902, 3386-88.

3430. Rost, H., und C. Sievert. Abhaengigkeit der Diurese und der Nieren-Clearance von der Schlaftiefe nach Applikation von Phenothiazin-derivaten allein und nach deren Kombination mit Barbituraten oder Morphin. Zbl. Gyn., 77:483-87, 1955.

3431. Rosvold, H. E., and J. M. R. Delgado. The effect on delayed-alternation test performance of stimulating or destroying electrically structures within the frontal lobes of the monkey's brain. J. Comp. Physiol. Psychol., 49:365-72, 1956.

3432. Roth, B. (Czech.) On some general characteristics of the vegetative regulation with special ref-

erence to sleep. Čas. Lék. Česk., 91:569-75, 1952. 272, 344

3433. _____. (Czech.) Narcolepsy. Prakt. Lék. (Praha), 33:9-12, 1953. 234

3434. _____. (Czech.) The vegetative system in narcolepsy. Neurol. Psychiat. Česk., 16:173-81, 1953. 240

3435. _____. (Czech.) Narcolepsy and epilepsy; clinical and electroencephalographic comparative study. Neurol. Psychiat. Česk., 17:303-11, 1954. 237, 238

3436. _____. (Czech.) On a case of familial essential narcolepsy. Čas. Lék. Česk., 93:127-29, 1954. 237, 242

3437. _____. (Czech.) Sleep drunkenness and sleep paralysis. Neurol. Psychiat. Česk., 19:48-58, 1956. 236, 271

3438. _____. (Czech.) Narcolepsy and Hypersomnia from the Aspect of the Physiology of Sleep. Praha: Státní Zdravotnické Nakladatelství, 1957. Pp. 332. 234

3439. _____. (Czech.) Disturbances of wakefulness, sleep and consciousness induced by deafferentation of the central nervous system. Česk. Psychiat., 54: 303-9, 1958. 234

3440. _____. The sleep-EEG-characteristics as indicator of chronic insufficiency of awareness. Proc. Fourth Internat. Congr. EEG Clin. Neurophysiol., Brussels, 1957. New York: Pergamon Press, 1959, pp. 321-22. 31, 271

3441. _____. Beitraege zum Studium der Narkolepsie. Schweiz. Arch. Neurol. Psychiat., 84:180-210, 1959. 234

3442. _____. The clinical and theoretical importance of EEG rhythms corresponding to states of lowered vigilance. EEG Clin. Neurophysiol., 13:395-99, 1961. 272

3443. _____, and J. Šimek. (Czech.) Electroencephalographic finding in essential and symptomatic narcolepsy. Neurol. Psychiat. Česk., 15:80-109, 1952. 30, 31, 238

3444. _____, and J. Šimon. (Czech.) Contributions to the clinic of narcolepsy. Čas. Lék. Česk., 91:1462-68, 1952. 234, 237, 242

3445. _____, and M. Tuháček. (Czech.)

Electroencephalographic findings in organic and so-called functional hypersomnias. Neurol. Psychiat. Česk., 17:235-44, 1954. 271 Roth, B., co-author: 930, 1371, 1984.

3446. Roth, M., and J. Green. The "lambda" wave as a normal physiological phenomenon in the human EEG. EEG Clin. Neurophysiol., 5:622, 1953.

3447. _____, J. Shaw, and J. Green. The form, voltage distribution and physiological significance of the K-complex. EEG Clin. Neurophysiol., 8:385-402, 1956. 26

3448. Roth, N. Some problems in narcolepsy: With a case report. Bull. Menninger Clin., 10:160-70, 1946. 237, 238

3449. _____. Sublimation in dreams. Am. J. Psychother., 8:32-42, 1954. 103

3450. Rothballer, A. B. Studies of the adrenaline sensitive component of the reticular activating system. EEG Clin. Neurophysiol., 8:603-22, 1956. 209

3451. Rothenberg, S. Psychoanalytic insight into insomnia. Psychoanal. Rev., 34:141-68, 1947. 275

3452. Rothfeld, J. Affektiver Tonus und Bewusstseinsverlust beim Lachen und Orgasmus (Gelo- und Orgasmolepsia). Z. ges. Neurol. Psychiat., 115:516-30, 1928. 235

3453. _____. Ueber Orgasmolepsie und ueber sexuelle Erregungen bei narkoleptischen Schlafzustaenden, nebst Bemerkungen zur Narkolepsiefrage. Z. ges. Neurol. Psychiat., 138:705-19, 1932. 235, 237

3454. Rothman, T., J. Goodman, and D. B. Tyler. Studies on experimental insomnia. Electroencephalographic changes during 112 hours of wakefulness. Trans. Am. Neurol. Ass., 71:173-74, 1946. Rothman T., co-author: 3998.

3455. Rothmann, H. Zusammenfassender Bericht ueber den Rothmannschen grosshirnlosen Hund nach klinischer und anatomischer Untersuchung. Z. ges. Neurol. Psychiat., 87:247-313, 1923. 21

3456. Rovetta, P. Electrocorticographic changes in temporal lobe epilepsy at rest and during induced sleep. EEG Clin. Neurophysiol., 11:521-38, 1959. 258, 260

3457. Rowe, A. H. The effect of venous stasis on the proteins of human blood serum. J. Lab. Clin. Med., 1:485-89, 1915. 38

3458. Rowe, E. C. The hygiene of sleep. Psychol. Rev., 18:425-32, 1911. 186, 314

3459. Rowe, S. N. Localization of the mechanism controlling sleep. Arch. Neurol. Psychiat., 33:440-41, 1935; also Brain, 58:21-43, 1935. 264, 265, 272

3460. Rowland, V. Differential electroencephalographic response to conditioned auditory stimuli in arousal from sleep. EEG Clin. Neurophysiol., 9:585-94, 1957. 29

3461. _____. Conditioning and brain waves. Sci. Am., 201(2):89-96, 1959.

3462. Royce, P. C., and G. Sayers. Blood ACTH: effects of ether, pentobarbital, epinephrin and pain. Endocrinology, 63:794-800, 1958. 356

3463. Rozhanski (Rojanski), N. A. (Russ.) Material on the Physiology of Sleep. St. Petersburg: Print. Office Imper. Acad. Sci., 1913. Pp. 94 + viii. Reissued, with changes, Moskva: State Publ. Med. Liter., 1954. Pp. 126. 344

3464. Rozner, E. Schlafzentrum und seine Beziehungen zur Diplopie bei Schlaftrunkenheit. Med. Klin., 31(I):205-7, 1935. 245, 246

3465. Rubenstein, B. B. The relation of cyclic changes in human vaginal smears to body temperatures and basal metabolic rates. Am. J. Physiol., 119:635-41, 1937. 185

3466. Rubenstein, L. Humming: a vocal standard with a diurnal variation. Science, 134:1519-20, 1961. 159

3467. Rubin, H. Ueber Agrypnia gastrica. Z. aerztl. Fortbild., 19:720-21, 1922. 294

3468. Rubin, M. A. The distribution of the alpha rhythm over the cerebral cortex of normal man. J. Neurophysiol., 1:313-23, 1938. 28

3469. Rubino, A. Interpretazione delle variazioni di coscienza nel ritmo sonno-veglia. Acta Neurol. (Napoli), 2:632-53, 1947. 31

3470. _____. Il Sonno. Napoli: Idelson, 1949. Pp. xii + 282. 100, 362

3471. _____. Nuove acquisizioni sulla

genesi del sonno. Acta Neurol.
(Napoli), Quaderno III:173-83,
1953. 34, 35

3472. _____, e R. Balbi. Fluttuazioni
nictemerali del magnesio in rapporto con il ritmo sonno-veglia.
Acta Neurol. (Napoli), 6:618-33,
1951. 163

3473. _____, e _____. Ricerche sulla
genesi del sonno—Fluttuazioni
nictemerali della colinesterasi.
Acta Neurol. (Napoli), 8:875-78,
1953. 162

3474. Rudolph, G. de M. Length of sleep
in adults. Med. Press, 233:324-
27, 1955. 121

3475. Rüdiger, K. Stoerungen des
Schlafes bei organischen Gehirn-
leiden, insbesondere bei Parkinsonismus. Rostock: Diss., 1937.
Pp. 24.

3476. Rütimeyer, W. Ueber postencephalitische Schlafstoerung.
Schweiz. med. Wschr., 51:7-12,
1921. 247

3477. Ruschke, C. Behandlung der
"Alltagsinsomnie" in der Heilan-
stalt. Med. Welt, 6(II):1316-17,
1932. 294

3478. _____. Schlafstoerungen und ihre
ambulante Behandlung. Z. aerztl.
Fortbild., 32:352-54, 1935. 294

3479. Rushton, J. G. Sleep paralysis:
report of two cases. Dis. Nerv.
Syst., 5:115-17, 1944; also Proc.
Staff Meet. Mayo Clin., 19:51-
54, 1944. 236

3480. Russell, J. S. R. The value of
sleep. Practitioner, 122:12-17,
1929. 294

3481. Rutenfranz, J., und T. Hellbruegge. Ueber Tagesschwankungen der Rechengeschwindig-
keit bei 11jaehrigen Kindern. Z.
Kinderheilk., 80:65-81, 1957. 158

3482. _____, _____, und W. Nigge-
schmidt. Ueber die Tagesryth-
mik des elektrischen Hautwider-
stand bei 11-jaehrigen Kindern.
Z. Kinderheilk., 78:144-57, 1956.
110
Rutenfranz, J., co-author: 1690-
92.

3483. Rycroft, C. A contribution to the
study of the dream screen. Internat. J. Psycho-anal., 32:178-84,
1951. 101

3484. Rynberk, G. van. Mouvements
rythmiques dans le rêve comme
symboles des mouvements du
coeur. Encéphale, 22:270-71,
1927. 105

3485. Saar, H., und W. Paulus. Experimentelle Untersuchungen ueber
die Ausscheidung des Alkohols
im Schlaf. Dsche Z. gerichtl.
Med., 35:28-36, 1942.

3486. Sabatini, G. Sui fenomeni d'inversione nell'encefalite epidemica. Policlinico (Sez. Prat.),
30:2-7, 1923. 247, 249

3487. Sabouraud, R. Sur la pelade,
l'hyperthyroïdisme latent, les
insomnies et sur l'hématoéthy-
roïdine employée comme hypnotique. Presse Méd., 38:757-
58, 1930. 294

3488. Saccheto, A. Sopra una sindrome fenomenica particolare
di encefalite epidemica. Boll.
Soc. Med.-Chir. Modena, 21/22:
421-39, 1921. 247

3489. Sagal, Z. Insomnia in the aged.
Geriatrics, 13:463-66, 1958.
312

3490. Sager, O. Experimentelle Untersuchungen ueber die Bulbo-
capninstarre (zugleich ein Beitrag zum Mechanismus der Katalepsie). Z. ges. exp. Med., 81:
543-58, 1932. 253, 254

3491. _____, A. Kreindler, et G. Stier.
L'hydrophilie des tissus pen-
dant le sommeil. C. R. Soc.
Biol., 102:150-51, 1929.

3492. _____, L. Goldhammer, and A.
Mareş. (Roum.) Researches on
the problems of sleep and muscle tonus. Bull. Ştiinţ. Acad.
Secţ. Med., 7:1281-99, 1955.
Sager, O., co-author: 976, 2679,
2681-86.

3493. Sahlgren, E. Experimentelle Untersuchungen ueber den Angriffs-
punkt des Luminals im Gehirn
bei Kaninchen. Acta Psychiat.
Neurol., 9:129-47, 1934. 295
Sahlgren, E., co-author: 2664.

3494. Sailer, S., und C. Stumpf. Weitere Hinweise auf den choliner-
gen Mechanismus der "arousal
reaction." Arch. exp. Path.
Pharmakol., 232:277-78, 1957.
209, 303

3495. Saito, Y., K. Maekawa, S. Take-
naka, and A. Kasamatsu. Single
cortical unit activity during
EEG arousal. EEG Clin. Neurophysiol., Suppl. 9:95-98, 1957.
211

3496. Sal y Rosas, F. Influence probable de l'état de veille et de sommeil sur les crises épileptiques.
Ann. Méd.-Psychol., 2:706-22,

1957. 260

3497. Salamone, F. P., S. Navarra, e G. Rodolico. Fisiopatologia del sonno artificiale protratto. Riv. Pat. Clin., 9:105-8, 1954. 206

3498. Salkind, E. (Russ.) On the pathogenesis of sleep, after observations in epidemic encephalitis. Soviet. Psikhonevrol., 1:32-44, 1925. 244, 245, 349, 361

3499. Salmon, A. Teoria ipofisaria e teoria infundibolare dell'ipersonno. Cervello, 2:281-301, 1923. 355

3500. ____. Il sistema vegetativo nel sonno. Quaderni Psichiat., 12: 137-47, 1925. 355

3501. ____. La narcolessia di Nape leoni. Riforma Med., 41:1157-80, 1925. 355

3502. ____. Les rapports du sommeil, considéré comme une fonction végétative avec le systême endocrino-sympathique. Rev. Neurol., I:841-46, 1927. 355

3503. ____. Il sistema diencefalo-ipofisario nel sonno. Cervello, 8: 124-32, 1929; also Riv. Pat. Nerv., 35:72-80, 1930. 355

3504. ____. Sul meccanismo del letargo dei mammiferi ibernanti. Riv. Biol., 12:80-92, 1930. 355

3505. ____. Il centro diencefalico regolatore del sonno. Scritti Med. in onore Gabbi, I:132-46, 1930. 355

3506. ____. La Fisiopatologia del Sonno. Bologna: Cappelli, 1930. Pp. 211. 113, 355

3507. ____. Le sommeil est-il déterminé par l'excitation d'un centre hypnique ou par la dépression fonctionelle d'un centre de la veille? Rev. Neurol., I:714-20, 1932. 355

3508. ____. Le attuali vedute sul sonno. Giorn. Psichiat. Neuropat., 61:56-66, 1933. 355

3509. ____. L'insonnia. Riforma Med., 52:1382-85, 1936. 355

3510. ____. L'incontinenza di sonno. Gazz. Osp., 57:1020-23, 1936. 355

3511. ____. Le rôle des corrélations cortico-diencéphaliques et diencéphalo-hypophysaires dans la régulation de la veille et du sommeil. Presse Méd., 45:509-12, 1937. 355

3512. ____. L'apparato diencefalo-ipofisario nella fisio-patologia del sonno. Riv. Pat. Nerv. Ment.,

69:178-90, 1948. 356, 358

3513. ____. Le rôle du système diencéphalo-hypophysaire dans la physiologie du sommeil. Presse Méd., 60:54-57, 1952. 356

3514. Samaan, A. La fréquence cardiaque du chien en différentes conditions expérimentales d'activité et de repos. C. R. Soc. Biol., 115:1383-88, 1934. 42

3515. Samuels, I. Reticular mechanisms and behavior. Psychol. Bull., 56:1-25, 1959. 209

3516. Sandler, S. A. Somnambulism in the Armed Forces. Ment. Hyg., 29:236-47, 1945. 283

3517. Sanz-Ibáñez, J. Estudio experimental sobre el sueño. Arch. Neurobiol., 13:793-803, 1933. 202

3518. Saper, A. L. (Russ.) The dynamics of sleep in old age. Fiziol. Zh. SSSR, 29:139-43, 1940. 14

3519. Sapir, M., M. Lévy, J. Stroun, H. Miller, et J.-P. Bailliart. Réflexions sur quatre ans de traitement par la cure de sommeil dans l'hypertension artérielle. In: La Cure de Sommeil, 1954 (3021), pp. 73-117. 207 Sapir, M., co-editor: 3021.

3520. Sarajas, H. S. S. Observations on the electrocardiographic alterations in the hibernating hedgehog. Acta Physiol. Scand., 32:28-38, 1954. 323

3521. Sarason, D., Ed. Der Schlaf. Mitteilungen und Stellungnahme zum derzeitigen Stande des Schlafproblems. Muenchen: J. F. Lehmanns, 1929. Pp. 107. 294, 312

3522. Sarbin, T. R. Contributions to role-taking theory: I. Hypnotic behavior. Psychol. Rev., 57: 255-70, 1950. 335 Sarbin, T. R., co-author: 1295, 2476.

3523. Sargant, W. Battle of the Mind. Garden City, N.Y.: Doubleday & Co., 1957. Pp. 263. 228 Sargant, W. W., co-author: 725.

3524. Sarton, G. Sleeping along the meridian. Isis, 22:525-29, 1935. 310

3525. Sarylowa, K. P. (Russ.) On the question of the sleep regimen of young children in institutions. Soviet. Pediat., (5):56-61, 1934. 305

3526. Sasaki, T. Some experiments on the mechanism of the diurnal variation in the human body temperature, with particular reference to some influence of the labyrinth. Bull. Res. Inst. Diathetic Med., 3:262-70, 1953. <u>174</u>

3527. Saul, L. J., H. Davis, and P. A. Davis. Psychologic correlations with the electroencephalogram. Psychosom. Med., 11:361-76, 1949. <u>29</u>

3528. _____, E. Sheppard, D. Selby, W. Lhamon, D. Sachs, and R. Master. The quantification of hostility in dreams with reference to essential hypertension. Science, 119:382-83, 1954. <u>103</u>

3529. Saunders, P. Disorders of sleep. Oxford Med., Part II, 6:1087-99, 1933.

3530. Savvateev, V. B. (Russ.) Effect of modification of daily rhythm on the functional properties of the nervous system in hens. Zh. Vysshei Nerv. Deiat., 9:776-81, 1959. <u>175</u>

3531. Sawyer, C. H., and M. Kawakami. Characteristics of behavioral and electroencephalographic after-reactions to copulation and vaginal stimulation in the female rabbit. Endocrinology, 65:622-30, 1959. <u>209</u>
Sawyer, C. H., co-author: 2095.

3532. Scantlebury, R. E., H. L. Frick, and T. L. Patterson. The effect of normal and hypnotically induced dreams on the gastric hunger movements of man. J. Appl. Psychol., 26:682-91, 1942. <u>333</u>, <u>334</u>

3533. Scarponi, E. La fisiologia dell'attività nervosa superiore e il problema della conoscenza. Rass. Clin. Terap. Sci. Affini, 56:31-38, 1957. <u>31</u>

3534. Schachter, M. Une observation de narcolepsie infantile. J. Méd. Paris, 60:231-32, 1940. <u>237</u>

3535. _____. Insomnie rebelle passagère, complication diencéphalique du brûlure intense, localisée. Méd. Infant. (Paris), 54:36-40, 1947.

3536. _____. Syndrome narcoleptique d'origine encéphalitique. Données biologiques et psychologiques. Praxis, 37:564-66, 1948. <u>237</u>

3537. _____. Etude sur les rythmes du jour ou du sommeil chez l'enfant. (Spasmus nutans, tic de Salaam, Jactatio capitis nocturna). Encéphale, 43:173-92, 1954. <u>285</u>

3538. Schack, J. A., and L. R. Goldbaum. The analeptic effect of sodium succinate in barbiturate anesthesia in rabbits. J. Pharmacol. Exp. Therap., 96:315-24, 1949. <u>297</u>

3539. Schaeffer, G., et O. Thibault. Recherches sur les facteurs hormonaux de la régulation thermique. Effets de l'adrénaline sur les échanges en fonction de l'activité thyroïdienne. C. R. Soc. Biol., 139:855-56, 1945.

3540. _____, et _____. Recherches sur les facteurs hormonaux de la régulation thermique. Variations de la température centrale du rat hypophysectomisé en fonction de la température extérieure. C. R. Soc. Biol., 140:765-66, 1946.

3541. Schaeffer, H. Les réflexes conditionnels chez l'homme. Presse Méd., 44:405-10, 1936. <u>362</u>

3542. Schär, O. Schlafstoerungen. Dresden: Verlag von Holze & Pahl, 1913. Pp. 76. <u>278</u>

3543. Schallek, W. The vertical migration of the copepod Acartia tonsa under controlled illumination. Biol. Bull., 82:112-26, 1942. <u>132</u>

3544. Schaltenbrand, G. Ueber die Beziehungen zwischen krankhaften Steigerungen des Muskeltonus und dem Schlaf. XII. Mitteilung zu den myographischen Untersuchungen in der Klinik. Pfluegers Arch., 244:610-21, 1941. <u>13</u>, <u>15</u>

3545. _____. Thalamus und Schlaf. Allg. Z. Psychiat., 125:48-62, 1949. <u>266</u>

3546. Schaper, G. Das Hirnstrombild des schlafenden Saeuglings im 2. Trimenon. Mschr. Kinderheilk., 101:258-62, 1953.

3547. Scharrer, E., and B. Scharrer. Secretory cells within hypothalamus. Res. Publ. Ass. Nerv. Ment. Dis., 20:170-94, 1940. <u>356</u>

3548. Scheer, W. M. van der. (Dutch) Sleep cures in psychoses. Ned. Tschr. Geneesk., 82:386-88, 1937. <u>206</u>

3549. Scheibel, M. E., and A. B. Scheibel. The physiology of consciousness. Am. J. Orthopsychiat., 30:10-14, 1960. <u>31</u>

3550. _____, _____, A. Mollica, and G. Moruzzi. Convergence and interaction of afferent impulses on single units of the reticular formation. J. Neurophysiol., 18: 309-31, 1955.

3551. Schein, E. H. The effects of sleep deprivation on performance in a simulated communication task. J. Appl. Psychol., 41: 247-52, 1957. 226
Schein, E. H., co-author: 2955.

3552. Schenk, P. Ueber das Schlaferleben. Mschr. Psychiat. Neurol., 72:1-23, 1929.

3553. _____. Ueber den Winterschlaf und seine Beeinflussung durch die Extrakte innersekretorischer Druesen. Pfluegers Arch., 197: 66-80, 1922. 324, 326

3554. _____. Versuch einer psychologischen Theorie des Schlafes. Leipzig: Diss., 1928. Pp. 111. 362

3555. Scherbakova (Shcherbakova), O. P (Russ.) Materials for the study of the diurnal periodicity of physiological processes in higher mammals. I. The normal diurnal periodicity of physiological processes. II. Bull. Eksp. Biol. Med., 4:335-37, 1937; 5: 167-70, 1938. 163, 167, 175
Shcherbakova, O. P., co-author: 3727.

3556. Schergna, E., e R. Zappoli. Considerazioni elettroencefalografiche sul sonno indotto dagli ipnotici della serie dei carbinoli insaturati (Con particolare riguardo al carbammato di feniletinil-carbinolo). Rass. Neurol. Veget., 11:199-220, 1955. 296

3557. Schiele, B. C. A clinical study of sleep disturbances. Am. J. Psychiat., 98:119-23, 1941. 286
Schiele, B. C., co-author: 1265.

3558. Schiff, P., et R. Simon. Erythrémie avec accès de cataplexie, de chorée et de confusion mentale. Ann. Méd.-Psychol., 91:616-19, 1933. 238, 240

3559. Schiff, S. K., W. E. Bunney, and D. X. Freedman. A study of ocular movements in hypnotically induced dreams. J. Nerv. Ment. Dis., 133:59-68, 1961. 98, 104, 334

3560. Schiller, F. Consciousness reconsidered. A.M.A. Arch. Neurol. Psychiat., 67:199-227, 1952. 30

3561. Schindler, J. A. How To Live 365 Days a Year. New York: Prentice-Hall, 1954. Pp. x + 222. 100, 312

3562. Schindler, R. Das Traumleben der Leukotomierten. Wien. A. Nervenheilk., 6:330-34, 1953. 103

3563. Schlag, J. A study of the action of nembutal on diencephalic and mesencephalic unit activity. Arch. Internat. Physiol., 64:470-88, 1956. 295

3564. _____, and J. Faidherbe. Recruiting responses in the brain stem reticular formation. Arch. Ital. Biol., 99:135-62, 1961. 210

3565. _____, F. Chaillet, and J.-P. Herzet. Thalamic reticular system and cortical arousal. Science, 134:1691-92, 1961. 210
Schlag, J., co-author: 922.

3566. Schlager, E., and T. Meier. A strange Balinese method of inducing sleep (with some notes about balyans). Acta Trop. (Basel), 4:127-34, 1947. 241

3567. Schlesinger, B. The study of the sleeping pulse-rate in rheumatic children. Q. J. Med., 1:67-77, 1932. 42

3568. Schlomer, G. M. Morphine withdrawal in addicts by the method of prolonged sleep. Dis. Nerv. Syst., 9:187-90, 1948. 207

3569. Schmeing, K. Flugtraeume und 'Exkursion des Ich.' Arch. gen. Psychol., 100:541-54, 1938. 101

3570. Schmidt, G. Die Verbrechen in der Schlaftrunkenheit. Z. ges. Neurol. Psychiat., 176:208-54, 1943. 271

3571. Schmidt, H., Jr. The reticular formation and behavioral wakefulness. Psychol. Bull., 54:75, 1957. 209

3572. Schmidt, M. (Danish) Hypnotic drug therapy. Ugesk. Laeger, 93:902-65, 1932.

3573. Schneck, J. M. The rôle of a dream in treatment with hypnosis. Psychoanal. Rev., 34:485-91, 1947. 335

3574. _____. Sleep paralysis: psychodynamics. Psychiat. Q., 22:462-69, 1948; also Am. J. Psychiat., 108:921-23, 1952. 236

3575. _____. A theory of hypnosis. J. Clin. Exp. Hypn., 1(3):16-17, 1953. 336

3576. _____. Dreams in self-hypnosis. Psychoanal. Rev., 41:1-8, 1954. 333

3577. _____. Sleep paralysis, a new evaluation. Dis. Nerv. Syst., 18:144-46, 1957. 236

3578. _____. Sleep paralysis without narcolepsy or cataplexy. J. Am. Med. Ass., 173:1129-30, 1960. 236

3579. ____, and M. Bergman. Auditory acuity for pure tones in the waking and hypnotic states. J. Speech Disord., 14:33-36, 1949. 331

3580. Schnedorf, G., and A. C. Ivy. An examination of the hypnotoxin theory of sleep. Am. J. Physiol., 125:491-505, 1939. 203
Schnedorf, G., co-author: 1926.

3581. Schneider, D. E. Time-space and the growth of the sense of reality: a contribution to the psychophysiology of the dream. Psychoanal. Rev., 35:229-52, 1948. 106

3582. Schneider, J., E. Woringer, G. Thomalske, et G. Brogly. Bases électrophysiologiques des mécanismes d'action du pentothal chez le chat. Rev. Neurol., 87:433-51, 1952. 362

3583. Schneider, M., und H. Hirsch. Neuere Untersuchungen zur Physiologie des Schlafes. Med. Klin. (Berlin), 54:933-37, 1959.

3584. Schneyer, W. P., L. Hanahan, and R. W. Gilmore. Salivary secretion in man during sleep. Am. J. Physiol., 179:671, 1954. 53

3585. Schnore, M. M. Individual patterns of physiological activity as a function of task differences and degree of arousal. J. Exp. Psychol., 58:117-28, 1959.

3586. Schoen, R. Schlafstoerungen und Schlafmitteltherapie. Muench. med. Wschr., I:12-15, 51-55, 1936. 294

3587. Schoetensack, W., und J. Hann. Zur Wirkung der Narkotica auf die Blutdruckregulation und zur Differenzierung zwischen Schlaf und Narkose (nach Untersuchungen beim Elektrokrampf). Arch. exp. Path. Pharmakol., 213:102-10, 1951. 295

3588. Scholander, T. The effects of moderate sleep deprivation on the habituation of the autonomic response elements. Acta Physiol. Scand., 51:325-42, 1961. 226, 229

3589. Scholten, C. Ueber experimentelle und therapeutische Grundlagen der Schlafmittelanwendung nach Erfahrungen bei Herzkranken. Med. Welt, 14:961-65, 1940. 294

3590. Schonbar, R. A. Some manifest characteristics of recallers and nonrecallers of dreams. J. Consult. Psychol., 23:414-18, 1959. 101

3591. Schottstaedt, W. W., W. J. Grace, and H. G. Wolff. Life situation, behavior patterns, and renal excretion of fluid and electrolytes. J. Am. Med. Ass., 157:1485-88, 1955. 167

3592. Schreiner, L., D. McK. Rioch, C. Pechtel, and J. H. Masserman. Behavioural changes following thalamic injury in cats. J. Neurophysiol., 16:234-46, 1953. 206
Schreiner, L. H., co-author: 2531.

3593. Schrumpf, A. Beitraege zur Beleuchtung des klinischen Wertes der Impedanzmessung. Z. klin. Med., 133:139-67, 1937. 158

3594. Schuetz, E. Induction of sleep by simultaneous administration of posterior pituitary extracts and water. Nature, 153:432-33, 1944. 204

3595. ____, and H. Caspers. On the provocation and activation of epileptic discharges by anesthesia and sleep induced by medicaments. EEG Clin. Neurophysiol., 5:118, 1953. 296

3596. ____, und H.-W. Mueller. Das kindliche Elektroencephalogramm. Klin. Wschr., 29:20-21, 1951. 27

3597. ____, ____, und H. Schoenenberg. Ueber die Entwicklung zentralnervoeser Rhythmen im Elektroencephalogramm des Kindes. Z. ges. exp. Med., 117:157-70, 1951. 28

3598. Schuetz, F. Position of the body during sleep. Lancet, 241:774-75, 1941. 9, 11

3599. Schulte, W. Temporaere homosexuelle Triebumkehr bei Stoerungen der Schlaf-Wachsteuerung. Nervenarzt, 15:68-76, 1942. 271

3600. ____. Ergaenzende Bemerkungen zur Behandlung der Brachialgia paraesthetica nocturna. Dsche med. Wschr., 74:366-68, 1949. 285

3601. ____. Der Schlafentzug und seine Folgen. Med. Klin. (Berlin), 54:969-73, 1959. 257

3602. Schultz, J. H. Psychotherapie der Schlafmangels. Dsche med. Wschr., 52:229-31, 1926. 294

3603. ____. Hypnose und Suggestion beim Menschen. Handb. norm. path. Physiol., 17:669-89, 1926. 329, 337

3604. _____. Die Psychopathologie und Psychotherapie des Schlafes. Z. aerztl. Fortbild., 30:225-28, 1933. 294, 308

3605. _____. Wachen und Schlafen. Dsche med. Wschr., 60:1827-30, 1934. 362

3606. _____. Neurose, Ermuedung und Schlaf. Mensch und Arbeit, 4:69-78, 1952.

3607. _____. Zur Psychotherapie der Schlafstoerungen. Med. Klin. (Berlin), 54:978-81, 1959. 286

3608. Schultz-Hencke, H. Lehrbuch der Traumanalyse. Stuttgart: G. Thieme, 1949. Pp. xii + 283. 103

3609. Schumacher, G. A., H. Goodell, J. D. Hardy, and H. G. Wolff. Uniformity of the pain threshold in man. Science, 92:110-12, 1940. 159

3610. Schumann, H.-J. von. Traeume in der Polarnacht. Polarforschung, 3:342-46, 1955. 102

3611. _____. Die Traeume der Blinden in Riten, Mythen, Sagen, Legenden, Maerchen, und im Folklore. Med. Mschr., 10:264-68, 1956. 102

3612. _____. Das Traumleben der Seeleblinden. Med. Mschr., 11:439-41, 1957. 102

3613. _____. Traeume der Blinden. Psychol. Praxis, Heft 25, 1959. Pp. 152. 102

3614. Schuster, U. Das Elektrodermatogramm und das Hypnokinegramm in ihrer Beziehung zur Schlaftiefe. Muenchen: Inaug. Diss., 1955. Pp. 34. 113

3615. Schutz, F. Some factors concerning sleep and wakefulness. Queen Med. Mag. (Birmingham), 38:104-5, 1945. 356

3616. Schwab, E. Zur Lokalisationsfrage des Schlafzentrums. Muench. med. Wschr., 79:94-95, 1932. 267, 359, 362

3617. Schwab, R. S. Method of measuring consciousness in attacks of petit mal epilepsy. Arch. Neurol. Psychiat., 41:215-17, 1939. 258

3618. _____. The influence of visual and auditory stimuli on the electroencephalographic tracing of petit mal. Am. J. Psychiat., 97:1301-12, 1941. 258

3619. _____, P. Passouant, et J. Cadilhac. Action des stimulations auditives rythmées sur le sommeil humain. Montpellier Méd., 45:501-14, 1954. 210

Schwab, R. S., co-author: 725, 3114.

3620. Schwartz, B. A. Endormissement et Réveil du Sommeil Nembutalique de l'Adulte. Paris: Copie-Comète, 1958. Pp. 62. 30, 296

3621. _____. EEG et mouvements oculaires dans le sommeil de nuit. EEG Clin. Neurophysiol., 14:126-28, 1962.

3622. _____, C. Dreyfus-Brisac, H. Fischgold. Polygraphie du sommeil. Souvenir du sommeil; signification des stimuli. Rev. Neurol., 101:273-75, 1959.

3623. _____, et H. Fischgold. Introduction à l'étude polygraphique du sommeil de nuit (Mouvements oculaires et cycles de sommeil). Vie Méd., 41, S1:39-46, 1960. 50, 98

Schwartz, B. A., co-author: 1183-85, 1686.

3624. Schwartz, J., R. Geiger, et Y. Kempf. Le métabolisme de base dans le sommeil. Sem. Hôp. (Paris), 33:586-89, 1957. 55

Schwartz, J., co-author: 2788.

3625. Schwartz, S. Encephalitis lethargica. New York Med. J. Med. Rec., 112:182-85, 1920. 246

3626. Schwarz, A. M. Ueber den Einfluss von Schlaflagen auf die Entstehung von Kieferanomalien. Z. Stomatol., 30:731-37, 1932. 11, 306

3627. Schwarz, B. E., and R. G. Bickford. Electroencephalographic changes in animals under the influence of hypnosis. J. Nerv. Ment. Dis., 124:433-39, 1956. 336

3628. _____, _____, and W. C. Rasmussen. Hypnotic phenomena, including hypnotically activated seizures, studied with the electroencephalogram. J. Nerv. Ment. Dis., 122:564-74, 1955. 333

3629. Schwarz, H. Zur Klinik der Schlafstoerung. Psychiat. Neurol. med. Psychol. (Leipzig), 7:102-12, 1955. 286

3630. Schweisheimer, W. Schlaf und Schlaflosigkeit—ein Weg zum Schlaflernen. Muenchen: J. F. Bergmann, 1925. Pp. 98. 294

3631. Scott, E. A study of the sleeping habits of twenty-nine children of pre-school age. Child Develop., 2:326-28, 1931. 9,

117, 186

3632. Scott, H. D. Hypnosis and the conditioned reflex. J. Gen. Psychol., 4:113-30, 1930. 332

3633. Scott, J. W. The EEG during hypothermia. EEG Clin. Neurophysiol., 7:466, 1955. 327

3634. Scott, T. H., W. H. Bexton, W. Heron, and B. K. Doane. Cognitive effects of perceptual isolation. Canad. J. Psychol., 13: 200-209, 1959. 198
Scott, T. H., co-author: 326.

3635. Scott, W. C. M. Sleep in psychoanalysis. Bull. Philadelphia Ass. Psychoanal., 6:72-83, 1956. 362

3636. Scripture, E. W. A case of defective sleep-shunt. Lancet, 199(II): 652, 1920.

3637. Sears, A. B., and J. M. Beatty. A comparison of the galvanic skin response in the hypnotic and waking state. J. Clin. Exp. Hypn., 4:49-60, 1956. 331

3638. Sears, R. R. An experimental study of hypnotic anesthesia. J. Exp. Psychol., 15:1-22, 1932. 332

3639. Seashore, C. E. The frequency of dreams. Sci. Monthly, 2:467-74, 1916. 283

3640. Sediari, F., e E. Moretti. Studio elettroencefalografico di 4 casi di narcolessia. Riv. Pat. Nerv. Ment., 77:609-11, 1956. 237

3641. See, P. La Cure de Sommeil dans la Maladie Ulcéreuse. Paris: Editions A.G.E.M.P., 1955. Pp. 54. 207

3642. Seeligmüller, A. Hyperventilation und Schlaf: kurze Mitteilung zur Technik der Hypnose. Therap. Gegenw., 75:286-87, 1934.

3643. Seguín, C. A. La producción de la hipnosis. Rev. As. Méd. Argentina, 56:593-94, 1942. 336

3644. ———. Un caso de insomnio rebelde. Rev. Neurol. Psiquiat. (S. Paulo), 10:354-56, 1947.

3645. Segundo, J. P. The reticular formation. A survey. Acta Neurol. Latinoam., 2:245-81, 1956. 209

3646. ———, R. Arana, and J. D. French. Behavioral arousal by stimulation of the brain in the monkey. J. Neurosurg., 12:601-13, 1955. 209

3647. ———, ———, E. Migliaro, J. E. Villar, A. Garcia Guelfi, and E. Garcia Austt, H. Respiratory responses from fornix and wall of third ventricle in man. J. Neurophysiol., 18:96-101, 1955.

3648. ———, R. Naquet, and P. Buser. Effect of cortical stimulation on electrocortical activity in monkeys. J. Neurophysiol., 18:236-45, 1955. 211
Segundo, J. P., co-author: 16, 3697.

3649. Seiger, H. W. Treatment of essential nocturnal enuresis. J. Pediat., 40:738-49, 1952. 285

3650. Selbach, H. Das Kippschwingungsprinzip in der Analyse der vegetativen Selbststeuerung. Fortschr. Neurol., 17(I):129-69, 1949. 358
Selbach, H., co-author: 2214.

3651. Selkirk, W. J. B. The night cap for insomnia. Brit. Med. J., II: 255, 1918. 294, 312

3652. Selling, L. S. Effect of conscious wish upon dream content. J. Abnorm. Soc. Psychol., 27: 172-78, 1932.

3653. Selsam, M. A Time for Sleep. How Animals Rest. New York: W. R. Scott, 1953. Unpaged. 307

3654. Sendrail, M. Hypoglycémie et sommeil. Gaz. Méd. France, 44: 587-91, 1937. 165, 359
Sendrail, M., co-author: 667.

3655. Serbescu, P., et G. A. Buttu. Quelques recherches sur le métabolisme du brome dans l'organisme humain. Bull. Acad. Méd. Paris, 111:232-38, 1934. 57

3656. Serejski, M., und S. Frumkin. Narkolepsie und Epilepsie. Z. ges. Neurol. Psychiat., 123:232-50, 1929. 237, 240

3657. Serog, M. New Light on Dreams; A New Approach to the Dream Problem. Boston: House of Edinboro, 1953. Pp. 159. 107

3658. Serota, H. M. Temperature changes in the cortex and hypothalamus during sleep. J. Neurophysiol., 2:42-47, 1939. 62
Serota, H. M., co-author: 1520.

3659. Serra, P. Una rara manifestazione di natura epilettica—automatismo-oniro-ambulatorio. Riv. Pat. Nerv., 44:666-77, 1934. 283

3660. Service, W. C. Insomnia in tuberculosis. Am. Rev. Tuberc., 23:440-54, 1931. 277

3661. Servít, Z. (Czech.) Some experimental data on the physiology of electric sleep. Fysiat. Vestn.

(Praha), 33:149-53, 1955. 299

3662. _____, J. Bureš, O. Burešová, and M. Petráň. (Czech.) Problem of electronarcosis and of electrically induced sleep. Česk. Fysiol., 2:345-54, 1953. 299
Servite, Z., co-author: 3913.

3663. Seymour, J. H. Some changes in psychometric, perceptual and motor performance as a function of sleep deprivation. New York Univ. Thesis, 1956. Pp. 196; also Diss. Abstr., 16:2216, 1956. 226, 228

3664. Sézary, A., et C. de Montet. Attaques de sommeil et narcolepsie épileptique. Rev. Méd., 28: 69-77, 1908. 256

3665. Shackel, M. A. Electro-oculography: the electrical recording of eye position. Proc. 3rd Internat. Conf. Med. Electronics, London, 1960, pp. 323-35.

3666. Shafer, J. N., and J. D. Baker. Factors related to sound precipitated convulsions. Proc. W. Va. Acad. Sci., 29:95-97, 1957. 219

3667. Shagass, C., and A. Kerenyi. The 'sleep' threshold. A simple form of sedation threshold for clinical use. Canad. Psychiat. Ass. J., 3:101-9, 1958. 295

3668. _____, K. Muller, and H. B. Acosta. The pentothal "sleep" threshold as an indicator of affective change. J. Psychosom. Res., 3: 253-70, 1959. 295
Shagass, C., co-author: 1969.

3669. Shakel, B. Pilot study in electro-oculography. Brit. J. Ophthalm., 44:89-113, 1960. 93

3670. Shapiro, W., E. H. Estes, and H. L. Hilderman. Diurnal variability in scrum cholesterol at normal and reduced levels. J. Lab. Clin. Med., 54:213-15, 1959.

3671. Sharp, G. W. G. Reversal of diurnal temperature rhythms in man. Nature, 190:146-48, 1961. 174

3672. Sharpless, S., and H. Jasper. Habituation of the arousal reaction. Brain, 79:655-80, 1956. 210

3673. Shastin, N.P. (Russ.) Toward the study of the mechanism of sleep in children. In: The Sleep Problem, 1954 (392), pp. 188-91. 197

3674. Shaw, A. F. B. The diurnal tides of the leucocytes of man. J. Path. Bacteriol., 30:1-19, 1927. 162

3675. Shchukina, G. I. (Russ.) Dynam-ics of indices of cutaneous temperature in hypertension during prolonged sleep therapy. Terap. Arkh. (Moskva), 30(5):48-54, 1958. 207

3676. Sheldon, W. H. The Varieties of Temperament. New York: Harpers, 1942. Pp. ix + 520. 120, 161, 308

3677. Shepard, J. F. The Circulation and Sleep. New York: Macmillan, 1914. Pp. 83. 40, 46, 47, 48, 342, 343

3678. Sherman, M. The afternoon sleep of young children: some influencing factors. J. Genet. Psychol., 38:114-26, 1930. 306

3679. Shevrin, H., and L. Luborsky. The measurement of preconscious perception in dreams and images: an investigation of the Poetzl phenomenon. J. Abnorm. Soc. Psychol., 56:285-94, 1958. 104
Shevrin, H., co-author: 2571.

3680. Shimamoto, T., and M. Verzeano. Relations between caudate and diffusely projecting thalamic nuclei. J. Neurophysiol., 17:278-88, 1954.

3681. Shimazono, Y., T. Okuma, T. Fukuda, T. Hirai, and E. Yamamasu. An electroencephalographic study of barbiturate anesthesia. EEG Clin. Neurophysiol., 5:525-32, 1953. 296
Shimazono, Y., co-author: 3049.

3682. Shinn, A. V. A study of sleep habits of two groups of preschool children, one in Hawaii and one on the mainland. Child Develop., 3:159-66, 1932. 117, 186

3683. Shiotsuki, M., and Y. Ichino. EEG and sleep (2nd report). Electroencephalographic study on types of the natural whole night sleep. Folia Psychiat. Neurol. Jap., 8:184-85, 1954. 26

3684. Shirley, H. F., and J. P. Kahn. Sleep disturbances in children. Pediat. Clin. North Am., 5:629-43, 1958. 282, 285

3685. Shliffer, R. I. (Russ.) The effect of the injection of adrenalin on blood pressure during experimental sleep (hypnosis). Psikhoterapia, pp. 167-72, 1930. 331

3686. Shore, P. A., and B. B. Brodie. Influence of various drugs on serotonin and norepinephrine in the brain. In: Psychotropic

Drugs, 1957 (1357), pp. 423-27. 302

Shore, P. A., co-author: 1730, 3215.

3687. Short, J. J. Diurnal variations in concentration of red blood cells and hemoglobin. J. Lab. Clin. Med., 20:708-13, 1935. 162

3688. Shpilberg, P. I. (Russ.) Human electroencephalogram in sleep and hypnosis. Fiziol. Zh. SSSR, 41:178-86, 1955. 296, 330

3689. Shure, G. H., and W. C. Halstead. Cerebral Localization of Intellectual Processes. Psychol. Monogr., 72(12), Whole No. 465, 1958. Pp. 40.

3690. Shurley, J. T. Profound experimental sensory isolation. Am. J. Psychiat., 117:539-45, 1960.

3691. Sidis, B. An experimental study of sleep. J. Abnorm. Psychol., 3:1-32, 63-96, 170-207, 1908. 195

3692. Siebeck H. Das Traumleben der Seele. Berlin: Carl Habel, 1877. Pp. 40. 106

3693. Siebenthal, W. von. Die Wissenschaft vom Traum, Ergebnisse und Probleme; eine Einfuehrung in die allgemeinen Grundlagen. Berlin: Springer-Verlag, 1953. Pp. xvi + 523. 106

3694. Siemerling, E. Schlaf und Schlaflosigkeit. Schwabachers med. Bibliothek, 1923. Pp. 38; abstr. Z. ges. Neurol. Psychiat., 34: 286, 1923-24. 312

3695. _____. Ueber den Schlaf. Kiel: Lipsius & Tischer, 1926. Pp. 28.

3696. Silbere, H. The dream: introduction to the psychology of dreams. Psychoanal. Rev., 42:361-87, 1955. 106

3697. Silva, E. E., C. Estable, and J. P. Segundo. Further observations on animal hypnosis. Arch. Ital. Biol., 97:167-77, 1959. 336

3698. Silverman, D. Sleep as a general activation procedure in electroencephalography. EEG Clin. Neurophysiol., 8:317-24, 1956. 29

3699. _____, and R. A. Groff. Brain tumor depth determination by electrographic recording during sleep. A.M.A. Arch. Neurol. Psychiat., 78:15-28, 1957. 29

3700. _____, and A. Morisaki. Re-evaluation of sleep electroencephalography. EEG Clin. Neurophysiol., 10:425-31, 1958. 29

3701. Silvestri, T. A proposito dei fenomeni di inversione nell encefalite letargica. Gazz. Osp., 44: 338-39, 1923. 247

3702. Simarro, J. Poliglobulia. Sobre un caso clínico con somnolencia, síntoma inicial y dominante. Sintomatología. Tratamiento. Ann. Hosp. Santa Creu Sant Pau, 8: 108-22, 1934. 238

3703. Simmel, E. Neurotic disturbances of sleep. Internat. J. Psycho-anal., 23:65-68, 1942. 237

3704. Simon, A., K. M. Bowman, and N. Halliday. Studies in electronarcosis therapy: II. Physiological effects in electronarcosis and electroshock. J. Nerv. Ment. Dis., 107:358-70, 1948. 298

Simon, A., co-author: 433.

3705. Simon, C. W. Some immediate effects of drowsiness and sleep on normal human performance. Human Factors, 3:1-17, 1961.

3706. _____, and W. H. Emmons. Considerations for research in a sleep-learning program. Project RAND Res. Mem. (RM-1222), Santa Monica, Calif., March, 1954. Pp. 68. 125

3707. _____, and _____. Responses to material presented during various levels of sleep. Project RAND Res. Mem. (RM-1442), Santa Monica, Calif., Dec., 1954. Pp. 51; also J. Exp. Psychol., 51:89-97, 1956. 125

3708. _____, and _____. Learning during sleep? Psychol. Bull., 52: 328-42, 1955. 125, 126

3709. _____, and _____. The EEG, consciousness, and sleep. Science, 124:1066-69, 1956. 26

Simon, C. W., co-author: 1073.

3710. Simonov, P. V. (Russ.) Experimental investigation of conditioned-reflex sleep in animals (rabbits). Zh. Vysshei Nerv. Deiat., 4:551-57, 1954. 297

3711. Simonson, E., and N. Enzer. Effect of pervitin (desoxyephedrine) on fatigue of the central nervous system. J. Industr. Hyg., 24:205-9, 1942. 300

3712. _____, _____, and S. S. Blankenstein. Effect of amphetamine (benzedrine) on fatigue of the central nervous system. War Med., 1:690-95, 1941. 300

3713. Simpson, G. E. Diurnal variations in the rate of urine excretion for two hour intervals: some associated factors. J. Biol. Chem., 59:107-22, 1924. <u>64</u>, <u>65</u>, <u>166</u>, <u>167</u>

3714. _____. Changes in the composition of the urine and blood as a result of sleep. Proc. Internat. Physiol. Congr., Stockholm, 1926, p. 153. <u>167</u>

3715. _____. The effect of sleep on urinary chlorides and pH. J. Biol. Chem., 67:505-16, 1926. <u>65</u>

3716. _____. Changes in composition of urine brought about by sleep and other factors. J. Biol. Chem., 84:393-411, 1929. <u>67</u>, <u>169</u>

3717. Simsarian, F. P., and P. A. McLendon. Feeding behavior of an infant during the first twelve weeks of life on a self-demand schedule. J. Pediat., 20:93-103, 1942. <u>133</u>

3718. Singh, B. Electroencephalographic study of 'bang' response during sleep in normal and epileptic individuals. Neurology (Madras), 6(2):425-31, 1958. <u>259</u>

3719. Sirna, A. A. An electroencephalographic study of the hypnotic dream. J. Psychol., 20:109-13, 1945. <u>333</u>, <u>334</u>

3720. Sirota, J. H., D. S. Baldwin, and H. Villarreal. Diurnal variations in renal function in man. J. Clin. Investig., 29:187-92, 1950. <u>64</u>, <u>166</u>, <u>167</u>
Sirota, J. H., co-author: 191.

3721. Sittig, O. Schlafsucht. Z. ges. Neurol. Psychiat., 39:324, 1924-25. <u>248</u>

3722. Skalweit, W. Narkolepsie und zentral-nervoese Regulationsstoerungen. Nervenarzt, 19:140-46, 1948. <u>240</u>

3723. Skliar, N. (Russ.) On the origin of sleep. Zh. Nevropat. Psikhiat., 21:621-43, 1928. <u>360</u>

3724. Slavina, E. E. (Russ.) On diurnal variations in the excitability of the cerebral hemispheres, and the influence on it of lack of sleep. Arkh. Biol. Nauk, 41(2):9-12, 1936. <u>158</u>

3725. Slight, D. Hypnagogic phenomena. J. Abnorm. Soc. Psychol., 19:274-82, 1924-25. <u>79</u>

3726. Slonim, A. D., and E. M. Cherkovich. (Russ.) The influence of therapeutic sleep on the 24-hour periodicity of physiological functions in monkeys. Trudy Pavlov Fiziol. Inst., 1:222-28, 1952; also

in: The Sleep Problem, 1954 (392), pp. 320-24. <u>173</u>

3727. _____, and O. P. Shcherbakova. (Russ.) Observations of night sleep in monkeys. In: The Sleep Problem, 1954 (392), pp. 312-19. <u>78</u>, <u>191</u>, <u>366</u>

3728. Small, M. L. Dreams. Psychol. Bull., 17:346-49, 1920, <u>99</u>

3729. Smirnov, A. A. (Russ.) Phosphorus metabolism in the dog's cerebral cortex in sleep and wakefulness. Doklady Akad. Nauk SSSR, 101:913-16, 1955.

3730. Smith, C. M. Comments and observations on psychogenic hypersomnia. A.M.A. Arch. Neurol. Psychiat., 80:619-24, 1958. <u>271</u>

3731. _____. Psychosomatic aspects of narcolepsy. J. Ment. Sci., 104:593-607, 1958. <u>237</u>

3732. _____, and J. Hamilton. Psychological factors in the narolepsy-cataplexy syndrome. Psychosom. Med., 21(1):40-49, 1959. <u>237</u>

3733. _____, and R. A. Schneider. Narcolepsy and hypoglycemia. J. Ment. Sci., 105:163-70, 1959. <u>237</u>

3734. Smith, F. O. The patellar tendon reflex as influenced by sleep, insomnia, nicotine and hypnosis. Proc. Ninth Internat. Congr. Psychol., 1929, pp. 399-400. <u>15</u>

3735. Smith, G. M. The effect of prolonged mild anoxia on sleepiness, irritability, boredom, and other subjective conditions. J. Gen. Psychol., 35:239-50, 1946; also 38:3-14, 1948. <u>197</u>

3736. Smith, H. M. Insomnia. J. Florida Med. Ass., 17:18-22, 1930. <u>362</u>

3737. _____. Sleep and cerebral mechanism. South. Med. Surg., 94:124-27, 1932.

3738. Smith, J. R. The electroencephalogram during normal infancy and childhood: I. Rhythmic activities present in the neonate and their subsequent development. II. The nature of the growth of the alpha waves. III. Preliminary observations on the pattern sequence during sleep. J. Genet. Psychol., 53:431-82, 1938; prelim. commun. Proc. Soc. Exp. Biol. Med., 36:384-86, 1937. <u>27</u>, <u>28</u>, <u>76</u>

3739. _____. The frequency growth of

the human alpha rhythms during normal infancy and childhood. J. Psychol., 11:177-98, 1941. 27, 28

3740. Smith, M. A contribution to the study of fatigue. Brit. J. Psychol., 8:327-50, 1916. 228

3741. Smith, M. A sleep campaign in the fourth grade. J. School Health, 22:200-205, 1952. 307

3742. Smith, S. W. Sleep in health and in illness. Practitioner, 155:161-69, 1945. 312

3743. Smith, W. K. The functional significance of the rostral cingular cortex as revealed by its responses to electrical stimulation. J. Neurophysiol., 8:241-55, 1945.

3744. Smitt, J. W. (Danish) Sleeplessness and Vitamin B. Ukeskr. Laeg., 103:845-50, 1941. 278

3745. Snyder, C. H. Epileptic equivalents in children. Pediatrics, 21:308-18, 1958. 257

3746. Sokolov, E. N. Neuronal models and the orienting reflex. In: The Central Nervous System and Behavior, III, M. A. B. Brazier, Ed., Josiah Macy Found., 1960, pp. 186-276. 74
Sokolov, E. N., co-author: 3389.

3747. Sollberger, A., and T. Petrén, Eds. Reports from 5th Internat. Confer., Soc. Biol. Rhythm, Stockholm, 1961. Pp. 186. 131
Sollberger, A., co-author: 1061.

3748. Solomon, A. P. Report of a case of periodic somnolence with major operation and hypnosis. Arch. Neurol. Psychiat., 20:595-602, 1928.

3749. Solomon, M. Shall hypnotics be used in the treatment of insomnia in the psychoneuroses? New York Med. J. Med. Rec., 138:22-26, 1933. 294

3750. Solomon, P. Narcolepsy in Negroes. Dis. Nerv. Syst., 6:179-83, 1945. 234, 236

3751. _____. Insomnia. New Engl. J. Med., 255:755-60, 1956. 274, 275

3752. _____, P. H. Leiderman, J. Mendelson, and D. Wexler. Sensory deprivation. A review. Am. J. Psychiat., 114:357-63, 1957. 198
Solomon, P., co-author: 2422, 2769, 4182.

3753. Soskin, S., and M. Taubenhaus. Sodium succinate as an antidote for barbiturate poisoning and in the control of the duration of barbiturate anesthesia (including its successful use in case of barbitu-

rate poisoning in a human). J. Pharmacol. Exp. Therap., 78:49-55, 1943. 297

3754. Souques, A., H. Baruk, et I. Bertrand. Tumeur de l'infundibulum avec léthargie isolée. Rev. Neurol., I:532-40, 1926. 263

3755. Soureau, M., H. Fischgold, et G. Capdevielle. L'EEG du nouveau-né: normal et pathologique. EEG Clin. Neurophysiol., 2:113-14, 1950.

3756. Spadolini, N. Alcune considerazioni sulla fisiologia e fisiopatologia del sonno. Note Riv. Psichiat., 55:283-90, 1930; also Atti XIX Congr. Soc. Freniat. Ital., 1931, pp. 1198-1205. 361

3757. Spealman, C. R., M. Newton, and R. L. Post. Influence of environmental temperature and posture on volume and composition of blood. Am. J. Physiol., 150:628-39, 1947. 38, 39

3758. Spear, A. B., and E. C. Turton. EEG findings in 100 cases of severe enuresis. EEG Clin. Neurophysiol., 5:324, 1953. 284
Spear, A. B., co-author: 3994.

3759. Speirs, R. S., and R. K. Meyer. Effects of stress, adrenal and adrenocorticotrophic hormones on the circulating eosinophils of mice. Endocrinology, 45:403-29, 1949. 170

3760. Spencer, L. T., and L. H. Cohen. The concept of the threshold and Heyman's law of inhibition. III. The relation of the threshold to estimates of daily variation in "freshness." J. Exp. Psychol., 11:281-92, 1928.

3761. Sperling, M. Neurotic sleep disturbances in children. Nervous Child, 8:28-46, 1949. 285

3762. _____. Etiology and treatment of sleep disturbances in children. Psychoanal. Q., 24:358-68, 1955. 285

3763. _____. Pavor nocturnus. J. Am. Psychoanal. Ass., 6:79-94, 1958. 281

3764. Spicer, D. G. Insomnia. Trained Nurse, 118:42-45, 77, 1947. 278

3765. Spiegel, E. A. Bemerkungen zur Theorie des Bewusstseins und zum Schlafproblem. Z. ges. exp. Med., 55:183-97, 1927. 360

3766. _____, und C. Inaba. Zur zentralen Localisation von Stoerungen des Wachzustandes. Klin. Wschr., 5:2408, 1926. 205

3767. ____, H. T. Wycis, and V. Reyes. Diencephalic mechanisms in petit mal epilepsy. EEG Clin. Neurophysiol., 3:473-75, 1951. 258 Spiegel, E. A., co-author: 2821.

3768. Spiegel, L. A., and C. P. Oberndorf. Narcolepsy as a psychogenic symptom. Psychosom. Med., 8:28-35, 1946. 237

3769. Spiller, W. Narcolepsy occasionally a post-encephalitic syndrome. J. Am. Med. Ass., 86:673-74, 1926. 250

3770. Spitta, H. Die Schlaf- und Traumzustaende der menschlichen Seele, mit besonderer Beruecksichtung ihres Verhaeltnisses zu den psychischen Alienationen. Tuebingen: Franz Fues, 1878. Pp. xvi + 294. 106

3771. Spitzer, B. Schlaflage und Zahnsystem. Z. Stomatol., 35:289-92, 1937. 11, 306

3772. Spock, B. Chronic resistance to sleep in infancy. Pediatrics, 4: 89-93, 1949. 278

3773. ____. Is your child getting enough sleep? How much sleep is enough? Ladies Home J., Aug. 1958, pp. 14, 100. 307

3774. Spohn, A. H. Discussion of disorders of sleep in childhood. Brit. Med. J., II,525, 1930. 307

3775. Srivastava, D. D. My personal conception about the nature of sleep. Antiseptic (Madras), 48: 274-80, 1951. 362

3776. Stadler, H. Zur Frage der Beziehung zwischen periodischen und episodischen Daemmer- und Schlafzustaenden und Hypophysenstoerungen. Zbl. ges. Neurol. Psychiat., 87:695-96, 1938. 269

3777. Stallard, H. A consideration of extraoral pressure in the etiology of malocclusions. Internat. J. Orthodont., 16(I):475-526, 1930. 10

3778. Stanbridge, R. H. Fatigue in aircrew observations in the Berlin airlift. Lancet, 261:1-3, 1951. 316

3779. Stanbury, S. W., and A. E. Thomson. Diurnal variations in electrolyte excretion. Clin. Sci., 10: 267-93, 1951. 167 Stanbury, S. W., co-author: 2830-32.

3780. Stanley, L. L., and G. L. Tescher. Sleep recording apparatus. New York Med. J. Med. Rec., 134:609, 1931. 87

3781. ____, and ____. The effects of coffee on sleep. Calif. West. Med., 34:359-61, 1931. 87

3782. ____, and ____. What to eat on going to bed. Calif. West. Med., 36:318-19, 1932. 309

3783. Stanojevic, L. Die ergographische Leistungsfaehigkeit nach dem physiologischen und nach dem mit verschiedenen hypnotischen Mitteln erzeugten Schlafe. Eine psychopharmakologische Studie. Mschr. Psychiat. Neurol., 74:121-28, 1929. 297

3784. Staples, R. Some factors influencing the afternoon sleep of young children. J. Genet. Psychol., 41:222-28, 1932.

3785. ____, and A. C. Anderson. A study of outdoor play, appetite and afternoon sleep of young children. Child Develop., 4: 191-95, 1933. 306

3786. Stark, H. Ueber humorale Verhaeltnisse im Schlaf und ihre Beziehungen zum epileptischen Krampfanfall. Arch. Psychiat., 91:489-92, 1930. 259

3787. Stark, L. The effects of visual blocking on theta rhythm. In: Rep. 5th Conf. Soc. Biol. Rhythm, 1961 (3747), p. 150. 259

3788. Starzl, T. E., C. W. Taylor, and H. W. Magoun. Ascending conduction in reticular activating system, with special reference to the diencephalon. J. Neurophysiol., 14:461-77, 1951. 209

3789. ____, ____, and ____. Collateral afferent excitation of reticular formation of brain stem. J. Neurophysiol., 14:479-96, 1951. 209

3790. ____, and D. G. Whitlock. Diffuse thalamic projection system in monkey. J. Neurophysiol., 15: 449-68, 1952. 210

3791. Staub, H. Die Ausscheidung von Barbitursaeuren bei der Dauerschlafbehandlung der Schizophrenie. Schweiz. Arch. Neurol., 65: 330-70, 1950. 207

3792. ____. Ueber die Verteilung von Barbitursaeuren im Organismus Geisteskranker waehrend der Schlafkur. Schweiz. Arch. Neurol., 65:371-80, 1950. 207

3793. Stauder, K. H. Anfall, Schlaf, Periodizitaet. Nervenarzt, 19: 107-19, 1948. 257

3794. Stechler, G., D. Gallant, and T.

Berry. Some aspects of the sleeping EEG in the human newborn. EEG Clin. Neurophysiol., 13:305, 1961. 27

3795. Steckelmacher. Schlaf und Schlaflosigkeit. Umschau, 6:104-7, 1920. 312

3796. Stegman, H. M. The nap as a pick-me-up. Hygeia (Chicago), 10:541-43, 1932. 307

3797. Stehle, H. C. Value of electroencephalography for the differential diagnosis of neurosis and organic brain disease. EEG Clin. Neurophysiol., 5:65-68, 1953. 29

3798. Steinhart, P. Der Schlaf des Pferdes. Seine Dauer, Tiefe, Bedingungen. Z. Vet., 49:145-57, 193-232, 1937. 10, 16, 113, 149

3799. Steinicke, G. Die Wirkungen von Laerm auf den Schlaf des Menschen. Koeln: Westdeutscher Verlag, 1957. Pp. 34. 113

3800. Steiniger, F. Die Bedeutung der sogenannten "tierischen Hypnose." Ergebn. Biol., 13:348-451, 1936. 335

3801. Steinkamp, G. R., W. R. Hawkins, G. T. Hauty, R. R. Burwell, and J. E. Ward. Human experimentation in the space cabin simulator: Development of life support systems and results of initial seven-day flights. USAF School Aviat. Med., Brooks AFB, Texas, Rep. 59-101, Aug. 1959. Pp. 88. 316

3802. Steinmetzer, K. Ueber die Beziehung der Stellreflexe zu Schlaf und Narkose nach Versuchen an Huehnern. Arch. exp. Path. Pharmakol., 180:37-51, 1935. 295

3803. Stennett, R. G. The relationship of alpha amplitude to the level of palmar conductance. EEG Clin. Neurophysiol., 9:131-38, 1957. 29

3804. ____. The relationship of performance level to level of arousal. J. Exp. Psychol., 54:54-61, 1957.

3805. Sterling, K., and J. G. Miller. Conditioning under anesthesia. Am. J. Psychol., 54:92-101, 1941; also Current Res. Anesth. Analg., 23:89-94, 1944. 297

3806. Sterling, W. (Polish) Attacks of sleep and fever in epilepsy. Polska Gaz. Lek., 5:587-90, 1926; abstr. Zbl. ges. Neurol. Psychiat., 45:906, 1926-27. 256

3807. Sterman, M. B., and C. D. Cle-

mente. Cortical recruitment and behavioral sleep induced by basal forebrain stimulation. Fed. Proc., 20:334, 1961. 204

3808. Stern, A. Blickkraempfe, Schlaf und psychische Stoerungen. Mschr. Psychiat. Neurol., 108:90-103, 1943.

3809. ____. (Hebrew) On the pathology of sleep. Harefuah (Tel Aviv), 44:268-70, 1953.

3810. Stern, K. Severe dementia associated with bilateral symmetrical degeneration of the thalamus. Brain, 62:157-71, 1939. 266

3811. Stern, L. S. (Russ.) The chemical basis for the transition from sleep to wakefulness—the role of the blood-cerebrospinal fluid barrier. Trudy Nauchn.-Issled. Inst. Fiziol., 2:27-38, 1936; abstr. Ber. ges. Physiol. exp. Pharmakol., 98:287-88, 1937. 217, 218, 353

3812. ____. (Russ.) On the alternation of sleep and wakefulness. Nevropat. Psikhiat., 6(2):189-200, 1937; abstr. Zbl. ges. Neurol. Psychiat., 86:58-59, 1937. 217, 218, 353

3813. ____, N. S. Voskressensky, E. S. Lokchina, Nikolskaya, et Outevskaya. Influence de l'insuline sur les changements de l'état fonctionnel de la barrière hémato-encéphalique correspondant aux périodes du sommeil et de la veille. Bull. Biol. Méd. Exp. U.R.S.S., 2:406-9, 1936. 217

3814. Stern, M. M. Pavor nocturnus. Internat. J. Psycho-anal., 32:302-9, 1951. 281

3815. Stern, P., N. Marijan, and V. Eisen. (Croat) The role of calcium in the activation of the cholinergic system during sleep. Acta Med. Jugoslav., 2:113-34, 1948. 353

3816. Sternberg, L. Seasonal somnolence, a possible pollen allergy. Case report. J. Allergy, 14:89-90, 1942. 267

3817. Sterz, G. Ueber den Anteil des Zwischenhirns an der Symptomgestaltung organischer Erkrankungen des Zentralnervensystems: Ein diagnostisch brauchbares Zwischensyndrom. Dsche Z. Nervenheilk., 117-19:630-71, 1931. 265, 276

3818. Stevenson, L., B. E. Christensen, and S. B. Wortis. Some experiments in intracranial pressure during sleep and under certain other conditions. Am. J. Med. Sci., 178:663-77, 1929. <u>40</u>, <u>45</u>, <u>46</u>, <u>47</u>

3819. Stewart, H. Discussion on hypnotism in general practice. Techniques. The main use of hypnosis. Practitioner, 180:597-98, 1958. <u>335</u>

3820. Stiefler, G. Zirkulaere Schlafstoerungen nach Encephalitis lethargica. Muench. med. Wschr., 73:981-82, 1926. <u>248</u>

3821. ____. Ueber postencephalitische periodische Schlafzustaende. Wien. klin. Wschr., 40:586-87, 1927. <u>248</u>

3822. Stier, T. J. B. Spontaneous activity of mice. J. Gen. Psychol., 4:67-99, 1930. <u>159</u>

3823. Stockert, F. G. Zur Pathophysiologie der Schlafausloesung mit besonderer Beruecksichtung der Blickbewegung. Dsche Z. Nervenheilk., 111:53-56, 1929. <u>244</u>, <u>286</u>

3824. ____. Ueber die Beziehungen der Augenmuskeln zum Schlaf, gleichzeitig ein Beitrag zur Diagnostik der Encephalitis lethargica. Dsche Z. Nervenheilk., 111:263-98, 1929. <u>244</u>, <u>286</u>

3825. ____. Die Physiologie der Hypnose. Nervenarzt, 3:462-67, 1930. <u>336</u>

3826. ____. Die Beziehungen der Augenmuskeln zum Schlafe. Med. Klin., 29:697-98, 1933. <u>361</u>

3827. ____. Pathophysiologie einer in 48-Stunden-Rhythmus verlaufenden periodischen Katatonie. Confinia Neurol. (Basel), 18:183-88, 1958. <u>251</u>

3828. Stockmann, H. Die Schlafdrucklaehmungen. Freiburg i. Br.: Diss., 1934. Pp. 67. <u>310</u>

3829. Stoeckle, J. D., and G. E. Davidson. Bodily complaints and other symptoms of depressive reaction. J. Am. Med. Ass., 180:134-39, 1962. <u>286</u>

3830. Stöckmann, T. Versuche ueber Verkuerzung und Verlegung der Schlafzeit. Muench. med. Wschr., 80:422-23, 618, 1933. <u>307</u>

3831. ____. Bericht ueber die Weiterentwickelung meiner Schlafzeitforschung. Muench. med. Wschr., 81:1353-54, 1934. <u>307</u>

3832. ____. Die Beziehungen zwischen Sonnenlauf und Schlafzeit. Fortschr. Med., 52:1141-43, 1934. <u>307</u>, <u>362</u>

3833. ____. Die Naturzeit als Ausgangspunkt der Gesundung, Ertruechtigung und Entwicklung. Stuttgart: Hippokrates-Verlag, 1933. Pp. 28. <u>307</u>

3834. ____. Die Naturzeit; der Schlaf vor Mitternacht als Kraft- und Heilquelle. Stuttgart: Marquardt, 1940. Pp. 86. <u>307</u>

3835. Stokes, A. B. Continuous sleep treatment. Occup. Therap. Rehabil., 23:132-35, 1944. <u>206</u>

3836. Stokvis, B. Etude de l'influence de l'hypnose sur la pression du sang, à l'aide d'une nouvelle méthode d'enregistrement automatique interrompu. J. Physiol. Path. Gén., 35:691-700, 1937. <u>331</u>

3837. ____. Medico-psychological viewpoints on narco- and hypnoanalysis. Mschr. Psychiat. Neurol. (Basel), 131:247-51, 1956. <u>335</u>

3838. Stopes, M. C. Sleep. London: Chatto & Windus, 1956. Pp. 154. <u>310</u>

3839. Stoupel, N. Etude électroencéphalographique de sept cas de narcolepsie-cataplexie. Rev. Neurol., 83:563-70, 1950. <u>237</u>, <u>238</u>, <u>241</u>
Stoupel, N., co-author: 487, 488.

3840. Stoyva, J. M. The effect of suggested dreams on the length of rapid eye movement periods. Univ. Chicago: Diss., 1961. <u>98</u>, <u>104</u>, <u>334</u>

3841. Stracker, O. Die aeusseren und statischen Bedingungen des Schlafes. Medizinische, (27-28): 1111-15, 1958. <u>312</u>

3842. Stradling, R., and D. A. Laird. Further data on the handedness of sleep. J. Abnorm. Soc. Psychol., 29:462-64, 1929. <u>8</u>

3843. Strambach, F. Ueber Schlafstoerungen, mit besonderer Beruecksichtung solcher, die vom Schlafsteuerungszentren ausgehen. Muenchen: Inaug. Diss., 1952. Pp. 69. <u>286</u>

3844. Straub, H. Alveolargasanalyse. I. Ueber Schwankungen in der Taetigkeit des Atemzentrums speziell im Schlaf. Dsch. Arch. klin. Med., 117:397-417, 1951. <u>51</u>, <u>351</u>

3845. Strauch, A. Psychogenic disturbances in childhood and their treatment. Am. J. Dis. Child., 16:165-79, 1918. 285

3846. _____. Sleep in children and its disturbances. Am. J. Dis. Child., 17:118-39, 1919.

3847. Straus, E. W. Some remarks about awakeness. Tschr. Philos., 18:381-400, 1956. 4, 362

3848. Strauss, E. B. Insomnia. St. Bart's Hosp. J., 52:163-68, 1948. 275, 278

3849. Strauss, J. F. A new approach to the treatment of snoring; a preliminary report. Arch. Otolaryngol., 38:225-29, 1943. 50

3850. Strelchuk, I. V. (Russ.) An attempt to employ prolonged sleep and the study of its influence on the higher nervous system in morphinism. Zh. Vysshei Nerv. Deiat., 1(3):383-91, 1951; also in: The Sleep Problem, 1954 (392), pp. 453-61. 207

3851. Strizek, F. (Czech.) Sleep disturbances in chronic encephalitis lethargica. Rev. Neurol. Psychiat. (Praha), 24(3):71-75, 1927. 248

3852. Ström-Olsen, R. Enuresis in adults and abnormality of sleep. Lancet, 259(II):133-35, 1950. 113, 284

3853. Struempell, A. Beobachtungen ueber ausgebreitete Anaesthesien und deren Folgen fuer die willkuerliche Bewegung and das Bewusstsein. Dsch. Arch. klin. Med., 22:321-61, 1878.

3854. _____. Ein Beitrag zur Theorie des Schlafes. Pfluegers Arch., 15:573-74, 1878. 199

3855. Strughold, H. The physiological day-night cycle in global flights. J. Aviat. Med., 23:464-73, 1952. 315

3856. _____. Medicine ready to keep man alive in trip up, around and down (Interview). J. Am. Med. Ass., 169:494-95, 1959. 315

3857. Strumwasser, F. Factors in the pattern, timing and predictability of hibernation in the squirrel, Citellus beecheyi. Am. J. Physiol., 196:8-14, 1959. 324

3858. _____. Thermoregulatory, brain and behavior mechanisms during entrance into hibernation in the squirrel, Citellus beecheyi. Am. J. Physiol., 196:15-22, 1959. 324, 328

3859. _____. Regulatory mechanisms,

brain activity and behavior during deep hibernation in the squirrel, Citellus beecheyi. Am. J. Physiol., 196:23-30, 1959. 324

3860. Stuckey, J., and R. M. Coco. A comparison of the blood pictures of active and hibernating ground squirrels. Am. J. Physiol., 137:431-35, 1942. 322, 323

3861. Sturt, M. The judgment of time in sleep. Proc. Internat. Congr. Psychol., 1924, pp. 120-25. 79

3862. Subirana, A., L. Oller Daurella y J. Monteys. Manifestaciones electroencefalográficas de la enuresis nocturna. EEG Clin. Neurophysiol., 3:114, 1951. 256, 284

3863. Suckling, E. E., E. H. Koenig, B. F. Hoffman, and C. McC. Brooks. The physiological effects of sleeping on hard or soft beds. Human Biol., 29:274-88, 1957. 110, 309
Suckling, E. E., co-author: 524, 1810.

3864. Sumbajew, I. (Russ.) On the effect of pharmacological substances on hypnotic sleep. Soviet. Nevropat. Psikhiat. Psikhogig., 4:83-94, 1935. 333, 336

3865. Sumner, F. C. Core and context in the drowsy state. Am. J. Psychol., 35:307-8, 1924. 99

3866. Sumner, J. W., Jr., R. R. Cameron, and D. B. Peterson. Hypnosis in differentiation of epileptic from convulsive-like seizures. Neurology, 2:395-402, 1952. 257, 335
Sumner, J. W., Jr., co-author. 3161.

3867. Sundell, C. E. Sleeplessness in infants. Practitioner, 109:89-92, 1922. 114, 305

3868. Suomalainen, P. Ueber den Winterschlaf des Igels. Mit besonderer Beruecksichtung der Enzymtaetigkeit und des Bromstoffwechsels. Ann. Acad. Sci. Fenn., A, 45:1-110, 1937. 323

3869. _____. Ueber den Winterschlaf des Igels. II. Der Adrenalingehalt der Nebennieren. Biochem. Z., 295:145-53, 1938. 325

3870. _____. Magnesium and calcium content of hedgehog serum during hibernation. Nature, 141:471, 1938. 323

3871. _____, and A.-M. Herlevi. The alarm reaction and the hibernating gland. Science, 114:300, 1951. 327

3872. ____, and S. Sarajas. Heart beat of the hibernating hedgehog. Nature, 168:211, 1951.

3873. ____, and L. Saure. Hibernation and the islets of Langerhans. In: Rep. 5th Conf. Soc. Biol. Rhythm, 1961 (3747), pp. 157-59. 322

3874. Sureau, M., H. Fischgold, et G. Capdevielle. Activité électrique du cerveau du nouveau-né. Sem. Hôp., 26:2642-48, 1950; prelim. commun. EEG Clin. Neurophysiol., 1:376, 1949; also Rev. Neurol., 81:543-45, 1949. 257

3875. Suslova, M. M. (Russ.) Experimental study of the dynamics of hypnotic sleep in man. Fiziol. Zh. SSSR, 29:144-50, 1940. 336

3876. ____. (Russ.) Investigation of the working capacity of the cerebral cortex during the somnambulistic phase of hypnosis. I. and II. Trudy Inst. Fiziol. Pavlova, 1:296-302, 303-15, 1952. Suslova, M. M., co-author: 2244.

3877. Sutherland, G. A. The pulse rate and range in health and disease during childhood. Q. J. Med., 22: 519-29, 1929. 41, 42

3878. Sutton, G. E. F. The ravelled sleave of care. Med. Illustr. (London), 10:470-74, 1956. 362

3879. Sutton, R. L., Jr. Acne vulgaris a pustular lipoidosis. South. Med. J., 34:1071-82, 1941; also J. Missouri Med. Ass., 38:50-55, 1941. 113, 121

3880. Suvorov, N. F. (Russ.) Vascular reflexes in dogs at varying depth of sleep. Trudy Inst. Fiziol. Pavlova, 3:412-18, 1954. 74

3881. Svorad, D. "Animal hypnosis" (Totstellreflex) as experimental model for psychiatry. Electroencephalographic and evolutionary aspect. A.M.A. Arch. Neurol. Psychiat., 77:533-39, 1957. 336

3882. ____. Reticular activating system of brain stem and "animal hypnosis." Science, 125:156, 1957. 336

3883. ____. (Czech.) The question of "inhibition susceptibility" (Inhibition susceptibility I). Physiol. Bohemosloven., 7:341-47, 1958. 336

3884. ____, und L. Kohout. Eine Methode der Ausloesung experimenteller Schlaflosigkeit auf Grund

bedingter Schutzreaktion. Z. ges. exp. Med., 132:342-45, 1959. 219

3885. ____, and V. Novikova. (Russ.) The effect of experimentally induced insomnia on the neurotic state of rats. Fiziol. Zh. SSSR, 46:57-63, 1960. 219 Svorad, D., co-author: 4161.

3886. Swan, T. H. A note on Kohlschütter's curve of the "depth of sleep." Psychol. Bull., 26: 607-10, 1929. 108 Swan, T. H., co-author: 2001-3.

3887. Swank, R. L. Synchronization of spontaneous electrical activity of cerebrum by barbiturate narcosis. J. Neurophysiol., 12:161-72, 1949. 296

3888. ____, and C. W. Watson. Effects of barbiturates and ether on spontaneous electrical activity of dog brain. J. Neurophysiol., 12:137-60, 1949. 296

3889. Sweetland, A., and H. Quay. An experimental investigation of the hypnotic dream. J. Abnorm. Soc. Psychol., 47:678-82, 1952. 333

3890. Swensson, Aa. The Swedish investigation on shift workers. In: Rep. 5th Conf. Soc. Biol. Rhythm, 1961 (3747), p. 160. 316 Swensson, Aa., co-author: 361, 362.

3891. Switzer, R. E., and A. D. Berman. Comments and observations on the nature of narcolepsy. Ann. Int. Med., 44:938-57, 1956. 237

3892. Symonds, C. P. Sleep and sleeplessness. Brit. Med. J., I:869-71, 1925. 361

3893. ____. Narcolepsy as a symptom of encephalitis lethargica. Lancet, 211(II):1214-15, 1926. 250

3894. Szatmari, A. Clinical and electroencephalogram investigation on largactil in psychosis. (Preliminary study). Am. J. Psychiat., 112:788-94, 1956. 302

3895. ____, and R. A. Schneider. Induction of sleep by autonomic drugs. J. Nerv. Ment. Dis., 121: 311-20, 1955. 304

3896. Széky, A. Schlafstoerungen und Schlaftypen bei Nerven- und Geisteskranken und deren Beeinflussbarkeit durch Arzneimittel. Mschr. Psychiat. Neurol., 96: 197-210, 1937. 362

3897. Szymanski, J. S. Eine Methode zur Untersuchung der Ruhe und

Aktivitaetsperioden bei Tieren. Pfluegers Arch., 158:343-85, 1914. 81, 148, 310

3898. ____. Versuche ueber Aktivitaet und Ruhe bei Saeuglingen. Pfluegers Arch., 172:424-30, 1918. 81, 88, 148

3899. ____. Aktivitaet und Ruhe bei Tieren und Menschen. Z. allg. Physiol., 18:105-62, 1919. 81, 148

3900. ____. Aktivitaet und Ruhe bei den Menschen. Z. angew. Psychol., 20:192-222, 1922. 82

3901. Tait, J. The heart of hibernating animals. Am. J. Physiol., 59: 467, 1922. 323, 327

3902. Talbert, G. A., F. L. Ready, and F. W. Kuhlman. Plethysmographic and pneumographic observations made in hypnosis. Am. J. Physiol., 68:113, 1924. 330, 331

3903. Tanaka, T., and K. Kadowaki. E.E.G. findings in cases of narcolepsy and periodic somnolence. Folia Psychiat. Neurol. Jap., 8: 187-88, 1954. 237, 238

3904. Tanner, J. M. The relationships between the frequency of the heart, oral temperature, and rectal temperature in man at rest. J. Physiol. (London), 115:391-409, 1951. 163

3905. Tapia, F., J. Werboff, and G. Winokur. Recall of some phenomena of sleep. A comparative study of dreams, somnambulism, orgasm, and enuresis in a control and neurotic population. J. Nerv. Ment. Dis., 127:119-23, 1958. 101, 102

3906. Tarchanoff, J. Quelques observations sur le sommeil normal. Arch. Ital. Biol., 21:318-21, 1894. 14, 42, 46

3907. Tarozzi, G. Sull'influenza dell'insonnio sperimentale sul ricambio materiale. Riv. Pat. Nerv. Ment., 4:1-23, 1899. 215

3908. Tatai, K., and S. Ogawa. A study of diurnal variation in circulating eosinophils especially with reference to sleep in healthy individuals. Jap. J. Physiol., 1:328-31, 1951. 169

3909. Tatibana, Y. Grundtypen der Traumfarben. Tohoku Psychol. Folia, 6:127-44, 1938. 102

3910. Taussig, L. (Czech.) Psychophysiological relationships between sleep and psychosis. Rev. Neurol. Psychiat. (Praha), 28: 387-98, 1931. 362

3911. Taylor, N. B. The physiology of sleep. Bull. Acad. Med. Toronto, 9:241-48, 1936.

3912. Taylor, R. Hunger in the infant. Am. J. Dis. Child., 14:233-57, 1917. 133

3913. Tchepelyak, Y., Z. Toumova, and Z. Servite. (Russ.) Therapeutic sleep induced by electrotone. Zh. Nevropat. Psikhiat., 58(2):163-70, 1958. 299

3914. Teitelbaum, H. A. Spontaneous rhythmic ocular movements. Their possible relationship to mental activity. Neurology, 4: 350-54, 1954.

3915. Teplitz, Z. An electroencephalographic study of dreams and sleep. Univ. Illinois: Master's thesis, Chicago, 1943. Pp. 22. 95, 100

3916. ____. The ego and motility in sleep-walking. Am. J. Psychoanal., 6:95-110, 1958. 283

3917. Terman, L. M. Genetic Studies of Genius. Mental and Physical Traits of 1000 Gifted Children. Stanford, Calif.: Stanford Univ. Press, 1925. Pp. xiii + 648. 118

3918. ____, and A. Hocking. The sleep of school children; its distribution according to age and its relation to physical and mental efficiency. J. Educ. Psychol., 4:138-47, 199-208, 269-82, 1913. 117, 118, 288

3919. Tersuolo, C. La formation réticulée du tronc cérébral et la physiologie du sommeil. Acta Neurol. Psychiat. Belg., 52:125-28, 1952. 209
Terzuolo, C., co-author: 122, 489-92.

3920. Thelander, H. E., and M. L. Fitzhugh. Posture habits in infancy affecting foot and leg alignments. J. Pediat., 21:306-14, 1942. 9

3921. Thigpen, C. H., and B. F. Moss. Unusual paranoid manifestations in a case of psychomotor epilepsy and narcolepsy. J. Nerv. Ment. Dis., 122:381-85, 1955. 237

3922. Thiis-Evensen, E. (Norw.) Shiftwork and Health. Eidanger Salpeterfabrikers Helsekontor, Norsk Hydro: Andreas Jacobsens Boktrykkeri, 1949. Pp. 112. 316

3923. ____. (Norw.) Shiftwork and gastric ulcer disease. Nord. Hyg. Tskr., 3-4:69-77, 1953. 316

3924. Thomas, S. Effects of change of posture on the diurnal renal excretory rhythm. J. Physiol. (London), 148:489-506, 1959. 65
Thomas, S., co-author: 2833, 2834.

3925. Thompson, E. R. An inquiry into some questions connected with imagery in dreams. Brit. J. Psychol., 9:300-318, 1914. 104

3926. Thompson, G. N. Cerebral area essential to consciousness. Bull. Los Angeles Neurol. Soc., 16: 311-34, 1951. 31

3927. _____, and J. M. Nielsen. Area essential to consciousness—cerebral localization of consciousness as established by neuropathological studies. J. Am. Med. Ass., 137:285, 1948. 31
Thompson, G. N., co-author: 3007, 3941, 3942.

3928. Thompson, H. Duration of periods of waking and sleeping in infancy. Psychol. Bull., 31:639, 1934. 115, 305

3929. _____. Sleep requirements during infancy. Psychol. Rev. Monogr., Suppl. 47:64-73, 1936. 305

3930. Thomson, J. Notes of a case of extreme recurrent drowsiness in a child apparently due to hepatic disturbance. Brit. J. Child. Dis., 20:23-25, 1923. 267

3931. Thomson, M. M., T. W. Forbes, and M. M. Bolles. Brain potential rhythms in a case showing self-induced apparent trance states. Am. J. Psychiat., 93:1313-14, 1937. 333

3932. Thomson, W. O., P. K. Thomson, and M. E. Dailey. The effect of posture upon the composition and volume of blood in man. Proc. Nat. Acad. Sci., 14:94-98, 1938. 37, 39

3933. Thooris, A. L'hypnose d'après les expériences de Pavloff. Rev. Métapsychique, 1929, pp. 1-20. 337, 344

3934. Thorn, G. W., D. Jenkins, and J. C. Laidlaw. The adrenal response to stress in man. Recent Adv. Horm. Res., 8:171-215, 1953. 170
Thorn, G. W., co-author: 1771, 3318.

3935. Thorne, F. C. The incidence of nocturnal enuresis after age five. Am. J. Psychiat., 100:686-89, 1944. 284

3936. Thorner, H. Die Koerperstellung im Schlafe. Nervenarzt, 4:

197-206, 1931. 8, 312

3937. Thornton, G. R., H. G. O. Holck, and E. L. Smith. The effect of benzedrine and caffeine upon performance in certain psychomotor tasks. J. Abnorm. Soc. Psychol., 34:96-113, 1939. 299, 300

3938. Tichenor, H. T. Sleep—A Simple Method for Inducing Sleep. Newark, N.J.: Sleep Publ. Co., 1929. Pp. 46. 312

3939. Tiegel, W. Nicht mehr schlaflos! Stuttgart: Paracelsus-Verlag, 1955. Pp. 70. 278

3940. _____. Schlaf und Hydrotherapie. Arch. phys. Therap. (Leipzig), 9:15-19, 1957. 278

3941. Tietz, E. B., G. N. Thompson, A. van Harreveld, and C. A. G. Wiersma. Electronarcosis—A therapy in schizophrenia. Am. J. Psychiat., 103:821-23, 1945. 298

3942. _____, _____, _____, and _____. Electronarcosis, its application and therapeutic effects in schizophrenia. J. Nerv. Ment. Dis., 103:144-63, 1946. 298

3943. Tihen, H. N. Narcolepsy and benzedrine. J. Kansas Med. Soc., 38:208, 1937. 239, 300

3944. Tilling, E. Ueber den Schlaf und das Einschlafen am Lenkrad. Muench. med. Wschr., 85: 1983-86, 1938. 315

3945. Timmerman, J. C., G. E. Folk, Jr., and S. M. Horvath. Day-night differences of body temperature and heart rate after exercise. Q. J. Exp. Physiol., 44:258-63, 1959. 163

3946. Tinant, M. A propos de narcolepsie et d'épilepsie. Rev. Méd. (Liège), 8:383-90, 1953. 237

3947. Tissot, R., et M. Monnier. Dualité du système thalamique de projection diffuse (Antagonisme du système thalamique recrutant et du système réticulaire ascendant). EEG Clin. Neurophysiol., 11:675-86, 1959. 210

3948. Titelbaum, S. The electrical skin resistance during sleep. Univ. Chicago: Thesis, 1941. Pp. 16. 19, 87, 110, 222
Titelbaum, S., co-author: 2200, 2205, 2206.

3949. Tizzano, A. Il sonno e le sue varie forme nell'uomo e negli animali (rivista sintetica). Ann. Neurol., 44:145-67, 1930. 360, 362

3950. Tochtermann, W. Was ist der Traum? Von Wegen, Sinn und Zweck der Traumforschung. Med. Mschr., 1:408-12, 1947. 106

3951. _____. Ist eine "wissenschaftliche Methode" der Traumforschung moeglich? Med. Mschr., 2:368-69, 1948. 333

3952. Todd, J. A case of the narcolepsy-cataplexy syndrome. Canad. Med. Ass. J., 77:592-97, 1957. 239

3953. Toman, J. E. P., I. M. Bush, and J. T. Chachkes. Conditional features of sound-evoked responses during sleep. Fed. Proc., 17:163, 1958. 29
Toman, J. E. P., co-author: 1123.

3954. Tomescu, P., et A. Vasilescu. Contribution à l'étude du syndrome catatonique dû à l'insuffisance ovarienne. Bull. Soc. Psychiat. Bucarest, 2:37-48, 1937. 252

3955. Tomura, M. (Jap.) Studies on sleep and narcosis from the view-point of blood water content. I. Diurnal change of water picture; II. Change of blood water content in sleep. Shkoku Acta Med., 10:423-29, 1957. 38

3956. Toni, G. de. I movimenti pendolari dei bulbi oculari dei bambini durante il sonno fisiologico, ed in alcuni stati morbosi. Pediatria, 41:489-98, 1933. 90, 112

3957. Tonkikh, A. V. (Russ.) Sleep produced by the injection of calcium chloride into hypothalamic region. Fiziol. Zh. SSSR, 30:191-94, 1941. 202
Tonkikh (Tonkih), A. V., co-author: 2811, 2858.

3958. Toole, J. F. Stimulation of the carotid sinus in man. I. The cerebral response. II. The significance of head positioning. Am. J. Med., 27:952-58, 1959. 242

3959. Toulouse, E., et H. Piéron. Le mécanisme de l'inversion, chez l'homme, du rythme nycthéméral de la température. J. Physiol. (Paris), 9:425-40, 1907. 173

3960. Tournay, A. Séméiologie du Sommeil—Essai de Neurologie Expliquée. Paris: Doin & Cie, 1934. Pp. 131. 17, 348

3961. _____. Sur mes propres visions du demi-sommeil. Rev. Neurol., 73:209-24, 1941. 79

3962. _____. Qu'est-ce que le sommeil? Rev. Prat. (Paris), 4: 1529-32, 1954.
Tournay, A., co-author: 2505.

3963. Tracy, D. F. The Sleep Secret. How to Sleep Without Pills. New York: Sterling Publ. Co., 1951. Pp. 62. 312

3964. Traina, S. Petrosite con vasta zona di rarefazione dell'apice, paralisi dell'abducente, assenza di sintomatologia dolorifica, ipersonnia recidivante; intervento, guarigione. Riv. Oto-Neuro-Oftal., 13:449-55, 1936. 267

3965. Traugott, N. N., and J. A. Poworinsky. (Russ.) Some peculiarities of cortical dynamics during hypnotic sleep. Arkh. Biol. Nauk, 44(II):5-21, 1936. 332

3966. Trautner, E. M., T. W. Murray, and C. H. Noack. Modification of barbiturate sleep treatment by the use of bemegride. Brit. Med. J., II:1514-18, 1957. 294

3967. Travis, L. E. Brain potentials and the temporal course of consciousness. J. Exp. Psychol., 21:302-9, 1937. 31

3968. Travis, R. C., and J. L. Kennedy. Prediction and automatic control of alertness. I. Control of lookout alertness. J. Comp. Physiol. Psychol., 40:457-61, 1947.
Travis, R. C., co-author: 2140, 2141.

3969. Trerotoli, P. Sul comportamento delle granulazioni lipidiche nelle capsule surrenali, nelle ipofisi e nel rene del riccio. Gazz. Osp., 57:208-9, 1936.

3970. Tretiakov, K. N. (Russ.) The symptom-complex of the aqueduct of Sylvius. Sovrem. Psikhopat., 8:271-87, 1929. 266

3971. _____. Une syndrome de l'aqueduc de Sylvius. Rev. Neurol., II: 31-45, 1934.

3972. Treves, M. Le rythme du sommeil et de la veille. Rev. Neurol., I:856-60, 1927.

3973. Trew, A., and R. Fischer. Faulty detoxication in schizophrenia. Lancet, I:402, 1955. 352

3974. Tribukait, B. Aktivitaetsperiodik der Maus im kuenstlich verkuerzten Tag. Naturwissenschaften, 41:92-93, 1954. 175

3975. _____. Die Aktivitaetsperiodik der weissen Maus im Kunsttag von 16-29 Stunden Laenge. Z.

vergl. Physiol., 38:479-90, 1956;
also Rep. 5th Conf. Soc. Biol.
Rhythm, 1961 (3747), pp. 163-66.
175

3976. Trimble, H. C., and S. J. Maddock. The fluctuations of the capillary blood sugar in normal young men during a 24 hour period, including a discussion on the effect of sleep and of mild exercise. J. Biol. Chem., 81:595-611, 1929. 34

3977. Trömner, E. Vorgaenge beim Einschlafen (Hypnogoge-Phaenomene). J. Psychol. Neurol., 17: 343-63, 1911.

3978. _____. Ueber motorische Schlafstoerungen—speziell Schlaftic, Somnambulismus, Enuresis nocturna. Z. ges. Neurol., 4:228-49, 1911. 349

3979. _____. Schlaf und Lethargica. Zbl. ges. Neurol. Psychiat., 33: 508, 1923. 246, 360

3980. _____. Schlaf und Enzephalitis. Z. ges. Neurol. Psychiat., 101: 786-97, 1926. 246, 360

3981. _____. Schlaffunktion und Schlaforgan. Dsche. Z. Nervenheilk., 105:191-204, 1928. 360

3982. _____. Funktion und Localisation des Schlafes. Arch. Psychiat., 86:184, 1929. 360

3983. _____. Schlafzwang. Arch. Psychiat., 88:816-19, 1929. 233, 235, 239, 360

3984. Troilo, E. B. Hipersomnia por heredo lues. Sem. Méd., I:1389-99, 1935. 267

3985. Trosman, H., A. Rechtschaffen, W. Offenkrantz, and E. Wolpert. Studies in psychophysiology of dreams. IV. Relations among dreams in sequence. A.M.A. Arch. Gen. Psychiat., 3:602-7, 1960. 98, 101
Trosman, H., co-author: 4269.

3986. True, R. M. Experimental control in hypnotic age regression states. Science, 110:583-84, 1945. 333

3987. _____, and C. W. Stephenson. Controlled experiments correlating electroencephalogram, pulse, and plantar reflexes with hypnotic age regression and induced emotional states. Personality, 1:252-63, 1951. 333

3988. Truslow, W. Tent-basket for outdoor sleeping of infants. Arch. Pediat., 30:779-80, 1913. 305

3989. Tsukamoto, H., H. Nagami, und

K. Tsunematsu. Beitraege zur Kenntnis des Schnarchens. Mschr. Ohrenheilk., 72:79-93, 1938. 49

3990. Tsutsui, H. Ein Beitrag zur Pathophysiologie des Mittel- und Zwischenhirns. Z. ges. Neurol. Psychiat., 157:717-33, 1937. 246, 359

3991. Tucci, J. H., M. A. B. Brazier, H. H. W. Miles, and J. E. Finesinger. A study of pentothal sodium anesthesia and a critical investigation of the use of succinate as an antidote. Anesthesiology, 10:25-39, 1949. 297
Tucci, J. H., co-author: 1169.

3992. Tüekel, K., and M. Tüekel. Dormison in electroencephalography. EEG Clin. Neurophysiol., 4:363-66, 1952. 296

3993. Turner, M. Electroneurofisiología de los estados de sueño y de vigilia. Día Méd. (Buenos Aires), 26:1628-32, 1954.

3994. Turton, E. C., and A. B. Spear. E.E.G. findings in 100 cases of severe enuresis. Arch. Dis. Childh., 28:316-20, 1953. 284
Turton, E. C., co-author: 3758.

3995. Tuttle, W. W. The effect of sleep upon the patellar tendon reflex. Am. J. Physiol., 68:345-48, 1924. 15, 113

3996. Tyler, D. B. The effect of amphetamine sulfate and some barbiturates on the fatigue produced by prolonged wakefulness. Am. J. Physiol., 150:253-62, 1947. 227, 228

3997. _____. Psychological changes during experimental sleep deprivation. Dis. Nerv. Syst., 16: 293-99, 1955. 225

3998. _____, J. Goodman, and T. Rothman. The effect of experimental insomnia on the rate of potential changes in the brain. Am. J. Physiol., 149:185-93, 1947. 229

3999. _____, W. Marx, and J. Goodman. Effect of prolonged wakefulness on the urinary excretion of 17-ketosteroids. Proc. Soc. Exp. Biol. Med., 62:38-40, 1946. 225
Tyler, D. B., co-author: 1480, 3454.

4000. Tyler, F. H., C. Migeon, A. A. Florentin, and L. T. Samuels. The diurnal variation of 17-hydroxycorticosteroid levels in plasma. J. Clin. Endocrinol., 14: 774, 1954. 170

Tyler, F. H., co-author: 2810, 3158.

4001. Uhlenbruck, P. Plethysmographische Untersuchung am Menschen. I. Ueber die Wirkung der Sinnesnerven der Haut auf den Tonus der Gefaesse. Z. Biol., 80:35-70, 1924. 47, 330, 331

4002. Uiberall, H. Zur Therapie der Schlaflosigkeit. Med. Klin., 27: 465-68, 1931. 294

4003. _____. Das Problem des Winterschlafes. Pfluegers Arch., 234: 78-97, 1934. 322
Uiberall, H., co-author: 412.

4004. Ukolova, M. A. (Russ.) Sleep and Dreams. Rostov-on-Don: Rostov Book Publ., 1955. Pp. 54, 114, 344, 345

4005. _____. (Russ.) Experimental neurosis evoked by sleep deprivation. Bull. Eksp. Biol. Med., 47(5):43-46, 1959. 219

4006. Ullman, M. Herpes simplex and second degree burn induced under hypnosis. Am. J. Psychiat., 103:828-30, 1947. 331, 335

4007. _____. The dream process. Psychotherapy, 1:30-60, 1955. 106

4008. _____. Physiological determinants of the dream process. J. Nerv. Ment. Dis., 124:45-48, 1956. 106

4009. _____. Dreams and arousal. Am. J. Psychother., 12:222-42, 1958. 106

4010. _____. The dream process. Am. J. Psychother., 12:671-90, 1958. 106

4011. _____. Dreams and the therapeutic process. Psychiatry, 21: 123-31, 1958. 106

4012. _____. Hypotheses on the biological roots of the dream. J. Clin. Exp. Psychopath., 19:128-33, 1958. 106

4013. _____. The adaptive significance of the dream. J. Nerv. Ment. Dis., 129:144-49, 1959. 106

4014. _____. Dream deprivation. Science, 132:1418-20, 1960. 106

4015. _____. Dreaming, altered states of consciousness and the problem of vigilance. J. Nerv. Ment. Dis., 133:529-35, 1961.

4016. _____. Dreaming, life style, and physiology: a comment on Adler's view of the dream. J. Indiv. Psychol., 18:18-25, 1962. 107

4017. Ulrich, H. Narcolepsy and its treatment with benzedrine sulfate. New Engl. J. Med., 217: 696-701, 1937. 239, 300

4018. _____, C. E. Trapp, and B. Vidgoff. Treatment of narcolepsy with benzedrine sulphate. Ann. Int. Med., 9:1213-21, 1936. 239, 300

4019. Umbach, W. Zur Elektrophysiologie des Caudatum der Katze: Elektrische Reizung und Krampfausloesung in verschiedenen Grosshirnstrukturen und ihre Beziehung zum Nucleus Caudatus. Arch. Psychiat., Z. ges. Neurol., 199:553-72, 1959. 212

4020. Unger, H. Schlafstoerungen und ihre naturgemaesse Behandlung im Lichte der Gehirnphysiologie. Hippokrates, 28:764-67, 1957. 286

4021. Urechia, C. I. Tumeur des lobes frontaux avec démence et hypersomnie. Arch. Internat. Neurol., 51:251-53, 1932.

4022. _____. Hypersomnie au debut de la paralysie générale. Arch. Internat. Neurol., 51:255-57, 1932. 267

4023. _____. Sur un cas de narcolepsie traumatique. Confinia Neurol., 5:132-34, 1942. 237

4024. _____. Sur un cas de cataplexie avec narcolepsie. Arch. Internat. Neurol., 66:13-14, 1947. 237

4025. _____, et M. Bumbacescu. Sur quelques cas de troubles du sommeil. Arch. Internat. Neurol., 52:107-13, 1933. 267

4026. _____, et S. Mihalescu. Troubles de la respiration, du sommeil et du caractère chez une fillette de neuf ans, avec encéphalite. Bull. Mém. Soc. Méd. Hôp. (Paris), 47: 210-15, 1923. 50, 278

4027. Ustvedt, H. J. Der Blutdruck waehrend des Schlafes bei diphtheriekranken Kindern. Acta Med. Scand., Suppl. 50:291-98, 1932. 43, 45

4028. Utterback, R. A., and G. D. Ludwig. A comparative study of schedules for standing watches aboard submarines based on body temperature cycles. Nav. Med. Res. Inst., Bethesda, Md., Rep. No. 1, Project NM 004 003,

March 1949. Pp. 11. <u>174</u>, <u>315</u>, <u>316</u>

4029. Vadász. J. Kombinierte, posten-cephalitische Anfaelle (Narkolep-sie, Kataplexie, Blickkraempfe). Schweiz. Arch. Neurol. Psychiat., 32:154-71, 1933. <u>238</u>, <u>250</u>, <u>300</u>

4030. Vaisrub, S. Nocturnal disorders of medical interest. Ann. Int. Med., 35:323-30, 1951. <u>285</u>

4031. Valerio, A. Durch uebermaes-sige Darmgase verursachte Hy-persomnolenz und pseudotuber-kuloese Syndrome. Muench. med. Wschr., 84:975-76, 1937. <u>267</u>

4032. Valkenburg, C. T. van. (Dutch) Treatment of pain in insomnia. Ned. Tschr. Geneesk., 81:3675-79, 1937. <u>294</u>

4033. _____. (Dutch) On the neurology of consciousness. Ned. Tschr. Geneesk., 102:1448-54, 1958. <u>30</u>

4034. Van der Heide, C., and J. Wein-berg. Sleep paralysis and combat fatigue. Psychosom. Med., 7:330-34, 1945. <u>236</u>

4035. Vandorfy, J. Studien ueber die interdigestive Phase des Magens beim Menschen. I. Die Bildung des Nuechterinhaltes. Arch. Ver-dauungskr., 38:198-202, 1926. <u>54</u>

4036. Vane, J. R., G. E. W. Wolsten-holme, and M. O'Connor, Eds. CIBA Symposium on Adrenergic Mechanisms. Boston: Little, Brown, 1960. Pp. xx + 632. <u>358</u>

4037. Van Epps, C. Narcolepsy and cataplexy. J. Iowa State Med. Soc., 20:476-77, 1930. <u>234</u>

4038. Van Ormer, E. B. Retention after intervals of sleep and of waking. Arch. Psychol., 137:5-49, 1932. <u>125</u>

4039. _____. Sleep and retention. Psy-chol. Bull., 30:415-39, 1933. <u>125</u>

4040. Vaschide, N. Le Sommeil et les Rêves. Paris: Ernest Flamma-rion, 1911. Pp. 305. <u>126</u>

4041. _____, et H. Piéron. La Psycho-logie du Rêve au Point de Vue Médical. Paris: J. B. Baillière et Fils, 1902. Pp. 96. <u>99</u>

4042. Vasilyev, I. G., L. P. Zimnits-kaya, E. L. Sklyarchik, K. M. Smirnov, B. G. Filippov, S. A. Khitun, and A. M. Shatalov. The diurnal rhythm of working effi-ciency in man. Sechenov J. Phys-iol. USSR (Engl. Ed.), 43:755-60, 1957.

4043. Veghelyi, P. V. Artificial hiber-nation. J. Pediat., 60:122-38, 1962. <u>328</u>

4044. Veit, H. Ueber elektrogastro-graphische Studien an nuechter-nen Magen. Z. ges. exp. Med., 56:61-75, 1927. <u>53</u>

4045. Velhagen, K. Ophthalmologische Bemerkungen zu den Untersu-chungen von Stockerts. Dsche Z. Nervenheilk., 111:56-60, 1929. <u>245</u>

4046. Verdeaux, G., et R. Marty. Ac-tion sur l'électroencéphalo-gramme de substances pharma-codynamiques d'intérêt clinique. Rev. Neurol., 91:405-27, 1954. <u>304</u>
Verdeaux, G., co-author: 881, 882, 2438.

4047. Vereby, G., F. Kékesi, und E. Grastyán. Vergleichende Unter-suchung der Aktivierungssys-teme des Hippocampus und des Hirnstammes durch Reizung und EEG-Analyse waehrend des na-tuerlichen Schlafes. Acta Phys-iol. Hungar., 11 Suppl.:21-22, 1957. <u>211</u>
Vereby, G., co-author: 2538.

4048. Vering, F. Einfluss der Tag-und Nachtschicht auf den Ar-beiter. Wien. med. Wschr., 100: 652-55, 1950. <u>317</u>

4049. Verkhutina, A. I., and V. V. Efi-mov. (Russ.) Electric sensitiv-ity of the eye as influenced by age, season, and time of day. Bull. Eksp. Biol. Med., 23:37-40, 1947. <u>159</u>

4050. Vernon, J., and J. Hoffman. Ef-fect of sensory deprivation on learning rate in human beings. Science, 123:1074-75, 1956. <u>198</u>

4051. Verzeano, M. Activity of cere-bral neurones in the transition from wakefulness to sleep. Sci-ence, 124:366-67, 1956. <u>211</u>

4052. _____, D. B. Lindsley, and H. W. Magoun. Nature of the recruit-ing response. J. Neurophysiol., 16:183-95, 1953. <u>210</u>

4053. _____, and K. Negishi. Neuronal activity in wakefulness and in sleep. In: A CIBA Found. Sym-posium on the Nature of Sleep, 1961 (4270), pp. 108-26. <u>76</u>, <u>211</u>
Verzeano, M., co-author: 1285-87, 3680.

4054. Vesely, L. (Czech.) Electroen-cephalographic recording of hyp-notic state. Neurol. Psychiat. Česk., 13:210-19, 1950. <u>270</u>, <u>271</u>

4055. Viallefont, et Boudet. La cure de sommeil en ophthalmologie. Ann.

Oculist., 188(II):1033-38, 1955. 207

4056. Viaud, G. Le pouvoir réparateur du sommeil et les variations diurnes de l'activité. C. R. Soc. Biol., 139:553-55, 1945. 314

4057. _____. Le pouvoir réparateur du sommeil et sa mesure. J. Psychol. Norm. Path., 40:195-231, 1947. 314

4058. Vidart, L., et E. Gasteau. La cure de sommeil en pratique neuro-psychiatrique. Rev. Prat. (Paris), 4:1583-88, 1954. 207

4059. Vidovic, V. L., and V. Popovic. Studies on the adrenal and thyroid glands of the ground squirrel during hibernation. J. Endocrinol. (London), 11:125-33, 1954. 325

4060. Vignes, J. Influence exercée par la gestation sur le sommeil. C. R. Soc. Biol., 97:235-36, 1927. 277

4061. Vihvelin, H. On the differentiation of some typical forms of hypnagogic hallucinations. Acta Psychiat. Neurol., 23:359-89, 1948. 79

4062. Vijnovsky, B. El Sueño Normal y Patológico en el Niño. Buenos Aires: "El Ateneo," 1944. Pp. 342.

4063. Villamil, A., J. Clavijo, R. J. Franco, R. M. Buzzi, and V. Abelardi. Circulatory function in artificial hibernation. Acta Physiol. Latino-Am., 5(2):104-13, 1955. 328

4064. Villaverde, J. M. de. Sobre las manifestaciones motoras que acompañan a la narcolepsia. A proposito de un caso observado en un niño. Arch. Españ. Pediat., 11:652-66, 1927.

4065. Visscher, M. B., and F. Halberg. Daily rhythms in numbers of circulating eosinophils and some related phenomena. Ann. New York Acad. Sci., 59:834-49, 1955. 169
Visscher, M. B., co-author: 1156, 1590, 1597, 1600, 1601.

4066. Visser. (Dutch) A case of narcolepsy. Ned. Tschr. Geneesk., 75: 1498-1500, 1931. 234, 235, 238

4067. Vitale, A. La reazione di risveglio nell'EEG umano patologico. Arch. Psicol. Neurol. Psichiat., 19:243-64, 1958.

4068. Vitenzon, A. S. (Russ.) Study of nervous processes in the course of visual trace reactions in sleep deficit. Zh. Vysshei Nerv. Deiat., 6:212-17, 1956. 121

4069. Vitte, N. K., J. A. Misrukhin, and E. P. Topchieva. (Russ.) Registration of bioelectric potentials of brain and heart in schizophrenics during sleep. Nevropat. Psikhiat., 59:416-21, 1959. 41

4070. Vizioli, R. Unusual sleep induced pattern: Suppression-burst activity. EEG Clin. Neurophysiol., 7:631-32, 1955. 298

4071. _____, and A. Giancotti. EEG findings in a case of narcolepsy. EEG Clin. Neurophysiol., 6: 307-9, 1954. 237, 238

4072. _____, e D. Merigliano. Narcolessia ed epilessia temporale. Riv. Neurol. (Napoli), 25:303-8, 1955. 237, 238

4073. _____, e F. Zappi. Contributo allo studio della sindrome narco-cataplettica. Riv. Neurol. (Napoli), 27:423-27, 1957. 239
Vizioli, R., co-author: 2662, 2884.

4074. Völker, H. Ueber die tagesperiodischen Schwankungen einiger Lebensvorgaenge des Menschen. Pfluegers Arch., 215: 43-77, 1927. 50, 163, 166, 167, 174

4075. Vogel, G. Studies in psychophysiology of dreams. III. The dream of narcolepsy. A.M.A. Arch. Gen. Psychiat., 3:421-28, 1960. 98, 103, 238

4076. Vogl, A. Ueber den Vorgang des Traeumens. Med. Mschr. (Stuttgart), 6:603-7, 1952. 106

4077. Vogl, M. Neurotische Schlafstoerungen im Kindesalter. Prax. Kinderpsychol. Kinderpsychiat., 4:33-37, 1955. 286

4078. Vogler, P. Die Prophylaxe der Schlafstoerung. Leipzig: Georg Thieme, 1959. 2nd ed. Pp. 130. 286, 294, 307, 312, 317

4079. Vogt, H. Die Atemzahl des gesunden Kindes. Mschr. Kinderheilk., 42:460-68, 1929. 50

4080. Vogt, J. H. Partial hypopituitarism, presumably of hypothalamic pathogenesis, associated with dilatation of the third ventricle. Acta Endocrinol., 28: 337-43, 1958.

4081. Vogtherr, K. Zur Psychotherapie der Schlafstoerungen. Nervenarzt, 27:309-15, 1956. 286

4082. Voitkevitch, V. I. (Russ.) The influence of sleep on the saturation of arterial blood with oxygen. Fiziol. Zh. SSSR, 40:269-73, 1954. 51

4083. Volkind, N. Ya. (Russ.) On changes in breathing during sleep in dogs. Trudy Fiziol. Lab. Pavlova, 16:351-59, 1950; also in: The Sleep Problem, 1954 (392), pp. 324-31. 48, 49, 308

4084. Vormittag, S. Untersuchungen ueber die Atmung des Kindes. I. Atemzahl und Atemform des gesunden Kindes. Mschr. Kinderheilk., 58:249-65, 1933. 50

4085. Vorwahl. Radiogefahren. Z. psychol. Hyg., 2:71-74, 1929. 311

4086. Vosburg, R. L. Sensory deprivation and isolation. Psychiat. Commun., 2:11-19, 1959. 199

4087. _____, N. G. Fraser, and J. J. Guehl. Sensory deprivation and image formation. Psychiat. Commun., 2:157-70, 1959. 199

4088. Votchal, B. E., U. A. Tupoleva, and S. G. Salimov. (Russ.) Conditioned reflex motor method for objective monitoring of the state of sleep. Klin. Med. (Moskva), 36(9):25-29, 1958. 72

4089. Vranski, V., V. Ivanov, I. Kasabov, V. Marinov, and L. Korueva. (Bulgar.) Experimental studies on the possibility of producing electrosleep and electronarcosis. (Preliminary communication). Suvrem. Med. (Sofia), 5(1):21-24, 1954. 299

4090. Vujic, V. Schlaf und Liquordruck. Jahresb. Psychiat. Neurol., 49:112-62, 1933. 46, 47

4091. Vulliamy, D. The day and night output of urine in enuresis. Arch. Dis. Child., 31:439-43, 1956. 285

4092. Wada, T. Experimental study of hunger in its relation to activity. Arch. Psychol., 8:1-65, 1922. 53, 87

4093. Wagner, C. P. Comment on the mechanism of narcolepsy. J. Nerv. Ment. Dis., 72:405-6, 1930. 235, 240

4094. Wagner, I. F. The establishment of a criterion of depth of sleep in the new born infant. J. Genet. Psychol., 51:17-59, 1937. 50, 88, 111

4095. _____. The sleeping posture of the neonate. J. Genet. Psychol., 52:235-39, 1938. 9

4096. _____. Curves of sleep depth in newborn infants. J. Genet. Psychol., 55:121-35, 1939. 50, 112

4097. Wagner, M. A. Day and night sleep in a group of young orphanage children. J. Genet. Psychol., 42:442-59, 1933. 117

4098. Wagner, R. Die Schlaflage und ihre Abhaengigkeit von Alter und Herzkrankheiten. Z. Altersforsch., 7:346-51, 1954. 11

4099. Wagner, W. Selbstmord in Schlaftrunkenheit. Nervenarzt, 26:298, 1955. 271

4100. Wahl, E. F. Narcolepsy. South. Med. J., 24:169-70, 1931. 235

4101. Wald, G., and B. Jackson. Activity and nutritional deprivation. Proc. Nat. Acad. Sci., 30:255-63, 1944. 149

4102. Walden, E. C. Plethysmographic study of the vascular conditions during hypnotic sleep. Am. J. Physiol., 4:124-61, 1900. 329, 330

4103. Walker, E., J. Merlis, and C. Henry, Eds. Symposia—III International Congress of EEG Clinical Neurophysiology, Cambridge, Mass., Aug. 1953. Table of Contents in EEG Clin. Neurophysiol., 6:502, 1954. 29

4104. Wallaszek, E. J., and L. G. Abood. Effect of tranquilizing drugs on fighting response of Siamese fighting fish. Science, 124:440-41, 1956. 302

4105. Wallgren, A. (Danish) Sleep disturbances and loss of appetite in children, and their treatment. Ugeskr. Laeg., 99:25-32, 1937. 274

4106. Walls, E. W. Specialized conduction tissue in the heart of the golden hamster (Cricetus auratus). J. Anat., 76:359-68, 1942.

4107. Walsh, W. S. Dreams of the feeble-minded. Med. Rec., 97:395-98, 1920. 103, 281

4108. Walshe, F. Topic "States of Consciousness in Neurology"—Discussion of report of Dr. P. Bailey. First Internat. Congr. Neurol. Sci., Seconde Journée Commune. Brussels: Acta Med. Belg., 1957, pp. 141-45. 30 Walshe, F., co-author: 1069.

4109. Walter, F. K. Ueber Schlafstoerungen nach Grippe. Med. Klin., 17:245-47, 1921.

4110. Walter, W. G. The Living Brain. New York: W. W. Norton & Co., 1953. Pp. 311. 100, 337, 362

4111. _____. Theoretical properties of diffuse projection systems in relation to behaviour and consciousness. In: Brain Mechanisms and Consciousness, 1954 (875), pp. 345-73. 210

4112. Walters, O. S. The erythrocyte count, quantity of hemoglobin and volume of packed cells in normal human subjects during muscular inactivity. Am. J. Physiol., 108: 118-24, 1934. 38

4113. Walton, D. The application of the learning theory to the treatment of a case of somnambulism. J. Clin. Psychol., 17:96-99, 1961.

4114. Wang, C. C. (Van-Tzin-Tzyan) (Russ.) Observations on daytime sleep of children in kindergarten setting. Pediatria (Moskva), No. 6:47-51, 1958. 90

4115. Wang, C. C., and R. Kern. Influence of sleep on basal metabolism in children. Proc. Inst. Med. Chicago, 6:253, 1927; also Am. J. Dis. Child., 36:83-88, 1928. 41, 56

4116. Wang, G. H. The galvanic skin reflex. A review of old and recent works from the physiologic point of view. Am. J. Phys. Med., 36: 295-320, 1957; 37:35-57, 1958.

4117. Wangh, M. Day residue in dream and myth. J. Am. Psychoanal. Ass., 2:446-52, 1954. 103

4118. Ward, A. A., Jr., and W. S. McCulloch. The projection of the frontal lobe on the hypothalamus. J. Neurophysiol., 10:309-14, 1947. 211

4119. Ward, C. H., A. T. Beck, and E. Rascoe. Typical dreams. A.M.A. Arch. Gen. Psychiat., 5:606-15, 1961. 101

4120. Warren, J. E. Diurnal plasma corticoid studies and their relation to morning stiffness in rheumatoid arthritis. Ann. Rheumat. Dis., 15:70, 1956. 170

4121. Warren, L. F., and F. Tilney. Tumor of the pineal body with invasion of the midbrain, thalamus, hypothalamus and pituitary body. J. Nerv. Ment. Dis., 45:74-75, 1917. 263

4122. Warren, N., and B. Clark. Blocking in mental and motor tasks during a 65 hour vigil. J. Exp. Psychol., 21:97-105, 1937; prelim. commun. Psychol. Bull., 33: 814-15, 1936. 225
Warren, N., co-author: 712, 713.

4123. Wartenberg, R. Brachialgia statica paresthetica (nocturnal arm dysesthesias). J. Nerv. Ment. Dis., 99:877-87, 1944. 285

4124. Washburn, R., and N. Putnam. A study of child care in the first two years of life. J. Pediat., 2: 517-37, 1933. 115

4125. Wassermann, M. (Czech.) Contribution to the treatment of insomnia. Čas. Lék. Česk., 63: 273, 1924; abstr. Med. Klin., 20:1018, 1924. 294

4126. Waterfield, R. L. The effects of posture on the circulating blood volume. J. Physiol. (London), 72:110-20, 1931. 37, 38

4127. _____. The effect of posture on the volume of the leg. J. Physiol. (London), 72:121-31, 1931. 38, 39

4128. Watson, C. W., and R. D. Adams. The electroencephalogram in its relation to consciousness and responsiveness in destructive lesions of the brain stem. A clinical pathological EEG study of brain stem disease particularly basilar artery occlusion. EEG Clin. Neurophysiol., 3:371, 1951. 31
Watson, C. W., co-author: 3888.

4129. Watts, C. A. H. Discussion on hypnotism in general practice. The disadvantages of hypnotism. Practitioner, 180:599-600, 1958. 335

4130. Wayne, H. L. Sleep records in electroencephalography. New York Med., 6(9): 16-19, 44-45, 1950. 29
Wayne, H. L., co-author: 2289.

4131. Webb, W. B. Antecedents of sleep. J. Exp. Psychol., 53:162-66, 1957. 219

4132. _____. An overview of sleep as an experimental variable. Science, 134:1421-23, 1961.

4133. _____, and H. W. Agnew, Jr. Sleep deprivation, age, and exhaustion time in the rat. Science, 136:1122, 1962. 219

4134. Wechsler. Discussion of tumors of the third ventricle. Arch. Neurol. Psychiat., 20:1404, 1928. 361

4135. Wechsler, I. S. The meaning of consciousness. A.M.A. Arch. Neurol. Psychiat., 67:554-56, 1952; also Bull. New York Acad. Med., 28:739-47, 1952; also J. Nerv. Ment. Dis., 116:260-62,

1952. 30

4136. Wechsler, R. L., R. D. Dripps, and S. S. Kety. Blood flow and oxygen consumption of the human brain during anestheia produced by thiopental. Anesthesiology, 12:308-14, 1951. 297

4137. Wedgwood, H. Sleep. Washington, D.C.: G.P.O. Bureau Educ., 1923. Pp. 21. 307

4138. Weech, A. A. Narcolepsy, a symptom complex. Am. J. Dis. Child., 32:672-81, 1926. 239

4139. Weed, S. C., and F. M. Hallam. A study of the dream-consciousness. Am. J. Psychol., 7:405-11, 1896. 106

4140. Wegierko, J. Le léger choc insulinique comme facteur hypnotique et analgésique. Paris Méd., 1:365-67, 1937. 294

4141. Wehmeyer, H., und H. Caspers. Bioelektrische Registrierung der Schlaf-Wach-Periodik beim Tier. Pfluegers Arch., 267:298-306, 1958. 148, 365

4142. Weidner, K. Schlaftherapie innerer Krankheiten. Klin. Wschr., 26:441-42, 1948. 207

4143. _____. Schlaftherapie der Influenza. Med. Klin., 45(II):958-59, 1950. 207

4144. _____. Was leistet der kuenstliche Schlaf? Med. Klin., 46(I): 240-41, 1951. 207

4145. _____. Schlafen ohne Tabletten. Stuttgart: Frank'sche Verlagshandlung, 1955. Pp. 27. 113

4146. _____. Die Schlaftherapie. Stuttgart: Hippokrates, 1956. Pp. 64. 206

4147. Weinberg, I. C. (Russ.) On the treatment of insomnia (difficulty in falling asleep) by oxygen baths. Soviet. Vrach. Gaz., (17):1348-52, 1935. 294

4148. Weiskotten, T. F. On the effects of loss of sleep. J. Exp. Psychol., 8:363-80, 1925. 225

4149. _____, and J. E. Ferguson. A further study of the effects of loss of sleep. J. Exp. Psychol., 13: 247-66, 1930. 225

4150. Weiskrantz, L., and W. A. Wilson, Jr. Effect of reserpine on learning and performance. Science, 123:1116-18, 1956. 302

4151. Weismann-Netter, R., R. Levy, H. Boileau, et C. Jarry. Les cures de sommeil dans l'hypertension artérielle: actualités et perspectives. In: La Cure de Sommeil, 1954 (3021), pp. 118-36. 207

4152. Weiss, S. Histopathologische Befunde im Zwischenhirn bei Tumoren mit "Zwischenhirn" Symptomen, mit Bemerkungen ueber das Schlafproblem. Z. ges. Neurol. Psychiat., 144:21-53, 1933. 349

4153. Weiss, S., and J. P. Baker. The carotid sinus in health and disease. Its rôle in the causation of fainting and convulsions. Medicine, 12:297-354, 1933. 241

4154. _____, R. B. Capps, E. B. Ferris, and D. Munro. Syncope and convulsions due to a hyperactive carotid sinus reflex. Arch. Int. Med., 58:407-17, 1936. 241

4155. Weitzenhoffer, A. M. The production of antisocial acts under hypnosis. J. Abnorm. Soc. Psychol., 44:420-22, 1949. 334

4156. _____. Hypnotism: An Objective Study in Suggestibility. New York: Wiley, 1953. Pp. 380. 336

4157. Weitzmann, E. D. A note on the EEG and eye movements during behavioral sleep in monkeys. EEG Clin. Neurophysiol., 13: 790-94, 1961. 102

4158. Weitzner, H. A. Sleep paralysis, successfully treated with insulin hypoglycemia. A.M.A. Arch. Neurol. Psychiat., 68:835-41, 1952.

4159. Welch, L. The space and time of induced hypnotic dreams. J. Psychol., 1:171-78, 1936. 334

4160. _____. A behavioristic explanation of the mechanism of suggestion and hypnosis. J. Abnorm. Soc. Psychol., 42:359-64, 1947. Welch, L.. co-author: 760.

4161. Wellnerová, J., and D. Svorad. (Czech.) Sleep deficiency (debt); its measurement and influence. Česk. Fysiol., 8(2):136-37, 1959. 219

4162. Wells, H., F. N. Briggs, and P. L. Munson. The inhibitory effect of reserpine on ACTH secretion in response to stressful stimuli. Endocrinology, 59: 571-79, 1956. 302

4163. Wells, W. R. Experiments in waking hypnosis for instructional purposes. J. Abnorm. Soc. Psychol., 18:389-404, 1924.

4164. _____. Experiments in the hypnotic production of crime. J. Psychol., 11:63-102, 1941; also in Modern Hypnosis, 1958 (2299), pp. 170-202. 334

4165. Welsh, J. H. Diurnal rhythms. Q. Rev. Biol., 13:123-39, 1938. 172

4166. ____, F. A. Chace, Jr., and R. F. Nunnemacher. The diurnal migration of deep-water animals. Biol. Bull., 73:185-96, 1937. 132

4167. ____, and C. M. Osborn. Diurnal changes in the retina of the catfish, Ameiurus nebulosis. J. Comp. Neurol., 66:349-59, 1937. 172

Welsh, J. H., co-author: 1515, 2466.

4168. Welte, E. Methode der Pruefung von Schlafmitteln. Therapiewoche, 8:329-31, 1958. 113

4169. Wenderowič, E. Hypnolepsie (Narcolepsie Gélineau) und ihre Behandlung. Arch. Psychiat., 72: 459-72, 1924-25. 233, 294

4170. Wendt, C. F. Ueber Wirkungen eines Extraktes aus dem braunen Fettgewebe des winterschlafenden Igels. IV. Z. physiol. Chem., 249:182IV, 1937. 326

4171. ____. Psychotherapie der Schlafstoerungen in der nervenaerztlichen Sprechstunde. Berlin: Springer, 1957. Pp. 24. 286

4172. Werner, G. Ueber den Bromgehalt der Hypophyse und des Blutes im experimentellen Schlaf. Vol. Jubil. en l'honneur du Prof. C. I. Parhon, Soc. Roum. Neurol. Psychiat. Psychol. Endocrinol., Jassy, 1934, pp. 540-45. 57

4173. Werner, J. Reizfreie Schlaftiefenmessung durch simultane Registrierung meherer Vorgaenge. Pfluegers Arch., 270:19, 1959. 26, 113

4174. ____. Methodik und erste Ergebnisse einer fortlaufenden Schlaftiefenmessung fuer Tier und Mensch. Zbl. Vet.-Med., 7: 180-82, 1960. 26, 113

4175. ____. Eine Methode zur weckreizfreien und fortlaufenden Schlaftiefenmessung beim Menschen mit Hilfe von Elektroencephalo-, Elektrooculo- und Elektrocardiographie (EEG, EOG und EKG). Z. ges. exp. Med., 134: 187-209, 1961. 26, 113

4176. Werre, P. F. The Relationships between Electroencephalographic and Psychological Data in Normal Adults. Leiden: Leiden Univ. Press, 1958. Pp. viii + 152. 29

4177. Wertheimer, P., et J. Angel. La cure de sommeil dans les douleurs irréductibles. In: La Cure de Sommeil, 1954 (3021), pp. 167-74. 207

4178. Weschke, C. Overcoming Sleeplessness. Saint Paul, Minn.: Book Masters, 1935. Pp. 76. 278

4179. West, L. J. Psychophysiology of hypnosis. J. Am. Med. Ass., 172:672-75, 1960. 336

West, L. J., co-author: 461.

4180. Westphal, A. Kurze Mitteilung ueber eigenartige Stoerung des Erwachens. Selbstbeobachtung. Arch. Psychiat., 94:268-72, 1931.

4181. Wexberg, L. E. Insomnia as related to anxiety and ambition. J. Clin. Psychopath., 10:373-75, 1949. 275, 358

4182. Wexler, D., J. Mendelson, H. Leiderman, and P. Solomon. Sensory deprivation. A technique for studying psychiatric aspects of stress. A.M.A. Arch. Neurol. Psychiat., 79:225-33, 1958. 198

Wexler, D., co-author: 2422, 3752.

4183. Weygandt, W. Experimentelle Beitraege zur Psychologie des Schlafes. Z. Psychol., 39:1-41, 1905. 120

4184. Wheeler, E. O., and P. D. White. Insomnia due to left ventricular heart failure unrecognized as such and inadequately treated. J. Am. Med. Ass., 129: 1158-59, 1945. 277

4185. Wheeler, R. H. Visual phenomena in the dreams of a blind subject. Psychol. Rev., 27:315-22, 1920. 102

4186. White, J. C. Autonomic discharges from stimulation of hypothalamus in man. Res. Publ. Ass. Nerv. Ment. Dis., 20:854-63, 1940. 358

4187. ____, E. Eidelberg, and J. D. French. Experimental assessment of epileptogenesis in the monkey cerebral cortex. A.M.A. Arch. Neurol., 2:376-83, 1960. 297

4188. White, K. L., and W. N. Long, Jr. The incidence of "psychogenic" fever in a university hospital. J. Chron. Dis., 8:567-86, 1958. 145

4189. White, M. R. Some factors affecting the night sleep of children. Child Develop., 2:234-35, 1931. 117, 307

4190. White, R. W. Prediction of hypnotic susceptibility from a knowledge of subjects' attitudes. J. Psychol., 3:265-77, 1937. 335

4191. _____. Two types of hypnotic trance and their personality correlates. J. Psychol., 3:279-89, 1937. 335

4192. _____. A preface to the theory of hypnotism. J. Abnorm. Soc. Psychol., 36:477-505, 1941.

4193. _____. An analysis of motivation in hypnosis. J. Gen. Psychol., 24:145-62, 1941. 335

4194. Whitehorn, J. C., H. Lundholm, E. L. Fox, and F. G. Benedict. The metabolic rate in "hypnotic sleep." New Engl. J. Med., 206: 777-81, 1932. 330

4195. _____, _____, and G. E. Gardner. The metabolic rate in emotional moods induced by suggestion in hypnosis. Am. J. Psychiat., 9: 661-66, 1930. 331

4196. Whitlock, D. G., A. Arduini, and G. Moruzzi. Microelectric analysis of pyramidal system during transition from sleep to wakefulness. J. Neurophysiol., 16:414-29, 1933. Whitlock, D. G., co-author: 3790.

4197. Whitman, R. M., M. Kramer, and B. Baldridge. Which dream does the patient tell? Arch. Gen. Psychiat., 8:277-82, 1963. 98, 103

4198. _____, C. M. Pierce, J. W. Maas, and B. Baldridge. Drugs and dreams. II: Imipramine and prochlorperazine. Comprehensive Psychiat., 2:219-26, 1961. 98, 105 Whitman, R. M., co-author: 3190.

4199. Wible, C. L., and A. Jenness. Electrocardiograms during sleep and hypnosis. J. Psychol., 1:235-45, 1936. 41, 329, 330 Wible, C. L., co-author: 1981.

4200. Wicke, H. Die Behandlung der Enuresis nocturna auf der Grundlage der fraktionierten Aktivhypnose. Nervenarzt, 22: 451-57, 1951. 284, 335

4201. Wickes, I. G. Treatment of persistent enuresis with the electric buzzer. Arch. Dis. Childh. (London), 33:160-64, 1958. 285

4202. Wiechmann, E. Koerper und Schlaf. Muench. med. Wschr., 71:1191-93, 1924. 45

4203. _____, und J. Bamberger. Puls und Blutdruck im Schlaf. Z. ges. exp. Med., 41:37-51, 1924. 40, 45, 297

4204. Wiersma, E. D. (Dutch) On sleep and hypnotic drugs. Ned. Tschr. Geneesk., 75:4752-66, 1931. Wiersma, E. D., co-author: 338.

4205. Wieser, S. Neurologische Untersuchungen ueber Bewusstseinsstoerungen. Dsche med. Wschr., 83:149-51, 1958. 31

4206. Wikler, A. Relationships between clinical effects of barbiturates and their neurophysiological mechanisms of action. Fed. Proc., 11:647-52, 1952. 295

4207. _____. Pharmacologic dissociation of behavior and EEG "sleep patterns" in dogs: Morphine, N-allylnormorphine, and Atropine. Proc. Soc. Exp. Biol. Med., 79: 261-65, 1952. 30, 304

4208. Wiktor, Z. (Polish) Effect of prolonged sleep on certain functions of the organism. Polski Tygod. Lek., 9:372-74, 1954. 206

4209. _____. (Polish) Clinical and Experimental Researches on the Effect of Prolonged Sleep on some Organic Functions. Warszawa: Pánstwowy Zaklad Wydawn. Lek., 1954. Pp. 74. 206

4210. Wilbur, D. L., A. R. Macleand, and E. V. Allen. Clinical observations on the effect of benzedrine sulphate: a study of patients with states of chronic exhaustion, depression and psychoneuroses. J. Am. Med. Ass., 109:549-54, 1937.

4211. Wilkinson, R. T. Lack of sleep and performance. Bull. Brit. Psychol. Soc., No. 34:5A-6A, 1958. 226

4212. _____. Rest pauses in a task affected by lack of sleep. Ergonomics (London), 2:373-80, 1959. 226

4213. _____. The effect of lack of sleep on visual watch-keeping. Q. J. Exp. Psychol., 12:36-40, 1960. 226

4214. _____. Interaction of lack of sleep with knowledge of results, repeated testing, and individual differences. J. Exp. Psychol., 62:263-71, 1961. 226

4215. Willcocks, G. C. Insomnia due to physical causes. Med. J. Australia, 22:170-73, 1935. 50, 275, 294

4216. Willey, M. M. Sleep as an escape mechanism. Psychoanal. Rev., 11:181-83, 1924. 270

4217. _____, and S. A. Rice. The psychic utility of sleep. J. Abnorm. Soc. Psychol., 19:174-78, 1924. 270

4218. William-Olsson, L. (Swed.) On sleep conditions in Swedish hospitals. Hygeia (Stockholm), 98: 750-65, 1936. 312

4219. Williams, D. Disorders of sleep. Practitioner, 164:135-42, 1950. 286

4220. Williams, D. E. The Influence of Sleep on the Energy Metabolism of Three and Four Year Old Children. New York: Columbia Univ. Diss., 1934. Pp. 28. 56

4221. Williams, E. H., and F. C. Harding. Morbid somnolence and narcolepsy. New York Med. J. Med. Rec., 137:71-74, 101-2, 1933. 240

4222. Williams, E. S. Sleep and wakefulness at high altitudes. Brit. Med. J., I:197-98, 1959. 120

4223. Williams, G. W. The effect of hypnosis on muscular fatigue. J. Abnorm. Soc. Psychol., 24:318-29, 1929. 331

4224. _____. A comparative study of voluntary and hypnotic catalepsy. Am. J. Psychol., 42:83-95, 1930.

4225. Williams, H. L., A. M. Granda, R. C. Jones, A. Lubin, and J. C. Armington. EEG frequency and finger pulse volume as predictors of reaction time during sleep loss. EEG Clin. Neurophysiol., 14:64-70, 1962. 226

4226. _____, and A. Lubin. Impaired performance in a case of prolonged sleep loss. Walter Reed Army Inst. Res., July, 1959. Pp. 15. 226

4227. _____, _____, and J. J. Goodnow. Impaired Performance with Acute Sleep Loss. Psychol. Monogr., 73, No. 14 (Whole No. 484), 1959. Pp. 26. 226
Williams, H. L., co-author: 1440, 1441, 2570, 2889, 2956, 2957.

4228. Williams, R. J., and R. C. Thompson. A device for obtaining a continuous record of body temperature from the external auditory canal. Science, 108:90-91, 1948.

4229. Williams, R. L. Effects of dormison compared to seconal for sleep electroencephalogram. EEG Clin. Neurophysiol., 6: 497-98, 1954. 296

4230. Willis, H. Narcolepsy. Med. J. Australia, II:119-20, 1928. 234

4231. Willoughby, R. R. A note on a child's dream. J. Genet. Psychol., 42:224-28, 1933. 102

4232. Wilson, D. C., and R. F. Watson. Narcolepsy with reference to carotid sinus reflex. South. Med. J., 27:754-59, 1934. 241, 242

4233. Wilson, S. A. K. The narcolepsies. Brain, 51:63-107, 1928. 234, 235

4234. Wilson, S. R. Physiologic basis of hypnosis and suggestion. Proc. Roy. Soc. Med. (Sect. on Anesthesia), 20:15-21, 1926-27. 333

4235. Wimmer, A. Epilepsy in chronic, epidemic encephalitis. Acta Psychiat. Neurol., 3:367-407, 1928. 256

4236. Winans, H. M. Insomnia. Internat. Clin., 1:39-55, 1935. 294

4237. Windholtz, E. Neurotic disturbances of sleep. Internat. J. Psycho-anal., 23:49-52, 1942. 106, 286

4238. Winkel, C. M. Can any significance be attributed to "sleep-patterns" in routine EEG-records? EEG Clin. Neurophysiol., 7:658, 1955.

4239. _____, and A. M. Hamoen. Sleep-patterns in routine E.E.G. records. Folia Psychiat. Neerl., 62:28-33, 1959. 192

4240. Winkelstein, A. 169 studies in gastric secretion during the night. Am. J. Digest. Dis. Nutrition, 1:778-82, 1935. 54

4241. Winkler, C. (Dutch) About sleep. Ned. Tschr. Geneesk., 76:5826-31, 1932. 362
Winkler, C., co-author: 3256.

4242. Winkler, W. Zur Behandlung der Brachialgia paraesthetica nocturna. Dsche med. Wschr., 74(I): 364-65, 1949. 285

4243. _____. Der Traum. Fortschr. Neurol. Psychiat., 22:227-54, 1954. 99

4244. Winnicott, D. W. Pathological sleeping. Proc. Roy. Soc. Med., 23(II):1109-10, 1930. 267

4245. Winterstein, H. Schlaf und Traum.

Berlin: Springer, 1953. 2nd ed.
Pp. vii + 135. 99

4246. Wittersheim, G., F. Grivel, et
B. Metz. Application d'une
épreuve de choix multiple avec
enregistrement continu des réponses, des erreurs et des
temps de réaction à l'étude des
effets sensori-moteurs de l'inversion du rythme nyctéméral
chez l'homme normal. C. R. Soc.
Biol., 152:1194-98, 1958. 174

4247. Wittstock, E. Schlafgewohnheiten
und Schlafverhaeltnisse Erzge-
birgischer Volksschueler. Ge-
sundh. Erziehung, 46:97-107,
1933. 118, 161, 305

4248. Witzleben, H. D. Die Behandlung der postencephalitischen
Hypersomnie mit Ephedrin.
Therap. Gegenw., 78:475-76,
1937. 300

4249. Wodoginskaja, S. (Russ.) Sleep
disturbance in brain tumors.
Soviet. Nevropat. Psikhiat., 5:
2069-73, 1936. 265

4250. Woehlisch, E. Zur Definition des
Begriffes der Schlaftiefe. Z.
Biol., 103:81-86, 1949. 113

4251. _____. Schlaf und Erholung.
Mensch und Arbeit, 4:31-45,
1952. 113

4252. _____. Gehirnvolum und Liquordruck im Schlafe. Klin. Wschr.,
31:620-21, 1953. 113

4253. _____. Die Schlaftiefenzahl und
der Schlaftiefenbegriff. Klin.
Wschr., 31:1010-11, 1953. 113

4254. _____. Eine Logarithmische Fas-
sung der Schlaftiefenzahl. Klin.
Wschr., 32:268-69, 1954. 113

4255. _____. Die absolute Schlaftiefenzahl. Klin. Wschr., 32:703-4,
1954. 113

4256. _____. Die Schlaftiefenzahl: Theorie und Anwendung. Z. Biol.,
106:330-76, 1954. 113

4257. _____. Die lincare und die logarithmische Schlaftiefenzahl. Z.
ges. inn. Med., 9:1047-52, 1954.
113

4258. _____. Schlaf und Erholung als
Probleme der Energetik und Ge-
faessversorgung des Gehirns.
Klin. Wschr., 34:720-29, 1956.
113

4259. _____. Der Schlaftiefenverlauf
und sein Erholungsaequivalent.
Klin. Wschr., 35:480-85, 1957.
113

4260. _____. Der Schlaftiefenverlauf
und sein Erholungsaequivalent.

II. Klin. Wschr., 35:705-14,
1957. 113

4261. _____, K. Reichert, und S. Jaeh-
nichen. Zur Methodik der
Schlaftiefenmessung. Klin.
Wschr., 35:195-96, 1957. 113
Woehlfahrt, E., co-author: 3304.

4262. Wohlfahrt, S. Quelques recherches cliniques sur la narcolepsie. Acta Psychiat. Neurol., 6:
277-92, 1931. 250

4263. Wolberg, L. R. Hypnoanalysis.
New York: Grune & Stratton,
1945. Pp. xviii + 342. 335

4264. _____. Medical Hypnosis. New
York: Grune & Stratton, 1948.
I, Pp. xii + 449; II, Pp. viii +
513. 335

4265. Wolff, H. G. The cerebral circulation. Physiol. Rev., 16:545-
86, 1936. 47
Wolff, H. G., co-author: 1237,
1777, 3591, 3609.

4266. Wolff, P. H. Observations on
newborn infants. Psychosom.
Med., 21:110-18, 1959. 88

4267. Wolff, W. The Dream—Mirror
of Conscience. A History of
Dream Interpretation from 2000
B.C. and a New Theory of Dream
Synthesis. New York: Grune &
Stratton, 1952. Pp. vi + 348. 106

4268. Wolpert, E. A. Studies in psychophysiology of dreams. II. An
electromyographic study of
dreaming. A.M.A. Arch. Gen.
Psychiat., 2:231-41, 1960. 96,
98

4269. _____, and H. Trosman. Studies
in psychophysiology of dreams.
I. Experimental evocation of se-
quential dream episodes. A.M.A.
Arch. Neurol. Psychiat., 79:
603-6, 1958. 98, 100
Wolpert, E. A., co-author: 903,
904, 3985.

4270. Wolstenholme, G. E. W., and M.
O'Connor, Eds. A CIBA Foundation Symposium on the Nature of
Sleep. Boston: Little, Brown,
1961. Pp. xii + 416.
Wolstenholme, G. E. W., co-editor: 4036.

4271. Wong, A. A case of insomnia in
pregnancy. Chinese Med. J., 49:
1146-48, 1935. 277

4272. Woodhead, G. S., and P. C. Var-
rier-Jones. Investigations on
clinical thermometry; continuous and quasi-continuous temperature records in man and
animals in health and disease.

IV. Temperature records in normal individuals. Lancet, I:450-53, 1916. 138

4273. Woods, R. L., Ed. The World of Dreams; An Anthology. New York: Random House, 1947. Pp. xxviii + 947. 99

4274. Woodworth, R. S. Note on the rapidity of dreams. Psychol. Rev., 4:524-26, 1897. 100

4275. _____. Psychology, A Study of Mental Life. New York: Henry Holt & Co., 1921. Pp. x + 579. 99

4276. Woolbert, C. H. A behavioristic account of sleep. Psychol. Rev., 27:420-28, 1920. 311

4277. Wooley, H. T. Eating, sleeping and elimination. In: A Handbook of Child Psychology. Worcester, Mass.: Clark Univ. Press, 1931, pp. 28-70. 307

4278. Worchel, P., and M. H. Marks. The effects of sleep prior to learning. J. Exp. Psychol., 42: 313-16, 1951. 125

4279. Worrall, R. L. Cerebral cortex during unconsciousness: a critical review of the theory of conditioned reflexes, with reference to the symptoms of epilepsy and narcolepsy. J. Neurol. Psychopath., 11:328-41, 1931.

4280. Worster-Drought, C. The treatment of insomnia. I. General considerations. Lancet, 213(II): 720-21, 1927. 275

4281. Wortis, S. B., and F. Kennedy. Narcolepsy. Am. J. Psychiat., 12:939-46, 1933. 238, 240, 300
Wortis, S. B., co-author: 3818.

4282. Wuth, O. Ueber den Saeurebasenaushalt im Schlaf, bei Schlaflosigkeit und im Schlafmittelschlaf. Z. Neurol., 118:447-50, 1929. 52, 352

4283. _____. Klinik und Therapie der Schlafstoerungen. Schweiz. med. Wschr., 12:833-37, 1931. 275, 294, 307

4284. _____. Ueber die Behandlung der Schlafstoerungen. Muench. med. Wschr., 81:387-90, 1934. 294, 362

4285. Wyatt, S., and R. Marriott. Night work and shift changes. Brit. J. Indust. Med., 10:164-72, 1953. 316

4286. Wyke, B. D. Electrical activity of the human brain during artificial sleep. 1. The cyclical pattern of response to barbiturate sedation. 2. Regional differentiation of response to barbiturate sedation. J. Neurol. Neurosurg. Psychiat., 13:288-95, 1950; 14: 137-46, 1951.
Wyke, B. D., co-author: 609.

4287. Wyss, R. Schlafstoerungen bei Kindern. Heilpaedag. Werkbl., 26:194-97, 1957. 286

4288. Yamamoto, K. Studies on the normal EEG of the cat. Annual Rep. Shionogi Res. Lab., 9: 1125-64, 1959. 27

4289. Yamawaki, S. Schlafmittelstudien. I. Ueber die Ursache der Weckwirkung der Kalksalze bei der Magnesiumnarkose. Arch. exp. Path. Pharmakol., 136:1-33, 1928. 295

4290. Yanischevsky, A. E. (Czech.) Biological conception of sleep. Rev. Neurol. Psychiat. (Praha), 28:141-51, 1931.

4291. Yates, A. J. Hypnotic age regression. Psychol. Bull., 58: 429-40, 1961. 333

4292. Yoshihara, H. (Jap.) Effects of inorganic salt solutions on the tuber cinereum. J. Chosen Med. Ass., 26:742-814, 1936. 201

4293. Yoshii, N., P. Pruvot, and H. Gastaut. Electrographic activity of the mesencephalic reticular formation during conditioning in the cat. EEG Clin. Neurophysiol., 9:595-608, 1957.

4294. Yoss, R. E., and D. D. Daly. Criteria for the diagnosis of the narcoleptic syndrome. Proc. Staff Meet. Mayo Clin., 32:320-28, 1957. 234

4295. _____, and _____. Treatment of narcolepsy with Ritalin. Neurology, 9:171-73, 1959. 239

4296. _____, and _____. Narcolepsy. Med. Clin. North Am., 44:953-68, 1960. 234, 237, 239, 242
Yoss, R. E., co-author: 815.

4297. Youde, M. H. (Pseud.) Invigorating and Revitalizing the Body by a New Method of Sleeping. The Key to Rejuvenation. Manchester: Fletcher, 1951. Pp. 42. 312

4298. Youmans, J. B., H. S. Wells, D. Donley, and D. G. Miller. The effect of posture (standing) on the serum protein concentration and colloid osmotic pressure of blood from the foot in relation to the formation of edema. J. Clin. Investig., 13:447-59, 1934. 38

4299. Young, P. C. An experimental study of mental and physical functions in the normal and hypnotic states. Am. J. Psychol., 36:214-32, 1925. 335

4300. _____. Hypnotic regression—fact or artifact? J. Abnorm. Soc. Psychol., 35:273-78, 1940. 333

4301. _____. Experimental hypnotism: a review. Psychol. Bull., 38:92-104, 1941. 336

4302. Young, T. L. Insomnia. New Orleans Med. Surg. J., 104:195-97, 1951. 274

4303. Yuasa, E. (Jap.) Effect of fatigue upon the sinking speed of red blood corpuscles. Kaigun Gun'i-Kai Zasshi, 25:777, 1936. 162

4304. Zacks, D., O. Pettingill, and A. H. Stanhope. Preliminary study of natural position in sleep and its relation to the more affected lung in pulmonary tuberculosis. Boston Med. Surg. J., 188:946-48, 1923. 11

4305. Zalesky, M., and L. J. Wells. Effects of low environmental temperature on the thyroid and adrenal glands of the ground squirrel, Citellus Tridecemlineatus. Physiol. Zool., 13:268-76, 1940. 325

4306. Zalla, M. I disturbi del sonno postumi di encefalite epidemica. Riv. Pat. Nerv., 25:375-83, 1921. 247

4307. Zanchetti, A., S. C. Wang, and G. Moruzzi. The effect of vagal afferent stimulation on the EEG pattern of the cat. EEG Clin. Neurophysiol., 4:357-61, 1952. 212

Zanchetti, A., co-author: 252-56, 523, 1375, 1376, 2350, 2618, 2619, 2901, 2902, 3427.

4308. Zanocco, G., e C. Alvisi. Contributo allo studio delle alterazioni della vigilanza. Rass. Stud. Psichiat., 45:1229-49, 1956. 272

4309. Zappi, F., M. L. Casorati, e F. Maccagnani. Abnorme presenza di acido paraossifenilpiruvico nelle urine di narcolettici. Riv. Neurol. (Napoli), 26:207-12, 1956. 237

Zappi, F., co-author: 4073.

4310. Zara, E., e E. Buondonno. Ricerche biologiche in ammalati di mente: fluttuazioni nictemerali della glutationemia. Neuropsichiatria, 11:541-58, 1955. 162

4311. _____, e _____. Ricerche sulla genesi del sonno—fluttuazioni nictemerali del colesterolo. Folia Psichiat. (Lecce), 1:43-112, 1958. 162

4312. Zeckel, A. (Dutch) Pathological induction of sleep and conditions equivalent to sleep. Ned. Tschr. Geneesk., 78:2071-83, 1934. 245, 250

4313. Zeiner-Henriksen. (Norw.) Encephalitis lethargica. Review of experiences in Vienna in 1921. Norsk Mag. Laegevidensk., 84: 229-43, 1923. 247

4314. Zeitlin, H., and B. W. Lichtenstein. Cystic tumor of the third ventricle containing colloid material. Arch. Neurol. Psychiat., 38:268-87, 1937. 264

4315. Zellweger, H. Narkolepsie und Epilepsie. Ein Fall von Narkolepsie mit Spikes and Waves im Elektroencephalogramm. Helvet. Paediat. Acta, 11:269-74, 1956. 237

4316. Zénope, B. L'insomnie dite nerveuse et son traitement par la galvano- et la roentgen-thérapie. Evol. Thérap., 8:182-85, 1927. 294

4317. Zickgraf, H. Untersuchungen ueber die Zusammenhaenge zwischen den Schlafbewegungen und der Tiefe des normalen Schlafes. Z. klin. Med., 152:96-117, 1953. 113

4318. Ziegler, L. H. Psychopathology and sleep. Colorado Med., 23: 141, 1926. 349

4319. _____. Disturbances of sleep and maniacal delirium associated with spontaneously low blood sugar. Med. Clin. North Am., 13:1363-65, 1930. 283

4320. Zimkina, A. M. (Russ.) The cerebellum and sleep. Fiziol. Zh. SSSR, 32:207-12, 1946.

4321. Zimny, M. L., and R. Gregory. High-energy phosphates during long-term hibernation. Science, 129:1363-64, 1959. 324

4322. Zingerle, H. Ueber einen bei Gehirnkranken kuenstlich ausloesbaren pathologischen Schlafzustand. Klin. Wschr., 11:2143-46, 1932. 267

4323. Ziskind, E. Isolation stress in

medical and mental illness. J. Am. Med. Ass., 168:1427-30, 1958. 198, 199

4324. _____, H. Jones, W. Filante, and J. Goldberg. Observations on mental symptoms of eye patched patients: hypnagogic symptoms in sensory deprivation. Am. J. Psychiat., 116:893-900, 1960. 199

4325. Zitowitsch, J. Ueber die Nierentaetigkeit. II. Die periodische Nierentaetigkeit. Pfluegers Arch., 224:562-68, 1930.

4326. Zobel-Nacca, R. F. Science looks at sleep. Hygeia (Chicago), 23:258-59, 283, 1945.

4327. Zondek, B. Untersuchungen ueber den Winterschlaf: ein Beitrag zum Wert Organextrakte. Klin. Wschr., 3:1529-30, 1924. 326

4328. Zondek, H. Entgegnung zu der Arbeit von Holtz und Roggenbau. Klin. Wschr., 12:1411-12, 1933.

4329. _____, und H. W. Bansi. Hormone und Narkotika. Klin. Wschr., 6:1319-21, 1927. 357

4330. _____, und A. Bier. Brom im Blute bei manisch-depressivem Irresein. Klin. Wschr., 11:633-36, 1932. 57, 355

4331. _____, und _____. Der Bromgehalt der Hypophyse und seine Beziehungen zum Lebensalter.

Klin. Wschr., 11:759-60, 1932. 56, 355

4332. _____, und _____. Hypophyse und Schlaf. Klin. Wschr., 11:760-62, 1932. 56, 57, 355

4333. Zubek, J. P., W. Sanson, and A. Prysiazniuk. Intellectual changes during prolonged perceptual isolation (darkness and silence). Canad. J. Psychol., 14:233-43, 1960. 198

4334. Zuckerbrod, M., and I. Graef. Clinical evaluation of disodium succinate, including report on its ineffectiveness in two cases of severe barbiturate poisoning and some toxicologic notes on other succinate salts. Ann. Int. Med., 32:905-16, 1950. 297

4335. Zung, W. K., and W. P. Wilson. Response to auditory stimulation during sleep. A.M.A. Arch. Gen. Psychiat., 4:548-52, 1961; prelim. commun. EEG Clin. Neurophysiol., 13:313, 1961. 113

4336. Zynkin, A. M. (Russ.) Blood pressure in hypnosis. Psikhoterapia, pp. 123-40, 1930; abstr., Psychol. Abstr., 9:249, 1935. 329

4337. _____. (Russ.) Pulse and respiration in waking and hypnotic states. Psikhoterapia, pp. 141-66, 1930; abstr., Psychol. Abstr., 9:249, 1935. 329